STEDMAN'S
MEDICAL
EPONYMS

Pat Forbis, CMT
Susan L. Bartolucci, CMT

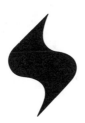

STEDMAN'S

MEDICAL

EPONYMS

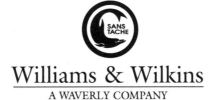

SANS
TACHE

Williams & Wilkins

A WAVERLY COMPANY

BALTIMORE • PHILADELPHIA • LONDON • PARIS • BANGKOK
HONG KONG • MUNICH • SYDNEY • TOKYO • WROCLAW

Series Editor: Maureen Barlow Pugh
Cover Designer: Tom Scheuerman
Typesetter: The PRD Group, Inc.
Copyright © 1998 Williams & Wilkins
351 West Camden Street
Baltimore, Maryland 21201-2436 USA

All rights reserved. This book is protected by copyright. No part of this book may be reproduced in any form or by any means, including photocopying, or utilized by any information storage and retrieval system without written permission from the copyright owner.

Printed in the United States of America

Library of Congress Cataloging-in-Publication Data
Forbis, Pat, 1940–
  Stedman's medical eponyms / by Pat Forbis and Susan L. Bartolucci.
     p.   cm.
  Includes bibliographical references.
  ISBN 0-683-07965-4
  1. Medicine—Abbreviations. 2. Eponyms—Dictionaries.
I. Stedman, Thomas Lathrop, 1853–1938. II. Bartolucci, Susan L.
III. Title. IV. Title: Medical eponyms.
  [DNLM: 1. Eponyms dictionaries. 2. Disease dictionaries.
3. Biography dictionaries.   WB 15 F696s 1998]
  R121.F67 1998
  610'.1'48—DC21
  DNLM/DLC
  for Library of Congress
                                                            98-17560
                                                                CIP
                                                              98 99
                                              2 3 4 5 6 7 8 9 10

Contents

Dedication

To the men with whom I share life's safari:
my husband, Bob, and
our sons, Robert, Tim, Rick, and Michael,

and to the memory of Kristen Noelle.

Pat Forbis, CMT

To my husband Gene and to my family for
their encouragement and support in this effort,
and to all medical transcriptionists who work
so hard to provide accurate records for
healthcare professionals and their patients.

Sue Bartolucci, CMT

Acknowledgments

Books are wonderful treasures. Those of us who love language can't get enough of them. And we all fantasize about writing one . . . some day. When some day arrives, it is all too easy to underestimate the magnitude of the project. How hard can it be, we say. Time? A snap, we think—six months should do it. Not! Books are the result of real team work. And this book is no exception.

Thanks to the remarkable staff of Williams & Wilkins, particularly Maureen Barlow Pugh, Senior Managing Editor, for her persistence and urging. It can't be an easy task to work with authors who consistently miss deadlines! She is greatly appreciated. Thanks also to Bonnie Montgomery, who copyedited the manuscript. Special thanks to Joan Caldwell, Vice President and Publisher, whose belief in and support of medical transcriptionists has resulted in valuable references never before available to the profession.

Hats off to the next team member, Barbara Ferretti, who patiently made the hundreds of corrections and insertions after each proofreading. Her help is greatly appreciated.

What would we do without reviewers? Those "fresh" sets of eyes that find things that we can't imagine how we missed. We want to especially thank Julie Moncrief, CMT, for the hours she contributed to helping us "get it right."

Special thanks to Claudia Tessier, CAE, CMT, RRA, our friend and colleague, for being among the first to define the use of eponyms.

And to family, friends, and colleagues—without your support we couldn't have done it.

Pat Forbis, CMT
Sue Bartolucci, CMT

Preface

Those who love the language of medicine never tire of exploring its uniqueness. Who else would spend hours assuring that something as simple as John Smith is spelled correctly? Or could it be Ian Smythe or Jon Smyth? Or, should it be the alternative spelling, Sean Smithe? Eponyms and terms and phrases that spring from them provide a nourishing substance for the curious minds of medical language specialists.

Although the use of eponyms has been controversial among some groups over the past few years, they continue to be important in distinguishing syndromes, instruments, phenomena, etc., from one another. And with the addition of new eponyms to burgeoning medical vocabularies, it does not appear likely that they will be extinct any time soon.

Many hours of searching for the correct spelling, the accurate place and date of birth and the appropriate definition have gone into this book. We found many variations in spelling and frequent disagreement in birth and death dates among references. Definitions, although usually similarly described, were also sometimes not the same. We've come to terms with what we believe to be closest to "right."

Some eponyms are confusing, to say the least. Names with von, van, de, la (or worse, dela), commonly used with and without the prefix, or full names, such as Marcus Gunn, were challenging to place. Those with variant spellings, such as Abrikossoff/Abrikossov, appear as we understand the preferred spelling.

Our book has been proofread several times. Nevertheless, it is possible that knowledgeable users will find errors that were not detected. We encourage suggestions; thus, the postpaid card at the back of the book. Recommendations from the medical language specialist are the inspiration for excellent libraries such as those provided by Williams & Wilkins.

Publisher's Preface

Stedman's Medical Eponyms offers authoritative assurance of quality and exactness to the wordsmiths of the healthcare professions—medical transcriptionists, medical writers, editors and copy editors, health information management personnel, court reporters, and the many other users and producers of healthcare documentation.

When the authors of this book submitted their proposal to us, we were immediately attracted to the idea of publishing a reference on eponyms and their associated terms. Despite the decline in the use of eponyms, many physicians and the public continue to use eponymic terms. Because the spelling of people's names is so difficult to predict, having a comprehensive reference that provides a user with one place to find these terms is important.

We also realized that medical language professionals needed to know more than just the spelling of the eponymic terms: they needed to have information about the individual as well. Biographical information about an individual helps the user make accurate spelling decisions. For example, how does one know whether the "Dukes test" the physician just dictated is spelled "Dukes" or "Duke's?" With this reference, the user will be able to find the answer. Also, if a physician dictates an eponymic term that isn't in this reference, the user may be able to identify the person on whom the term is based and thus determine the spelling of the term in question.

This resource offers thousands of equipment names, diagnostic and therapeutic procedures, operations, new techniques and maneuvers, incisions, methods and approaches, syndromes and diseases, anatomy terms, and more from all the major specialties and subspecialties of medicine.

This compilation contains over 15,000 eponyms and their associated terms. The extensive A-Z list was developed from the database of *Stedman's Medical Dictionary* and supplemented by the authors with terminology found in current medical literature (please see the list of References on page xix).

Explanatory Notes

Medical transcription is an art as well as a science. Both are needed to correctly interpret the dictation of a healthcare provider, whose language is a product of education, training, and experience. This variety in medical language yields several acceptable ways to express certain terms, including jargon, slang, backformations, coined words and phrases, etc. *Stedman's Medical Eponyms* provides variant spellings and phrasings for many eponymic terms. *Stedman's Medical Eponyms* is a valuable resource for determining the validity of terms as they are encountered.

Alphabetical Organization
Eponyms are listed in alphabetical order by last name. Subentered under the eponym are any eponymic terms associated with that individual. The alphabetization of both names and their associated terms is word by word as spelled, ignoring punctuation, spaces, prefixes, accented letters, or other characters. For example:

Debré, Robert, French pediatrician and bacteriologist, *1882.
> **Debré phenomenon**
> **Debré-De Toni-Fanconi syndrome**
> **Debré-Marie syndrome**

de Clérambault, G., French psychiatrist, 1872–1934.

Deetjen, Hermann, German physician, 1867–1915.

Format and Style
As often as possible, the style of the book follows the style recommended by the American Association for Medical Transcription (AAMT) in *The AAMT Book of Style for Medical Transcription.*

Main entries and subentries are in **boldface** to speed location of a sought-after entry, to enhance distinction between the entries and their associated explanatory information, and to relieve the textual density of the pages.

Biographical/Geographical Information

Both the authors and the publisher have made every attempt to provide comprehensive biographical and geographical information about the individuals listed in this text. In some cases, when we could not find or verify information, only partial information has been provided. When the birth date or death dates are not known or the death date is not yet applicable, the following conventions are used:

Date of birth is represented by an asterisk "*" followed by a date. For example, *1896 indicates the person was born in 1896 and that he or she is either still living or that the date of death is unknown.

Date of death is represented by "d." followed by a date. For example, d. 1896 indicates the person died in 1896 and that his or her birth date is unknown.

Variant Forms

Variant spellings of eponyms are listed alphabetically, and refer the user to the preferred spelling. For example:

> **Abrikossoff,** var. of Abrikossov
> **Abrikossov,** Aleksei I., Russian physician, 1875–1955.

American spellings are used for words with variant spellings, such as orthopedic/orthopaedic and curet/curette, with the understanding that popular variant spellings remain a matter of preference.

Accent Marks

Accent marks, which show pronunciation and syllabic emphasis, occur frequently in proper names. Per *The AAMT Book of Style,* it is acceptable to omit these accents when wordprocessing software does not accommodate special characters or employers permit their omission.

Possessives

Possessive forms have been dropped in this reference for the sake of consistency and for conformance with the guidelines outlined by the AAMT and other groups.

Cross-indexing

Multiple eponymic terms are cross-referenced under all names listed in the term. For example, Dollinger-Bielschowsky syndrome is listed both under Max Bielschowsky and Albert Dollinger. This format provides the user with more than one way to locate and identify a multiple eponymic term. It also allows the user to see together all terms that contain a certain name.

In some cases, the order of the names within a term can vary. Based on the medical literature, a preferred order for that term has been identified. Any explanatory information about the term will only appear under the *first* name of the *preferred* term.

See under

Consider the example above of Bielschowsky and Dollinger. Bielschowsky-Dollinger syndrome is the nonpreferred term, so its entry reads, "Syn: Dollinger-Bielschowsky syndrome." A little further down the list is "Dollinger-Bielschowsky syndrome," the preferred term. Since it is not under Dollinger, but under Bielschowsky, no explanatory material appears here. Instead, a "see under Dollinger" reference points the user to Dollinger for any necessary explanatory material. Where more than one entry shares the same surname, the first name also appears at "see under."

Synonyms

Explanatory information about a term can be of several types. When the eponymic term is the preferred term in *Stedman's Medical Dictionary,* a brief definition and any applicable synonyms follow it. These synonyms can be other eponyms, or they can be noneponymic terms. For example:

Marjolin, Jean N., French physician, 1780–1850.
    Marjolin syndrome—*SYN:* Marjolin ulcer
    Marjolin ulcer—well-differentiated but aggressive squamous cell carcinoma occurring in cicatricial tissue at the epidermal edge of a sinus draining underlying osteomyelitis. *SYN:* Marjolin syndrome; epidermoid ulcer

In other cases, a noneponymic term is the preferred term in *Stedman's Medical Dictionary.* Where the noneponymic synonym is sufficient for the user to determine that the appropriate condition, anatomical structure, or procedure is being discussed, the noneponymic synonym will stand for all eponymic entries. For example:

Keith, Sir Arthur, Scottish anatomist, 1866–1955.
    Keith and Flack node—*SYN:* sinuatrial node
    Keith bundle—*SYN:* atrioventricular bundle
    Keith node—*SYN:* sinuatrial node

Flack, Martin, English physiologist, 1882–1931.
    Flack node—*SYN:* sinuatrial node
    Keith and Flack node—*SYN:* sinuatrial node

Using synonyms alone saves the user time flipping back and forth to find explanatory material. If Flack node is transcribed, that is the only place the user needs to look; there is no need to flip ahead to Keith.

On the other hand, at times the preferred noneponymic synonym in *Stedman's Medical Dictionary* is ambiguous anatomically or contains uncommon medical vocabulary. In those cases, explanatory material appears at an eponymic term and all eponymic synonyms refer back to that term.

References

American Medical Association. Directory of deceased American physicians 1804–1929, vol. I & II. Chicago: American Medical Association, 1993.

Dorland's illustrated medical dictionary, 28th ed. Philadelphia: WB Saunders Company, 1994.

Firkin BG, Whitworth JA, eds. Dictionary of medical eponyms. Park Ridge, NJ: Parthenon Publishing Group Inc, 1990.

Goldenson, RM. Longman dictionary of psychology and psychiatry. White Plains: Longman Inc. 1984.

Jablonski S. Jablonski's dictionary of syndromes & eponymic diseases, 2nd ed. Malabar, FL: Krieger Publishing Company, 1991.

Lourie, JA. Medical eponyms: who was Coudé? London: Pitman Publishing Limited, 1982.

Magalini SI, Magalini SC, de Francisci G. Dictionary of medical syndromes, 3rd ed. Philadelphia: JB Lippincott Company, 1990.

Merriam-Webster's collegiate dictionary, 10th ed. Springfield: Merriam-Webster Inc., 1996.

Random house dictionary of the English language, 2nd ed. New York: Random House Inc., 1994.

Sloane SB. Medical abbreviations & eponyms, 2nd ed. Philadelphia: WB Saunders Company, 1991.

Stedman's abbreviations, acronyms & symbols. Baltimore: Williams & Wilkins, 1992.

Stedman's cardiology & pulmonary words, 2nd ed. Baltimore: Williams & Wilkins, 1997.

Stedman's dentistry words. Baltimore: Williams & Wilkins, 1993.

Stedman's dermatology & immunology Words. Baltimore: Williams & Wilkins, 1997.

Stedman's ENT words. Baltimore: Williams & Wilkins, 1993.

Stedman's GI & GU words, 2nd ed. Baltimore: Williams & Wilkins, 1996.

Stedman's medical dictionary, 26th ed. Baltimore: Williams & Wilkins, 1995.

Stedman's medical & surgical equipment words. Baltimore: Williams & Wilkins, 1996.

Stedman's neurosurgery words. Baltimore: Williams & Wilkins, 1993.

Stedman's OB-GYN words, 2nd ed. Baltimore: Williams & Wilkins, 1995.

Stedman's ophthalmology words. Baltimore: Williams & Wilkins, 1993.

Stedman's orthopaedic & rehab words, 2nd ed. Baltimore: Williams & Wilkins, 1995.

Stedman's pathology & lab medicine words, 2nd ed. Baltimore: Williams & Wilkins, 1997.

Stedman's psychiatry words. Baltimore: Williams & Wilkins, 1992.

Stedman's radiology & oncology words, 2nd ed. Baltimore: Williams & Wilkins, 1995.

Tessier C. The surgical word book, 2nd ed. Philadelphia: WB Saunders Company, 1991.

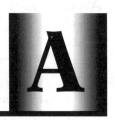

Aagenaes, Oystein, Norwegian pediatrician, *1925.
    Aagenaes syndrome—inherited condition of lymphedema and arrested bile flow.

Aaron, Charles Dettie, U.S. physician, 1866–1951.
    Aaron sign—in acute appendicitis, a referred pain or feeling of distress in the epigastrium or precordial region on continuous firm pressure over McBurney point.

Aarskog, Dagfinn, Norwegian pediatrician, *1928.
    Aarskog-Scott syndrome—*SYN:* faciodigitogenital dysplasia

Aase, Jon Morton, U.S. pediatrician, *1936.
    Aase syndrome—affiliated with multiple birth defects; may be inherited recessive.

Abadie, Charles A., French ophthalmologist, 1842–1932.
    Abadie sign of exophthalmic goiter—spasm of the musculus levator palpebrae superioris in Graves disease.

Abadie, Joseph Louis Irénée Jean, French neurosurgeon, 1873–1946.
    Abadie sign of tabes dorsalis—insensibility to pressure over the Achilles tendon.

Abbe, Robert, U.S. surgeon, 1851–1928.
    Abbe flap—a full-thickness flap of the middle portion of the lower lip that is transferred into the upper lip, or vice versa.
    Abbe intestinal anastomosis
    Abbe neurectomy
    Abbe operation—use of an Abbe flap in plastic surgery of the lips.
    Abbe refractometer
    Abbe repair
    Abbe ring
    Abbe small-bowel operation
    Abbe stage I cheiloplasty
    Abbe stage II cheiloplasty
    Abbe-Estlander cheiloplasty

Abbé, Ernst Karl, German physicist, 1840–1905.
    Abbé condenser—a system of two or three wide-angle, achromatic, convex, and planoconvex lenses.

Abbott, Alexander C., U.S. bacteriologist, 1860–1935.
    Abbott stain for spores

Abbott, Edville Gerhardt, U.S. orthopedic surgeon, 1871–1938.
    Abbott approach
    Abbott arthrodesis
    Abbott elevator
    Abbott method—a method of treatment for scoliosis.

Abbott, William Osler, U.S. physician, 1902–1943.
    Abbott tube—*SYN:* Miller-Abbott tube
    Miller-Abbott catheter—*SYN:* Miller-Abbott tube
    Miller-Abbott tube—see under Miller, Thomas

Abegg, Richard, Danish chemist, 1869–1910.
    Abegg rule—sometimes loosely stated as all atoms have the same number of valences, a consequence of the tendency of valence electron shells to be filled to 8.

Abel, Rudolf, German bacteriologist, 1868–1942.
    Abel bacillus—*Klebsiella pneumoniae* subspecies ozaenae.

Abelson, Herbert T., U.S. pediatrician, *1941.
    Abelson murine leukemia virus—a retrovirus belonging to the type C retrovirus group subfamily (family Oncovirinae), which is associated with leukemia.

Aberhalden, E., Swiss physiologist and biochemist, 1877–1950.
    Aberhalden-Kauffman-Lignac syndrome—renal rickets with widespread deposits of cystine crystals throughout the body.

Abernethy, John, English surgeon and anatomist, 1764–1831.
    Abernethy fascia—a layer of subperitoneal areolar tissue in front of the external iliac artery.
    Abernethy operation

Abrahams, Robert, U.S. physician, 1861–1935.
    Abrahams sign—rales and other adventitious sounds indicating progress from incipient to advanced tuberculosis.

Abrams, Albert, U.S. physician, 1863–1924.
    Abrams heart reflex—a contraction of the myocardium when the skin of the precordial region is irritated.

Abrikosov, Aleksei I., Russian physician, 1875–1955.
    Abrikosov myoblastoma—generally benign skin tumor. *SYN:* Abrikosov tumor
    Abrikosov tumor—*SYN:* Abrikosov myoblastoma

Abrikossoff, var. of Abrikosov

Abt, Arthur F., U.S. physician, 1867–1955.
    Abt-Letterer-Siwe syndrome—acute disease affecting liver, spleen, lymph nodes; occurs most often in infants and children. *SYN:* Letterer-Siwe syndrome; Letterer reticulosis; Letterer-Siwe disease

Achard, Émile Charles, French physician, 1860–1941.
    Achard syndrome—arachnodactyly with small, receding mandible, broad skull, and joint laxity limited to the hands and feet.
    Achard-Thiers syndrome—one form of a virilizing disorder of adrenocortical origin in women.

Achenbach, Walter, 20th century German internist.
Achenbach syndrome—hematoma of the finger pad with accompanying edema.

Achilles, mythical Greek warrior who was vulnerable only in the heel.
Achilles bursa—bursa between the tendo calcaneus and the upper part of the posterior surface of the calcaneum. *SYN:* bursa of tendo calcaneus
Achilles reflex—a contraction of the calf muscles when the tendo calcaneus is sharply struck. *SYN:* ankle jerk; ankle reflex; tendo Achillis reflex; triceps surae reflex
Achilles tendon—the tendon of insertion of the triceps surae (gastrocnemius and soleus) into the tuberosity of the calcaneus. *SYN:* tendo calcaneus

Achor, Richard W.P., U.S. physician, *1922.
Achor-Smith syndrome—potassium deficiency leading to pernicious anemia, severe diarrhea, muscle wasting, renal insufficiency. *SYN:* nutritional deficiency syndrome with hypopotassemia

Achúcarro, Nicolás, Spanish histologist, 1881–1918.
Achúcarro stain—stain for impregnating connective tissue.

Ackerman, Lauren V., contemporary U.S. histopathologist.
Ackerman tumor—rare verrucous carcinoma of the larynx.

Acosta, Joseph (José) de, Spanish Jesuit missionary, 1539–1600.
Acosta disease—*SYN:* altitude sickness

Acrel, Olof, Swedish surgeon, 1717–1806.
Acrel ganglion—a cyst on a tendon of an extensor muscle at the level of the wrist.

Adam, first man, according to the Bible.
Adam's apple—*SYN:* laryngeal prominence.

Adamkiewicz, Albert, Polish pathologist, 1850–1921.
artery of Adamkiewicz—largest of the medullary arteries which supply the spinal cord by anastomosing with the anterior (longitudinal) spinal artery. *SYN:* arteria radicularis magna

Adams, James Alexander, Scottish gynecologist, 1857–1930.
Alexander-Adams operation—*SYN:* Alexander operation

Adams, Robert, Irish physician, 1791–1875.
Adams-Stokes disease—*SYN:* Adams-Stokes syndrome
Adams-Stokes syncope—syncope due to complete atrioventricular block.
Adams-Stokes syndrome—characterized by slow or absent pulse, vertigo, syncope, convulsions, and sometimes Cheyne-Stokes respiration. *SYN:* Adams-Stokes disease; Morgagni disease; Stokes-Adams disease; Morgagni-Adams-Stokes syndrome; Spens syndrome
Morgagni-Adams-Stokes syndrome—*SYN:* Adams-Stokes syndrome

(continued)

NOTES

Adams *(continued)*
    Stokes-Adams disease—*Syn:* Adams-Stokes syndrome
    Stokes-Adams syndrome—*Syn:* Adams-Stokes syndrome

Adams, Sir William, English surgeon, 1760–1829.
    Adams operation
    Adams saw

Adanson, Michel, French naturalist, 1727–1806.
    adansonian classification—the classification of organisms based on giving equal weight to every characteristic of the organism.

Addis, Thomas, U.S. internist, 1881–1949.
    Addis count—a quantitative enumeration of the red and white blood counts, and casts in a 12-hour urine specimen, used to follow the progress of renal disease.

Addison, Christopher, English anatomist, 1869–1951.
    Addison clinical planes—a series of planes used as landmarks in thoracoabdominal topography.

Addison, Thomas, English physician, 1793–1860.
    Addison anemia—a chronic, progressive anemia of older adults due to failure of absorption of Vitamin B_{12}. *Syn:* pernicious anemia; Addison-Biermer disease; addisonian anemia; Biermer anemia; Biermer disease
    Addison disease—*Syn:* chronic adrenocortical insufficiency
    Addison-Biermer disease—*Syn:* Addison anemia
    Addison-Schilder disease—*Syn:* Schilder disease
    addisonian anemia—*Syn:* Addison anemia
    addisonian crisis—*Syn:* acute adrenocortical insufficiency

Adie, William John, Australian physician, 1886–1935.
    Adie pupil—*Syn:* Adie syndrome
    Adie syndrome—an idiopathic postganglionic denervation of the parasympathetically innervated intraocular muscles. *Syn:* Adie pupil; pupillotonic pseudotabes; Holmes-Adie pupil; Holmes-Adie syndrome; Weill syndrome
    Holmes-Adie pupil—*Syn:* Adie syndrome
    Holmes-Adie syndrome—*Syn:* Adie syndrome

Adler, Alfred, Austrian psychiatrist, 1870–1937.
    adlerian psychoanalysis—a theory of human behavior emphasizing humans' social nature, strivings for mastery, and drive to overcome, by compensation, feelings of inferiority. *Syn:* individual psychology; adlerian psychology
    adlerian psychology—*Syn:* adlerian psychoanalysis

Adler, Oscar, German physician, 1879–1932.
    Adler test—a test to detect the presence of blood. *Syn:* benzidine test

Adrian, Lord Edgar Douglas, English physiologist, 1889–1977, 1932 joint winner of Nobel Prize for discovery of neuron functions.

Adrian of Cambridge, var. of Adrian, Lord Edgar Douglas

Adson, Alfred Washington, U.S. neurosurgeon, 1887–1951.
    Adson aneurysm needle

Adson angular hook
Adson brain clip
Adson brain forceps
Adson brain hook
Adson brain retractor
Adson brain suction tip
Adson brain suction tube
Adson brain-exploring cannula
Adson cerebellar retractor
Adson cranial rongeur
Adson drainage cannula
Adson dural hook
Adson dural knife
Adson dural protector
Adson forceps
Adson Gigli saw
Adson Gigli-saw guide
Adson head rest
Adson maneuver—*SYN:* Adson test
Adson microbipolar forceps
Adson microdressing forceps
Adson microtissue forceps
Adson procedure—*SYN:* Adson test
Adson scalp clip
Adson scalp clip-applying forceps
Adson syndrome—(1) *SYN:* Naffziger syndrome; (2) cerebral sphingolipidosis.
Adson test—a test for thoracic outlet syndrome. *SYN:* Adson maneuver; Adson procedure
Brown-Adson forceps—see under Brown, James

Aeby, Christopher Theodore, Swiss anatomist, 1835–1885.
   Aeby muscle—a labial muscle formed by sagittal fibers running from the skin to the mucous membrane. *SYN:* cutaneomucous muscle
   Aeby plane—in craniometry, a plane perpendicular to the median plane of the cranium.

Afzelius, Arvid, Swedish physician.
   Afzelius erythema—*SYN:* Lipschütz erythema; erythema chronicum migrans

Ahumada, Juan Carlos, 20th century Argentinian physician.
   Ahumada-del Castillo syndrome—unphysiological lactation and amenorrhea not following pregnancy characterized by hyperprolactinemia and a pituitary adenoma. *SYN:* Argonz-del Castillo syndrome

Aicardi, J. Dennis, 20th century French neurologist.
   Aicardi syndrome—agenesis of the corpus callosum with infantile spasms in female babies.

NOTES

Aird, Robert B., U.S. neurologist, *1903.
  Flynn-Aird syndrome—see under Flynn

Åkerlund, A. Olof, Swedish radiologist, 1885–1958.
  Åkerlund deformity—indentation (incisura) with niche of duodenal cap as demonstrated radiographically.
  Åkerlund diaphragm

Akureyri, a town in Iceland.
  Akureyri disease—epidemic neuromyasthenia. Akureyri, Iceland, reported approximately 1,000 cases in 1948.

Alagille, Daniel B., French pediatrician, *1925.
  Alagille syndrome—*SYN:* syndromatic paucity of interlobular bile ducts

Alajouanine, Théophile, French neurologist, 1890–1980.
  Foix-Alajouanine myelitis—see under Foix
  Foix-Alajouanine syndrome—see under Foix

Alanson, Edward, English surgeon, 1747–1823.
  Alanson amputation—a circular amputation, the stump shaped like a cone.

Albarran y Dominguez, Joaquin, Cuban urologist, 1860–1912.
  Albarran bridge
  Albarran cystoscope
  Albarran glands—minute submucosal glands or branching tubules in the subcervical region of the prostate gland. *SYN:* Albarran y Dominguez tubules
  Albarran test—a test for renal insufficiency. *SYN:* polyuria test
  Albarran urethroscope
  Albarran y Dominguez tubules—*SYN:* Albarran glands

Albee, Fred H., U.S. surgeon, 1876–1945.
  Albee acetabuloplasty
  Albee arthrodesis
  Albee bone graft
  Albee bone graft calipers
  Albee bone saw
  Albee drill
  Albee fracture table
  Albee fusion
  Albee graft
  Albee hip reconstruction
  Albee operation—orthopedic hip procedure.
  Albee orthopedic table
  Albee osteotome
  Albee osteotomy
  Albee shelf procedure
  Albee spinal fusion

Albers-Schönberg, Heinrich E., German radiologist, 1865–1921.
  Albers-Schönberg disease—excessive formation of dense trabecular bone and calcified cartilage. *SYN:* osteopetrosis

Albert, Eduard, Austrian surgeon, 1841–1900.
    Albert disease—inflammation of the bursa between the Achilles tendon and the os calcis. *SYN:* Swediauer disease
    Albert suture—a modified Czerny suture, the first row of stitches passing through the entire thickness of the wall of the gut.

Albert, Henry, U.S. physician, 1878–1930.
    Albert stain—a stain for diphtheria bacilli.

Albini, Giuseppe, Italian physiologist, 1827–1911.
    Albini nodules—minute fibrous nodules on the margins of the mitral and tricuspid valves of the heart, representing fetal tissue rests.

Albinus, Bernhard Siegfried, German anatomist and surgeon, 1697–1770.
    Albinus muscle—a facial muscle that draws angle of mouth laterally. *SYN:* risorius muscle; scalenus minimus muscle

Albrecht, Karl Martin Paul, German anatomist, 1851–1894.
    Albrecht bone—a small bone between the basioccipital and basisphenoid.
    Albrecht syndrome

Albright, Fuller, U.S. physician, 1900–1969.
    Albright disease—*SYN:* McCune-Albright syndrome
    Albright hereditary osteodystrophy—an inherited form of hyperparathyroidism associated with ectopic calcification and ossification and skeletal defects. *SYN:* Albright syndrome (2)
    Albright IV syndrome—*SYN:* Martin-Albright syndrome
    Albright syndrome—(1) *SYN:* McCune-Albright syndrome; (2) *SYN:* Albright hereditary osteodystrophy.
    Albright synovectomy
    Albright-Hadorn syndrome—softening and bending of bones associated with abnormally small concentration of potassium in blood.
    Forbes-Albright syndrome—see under Forbes, A. P.
    Martin-Albright syndrome—see under Martin, D.
    McCune-Albright syndrome—see under McCune

Alcock, Benjamin, Irish anatomist, *1801.
    Alcock bag
    Alcock bladder syringe
    Alcock canal—the space within the obturator internis fascia lining the lateral wall of the ischiorectal fossa that transmits the pudendal vessels and nerves. *SYN:* pudendal canal; canalis pudendalis
    Alcock catheter
    Alcock catheter adapter
    Alcock catheter plug
    Alcock hemostatic bag
    Alcock hemostatic catheter
    Alcock lithotrite
    Alcock obturator

NOTES

Alder, Albert von.
> **Alder anomaly**—coarse azurophilic granulation of leukocytes, especially granulocytes, which may be associated with gargoylism and Morquio disease.
> **Alder bodies**—granular inclusions in polymorphonuclear leukocytes.
> **Alder-Reilly anomaly**

Aldrich, Robert Anderson, U.S. pediatrician, *1917.
> **Aldrich syndrome**—*SYN:* Wiskott-Aldrich syndrome
> **Wiskott-Aldrich syndrome**—see under Wiskott

Aleutian Islands, chain of islands in the North Pacific Ocean.
> **Aleutian disease**—plasma cell disorder of minks with characteristics similar to multiple myeloma.

Alexander, F. Matthias, Australian elocutionist, 1869–1955.
> **Alexander technique**—used to develop kinesthetic sense of normal movements and posture.

Alexander, Gustav, Austrian otolaryngologist, *1873.
> **Alexander antrostomy punch**
> **Alexander deafness**—high-frequency deafness due to membranous cochlear dysplasia.
> **Alexander mastoid bone gouge**
> **Alexander mastoid chisel**
> **Alexander otoplasty**
> **Alexander tonsil needle**

Alexander, W. Stewart, 20th century New Zealand pathologist.
> **Alexander disease**—a rare, fatal, central nervous system degenerative disease of infants.

Alexander, William, English surgeon, 1844–1919.
> **Alexander operation**—repair of uterine displacement. *SYN:* Alexander-Adams operation
> **Alexander-Adams operation**—*SYN:* Alexander operation

Alezzandrini, Arturo Alberto, Argentinian ophthalmologist, *1932.
> **Alezzandrini syndrome**—a rare syndrome appearing in adolescents and young adults, characterized by unilateral degenerative retinitis, followed by ipsilateral poliosis and facial vitiligo, and occasionally bilateral perceptive deafness.

Alfidi, Ralph J., U.S. physician.
> **Alfidi syndrome**—occlusion of the celiac axis leading to hypertension. *SYN:* renal-splanchnic steal

Allemann, Richard, Swiss physician, 1893–1958.
> **Allemann syndrome**—hereditary double kidney, clubbing of fingers; may be associated with facial asymmetry and motor nerve degeneration.

Allen, Alfred Henry, U.S. chemist, 1846–1904.
> **Allen test**—a test for phenol.

Allen, Arthur W., U.S. surgeon, 1887–1958.
> **Buerger-Allen exercises**—see under Buerger, Leo

Allen, Edgar Van Nuys, U.S. physician, 1900–1961.
Allen test—a test for radial or ulnar patency.

Allen, Edgar, U.S. endocrinologist, 1892–1943.
Allen-Doisy test—a test for estrogenic activity.
Allen-Doisy unit—the quantity of estrogen capable of producing in a spayed mouse a characteristic change in the vaginal epithelium. *SYN:* mouse unit

Allen, Frederick Madison, U.S. physician, 1879–1964.
Allen paradoxic law—that more sugar is utilized by nondiabetics as more is given; the opposite in those with diabetes.

Allen, Willard Myron, U.S. gynecologist, *1904.
Allen fetal stethoscope
Allen uterine forceps
Allen-Masters syndrome—pelvic pain resulting from old lacerations of the broad ligament during delivery.
Corner-Allen test—see under Corner, George
Corner-Allen unit—see under Corner, George

Allingham, William, English physician, 1829–1908.
Allingham colotomy
Allingham rectal speculum
Allingham rectum excision
Allingham ulcer—anal ulcer. *SYN:* fissure in ano

Allis, Oscar Huntington, U.S. surgeon, 1836–1921.
Allis forceps—a straight grasping forceps.
Allis hemostat
Allis intestinal forceps
Allis Micro-Line pediatric forceps
Allis sign—in fracture of the neck of the femur, the trochanter rides up, relaxing the fascia lata, so that the finger can be sunk deeply between the great trochanter and the iliac crest.

Allport, Gordon Willard, U.S. psychologist, 1897–1967.
Allport A-S Reaction Study—a personality test designed to determine whether a subject is dominant or submissive in dealing with situations.
Allport personality-trait theory—theory that personality traits are the key to individuality and consistency of behavior.

Almeida, Floriano Paulo de, Brazilian physician, *1898.
Almeida disease—a chronic mycosis caused by *Paracoccidioides brasiliensis. SYN:* paracoccidioidomycosis
Lutz-Splendore-Almeida disease—see under Lutz

Almén, August Teodor, Swedish physiologist, 1833–1903.
Almén test for blood—a test for occult blood. *SYN:* guaiac test; Schönbein test; van Deen test

NOTES

Alpers, Bernard J., U.S. neurologist, 1900–1981.
 Alpers disease—familial progressive spastic paresis of extremities with destruction and disorganization of nerve cells of the cerebral cortex. *Syn:* poliodystrophia cerebri progressiva infantalis

Alport, Arthur Cecil, South African physician, 1880–1959.
 Alport syndrome—progressive microscopic hematuria.

Alström, Carl-Henry, Swedish geneticist, *1907.
 Alström syndrome—retinal degeneration with nystagmus and loss of central vision.

Altherr, Franz.
 Meyenburg-Altherr-Uehlinger syndrome—*Syn:* Meyenburg disease

Altmann, Richard, German histologist, 1852–1900.
 Altmann anilin-acid fuchsin stain—a mixture of picric acid, anilin, and acid fuchsin which stains mitochondria crimson against a yellow background.
 Altmann fixative—a bichromate-osmic acid fixative.
 Altmann granule—a granule that has an affinity for fuchsin. *Syn:* fuchsinophil granule; mitochondrion
 Altmann theory—a theory that protoplasm consists of granular particles that are clustered and enclosed in indifferent matter.
 Altmann-Gersh method—the method of rapidly freezing a tissue and dehydrating it in a vacuum.

Alvarez, Walter C., U.S. physician.
 Alvarez syndrome—neurotic or hysterical bloating of the abdomen without clinical cause. *Syn:* pseudoileus; accordion abdomen; hysterical nongaseous abdominal bloating

Alzheimer, Alois, German neurologist, 1864–1915.
 Alzheimer dementia—*Syn:* Alzheimer disease
 Alzheimer disease—progressive mental deterioration. *Syn:* primary neuronal degeneration; Alzheimer dementia; presenile dementia; primary senile dementia
 Alzheimer sclerosis—hyaline degeneration of the medium and smaller blood vessels of the brain.

Ambard, Léon, French pharmacologist, 1876–1962.
 Ambard constant
 Ambard laws—laws for output of urea.

Amberg, Emil, U.S. otologist, 1868–1948.
 Amberg lateral sinus line—a line dividing the angle formed by the anterior edge of the mastoid process and the temporal line.

Ames, Adelbert, Jr., U.S. educator, 1880–1955.
 Ames demonstrations—series of illusions designed to test depth perception.

Ames, Bruce N., U.S. molecular geneticist, *1928.
 Ames assay—a screening test for possible carcinogens. *Syn:* Ames test
 Ames test—*Syn:* Ames assay

Amici, Giovanni Battista, Italian physicist, 1786–1863.
 Amici disk—thin membrane seen as a line which serves as delimiter of sarcomeres in striated muscle. *Syn:* Amici striae; Z band

Amici line
Amici striae—*Syn:* Amici disk

Ammon, Friedrich von, German ophthalmologist and pathologist, 1799–1861.
Ammon blepharoplasty
Ammon blue dye
Ammon canthoplasty
Ammon dacryocystotomy
Ammon eyelid repair
Ammon fissure—a pear-shaped opening in the sclera during early embryogenesis.
Ammon prominence—an external prominence in the posterior pole of the eyeball during early embryogenesis.

Ammon, Greek name of Egyptian god, Amun.
Ammon horn—one of the two interlocking gyri composing the hippocampus, the other being the dentate gyrus. *Syn:* cornu ammonis

Ammons, Henry R., U.S. physician, 1857–1923.
Ammons Full Range Picture Vocabulary Test

Amoss, Harold Lindsay, U.S. physician, 1886–1956.
Amoss sign—in painful flexion of the spine, it is necessary to support a sitting position by extending the arms behind the torso with the weight placed on the hands.

Ampère, André-Marie, French physicist, 1775–1836.
ampere—the practical unit of electrical current.
Ampère postulate—*Syn:* Avogadro law
statampere—the electrostatic unit of current, equal to 3.335641×10^{-10} ampere.

Amplatz, Kurt, 20th century U.S. cardiologist.
Amplatz angiography needle
Amplatz aortography catheter
Amplatz cardiac catheter
Amplatz coronary catheter
Amplatz fascial dilator
Amplatz femoral catheter
Amplatz guide
Amplatz II curve
Amplatz injector
Amplatz Super Stiff guide wire
Amplatz torque wire
AMPLATZER septal occluder

Amsler, Marc, Swiss ophthalmologist, 1891–1968.
Amsler chart—a 10-cm square divided into 5-mm squares upon which an individual may project a defect in the central visual field.
Amsler chart marker

(continued)

NOTES

Amsler *(continued)*
    Amsler corneal graft operation
    Amsler needle
    Amsler operation
    Amsler scleral marker
    Amsler test—projection of a visual field defect onto an Amsler chart.

Amussat, Jean Z., French surgeon, 1796–1856.
    Amussat incision
    Amussat operation
    Amussat probe
    Amussat valve—a series of crescentic folds of mucous membrane in the upper part of the cystic duct. *Syn:* spiral fold of cystic duct
    Amussat valvula—anomalous folds occurring at the level of the seminal colliculus. *Syn:* posterior urethral valves

Anagnostakis, Andrei, Cretan ophthalmologist, 1826–1897.
    Anagnostakis operation—(1) a procedure for entropion; (2) a procedure for trichiasis.

Andermann, Frederick, Canadian physician.
    Andermann syndrome—recessive gene causing agenesis of the corpus callosum. *Syn:* Charlevoix disease

Andernach, Johann Winther von (Guenther von Andernach), German physician, 1505–1574.
    Andernach ossicles—small irregular bones found along the sutures of the cranium. *Syn:* sutural bones

Anders, James Meschter, U.S. physician, 1854–1936.
    Anders disease—a condition characterized by a deposit of symmetrical nodular or pendulous masses of fat in various regions of the body, with discomfort or pain. *Syn:* adiposis dolorosa; adiposis tuberosa simplex

Andersch, Carolus Samuel, German anatomist, 1732–1777.
    Andersch ganglion—the lower of two sensory ganglions on the glossopharyngeal nerve as it traverses the jugular foramen. *Syn:* inferior ganglion of glossopharyngeal nerve
    Andersch nerve—*Syn:* tympanic nerve

Andersen, Dorothy Hansine, U.S. pediatrician, 1901–1963.
    Andersen disease—familial cirrhosis of the liver with storage of abnormal glycogen. *Syn:* type 4 glycogenosis
    Andersen syndrome—cystic fibrosis of the pancreas, vitamin A deficiency, and disease of the abdominal cavity. *Syn:* Andersen triad
    Andersen triad—*Syn:* Andersen syndrome

Anderson, Evelyn, U.S. physician, *1899.
    Anderson-Collip test—a procedure for evaluating the thyrotropic activity of an extract of the anterior lobe of the pituitary gland.

Anderson, James C., English urologist, *1899.
    Anderson-Hynes pyeloplasty—disjoined or dismembered pyeloplasty.

Anderson, Roger, U.S. orthopedic surgeon, 1891–1971.
    Anderson splint—a skeletal traction splint.

Anderson tibial lengthening
Anderson traction bow

Anderson, Rose G., U.S. psychologist, *1893.
Kuhlmann-Anderson tests—see under Kuhlmann

Anderson, W., English surgeon and dermatologist, 1842–1900.
Anderson-Fabry disease—*SYN:* Fabry disease

Andes, mountains in Peru.
Andes disease—chronic altitude sickness.

Andogskii, var. of Andogsky

Andogsky, N., Russian physician.
Andogsky syndrome—development of total soft cataracts in adults who have a history of chronic dermatologic eczema. *SYN:* cataracta dermatogenes; dermatogenic cataract; cataracta syndermatotica

Andrade, Corino M. de, 20th century Portuguese physician.
Andrade syndrome—accumulation of amyloid in organs and tissues of the body.

Andrade, Eduardo Penny, U.S. bacteriologist, 1872–1906.
Andrade indicator—solution used to culture acid-producing organisms.

Andral, Gabriel, French physician, 1797–1876.
Andral decubitus—position assumed by a patient who lies on the sound side in cases of beginning pleurisy.

Andresen, Viggo, Norwegian orthodontist, 1870–1950.
Andresen removable orthodontic appliance
Andresen activator
Andresen monoblock appliance

Andrews, C.J., U.S. surgeon.
Andrews gouge
Andrews iliotibial band reconstruction
Andrews iliotibial band tenodesis
Andrews knee reconstruction
Andrews lateral tenodesis
Andrews spinal surgery table
Andrews technique
Brandt-Andrews maneuver—see under Brandt, Thure

Anel, Dominique, French surgeon, 1679–1725.
Anel lacrimal duct dilation
Anel method—ligation of an artery immediately above (on the proximal side of) an aneurysm.
Anel probe
Anel syringe

NOTES

Angelman, Harry, 20th century English physician.
Angelman syndrome—recessive gene causing motor dysfunction, mental retardation, hypotonia. *SYN:* happy puppet syndrome

Angelucci, Arnaldo, Italian ophthalmologist, 1854–1934.
Angelucci syndrome—extreme excitability, vasomotor disturbances, and palpitation associated with vernal conjunctivitis.

Anger, Hal, U.S. electrical engineer, *1920.
Anger camera—a scintigraphic imaging system or type of gamma camera.

Anghelescu, Constantin, Romanian surgeon, 1869–1948.
Anghelescu sign—in vertebral tuberculosis, painful or impossible flexion of the spine when the patient attempts to rest weight on the heels and occiput.

Angle, Edward Hartley, U.S. orthodontist, 1855–1930.
Angle classification of malocclusion

Anglesey, designed for Henry William Paget, first marquis of Anglesey, 1768–1854.
Anglesey leg—first prosthetic wooden leg.

Ångström, Anders J., Swedish physicist, 1814–1874.
ångström—a unit of wavelength, 10^{-10} m, roughly the diameter of an atom; equivalent to 0.1 nm.
Ångström law—a substance absorbs light of the same wavelength as it emits when luminous.
Ångström scale—a table of wavelengths of a large number of light rays corresponding to as many Fraunhofer lines in the spectrum.
Ångström unit

Anichkov, var. of Anitschkow

Anitschkow, Nikolai, Russian pathologist, 1885–1964.
Anitschkow cell—a large mononuclear cell found in connective tissue of the heart wall in inflammatory conditions. *SYN:* cardiac histiocyte; Anitschkow myocyte
Anitschkow myocyte—*SYN:* Anitschkow cell

Anrep, G.V., 20th century Lebanese physiologist in Britain.
Anrep phenomenon—homeometric autoregulation of the heart whereby cardiac performance improves as the aortic pressure is increased.

Anton, Gabriel, German neuropsychiatrist, 1858–1933.
Anton syndrome—in cortical blindness, lack of awareness of being blind.

Antoni, Nils, Swedish neurologist, 1887–1968.
Antoni type A neurilemoma—relatively solid or compact arrangement of neoplastic tissue that consists of Schwann cells arranged in twisting bundles associated with delicate reticulin fibers.
Antoni type B neurilemoma—relatively soft or loose arrangement of neoplastic tissue that consists of Schwann cells in a nondescript arrangement among reticulin fibers and tiny cystlike foci.

Antopol, William, U.S. physician.
Antopol disease—cardiomegaly caused by glycogen deposits in the heart, thought to be caused by recessive transmission.

Antyllus, Greek physician, ca. 150 A.D.
    Antyllus method—ligation of the artery above and below an aneurysm, followed by incision into and emptying of the sac.

Apert, Eugène, French pediatrician, 1868–1940.
    Apert hirsutism—excessive body or facial hair caused by a virilizing disorder of adrenocortical origin.
    Apert syndrome—*SYN:* Crouzon-Apert disease; type I acrocephalosyndactyly
    Crouzon-Apert disease—*SYN:* Apert syndrome

Apgar, Virginia, U.S. anesthesiologist, 1909–1974.
    Apgar score—evaluation of a newborn infant's physical status by assigning numerical values to each of 5 criteria.
    Apgar timer

Apley, Alan G., English orthopedic surgeon.
    Apley grinding test—orthopedic test related to a meniscal tear.
    Apley knee test
    Apley maneuver
    Apley sign
    Apley traction

Applebaum, L., 20th century German physician.
    Recklinghausen-Applebaum disease—see under Recklinghausen

Aran, François, French physician, 1817–1861.
    Aran-Duchenne disease—*SYN:* Lou Gehrig disease
    Aran-Duchenne dystrophy—*SYN:* Lou Gehrig disease
    Duchenne-Aran disease—*SYN:* Lou Gehrig disease

Arantius, (Aranzio), Giulio C., Italian anatomist and physician, 1530–1589.
    Arantius ligament—a thin fibrous cord, lying in the fissure of the ligamentum venosum; the remains of the ductus venosus of the fetus. *SYN:* ligamentum venosum
    Arantius nodule—a nodule at the center of the free border of each semilunar valve at the beginning of the pulmonary artery and aorta. *SYN:* nodule of semilunar valve; corpus arantii
    Arantius ventricle—inferior part of the rhomboid fossa. *SYN:* calamus scriptorius
    corpus arantii—*SYN:* Arantius nodule
    ductus venosus arantii—rarely used term for ductus venosus.

Arber, Werner, Swiss microbiologist, *1929, 1978 joint winner of the Nobel Prize for medicine and physiology for his work on restriction enzymes.

Archambault, LaSalle, U.S. neurologist, 1879–1940.
    Meyer-Archambault loop—see under Meyer, Adolf

Arey, Leslie B., U.S. anatomist, 1891–1988.
    Arey rule—rule related to size of embryo or fetus.

NOTES

Argand, Aimé, Swiss physicist, 1755–1803.
    Argand burner—oil or gas burner with air supplied to flame by an inner tube.

Argonz, J., Argentinian physician.
    Argonz-del Castillo syndrome—*Syn:* Ahumada-del Castillo syndrome

Argyll Robertson, Douglas M.C.L., see under Robertson.

Arias-Stella, Javier, Peruvian pathologist, *1924.
    Arias-Stella effect—focal, unusual, decidual changes in endometrial epithelium that may be associated with ectopic or uterine pregnancy. *Syn:* Arias-Stella phenomenon; Arias-Stella reaction
    Arias-Stella phenomenon—*Syn:* Arias-Stella effect
    Arias-Stella reaction—*Syn:* Arias-Stella effect

Aristotle, Greek philosopher and scientist, 384–322 B.C.
    aristotellian method
    Aristotle anomaly

Arlt, Carl Ferdinand von, Austrian ophthalmologist, 1812–1887.
    Arlt epicanthus repair
    Arlt eyelid repair
    Arlt fenestrated lens scoop
    Arlt lens loupe
    Arlt operation—transplantation of the eyelashes back from the edge of the lid in trichiasis.
    Arlt pterygium excision
    Arlt recess
    Arlt sinus—an inconstant depression on the lower portion of the internal surface of the lacrimal sac.
    Arlt sutures
    Arlt trachoma

Armanni, Luciano, Italian pathologist, 1839–1903.
    Armanni-Ebstein change—glycogen vacuolization of the loops of Henle, seen in diabetics before the introduction of insulin. *Syn:* Armanni-Ebstein kidney
    Armanni-Ebstein kidney—*Syn:* Armanni-Ebstein change
    Armanni-Ebstein nephropathy—diabetic glycogen vacuolization of renal convoluted tubules.; related to glycosuria.

Armstrong, Arthur Riley, Canadian physician, *1904.
    King-Armstrong unit—see under King, Earl J.

Arndt, G., German physician, 1874–1929.
    Arndt-Gottron syndrome—generalized lichen myxedematosus with diffuse thickening of the skin underlying the papules. *Syn:* scleromyxedema

Arndt, Rudolph, German psychiatrist, 1835–1900.
    Arndt law—obsolete law stating that weak stimuli excite physiologic activity, moderately strong ones favor it, strong ones retard it, and very strong ones arrest it.

Arneth, Joseph, German physician, 1873–1955.
    Arneth classification—a classification of the polymorphonuclear neutrophils according to the number of their nuclear lobes.

Arneth count—the percentage distribution of polymorphonuclear neutrophils, based on the number of lobes in the nuclei (from 1 to 5).

Arneth formula—the normal, approximate ratio of polymorphonuclear neutrophils, based on the number of lobes in the nuclei.

Arneth index—an expression based on adding percentages of polymorphonuclear neutrophils.

Arneth stages—a differential grouping of polymorphonuclear neutrophils in accordance with the number of lobes in their nuclei.

Arning, Eduard, German physician, *1855.

Arning carcinoid—multiple flat skin tumors that heal spontaneously over time, found on face and trunk.

Arnold, Friedrich, German anatomist, 1803–1890.

Arnold bundle—a fiber group originating in the cerebral cortex of the temporal lobe and terminating in the pontine nuclei or the ventral part of the pons. *SYN:* temporopontine tract; Arnold tract

Arnold canal—the small opening in the petrous bone lateral to the hiatus of facial canal that gives passage to the lesser petrosal nerve. *SYN:* hiatus of canal of lesser petrosal nerve

Arnold ganglion—an autonomic ganglion situated below the foramen ovale medial to the mandibular nerve. *SYN:* otic ganglion

Arnold nerve—a branch of the superior ganglion of the vagus, supplying the back of the pinna and the external acoustic meatus. *SYN:* auricular branch of vagus nerve

Arnold tract—*SYN:* Arnold bundle

foramen of Arnold—an occasional opening in the greater wing of the sphenoid bone, between the foramen spinosum and foramen ovale, which transmits the lesser petrosal nerve. *SYN:* petrosal foramen

Arnold, Julius, German pathologist, 1835–1915.

Arnold bodies—small portions or minute fragments of erythrocytes.

Arnold-Chiari deformity—*SYN:* Arnold-Chiari malformation

Arnold-Chiari malformation—malformed posterior fossa structures. *SYN:* Arnold-Chiari deformity; Arnold-Chiari syndrome; cerebellomedullary malformation syndrome

Arnold-Chiari syndrome—*SYN:* Arnold-Chiari malformation

Arnott, Neil, Scottish physician, 1788–1874.

Arnott bed—a type of waterbed used to treat bed sores.

Arrhenius, Svante, Swedish chemist and Nobel laureate, 1859–1927.

Arrhenius doctrine—the theory of electrolytic dissociation that became the basis of modern understanding of electrolytes. *SYN:* Arrhenius law

Arrhenius equation—an equation relating chemical reaction rate to the absolute temperature.

Arrhenius law—*SYN:* Arrhenius doctrine

Arrhenius-Madsen theory—that the reaction of an antigen with its antibody is a reversible reaction.

NOTES

Arrillaga, student of A. Ayerza who wrote thesis correlating clinical findings of Ayerza syndrome with pulmonary artery sclerosis.
   Ayerza-Arrillaga disease—*Syn:* Ayerza syndrome

Arroyo, Carlos F., U.S. physician, 1892–1928.
   Arroyo expressor
   Arroyo implant
   Arroyo protector
   Arroyo sign—sluggish pupillary reaction to light. *Syn:* asthenocoria

Arruga, Count Hermenegildo, Spanish ophthalmologist, 1886–1972.
   Arruga capsular forceps
   Arruga cataract extraction
   Arruga eye expressor
   Arruga eye implant
   Arruga eye retractor
   Arruga eye speculum
   Arruga eye trephine
   Arruga forceps—for the intracapsular extraction of a cataract.
   Arruga globe retractor
   Arruga keratoplasty
   Arruga lacrimal trephine
   Arruga needle holder
   Arruga protector
   Arruga retinal detachment operation

Arthur, Mary Grace, U.S. psychologist, 1883–1967.
   Arthur Point Scale of Performance—nonverbal test of intellectual performance.

Arthus, Nicolas Maurice, French bacteriologist, 1862–1945.
   Arthus phenomenon—a form of immediate hypersensitivity observed in rabbits after injection of antigen to which the animal has already been sensitized and has specific IgG antibodies. *Syn:* Arthus reaction
   Arthus reaction—*Syn:* Arthus phenomenon

Asch, Solomon E., U.S. psychologist, *1907.
   Asch situation—a test designed to determine the degree to which subject conforms to group opinion.

Ascher, Karl W., U.S. ophthalmologist, 1887–1971.
   Ascher aqueous influx phenomenon—the filling of the aqueous vein, which normally carries blood and aqueous, with aqueous, when the junction of the aqueous vein and the recipient vein is partially occluded. *Syn:* aqueous influx phenomenon
   Ascher syndrome—a condition in which a congenital double lip is associated with blepharochalasis and nontoxic thyroid gland enlargement.
   Laffer-Ascher syndrome

Ascherson, Ferdinand Moritz, German physician, 1798–1879.
   Ascherson membrane—casein covering enclosing milk globules.

Aschheim, Selmar, German obstetrician and gynecologist, 1878–1965.
   Aschheim-Zondek test—an obsolete test for pregnancy. *Syn:* A-Z test; Zondek-Aschheim test
   Zondek-Aschheim test—*Syn:* Aschheim-Zondek test

Aschner, Bernhard, Austrian gynecologist, 1883–1960.

Aschner phenomenon—decrease in pulse rate associated with traction on extraocular muscles or compression of the eyeball; may produce asystolic cardiac arrest. *Syn:* Aschner reflex; Aschner-Dagnini reflex; oculocardiac reflex

Aschner reflex—*Syn:* Aschner phenomenon

Aschner-Dagnini reflex—*Syn:* Aschner phenomenon

Aschoff, Karl Ludwig, German pathologist, 1866–1942.

Aschoff bodies—a form of granulomatous inflammation characteristically observed in acute rheumatic carditis. *Syn:* Aschoff nodules

Aschoff cell—a large-cell component of rheumatic nodules in the myocardium.

Aschoff nodules—*Syn:* Aschoff bodies

node of Aschoff and Tawara—a small node of modified cardiac muscle that gives rise to the atrioventricular bundle of the conduction system of the heart. *Syn:* atrioventricular node; Tawara node

Rokitansky-Aschoff sinuses—see under Rokitansky

Ascoli, Alberto, Italian serologist, 1877–1957.

Ascoli reaction—a method for confirming the diagnosis of anthrax.

Ascoli test—a precipitin test for anthrax using a tissue extract and anthrax antiserum.

Aselli, Gasparo, Italian anatomist, 1581–1626.

Aselli gland—a single large lymph node ventral to the abdominal aorta that receives all the lymph from the intestines in many smaller mammals. *Syn:* Aselli pancreas

Aselli pancreas—*Syn:* Aselli gland

Asellio, var. of Aselli

Asellius, var. of Aselli

Ashby, Winifred, 20th century hematologist.

Ashby method—a differential agglutination method for estimating erythrocyte life span.

Asherman, Joseph G., Czech gynecologist, *1889.

Asherman syndrome—synechiae within the endometrial cavity, often causing amenorrhea and infertility.

Asherson, Nehemiah, English physician, *1897.

Asherson syndrome—dysphagia caused by neuromuscular incoordination, resulting in liquids entering air passages during swallowing.

Ashman, R., 20th century U.S. physiologist.

Ashman phenomenon—aberrant ventricular conduction of a beat ending a short cycle that is preceded by a longer cycle most commonly during atrial fibrillation.

NOTES

Ask-Upmark, E., 20th century Swedish pathologist.
Ask-Upmark kidney—true renal hypoplasia with decreased lobules and deep transverse grooving of the cortical surfaces of the kidney.

Askanazy, Max, German pathologist, 1865–1940.
Askanazy cell—*Syn:* Hürthle cell

Asperger, Hans, Austrian physician, 1844–1954.
Asperger syndrome—personality disorder characterized by insensitivity to others and speaking in a manner which is one-sided. *Syn:* autistic psychopathy

Assézat, Jules, French anthropologist, 1832–1876.
Assézat triangle—a triangle formed by lines connecting the nasion with the alveolar and nasal point; used to indicate prognathism in comparative craniology.

Assmann, Herbert, German internist, 1882–1950.
Assmann tuberculous infiltrate—an incipient lesion of tuberculous infection. *Syn:* infraclavicular infiltrate

Astrup, Poul, Danish clinical chemist, *1915.
micro-Astrup method—an interpolation technique for acid-base measurement.

Astwood, Edwin B., U.S. endocrinologist, 1909–1976.
Astwood test—a test for the assay of estrogenic substances. *Syn:* metrotrophic test

Aub, Joseph C., U.S. physician, 1890–1973.
Aub-DuBois table—table of basal metabolic rates in calories per square meter of body surface per hour or day for different ages.

Auberger, name of a French woman in whom this blood group was detected.
Auberger blood group—blood group found in 82% of Caucasians.

Aubert, Hermann, German physiologist, 1826–1892.
Aubert phenomenon—a bright perpendicular line appearing to incline to one side when the observer turns the head to the opposite side in a dark room.

Audouin, Jean-Victor, French physician, 1797–1841.
Audouin microsopron—ringworm fungus causing tinea capitis.

Audry, Charles, French physician, 1865–1934.
Audry syndrome—digital clubbing, coarsening of facial features, hyperostosis of hands and feet; genetic disorder. *Syn:* pachydermoperiostosis syndrome

Auenbrugger, Leopold, Austrian physician, 1722–1809.
Auenbrugger sign—an epigastric prominence seen in cases of marked pericardial effusion.

Auer, John, U.S. physician, 1875–1948.
Auer bodies—rod-shaped structures of uncertain nature in the cytoplasm of immature myeloid cells in acute myelocytic leukemia. *Syn:* Auer rods
Auer rods—*Syn:* Auer bodies

Auerbach, Leopold, German anatomist, 1828–1897.
 Auerbach ganglia—collections of parasympathetic nerve cells in the myenteric plexus.
 Auerbach plexus—a plexus of unmyelinated fibers and postganglionic autonomic cell bodies lying in the muscular coat of the esophagus, stomach, and intestines. *Syn:* myenteric plexus

Aufrecht, Emanuel, German physician, 1844–1933.
 Aufrecht sign—diminished breath sounds in the trachea just above the jugular notch, in cases of stenosis.

Aujeszky, Aládar, Hungarian pathologist, 1869–1933.
 Aujeszky disease—a highly contagious disease caused by porcine herpesvirus. *Syn:* pseudorabies
 Aujeszky disease virus—a herpesvirus causing pseudorabies in swine. *Syn:* pseudorabies virus

Australia, a continent commonly referred to as "the land down under."
 Australian antigen—hepatitis B antigen first identified in serum of Australian aborigines.

Avellis, Georg, German laryngologist, 1864–1916.
 Avellis syndrome—unilateral paralysis of the larynx and velum palati, with contralateral loss of pain and temperature sensibility in the parts below. *Syn:* jugular foramen syndrome

Avogadro, Amadeo, Italian physicist, 1776–1856.
 Avogadro constant—*Syn:* Avogadro number
 Avogadro hypothesis—*Syn:* Avogadro law
 Avogadro law—equal volumes of gases contain equal numbers of molecules, the conditions of pressure and temperature being the same. *Syn:* Ampère postulate; Avogadro postulate; Avogadro hypothesis
 Avogadro number—the number of molecules in one gram-molecular weight (1 mol) of any compound. *Syn:* Avogadro constant
 Avogadro postulate—*Syn:* Avogadro law

Axelrod, Julius, joint winner of 1970 Nobel Prize for work related to neural transmittors.

Axenfeld, K. Theodor P.P., German ophthalmologist, 1867–1930.
 Morax-Axenfeld conjunctivitis—see under Morax
 Morax-Axenfeld diplobacillus—*Syn: Moraxella lacunata*

Ayala, G., Italian neurologist, 1878–1943.
 Ayala index—the cerebrospinal index when 10 ml of cerebrospinal fluid has been removed. *Syn:* Ayala quotient; spinal quotient
 Ayala quotient—*Syn:* Ayala index

Ayer, James Bourne, U.S. neurologist, 1882–1963.
 Ayer test—used with spinal block to test pressure in lumbar puncture.
 Ayer-Tobey test
 Tobey-Ayer test

NOTES

Ayerza, L., Argentinian physician, 1861–1918.
    Ayerza disease—*SYN:* Ayerza syndrome
    Ayerza syndrome—sclerosis of the pulmonary arteries in chronic cor pulmonale. *SYN:* plexogenic pulmonary arteriopathy; cardiopathia nigra; Ayerza disease; Ayerza-Arrillaga disease
    Ayerza-Arrillaga disease—*SYN:* Ayerza syndrome

Ayre, J. Ernest, U.S. gynecologist, *1910.
    Ayre brush—a device for collecting gastric mucosal cells in cancer detection studies.

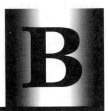

Baastrup, Christian Ingerslev, Danish physician, 1885–1950.

    Baastrup syndrome—compression of spinous processes related to various degenerative diseases. *SYN:* kissing osteophytes; kissing spine; Michotte syndrome

Babbitt, Isaac, U.S. inventor, 1799–1862.

    Babbitt metal—an alloy used occasionally in dentistry.

Babcock, Stephen M., U.S. chemist, 1843–1931.

    Babcock tube—a tube in which milk, after treatment with sulfuric acid, is centrifuged and its fat content then determined in a graduated neck.

Babès, Victor, Romanian bacteriologist, 1854–1926.

    Babès nodes—collections of lymphocytes in the central nervous system found in rabies.

    Babès nodules—*SYN:* Babès tubercles

    Babès tubercles—cellular aggregations found around medulla oblongata and spinal ganglia in the presence of rabies or encephalitis. *SYN:* Babès nodules

    Babès-Ernst bodies—intracellular granules present in many species of bacteria, which possess a strong affinity for nuclear stains. *SYN:* Ernst-Babès granules; Babès-Ernst granules

    Babès-Ernst granules—*SYN:* Babès-Ernst bodies

    Babesia—a protozoan parasite.

    Ernst-Babès granules—*SYN:* Babès-Ernst bodies

Babington, B.G., English physician, 1794–1866.

    Babington disease—hereditary telangiectasia.

Babinski, Joseph F., French neurologist, 1857–1932.

    Babinski phenomenon—*SYN:* Babinski sign (1)

    Babinski reflex—*SYN:* Babinski sign (1)

    Babinski sign—(1) extension of great toe and abduction of other toes instead of normal flexion reflex to plantar stimulation. *SYN:* Babinski phenomenon; Babinski reflex; Babinski test. (2) In hemiplegia, weakness of platysma muscle on affected side. (3) When patient is in supine position with hands crossed on chest and attempts to sit up, the thigh on the side of an organic paralysis is flexed and heel raised, whereas unaffected side remains flat. (4) In hemiplegia, the forearm on the affected side turns to a pronated position when placed in a position of supination.

    Babinski syndrome—the combination of cardiac, arterial, and central nervous system manifestations of tertiary syphilis.

    Babinski test—*SYN:* Babinski sign (1)

    Babinski-Nageotte syndrome—brain lesions resulting in Horner syndrome.

Baccelli, Guido, Italian physician, 1832–1916.
Baccelli sign—an obsolete sign; good conduction of the whisper in nonpurulent pleural effusions. *Syn:* aphonic pectoriloquy

Bachman, George W., U.S. parasitologist, *1890.
Bachman-Pettit test—modification of the Kober test for the detection of estrogenic hormones in the urine.

Bachmann, Jean George, U.S. physiologist, 1877–1959.
Bachmann bundle—division of the anterior internodal tract that continues into the left atrium providing a specialized path for interatrial conduction.

Bacon, Harry E., U.S. proctologist, *1900.
Bacon anoscope—an instrument resembling a rectal speculum, with a long slit on one side and an electric light opposite.
Bacon proctoscope

Baehr, George, U.S. physician, 1887–1978.
Baehr-Lohlein lesion—focal embolic glomerulonephritis occurring in bacterial endocarditis. *Syn:* Lohlein-Baehr lesion

Baelz, Erwin, German physician in Tokyo, 1849–1913.
Baelz disease—an acquired disorder of unknown etiology of the lower lip characterized by swelling, ulceration, crusting, mucous gland hyperplasia, abscesses, and sinus tracts. *Syn:* cheilitis glandularis

Baer, Karl E. von, German-Russian embryologist, 1792–1876.
Baer law—concept of embryonic recapitulation.
Baer vesicle—obsolete term for vesicular ovarian follicle.

Baeyer, Johann F.W.A. von, German chemist and Nobel laureate, 1835–1917.
Baeyer theory—that carbon bonds are set at fixed angles and that those carbon rings are most stable that least distort those angles.

Baggenstoss, Archie H., U.S. pathologist, *1908.
Baggenstoss change—distention of pancreatic acini by proteinaceous secretion, seen in dehydration.

Baghdad, capital of Iraq.
Baghdad boil—acute rapidly developing dermal lesion with moist necrotizing sores.

Bagolini, 20th century Italian ophthalmologist.
Bagolini lens
Bagolini test—a test for retinal correspondence with the subject observing a figure through two striated lenses.

Bahima, "Hamitic" Bahima people of Uganda.
Bahima disease—disease seen in Africa; may be due to iron deficiency when cow's milk is the exclusive diet.

Bailey, Charles, U.S. cardiac surgeon.
Bailey aortic clamp
Bailey aortic valve rongeur
Bailey aortic valve-cutting forceps
Bailey catheter

Baillarger, Jules Gabriel François, French neurologist, 1809–1890.
Baillarger bands—*SYN:* Baillarger lines
Baillarger lines—two laminae of white fibers that course parallel to the surface of the cerebral cortex. *SYN:* Baillarger bands
Baillarger sign—in cases of partial or incomplete paralysis, inequality of the pupils may occur.
Baillarger striae
Baillarger stripes
Baillarger syndrome

B

Bailliart, Paul, French ophthalmologist, 1877–1969.
Bailliart goniometer
Bailliart ophthalmodynamometer—an instrument used to measure the blood pressure of the central retinal artery.
Bailliart tonometer

Bainbridge, Francis A., English physiologist, 1874–1921.
Bainbridge clamp
Bainbridge hemostatic forceps
Bainbridge reflex—rise in right atrial pressure causing increased heart rate.
Bainbridge vessel clamp

Bairnsdale, Australian town.
Bairnsdale ulcer—infection due to Mycobacterium.

Baker, Henry A., U.S. surgeon, 1848–1934.
Baker velum—cleft palate obturator.

Baker, James Porter, U.S. physician, *1902.
Charcot-Weiss-Baker syndrome—see under Charcot

Baker, John Randal, English zoologist, *1900.
Baker acid hematein—an acidic solution of oxidized hematoxylin used on frozen sections for staining phospholipids.
Baker pyridine extraction—hot pyridine treatment of tissues fixed in dilute Bouin fixative.

Baker, William M., English surgeon, 1839–1896.
Baker cyst—a collection of synovial fluid seen in degenerative or other joint diseases.

Balbiani, Edouard G., French embryologist, 1823–1899.
Balbiani rings—*SYN:* chromosome puffs

Baldy, John M., U.S. gynecologist, 1860–1934.
Baldy operation—an obsolete operation for retrodisplacement of the uterus. *SYN:* Webster operation

Balestra, G., Italian physician.
De Martini-Balestra syndrome—*SYN:* Burke syndrome

NOTES

Balint, Rudolph, Hungarian neurologist and psychiatrist, 1874–1929.
   Balint syndrome—an entity characterized by optic ataxia and
   simultanagnosia.

Balkan, the countries of Romania, Bulgaria, and Yugoslavia.
   Balkan frame—metal frame above a bed which provides for limb
   suspension, named for the Balkan wars, 1908–1913.
   Balkan nephropathy—interstitial nephritis occurring in the Balkan
   countries.

Ball, Sir Charles, Irish surgeon, 1851–1916.
   Ball operation—division of the sensory nerve trunks supplying the anus,
   for relief of pruritus ani.

Ballance, Sir Charles A., English surgeon, 1856–1936.
   Ballance sign—the presence of a dull percussion note in both flanks,
   constant on the left side but shifting with change of position on the right,
   said to indicate ruptured spleen; the dullness is due to the presence of
   blood, fluid on the right side but coagulated on the left.
   Koerte-Ballance operation—see under Koerte

Baller, Friedrich, 20th century German physician.
   Baller-Gerold syndrome—autosomal recessive syndrome resulting in
   premature closing of skull sutures. *SYN:* Gerold-Baller syndrome
   Gerold-Baller syndrome—*SYN:* Baller-Gerold syndrome

Ballet, Gilbert, French neurologist, 1853–1916.
   Ballet sign—the appearance of partial or complete external
   ophthalmoplegia in Graves disease.

Balme, Paul Jean, French physician, *1857.
   Balme cough—nasopharyngeal obstruction causing coughing when patient
   lies down.

Balmoral, named for Balmoral Castle in Scotland.
   Balmoral shoe—a type of laced shoe.

Baló, Jozsef Matthias, Hungarian neurologist, *1896.
   Baló disease—encephalitis that is clinically similar to
   adrenoleukodystrophy, but pathologically characterized by concentric
   globes or circles of demyelination of cerebral white matter separated by
   normal tissue. *SYN:* encephalitis periaxialis concentrica

Balser, Wilhelm A., German physician, d. 1892.
   Balser fatty necrosis—fat necrosis accompanying pancreatitis.

Baltimore, David, joint winner of 1975 Nobel Prize for work related to tumor
   viruses and cell material.

Bamatter,, Fred, Swiss physician.
   Bamatter syndrome—genetic trait causing birdlike facies, alopecia,
   premature dryness, and wrinkling of the skin in children after the first
   year of normal development. *SYN:* premature senility syndrome

Bamberger, Eugen, Austrian physician, 1858–1921.
   Bamberger disease—chronic inflammation with effusions in several serous
   cavities resulting in fibrous thickening of serosa and constrictive
   pericarditis.

Bamberger sign—jugular pulse in tricuspid insufficiency. *Syn:* allochiria
Bamberger-Marie disease—*Syn:* Bamberger-Marie syndrome
Bamberger-Marie syndrome—expansion of the distal ends, or the entire shafts, of the long bones that occurs in chronic pulmonary disease, heart disease, and other acute and chronic disorders. *Syn:* hypertrophic pulmonary osteoarthropathy; Bamberger-Marie disease

Bamberger, Heinrich von, Austrian physician, 1822–1888.
Bamberger albuminuria—obsolete term for hematogenous albuminuria that is sometimes observed during the later phases of advanced anemia.
Bamberger disease—a spasmodic affection of the muscles of the lower extremities.

Bancroft, Sir Joseph, English physician in Australia, 1836–1894.
Bancroft filariasis—nematode which lives in body tissues and cavities; upon death of adult worm, granulomatous inflammation and permanent fibrosis develop.

Bandl, Ludwig, German obstetrician, 1842–1892.
Bandl obstetric ring—*Syn:* Bandl ring
Bandl ring—a constriction of the uterus resulting from obstructed labor. *Syn:* pathologic retraction ring; Bandl obstetric ring

Bang, Bernhard L.F., Danish veterinarian and physician, 1848–1932.
Bang bacillus—*Syn: Brucella abortus*
Bang disease—a disease in cattle caused by *Brucella abortus*. *Syn:* bovine brucellosis

Bankart, Arthur S.B., English surgeon, 1876–1951.
Bankart dislocation
Bankart lesion—related to shoulder dislocation.
Bankart procedure—surgical repair of Bankart lesion.
Bankart reconstruction
Bankart repair
Bankart retractor
Bankart shoulder repair set

Bannister, Henry M., U.S. physician, 1844–1920.
Bannister disease—recurrent large circumscribed areas of subcutaneous edema, frequently an allergic reaction to foods or drugs. *Syn:* angioedema

Bannwarth, Alfred, German neurologist, 1903–1970.
Bannwarth syndrome—neurologic manifestations of Lyme disease.

Banti, Guido, Italian physician, 1852–1925.
Banti disease—*Syn:* Banti syndrome
Banti syndrome—chronic congestive splenomegaly occurring primarily in children as a sequel to hypertension in the portal or splenic veins. *Syn:* Banti disease; splenic anemia

NOTES

Banting, Sir Frederick G., Canadian physician, 1891–1941, co-winner of the 1941 Nobel Prize for isolating insulin from the pancreas.

Bar, Paul, French obstetrician, 1853–1945.
Bar incision

Bárány, Robert, Austrian-Hungarian otologist and Nobel laureate, 1876–1936.
Bárány alarm apparatus
Bárány apparatus
Bárány box
Bárány caloric test—a test for vestibular function. *SYN:* caloric test; nystagmus test
Bárány chair
Bárány noise apparatus
Bárány noise apparatus whistle
Bárány sign—nystagmus induced by injecting either hot or cold water into the external ear canal in the caloric test.
Bárány syndrome—the direction of a fall is influenced by changing head position in the presence of equilibrium disturbance.
Bárány test
positional vertigo of Bárány—brief attacks of paroxysmal vertigo and nystagmus due to labyrinthine dysfunction. *SYN:* benign positional vertigo

Barbeau, Andre, Canadian physician.
Giroux-Barbeau syndrome—see under Giroux

Barber, Glenn, 20th century U.S. orthopedic surgeon.
Blount-Barber disease—*SYN:* Blount disease

Barber, Harold W., English dermatologist, 1886–1955.
Barber psoriasis

Barclay, Alfred E., English physician, 1877–1949.
Barclay-Baron disease—dysphagia caused by food becoming lodged above the epiglottis. *SYN:* vallecular dysphagia

Barcroft, Sir Joseph F., English physiologist, 1872–1947.
Barcroft-Warburg apparatus—*SYN:* Warburg apparatus
Barcroft-Warburg technique—*SYN:* Warburg apparatus

Bard, Louis, French physician, 1857–1930.
Bard sign—eye oscillations related to nystagmus.

Bard, Philip, U.S. physiologist, 1898–1945.
Cannon-Bard theory—see under Cannon

Bardet, Georges, French physician, *1885.
Bardet-Biedl syndrome—mental retardation, pigmentary retinopathy, polydactyly, obesity, and hypogenitalism.

Bardinet, Barthélemy A., French physician, 1809–1874.
Bardinet ligament—the posterior band of the ulnar collateral ligament of the elbow.

Barkan, Otto, U.S. ophthalmologist, 1887–1958.
Barkan cyclodialysis
Barkan forceps
Barkan goniolens

B

Barkan gonioscope
Barkan illuminator
Barkan implant
Barkan iris forceps
Barkan knife
Barkan lens
Barkan operation—goniotomy for congenital glaucoma under direct observation of the anterior chamber angle.
Barkan scissors

Barkman, Åke, 20th century Swedish internist.
   Barkman reflex—contraction of the ipsilateral rectus muscle in response to a stimulus applied to the skin below a nipple.

Barkow, Hans K.L., German anatomist, 1798–1873.
   Barkow ligaments—the anterior and posterior portions of the fibrous capsule of the elbow joint.

Barlow, John, 20th century South African cardiologist.
   Barlow syndrome—late apical systolic murmur or (so-called "mid-late") systolic click, or both, due to massive billowing of the anterior and/or posterior (mural) mitral valvular leaflet into the left atrial cavity.

Barlow, Sir Thomas, English physician, 1845–1945.
   Barlow disease—a cachectic condition in infants, resulting from malnutrition. *Syn:* infantile scurvy

Barnard, Christiaan, South African surgeon who performed first successful heart transplant in 1967.

Barnes, Robert, English obstetrician, 1817–1907.
   Barnes curve—a curve corresponding in general with Carus curve, being the segment of a circle whose center is the promontory of the sacrum.
   Barnes zone—the lower fourth of the pregnant uterus, attachment of the placenta to any part of which may cause dangerous hemorrhage. *Syn:* cervical zone

Barr, Murray L., Canadian microanatomist, *1908.
   Barr body—*Syn:* sex chromatin
   Barr chromatin body—a small condensed mass of the inactivated X-chromosome usually located just inside the nuclear membrane of the interphase nucleus. *Syn:* sex chromatin

Barr, Yvonne M., English virologist, *1932.
   Epstein-Barr virus—see under Epstein, Michael

Barraquer, Hignacio, Spanish ophthalmologist, 1884–1965.
   Barraquer ciliary forceps
   Barraquer corneal forceps
   Barraquer hemostatic mosquito forceps
   Barraquer irrigator spatula

(continued)

NOTES

Barraquer *(continued)*
Barraquer keratoplasty knife
Barraquer method—dissolution of the zonula ciliaris by enzymes (α-chymotrypsin) to facilitate surgical removal of a cataract. *SYN:* zonulolysis
Barraquer microkeratome
Barraquer needle carrier
Barraquer shield

Barraquer Roviralta, Luis, Spanish physician, 1855–1928.
Barraquer disease—a condition characterized by a complete loss of the subcutaneous fat of the upper part of the torso, the arms, neck, and face. *SYN:* Barraquer-Simons disease; progressive lipodystrophy; Simons disease
Barraquer-Simons disease—*SYN:* Barraquer disease

Barré, Jean A., French neurologist, 1880–1971.
Barré sign—a hemiplegic placed in the prone position with the limbs flexed at the knees is unable to maintain the flexed position on the side of the lesion but extends the leg.
Barré-Liéou syndrome—irritation of a nerve plexus around a vertebral artery produces symptoms of dizziness, headache, tinnitus. *SYN:* Liéou-Barré syndrome
Guillain-Barré reflex—see under Guillain
Guillain-Barré syndrome—see under Guillain
Landry-Guillain-Barré syndrome—*SYN:* Landry syndrome
Liéou-Barré syndrome—*SYN:* Barré-Liéou syndrome

Barrett, Norman R., English surgeon, 1903–1979.
adenocarcinoma in Barrett esophagus—an adenocarcinoma arising in the lower third of the esophagus that has become columnar cell lined (Barrett mucosa) due to gastroesophageal reflux.
Barrett epithelium—columnar esophageal epithelium seen in Barrett syndrome.
Barrett esophagus—chronic peptic ulceration of the lower esophagus acquired as a result of long-standing chronic esophagitis. *SYN:* Barrett syndrome; Barrett ulcer
Barrett syndrome—*SYN:* Barrett esophagus
Barrett ulcer—*SYN:* Barrett esophagus

Bart, Bruce Joseph, U.S. dermatologist, *1936.
Bart hemoglobin—abnormal hemoglobin with affinity for oxygen.
Bart syndrome—autosomal dominant trait resulting in extremity blistering, mouth erosions, and deformed nails, often with spontaneous improvement and no residual scarring.

Bart, nickname of St. Bartholomew's Hospital in London, England.
Bart hemoglobin—named for hospital where this hemoglobin was first isolated from a patient.

Bartenwerfer, Kurt, German physician, 1892–1942.
Bartenwerfer syndrome—a form of dwarfism.

Barth, Jean, French physician, 1806–1877.
Barth hernia—a loop of intestine between a persistent vitelline duct and the abdominal wall.

Bartholin, Casper, Danish anatomist, 1655–1738.
    Bartholin abscess—an abscess of the vulvovaginal gland.
    Bartholin cyst—a cyst arising from the major vestibular gland or its ducts.
    Bartholin cystectomy—removal of a cyst of a major vestibular gland. *SYN:* vulvovaginal cystectomy
    Bartholin duct—the duct that drains the anterior portion of the sublingual gland. *SYN:* major sublingual duct
    Bartholin gland—one of two mucoid-secreting tubuloalveolar glands on either side of the lower part of the vagina. *SYN:* greater vestibular gland

B

Bartholin, Thomas, Danish anatomist, 1616–1680.
    Bartholin anus—entrance to the cerebral aqueduct (of Sylvius) from the caudal part of the third ventricle. *SYN:* anus cerebri

Bartley, Samuel H., U.S. psychologist, *1901.
    Brücke-Bartley phenomenon—see under Brücke

Barton, A.L., Peruvian physician, 1871–1950.
    Bartonella—bacterium transmitted by Andean sandflies, causing bartonellosis.
    bartonellosis—infection with *Bartonella bacilliformis* causing acute febrile illness followed by benign skin eruptions.

Barton, John Rhea, U.S. surgeon, 1794–1871.
    Barton bandage—a figure-of-eight bandage supporting the mandible below and anteriorly.
    Barton blade
    Barton dressing
    Barton forceps—obstetrical forceps with one fixed curved blade and a hinged anterior blade for application to a high transverse head.
    Barton fracture—fracture of the distal radius with dislocation of the radiocarpal joint.
    Barton hook
    Barton operation
    Barton sling
    Barton tongs
    Barton traction handle

Bartsocas, Christos S., Greek physician.
    Bartsocas-Papas syndrome—severe autosomal recessive trait causing bone abnormalities, microcephaly, facial abnormalities.

Bartter, Frederic C., U.S. physician, 1914–1983.
    Bartter syndrome—primary juxtaglomerular cell hyperplasia with secondary hyperaldosteronism, reported in children with hypokalemic alkalosis and elevated renin or angiotensin levels.

Baruch, Simon, U.S. physician, 1840–1921.
    Baruch law—the effect of any hydriatric procedure is in direct proportion to the difference between the temperature of the water and that of the skin.

NOTES

Basedow, Karl A. von, German physician, 1799–1854.
  Basedow disease—*SYN:* Graves disease; thyrotoxicosis
  Basedow goiter—colloid goiter which becomes hyperfunctional after the ingestion of excess iodine, causing Jod-Basedow phenomenon.
  Basedow pseudoparaplegia—weakness of the thigh muscles in thyrotoxicosis.
  Basedow syndrome—myeloneuropathy seen in the presence of thyrotoxicosis.
  Jod-Basedow phenomenon—induction of thyrotoxicosis in a previously euthyroid individual as a result of exposure to large quantities of iodine. *SYN:* iodine-induced hyperthyroidism

Bassen, Frank A., U.S. physician, *1903.
  Bassen-Kornzweig disease—*SYN:* Bassen-Kornzweig syndrome
  Bassen-Kornzweig syndrome—autosomal recessive trait causing retinal pigmentary degeneration, malabsorption, engorgement of upper intestinal absorptive cells with dietary triglycerides, and neuromuscular abnormalities. *SYN:* Bassen-Kornsweig disease; abetalipoproteinemia

Basset, Antoine, French surgeon, 1882–1951.
  Basset operation—dissection of inguinal glands during surgery for vulvar cancer.

Bassini, Edoardo, Italian surgeon, 1844–1924.
  Bassini herniorrhaphy
  Bassini operation—an operation for an inguinal hernia repair.

Bassler, Anthony, U.S. physician, 1874–1959.
  Bassler sign—in chronic appendicitis, pinching the appendix between the thumb and the iliacus muscle causes sharp pain.

Bastedo, Walter A., U.S. physician, 1873–1952.
  Bastedo sign—an obsolete sign: in chronic appendicitis, pain and tenderness in the right iliac fossa on inflation of the colon with air.

Bastian, H.C., English neurologist, 1837–1915.
  Bastian aphasia—*SYN:* Wernicke aphasia
  Bastian-Bruns law—deep-reflex loss in lower limbs due to disruption of spinal cord above lumbar enlargement. *SYN:* Bastian-Bruns sign
  Bastian-Bruns sign—*SYN:* Bastian-Bruns law

Batson, Oscar V., U.S. otolaryngologist, 1894–1979.
  Batson plexus—any of four interconnected venous networks surrounding the vertebral column. *SYN:* vertebral venous system
  Carmody-Batson operation—see under Carmody

Batten, Frederick E., English ophthalmologist, 1865–1918.
  Batten disease—cerebral sphingolipidosis, late infantile and juvenile types. *SYN:* Batten-Mayou disease; Spielmeyer-Vogt disease; Vogt-Spielmeyer disease
  Batten-Mayou disease—*SYN:* Batten disease
  Curschmann-Batten-Steinhert syndrome—see under Curschmann

Battey, Battey State Hospital, Georgia, USA
  Battey bacillus—mycobacterium causing lung disease similar to tuberculosis; first isolated at Battey State Hospital in Georgia.
  Battey-type mycobacterium

Battle, William H., English surgeon, 1855–1936.
Battle incision
Battle operation
Battle sign—postauricular ecchymosis in cases of fracture of the base of the skull.

Baudelocque, Jean L., French obstetrician, 1746–1810.
Baudelocque diameter—the distance in a straight line between the depression under the last spinous process of the lumbar vertebrae and the upper edge of the pubic symphysis. *SYN:* external conjugate
Baudelocque uterine circle—a constriction of the uterus resulting from obstructed labor, one of the classic signs of threatened rupture of the uterus. *SYN:* pathologic retraction ring

Baudelocque, Louis A., French obstetrician, 1800–1864.
Baudelocque operation—an incision through the posterior cul-de-sac of the vagina for the removal of the ovum, in extrauterine pregnancy.

Bauer, Hans, 20th century German anatomist.
Bauer chromic acid leucofuchsin stain—a stain for glycogen and fungi.

Bauer, Walter, U.S. internist, *1898.
Bauer reaction
Bauer syndrome—aortitis and aortic endocarditis as a little recognized manifestation of rheumatoid arthritis.

Bauhin, Gaspard, Swiss anatomist, 1560–1624.
Bauhin gland—one of the small mixed glands deeply placed near the apex of the tongue on each side of the frenulum. *SYN:* anterior lingual gland
Bauhin valve—*SYN:* ileocecal valve

Baumé, Antoine, French chemist and pharmacist, 1728–1805.
Baumé scale—a hydrometer scale for determining the specific gravity of liquids.

Baumgarten, P. Clemens von, German pathologist, 1848–1928.
Baumgarten glands—*SYN:* Henle glands
Baumgarten veins—nonobliterated remnants of the vena umbilicalis.
Cruveilhier-Baumgarten disease—*SYN:* Cruveilhier-Baumgarten syndrome
Cruveilhier-Baumgarten murmur—see under Cruveilhier
Cruveilhier-Baumgarten sign—see under Cruveilhier
Cruveilhier-Baumgarten syndrome—see under Cruveilhier

Bayes, Thomas, English mathematician, 1702–1761.
Bayes theorem—to determine the impact of new data on the evidential merits of competing scientific hypotheses.

Bayle, Antoine L.J., French physician, 1799–1858.
Bayle disease—a disease of the brain, syphilitic in origin.

Bayle, Gaspard Laurent, French physician, 1774–1816.
Bayle granulations—tubercular lung nodules.

NOTES

Bayley, Nancy, U.S. psychologist, *1899.
    Bayley Scales of Infant Development—a psychological test used to measure the developmental progress of infants.

Bazett, Henry, English cardiologist, *1885.
    Bazett formula—used for correcting the observed Q-T interval in the electrocardiogram for cardiac rate.

Bazex, A., 20th century French physician.
    Bazex syndrome—lesions of an eczematous or psoriatic nature seen in patients with upper respiratory tract or digestive tract carcinomas. *Syn:* paraneoplastic acrokeratosis

Bazin, Antoine P.E., French dermatologist, 1807–1878.
    Bazin disease—recurrent, hard, subcutaneous nodules that frequently break down and form necrotic ulcers, usually on the calves; lesions are sterile and probably a form of nodular vasculitis. *Syn:* erythema induratum; nodular tuberculid

Beadle, George Wells, joint winner of 1958 Nobel Prize for work related to genetics.

Beale, Lionel S., English physician, 1828–1906.
    Beale cell—a bipolar ganglion cell of the heart with one spiral and one straight prolongation.

Beals, Rodney Kenneth, U.S. orthopedic surgeon, *1931.
    Beals syndrome—congenital condition resulting in abnormally long hands and fingers and often feet and toes. *Syn:* arachnodactyly

Beard, George Miller, U.S. physician.
    Beard disease—*Syn:* Beard syndrome
    Beard syndrome—may be associated with chronic fatigue syndrome. *Syn:* Beard disease; nervous exhaustion
    Beard test

Bearn, Alexander Gordon, English-U.S. physician, 1923–1983.
    Bearn-Kunkel syndrome—lupoid hepatitis. *Syn:* Kunkel-Bearn syndrome; Bearn-Kunkel-Slater syndrome; Kunkel syndrome
    Bearn-Kunkel-Slater syndrome—*Syn:* Bearn-Kunkel syndrome

Beau, Joseph H.S., French physician, 1806–1865.
    Beau disease—*Syn:* Beau syndrome
    Beau lines—transverse depressions on the fingernails following severe febrile disease, malnutrition, trauma, myocardial infarction, etc.
    Beau syndrome—*Syn:* Beau disease

Bechterew, var. of Bekhterev

Beck, var. of Bek

Beck, Carl, U.S. surgeon, 1856–1911.
    Beck gastrostomy
    Beck gastrostomy scoop

Beck, Claude S., U.S. surgeon, 1894–1971.
    Beck triad—the rising venous pressure, falling arterial pressure, and decreased heart sounds of pericardial tamponade. *Syn:* acute compression triad

Beck, Emil G., U.S. surgeon, 1866–1932.
Beck method—a permanent opening into the stomach made from its greater curvature.

Becker, J.P.
Becker disease—an obscure South African cardiomyopathy leading to rapidly fatal congestive heart failure and idiopathic mural endomyocardial disease.

Becker, Peter Emil, German geneticist, *1908.
Becker-type muscular dystrophy—a muscular dystrophy that has many of the clinical features of Duchenne muscular dystrophy. *SYN:* adult pseudohypertrophic muscular dystrophy
Becker-type tardive muscular dystrophy—*SYN:* adult pseudohypertrophic muscular dystrophy

Becker, Samuel W., U.S. dermatologist, 1894–1964.
Becker nevus—a nevus first seen as an irregular pigmentation of the shoulders, upper chest, or scapular area, gradually enlarging irregularly and becoming thickened and hairy. *SYN:* pigmented hair epidermal nevus

Beckmann, Ernst O., German chemist, 1853–1923.
Beckmann apparatus—apparatus for the accurate measurement of melting points and boiling points in connection with molecular weight determinations.
Beckmann thermometer

Beckwith, John Bruce, U.S. pediatric pathologist, *1933.
Beckwith syndrome—*SYN:* Beckwith-Wiedemann syndrome
Beckwith-Wiedemann syndrome—exomphalos, macroglossia, and gigantism, often with neonatal hypoglycemia; autosomal recessive inheritance. *SYN:* EMG syndrome; Beckwith syndrome

Béclard, Pierre A., French anatomist, 1785–1825.
Béclard anastomosis—an anastomosis between the right and the left end-branch of the deep lingual artery. *SYN:* arcus raninus
Béclard hernia—a hernia through the opening for the saphenous vein.
Béclard triangle—area bounded by the posterior border of the hyoglossus muscle, the posterior belly of the digastric and the greater horn of the hyoid bone.

Becquerel, Antoine H., French physicist and Nobel laureate, 1852–1908.
becquerel—the SI unit of measurement of radioactivity.
Becquerel rays—obsolete term for radiations given off by uranium and other radioactive substances.

Bednar, Alois, Austrian physician, 1816–1888.
Bednar aphthae—traumatic ulcers located bilaterally on either side of the midpalatal raphe in infants.
Bednar-Parrot syndrome—*SYN:* Parrot I syndrome

NOTES

Bednar, Blahoslav, 20th century Czech pathologist.
    Bednar tumor—an uncommon variant of dermatofibrosarcoma protuberans containing heavily pigmented dendritic melanocytes scattered between spindle cells of the tumor. *SYN:* pigmented dermatofibrosarcoma protuberans

Beer, August, German physicist, 1825–1863.
    Beer law—the intensity of a color or of a light ray is inversely proportional to the depth of liquid through which it is transmitted.
    Beer-Lambert law—the absorbance of light is directly proportional to the thickness of the ligand through which the light is being transmitted multiplied by the concentration of absorbing chromophore.

Beer, Georg J., Austrian ophthalmologist, 1763–1821.
    Beer canaliculus knife
    Beer cataract flap operation
    Beer cataract knife
    Beer cilia forceps
    Beer knife—a triangular knife with a sharp point and one sharp edge, formerly used for incision for cataract.

Beevor, Charles E., English neurologist, 1854–1908.
    Beevor phenomenon
    Beevor sign—with paralysis of the lower portions of the recti abdominis muscles, the umbilicus moves upward.

Begbie, James, Scottish physician, 1798–1869.
    Begbie disease—localized chorea.

Begg, P. Raymond, Australian orthodontist, *1898.
    Begg appliance
    Begg light wire differential force technique
    Begg paralleling
    Begg slots
    Begg straight-wire combination bracket
    Begg technique
    Begg theory
    Begg torquing

Béguez César, Antonio, 20th century Cuban pediatrician.
    Béguez César disease—*SYN:* Chédiak-Steinbrinck-Higashi syndrome

Behçet, Hulusi, Turkish dermatologist, 1889–1948.
    Behçet disease—*SYN:* Behçet syndrome
    Behçet syndrome—severe uveitis with ulceration of mouth and genitalia. *SYN:* triple symptom complex; Behçet disease; recurrent hypopyon; iridocyclitis septica; cutaneomucouveal syndrome

Behn-Eschenburg, H., German psychologist.
    Behn-Rorschach Test—alternative to standard Rorschach test.

Behr, Carl, German ophthalmologist, 1874–1943.
    Behr disease—adult or presenile form of heredomacular degeneration. *SYN:* Behr syndrome
    Behr syndrome—*SYN:* Behr disease

Behring, Emil A. von, German bacteriologist and Nobel laureate, 1854–1917.
  Behring law—parenteral administration of serum from an immunized person provides a relative, passive immunity to that disease.

Beigel, Hermann, German physician, 1830–1879.
  Beigel disease—fungal disease which affects hair shafts. *SYN:* tinea nodosa

Bek, E.V.V., Russian physician.
  Kashin-Bek disease—see under Kashin

Békésy, Georg von, Hungarian biophysicist in U.S. and Nobel laureate, 1899–1972.
  Békésy audiometer—an automatic audiometer.
  Békésy audiometry—automatic audiometry.

B

Bekhterev, Vladimir M., Russian neurologist, 1857–1927.
  band of Kaes-Bekhterev—see under Kaes
  Bekhterev band—*SYN:* band of Kaes-Bekhterev
  Bekhterev disease—arthritis and osteitis deformans involving the spinal column. *SYN:* spondylitis deformans
  Bekhterev nucleus—one of the nuclei raphes. *SYN:* nucleus centralis tegmenti superior
  Bekhterev sign—paralysis of automatic facial movements, the power of voluntary movement being retained.
  Bekhterev-Mendel reflex—percussion of the dorsum of the foot causes flexion of the toes in a pyramidal lesion. *SYN:* dorsum pedis reflex; Mendel-Bekhterev reflex
  layer of Bekhterev—*SYN:* band of Kaes-Bekhterev
  line of Bekhterev—*SYN:* band of Kaes-Bekhterev
  Mendel-Bekhterev reflex—*SYN:* Bekhterev-Mendel reflex

Bell, John, Scottish surgeon and anatomist, 1763–1820.
  Bell muscle—a band of muscular fibers forming a slight fold in the wall of the bladder.

Bell, Sir Charles, Scottish surgeon, anatomist, and physiologist, 1774–1842.
  Bell law—the ventral spinal roots are motor, the dorsal are sensory. *SYN:* Bell-Magendie law; Magendie law
  Bell palsy—paresis or paralysis, usually unilateral, of the facial muscles, caused by dysfunction of the 7th cranial nerve. *SYN:* peripheral facial paralysis
  Bell phenomenon—upward movement of the eye on attempted eyelid closure in a patient with peripheral facial paralysis.
  Bell respiratory nerve—*SYN:* long thoracic nerve
  Bell spasm—involuntary twitching of the facial muscles. *SYN:* facial tic
  Bell-Magendie law—*SYN:* Bell law
  external respiratory nerve of Bell—*SYN:* long thoracic nerve

Bellini, Lorenzo, Italian physician and anatomist, 1643–1704.
  Bellini ducts—the largest straight excretory ducts in the kidney medulla

(continued)

NOTES

Bellini *(continued)*
and papillae whose openings form the area cribrosa. *SYN:* papillary
ducts
Bellini ligament—a fasciculus from the ischiofemoral portion of the
articular fibrous capsule of the hip which extends to the greater
trochanter.
Bellini tubules

Belsey, Ronald, 20th century English surgeon.
Belsey esophagoplasty
Belsey antireflux operation
Belsey herniorrhaphy
Belsey hiatal hernia repair
Belsey Mark II fundoplication
Belsey Mark IV operation—a transthoracic antireflux procedure.
Belsey Mark IV procedure—a transthoracic hiatal hernia repair that
restores the lower esophageal sphincter zone to the high pressure region
below the diaphragm.
Belsey Mark V procedure—a modified Belsey Mark IV procedure.
Belsey perfusor

Benacerraf, Baruj, joint winner of 1980 Nobel Prize for work related to cell
structures and regulation of immunological reactions.

Bence Jones, Henry, English physician, 1814–1873.
Bence Jones albumin
Bence Jones cylinders—slightly irregular, relatively smooth, rod-shaped or
cylindroid bodies of fairly tenacious, viscid proteinaceous material in the
fluid of the seminal vesicles.
Bence Jones myeloma—multiple myeloma in which the malignant plasma
cells excrete only light chains of one type (either kappa or lambda). *SYN:*
L-chain myeloma; L-chain disease
Bence Jones proteins—proteins with unusual thermosolubility found in
the urine of patients with multiple myeloma, consisting of monoclonal
immunoglobulin light chains.
Bence Jones reaction—the classic means of identifying Bence Jones
protein.
Bence Jones test

Bender, Lauretta, U.S. psychiatrist, 1897–1987.
Bender gestalt test—a psychological test used for measuring visuospatial
and visuomotor coordination to detect brain damage. *SYN:* Bender Visual
Motor Gestalt test
Bender Visual Motor Gestalt test—*SYN:* Bender gestalt test

Benedek, Ladislaus (László), Austrian neurologist, 1887–1945.
Benedek reflex—plantar flexion of the foot by tapping the anterior margin
of the lower part of the fibula, while the foot is slightly dorsiflexed.

Benedict, Francis G., U.S. metabolist, 1870–1957.
Benedict-Roth apparatus—a device to measure the amount of oxygen
utilized in quiet breathing for the estimation of the basal metabolic rate.
Benedict-Roth calorimeter

Benedict, Stanley R., U.S. chemist, 1884–1936.
    Benedict solution—used to demonstrate a reducing sugar such as glucose in the urine.
    Benedict test for glucose—a copper reduction test for glucose in the urine.
    Benedict-Hopkins-Cole reagent—magnesium glyoxalate, made from a mixture of oxalic acid and magnesium, used for testing proteins for the presence of tryptophan.

Benedikt, Moritz, Austrian physician, 1835–1920.
    Benedikt syndrome—hemiplegia with clonic spasm or tremor and oculomotor paralysis on the opposite side.

B

Benjamin, E., German pediatrician.
    Benjamin binocular slimline laryngoscope
    Benjamin pediatric operating laryngoscope
    Benjamin syndrome—genetic trait resulting in hypochromic anemia and other abnormalities: megalocephaly, carious lesions, cardiac murmur, splenic tumors.

Bennett, Edward H., Irish surgeon, 1837–1907.
    Bennett fracture—fracture dislocation of the first metacarpal bone at the carpometacarpal joint.
    Bennett lesion
    Bennett nail biopsy
    Bennett posterior shoulder approach
    Bennett retractor

Bennett, George Kettner, U.S. psychologist, *1904.
    Bennett Differential Aptitude Test—aptitude test administered to children in grades 8 through 12.

Bennett, Norman G., English dentist, 1870–1947.
    Bennett angle—the angle formed by the sagittal plane and the path of the advancing condyle during lateral mandibular movement as viewed in the horizontal plane.
    Bennett movement—the bodily lateral movement or lateral shift of the mandible during a laterotrusive movement.

Bennhold, H., German physician, *1893.
    Bennhold Congo red stain—a stain for amyloid detection in pathologic tissue.

Bensley, Robert R., U.S.-Canadian anatomist, 1867–1956.
    Bensley osmic dichromate fluid
    Bensley specific granules—granules in the cells of the islets of Langerhans in the pancreas.

Benson, Alfred Hugh, Irish ophthalmologist, 1852–1912.
    Benson disease—small spherical bodies in corpus vitreum, a unilateral age change which does not affect vision. *SYN:* asteroid hyalosis

NOTES

Benton, Arthur Lester, U.S. psychologist, *1909.
Benton Visual Retention Test—test of ability to reproduce geometric designs from memory.

Beradinelli, Waldemar, Argentinian physician, 1903–1956.
Beradinelli syndrome—accelerated growth, lipodystrophy with muscular hypertrophy, hepatomegaly, and lipemia.

Bérard, Auguste, French surgeon, 1802–1846.
Bérard aneurysm—an arteriovenous aneurysm in the tissues outside the injured vein.

Béraud, Bruno J., French surgeon, 1825–1865.
Béraud valve—a small fold in the interior of the lacrimal sac at its junction with the lacrimal duct. *Syn:* Krause valve

Berenberg, William, U.S.physician, *1915.
Neuhauser-Berenberg syndrome—see under Neuhauser

Berger, Emil, Austrian ophthalmologist, 1855–1926.
Berger space—the space between the patellar fossa of the vitreous and the lens.

Berger, Hans, German neurologist, 1873–1941.
Berger rhythm—a wave pattern in the encephalogram in the frequency band of 8 to 13 Hz. *Syn:* alpha rhythm; Berger wave
Berger wave—*Syn:* Berger rhythm

Berger, Jean, 20th century French nephrologist.
Berger disease—*Syn:* focal glomerulonephritis
Berger focal glomerulonephritis—*Syn:* focal glomerulonephritis

Bergeron, E. J., French physician, 1817–1900.
Bergeron chorea—involuntary and usually self-limiting muscle spasm occurring at long intervals; may follow Syndenham chorea. *Syn:* Bergeron disease
Bergeron disease—*Syn:* Bergeron chorea

Bergmann, Gottlieb H., German neurologist and anatomist, 1781–1861.
Bergmann cords—*Syn:* medullary striae of fourth ventricle
Bergmann fibers—filamentous glia fibers traversing the cerebellar cortex perpendicular to the surface.

Bergmeister, O., Austrian ophthalmologist, 1845–1918.
Bergmeister papilla—a small mass of glial tissue that forms in the hyaloid artery during fetal life.

Bergström, Sune K., joint winner of 1982 Nobel Prize for work related to prostaglandins.

Berke, Raynold N., U.S. ophthalmologist, *1901.
Berke cilia forceps
Berke clamp
Berke forceps
Berke operation—correction of eyelid ptosis.
Berke ptosis clamp
Berke ptosis correction
Berke ptosis forceps

Berkefeld, name of a mine owner from which material to make filter was taken.
Berkefeld filter—filter for bacteria.

Berlin, Rudolf, German ophthalmologist, 1833–1897.
Berlin disease
Berlin edema—retinal edema after blunt trauma to the globe.

Bernard, Claude, French physiologist, 1813–1878.
Bernard canal—the excretory duct of the head of the pancreas. *SYN:* accessory pancreatic duct; Bernard duct
Bernard duct—*SYN:* Bernard canal
Bernard puncture—a puncture at a point in the floor of the fourth ventricle of the brain which causes glycosuria. *SYN:* diabetic puncture
Bernard syndrome—*SYN:* Horner syndrome
Bernard-Cannon homeostasis—the set of mechanisms responsible for the cybernetic adjustment of physiological and biochemical states in postnatal life. *SYN:* physiological homeostasis
Bernard-Horner syndrome—*SYN:* Horner syndrome
Bernard-Sergent syndrome—*SYN:* acute adrenocortical insufficiency

Bernard, Jean, 20th century French physician.
Bernard-Soulier syndrome—a coagulation disorder characterized by thrombocytopenia, giant platelets, and a bleeding tendency.

Bernays, Augustus C., U.S. surgeon, 1854–1907.
Bernays sponge—a compressed disk of aseptic cotton used in packing cavities.

Berndorfer, Alfred, Hungarian physician.
Berndorfer syndrome—syndrome of unknown etiology that causes cleft palate, harelip, and cleft hands and feet.

Bernhardt, Martin, German neurologist, 1844–1915.
Bernhardt disease—tingling, formication, itching, and other forms of paresthesia in the outer side of the lower thigh in the area of distribution of the lateral femoral cutaneous nerve. *SYN:* meralgia paraesthetica; Bernhardt-Roth syndrome; Roth-Bernhardt disease
Bernhardt-Roth syndrome—*SYN:* Bernhardt disease
Roth-Bernhardt disease—*SYN:* Bernhardt disease

Bernheim, Hippolyte-Marie, French psychologist, 1840–1919.
Bernheim therapy—obsolete term for hypnotic psychotherapy.

Bernheim, P., early 20th century French physician.
Bernheim syndrome—systemic congestion resembling consequences of right heart failure without pulmonary congestion in subjects with left ventricular enlargement from any cause.

Bernoulli, Daniel, Swiss mathematician, 1700–1782.
Bernoulli effect—the decrease in fluid pressure that occurs in converting

(continued)

NOTES

Bernoulli *(continued)*

potential to kinetic energy when motion of the fluid is accelerated in accordance with Bernoulli law.

Bernoulli law—when friction is negligible, the velocity of flow of a gas or fluid through a tube is inversely related to its pressure against the side of the tube. *Syn:* Bernoulli principle; Bernoulli theorem

Bernoulli principle—*Syn:* Bernoulli law

Bernoulli theorem—*Syn:* Bernoulli law

Bernreuter, Robert G., U.S. psychologist, *1901.

Bernreuter Personal Adjustment Inventory—test designed to measure personality and behavior.

Bernstein, Lionel M., U.S. internist, *1923.

Bernstein test—a test to establish that substernal pain is due to reflux esophagitis. *Syn:* acid perfusion test

Berry, Sir James, Canadian surgeon, 1860–1946.

Berry ligaments—thickened elastic bundle connecting the superior horn of thyroid cartilage to the tip of the greater horn of hyoid cartilage. *Syn:* lateral thyrohyoid ligament

Berson, Solomon A., U.S. internist, 1918–1972.

Berson test—a test of thyroid clearance of ^{131}I from the plasma by the thyroid gland.

Berthelot, Pierre Eugene Marcellin, French chemist, 1827–1907.

Berthelot reaction—the reaction of ammonia with phenol-hypochlorite, used to analyze ammonia concentration in body fluids.

Berthollet, Claude L., French chemist, 1748–1822.

Berthollet law—salts in solution will always react with each other so as to form a less soluble salt, if possible.

Bertin, Exupère Joseph, French anatomist, 1712–1781.

Bertin bones—paired ossicles of pyramidal shape, the bases forming the roof of the nasal cavity. *Syn:* sphenoidal conchae; Bertin ossicles

Bertin columns—the prolongations of cortical substance separating the pyramids of the kidney. *Syn:* renal columns

Bertin ligament—among the strongest of the body's ligaments, it limits extension at the hip joint. *Syn:* iliofemoral ligament

Bertin ossicles—*Syn:* Bertin bones

Bertolotti, Mario, Italian physician, *1876.

Bertolotti syndrome—fifth lumbar vertebra sacralization with concomitant scoliosis and sciatica.

Bertrand, Ivan Georges, 20th century French neurologist.

Canavan-van Bogaert-Bertrand disease—*Syn:* Canavan disease

Besnier, Ernest, French dermatologist, 1831–1909.

Besnier prurigo—an atopic form which may be associated with asthma, hay fever, or other allergic conditions.

Besnier-Boeck disease—systemic granulomatous disease of unknown cause which involves lungs with resulting fibrosis; also involving lymph nodes, skin, liver, spleen, eyes, phalangeal bones, and parotid glands. *Syn:*

sarcoidosis; Besnier-Boeck-Schaumann syndrome; Boeck sarcoid; Besnier-Boeck-Schaumann disease; Boeck disease; Schaumann syndrome

Besnier-Boeck-Schaumann disease—*SYN:* Besnier-Boeck disease

Besnier-Boeck-Schaumann syndrome—*SYN:* Besnier-Boeck disease

Best, Franz, German pathologist, 1878–1920.

Best carmine stain—a method for the demonstration of glycogen in tissues.

Best disease—autosomal dominant retinal degeneration beginning during the first years of life.

Bettendorff, Anton J., German chemist, 1839–1902.

Bettendorff test—a test for arsenic.

Betz, Vladimir A., Russian anatomist, 1834–1894.

Betz cells—large pyramidal cells in the motor area of the precentral gyrus of the cerebral cortex. *SYN:* Bevan-Lewis cells

Beuermann, Charles Lucien, French physician, 1851–1923.

Beuermann disease—*SYN:* Schenck disease

Beuermann-Gougerot disease—*SYN:* Schenck disease

Beuren, Alois J.

Beuren syndrome—supravalvular aortic stenosis with multiple areas of peripheral pulmonary arterial stenosis, mental retardation, and dental anomalies.

Bevan-Lewis, William, English physician and physiologist, 1847–1929.

Bevan-Lewis cells—*SYN:* Betz cells

Bezold, Albert von, German physiologist, 1836–1868.

Bezold ganglion—an aggregation of nerve cells in the interatrial septum.

Bezold-Jarisch reflex—a reflex with afferent and efferent pathways in the vagus, originating in unidentified chemoreceptors in the heart and resulting in sinus bradycardia, hypotension, and probable peripheral vasodilation.

Bezold, Friedrich, German otologist, 1842–1908.

Bezold abscess—an abscess deep in the neck's parapharyngeal space associated with suppuration in the mastoid tip cells.

Bezold mastoiditis—mastoiditis with perforation medially into the digastric groove, forming a deep neck abscess.

Bezold sign—inflammatory edema at the tip of the mastoid process in mastoiditis. *SYN:* Bezold symptom

Bezold symptom—*SYN:* Bezold sign

Bezold triad—diminished perception of the deeper tones, retarded bone conduction, and negative Rinne test, pointing, in the absence of objective signs, to otosclerosis.

Bial, Manfred, German physician, 1869–1908.

Bial reagent

Bial test—a test for pentoses with orcinol. *SYN:* orcinol test

NOTES

Bianchi, Giovanni, Italian anatomist, 1681–1761.
    Bianchi nodule—a nodule at the center of the free border of each semilunar valve at the beginning of the pulmonary artery and aorta. *Syn:* nodule of semilunar valve
    Bianchi valve—a fold of mucous membrane guarding the lower opening of the nasolacrimal duct. *Syn:* lacrimal fold

Bichat, Marie F.X., French anatomist, physician, and biologist, 1771–1802.
    Bichat canal—*Syn:* cistern of great cerebral vein.
    Bichat fat-pad—an encapsuled mass of fat in the cheek on the outer side of the buccinator muscle. *Syn:* buccal fat-pad
    Bichat fissure—the nearly circular fissure corresponding to the medial margin of the cerebral (pallial) mantle, marking the hilus of the cerebral hemisphere.
    Bichat foramen—*Syn:* cistern of great cerebral vein
    Bichat fossa—sphenomaxillary fossa, a small pyramidal space, housing the pterygopalatine ganglion, between the pterygoid process, the maxilla, and the palatine bone. *Syn:* pterygopalatine fossa
    Bichat ligament—the lower fasciculus of the posterior sacroiliac ligament.
    Bichat membrane—the inner elastic membrane of arteries.
    Bichat protuberance—*Syn:* buccal fat-pad
    Bichat tunic—the tunica intima of the blood vessels.

Bickel, Gustav, 19th century German physician.
    Bickel ring—the broken ring of lymphoid tissue, formed of the lingual, faucial, and pharyngeal tonsils. *Syn:* lymphoid ring

Bickers, D.S., U.S. physician.
    Bickers-Adams syndrome—congenital hydrocephalus caused by recessive gene. *Syn:* X-linked hydrocephalus

Bickerstaff, Edward R., English physician, *1920.
    Bickerstaff encephalitis—*Syn:* brainstem encephalitis
    Bickerstaff migraine

Bidder, Heinrich Friedrich, Estonian anatomist, 1810–1894.
    Bidder ganglia—cardiac nerve ganglia found at the atrial septum. *Syn:* Bidder organ
    Bidder organ—*Syn:* Bidder ganglia

Bidwell, Shelford, English physicist, 1848–1909.
    Bidwell ghost—visual afterimage in response to stimulus. *Syn:* Purkinje afterimage

Biebl, M.
    Biebl loop—a continuous loop of small intestine brought through the abdominal wall to a subcutaneous location, for observation of motility.

Biederman, Joseph, U.S. physician, *1907.
    Biederman sign—a dusky redness of the lower portion of the anterior pillars of the fauces in certain cases of syphilis.

Biedl, Artur, Austrian physician, 1869–1933.
    Bardet-Biedl syndrome—see under Bardet
    Biedl disease
    Laurence-Moon-Biedl syndrome—see under Laurence

B

Bielschowsky, Alfred, German ophthalmologist, 1871–1940.

Bielschowsky sign—in paralysis of a superior oblique muscle, tilting the head to the side of the involved eye causes that eye to rotate upward.

Roth-Bielschowsky syndrome—see under Roth, W.

Bielschowsky, Max, German neuropathologist, 1869–1940.

Bielschowsky disease—early childhood type of lipofuscinosis.

Bielschowsky head tilt test

Bielschowsky method

Bielschowsky stain—a method of treating tissues with silver nitrate to demonstrate reticular fibers, neurofibrils, axons, and dendrites.

Bielschowsky syndrome—*Syn:* Dollinger-Bielschowsky syndrome

Bielschowsky-Dollinger syndrome—*Syn:* Dollinger-Bielschowsky syndrome

Bielschowsky-Jansky disease—*Syn:* Jansky-Bielschowsky disease

Dollinger-Bielschowsky syndrome—see under Dollinger

Jansky-Bielschowsky disease—see under Jansky

Biemond, A., French neurologist, *1902.

Biemond ataxia—*Syn:* Friedreich ataxia

Biemond syndrome—iris coloboma, mental retardation, obesity, hypogenitalism, and postaxial polydactyly.

Bier, August K.G., German surgeon, 1861–1949.

Bier amputation—osteoplastic amputation of the tibia and fibula.

Bier amputation saw

Bier block anesthesia

Bier combined treatment

Bier hyperemia

Bier method—(1) *Syn:* intravenous regional anesthesia; (2) treatment of various surgical conditions by reactive hyperemia.

Bier spots—*Syn:* Marshall-White syndrome

Bier syndrome—*Syn:* Marshall-White syndrome

Biermer, Anton, German physician, 1827–1892.

Addison-Biermer disease—*Syn:* Addison anemia

Biermer anemia—*Syn:* Addison anemia

Biermer disease—*Syn:* Addison anemia

Biermer sign—*Syn:* Gerhardt sign

Biernacki, Edmund A., Polish pathologist, 1866–1912.

Biernacki sign—analgesia to percussion of the ulnar nerve in tabes dorsalis and dementia paralytica.

Biesiadecki, Alfred von, Polish physician, 1839–1888.

Biesiadecki fossa—a peritoneal recess between the psoas muscle and the crest of the ilium. *Syn:* iliacosubfascial fossa

Bigelow, Henry J., U.S. surgeon, 1818–1890.

Bigelow calvarium clamp

(continued)

NOTES

Bigelow *(continued)*
    Bigelow clamp
    Bigelow evacuator—instrument used to remove fragments of bladder calculi.
    Bigelow forceps
    Bigelow ligament—among the strongest of the body's ligaments, it limits extension at the hip joint. *Syn:* iliofemoral ligament
    Bigelow litholapaxy—process of crushing a bladder stone and using a catheter to wash out fragments.
    Bigelow lithotrite
    Bigelow septum—a bony spur springing from the underside of the neck of the femur above and anterior to the lesser trochanter. *Syn:* calcar femorale
    Bigelow sutures

Bignami, Amico, Italian physician, 1862–1929.
    Marchiafava-Bignami disease—see under Marchiafava

Bilharz, T.M., German parasitologist, 1825–1862.
    Bilharzia—schistosomiasis; tumor-like swelling of the skin due to infection by Schistosoma organism. *Syn:* Schistosoma

Bill, Arthur H., U.S. obstetrician, 1877–1961.
    Bill maneuver—forceps rotation of the fetal head at mid-pelvis before extraction of the head.

Billig, Harvey E., Jr., U.S. orthopedic surgeon.
    Billig exercise—an exercise for dysmenorrhea; used to counteract tendency toward lordosis and to stretch tight fascia around the pelvis.

Billroth, C.A. Theodor, Austrian surgeon, 1829–1894.
    Billroth anastomosis
    Billroth cords—the tissue occurring between the venous sinuses in the spleen. *Syn:* splenic cords
    Billroth disease
    Billroth forceps
    Billroth gastrectomy—(1) excision of pylorus with end-to-end anastomosis of stomach and duodenum; (2) resection of pylorus with greater part of lesser curvature of stomach, closure of cut ends of duodenum and stomach, followed by gastrojejunostomy. *Syn:* Billroth operation I and II
    Billroth gastroduodenoscopy
    Billroth gastroenterostomy
    Billroth gastrojejunostomy
    Billroth hypertrophy
    Billroth I anastomosis—*Syn:* Billroth operation I
    Billroth II anastomosis—*Syn:* Billroth operation II
    Billroth operation I—excision of the pylorus with end-to-end anastomosis of stomach and duodenum. *Syn:* Billroth I anastomosis
    Billroth operation II—resection of the pylorus with the greater part of the lesser curvature of the stomach, closure of the cut ends of the duodenum and stomach, followed by a gastrojejunostomy. *Syn:* Billroth II anastomosis
    Billroth ovarian retractor

Billroth venae cavernosae—small tributaries of the splenic vein in the pulp of the spleen. *Syn:* venae cavernosae of spleen

Binder, K.H., German dentist.
Binder syndrome—*Syn:* nasomaxillary hypoplasia; maxillonasal dysplasia

Binet, Alfred, French psychologist, 1857–1911.
Binet age—the age of the normal child with whose intelligence (as measured by the Stanford-Binet scale) the intelligence of the abnormal child corresponds.
Binet scale—a measure of intelligence designed for children and adults.
Binet test—*Syn:* Stanford-Binet intelligence scale
Binet-Simon scale—forerunner of individual intelligence tests, sometimes referred to as the Binet scale.
Stanford-Binet intelligence scale—a standardized test for the measurement of intelligence. *Syn:* Binet test

Bing, J., Scandinavian physician.
Bing-Neel syndrome—central nervous system response to macroglobulinemia.

Bing, Paul Robert, German neurologist, 1878–1956.
Bing reflex—when the foot is passively dorsiflexed, plantar flexion occurs if any point on the ankle between the two malleoli is tapped. *Syn:* Bing sign
Bing sign—*Syn:* Bing reflex

Bing, Richard J., U.S. physician, *1909.
Taussig-Bing disease—*Syn:* Taussig-Bing syndrome
Taussig-Bing syndrome—see under Taussig

Bingham, E.C., U.S. chemist, 1878–1945.
Bingham flow—the flow characteristics exhibited by a Bingham plastic.
Bingham model—a model representing the flow behavior of a Bingham plastic, in the idealized case.
Bingham plastic—a material that, in the idealized case, does not flow until a critical stress (yield stress) is exceeded, and then flows at a rate proportional to the excess of stress over the yield stress.

Binswanger, Otto Ludwig, German neurologist, 1852–1929.
Binswanger dementia—*Syn:* Binswanger disease
Binswanger disease—one of the causes of multiinfarct dementia, in which there are many infarcts and lacunes in the white matter, with relative sparing of the cortex and basal ganglia. *Syn:* encephalitis subcorticalis chronica; Binswanger encephalopathy; subcortical arteriosclerotic encephalopathy; Binswanger dementia
Binswanger encephalopathy—*Syn:* Binswanger disease

Binz, Carl, German pharmacologist, 1832–1913.
Binz test—a qualitative test for the presence of quinine in the urine.

NOTES

Biondi, Aldolpho, Italian pathologist, 1846–1917.
    Biondi-Heidenhain stain—an obsolete stain for spirochetes, using acid fuchsin and orange G.

Biot, Camille, French physician, *1878.
    Biot breathing—*SYN:* Biot respiration
    Biot breathing sign—irregular periods of apnea alternating with four or five deep breaths, seen with increased intracranial pressure.
    Biot respiration—abrupt, irregular alternating periods of apnea with constant rate and depth of breathing, as that resulting from lesions due to increased intracranial pressure. *SYN:* Biot breathing; ataxic breathing; respiratory ataxia
    Biot sign—abnormal breathing pattern characterized by periods of apnea and periods in which several breaths of similar volume are taken; seen with increased intracranial pressure.

Birbeck, Michael S., English cancer researcher.
    Birbeck granule—*SYN:* Langerhans granule

Birch-Hirschfeld, Felix V., German pathologist, 1842–1899.
    Birch-Hirschfeld stain—an obsolete stain for demonstrating amyloid.

Bird, Golding, English physician, 1814–1854.
    Bird formula—formula related to specific gravity of urine.

Bird, Samuel D., Australian physician, 1833–1904.
    Bird sign—the presence of a zone of dullness on percussion with absence of respiratory signs in hydatid cyst of the lung.

Birkett, John, English physician, 1815–1904.
    Birkett forceps
    Birkett hemostatic forceps
    Birkett hernia—inguinal hernia with sac extending into the anterior or inferior wall. *SYN:* intermuscular hernia; ascending hernia

Bischof, W., 20th century German neurosurgeon.
    Bischof corona
    Bischof myelotomy—longitudinal incision of the spinal cord through the lateral column for treatment of spasticity of the lower extremities.
    Bischof operation

Bishop, J. Michael, joint winner of 1989 Nobel Prize for work related to oncogenes.

Bishop, Louis F., U.S. physician, 1864–1941.
    Bishop sphygmoscope—an instrument for measuring the blood pressure.

Bitot, Pierre A., French physician, 1822–1888.
    Bitot patches—*SYN:* Bitot spots
    Bitot spots—small, circumscribed, lusterless, grayish white, foamy, greasy, triangular deposits on the bulbar conjunctiva adjacent to the cornea; occurs in vitamin A deficiency. *SYN:* Bitot patches

Bittner, John J., U.S. oncologist, 1904–1961.
    Bittner agent—member of the retrovirus subfamily Oncornavirinae. *SYN:* mammary tumor virus of mice; Bittner milk factor; Bittner factor

Bittner factor—*Syn:* Bittner agent
Bittner milk factor—*Syn:* Bittner agent

Bittorf, Alexander, German physician, 1876–1949.
Bittorf reaction—in cases of renal colic, pain radiating to the kidney upon squeezing the testicle or pressing the ovary.

Bizzozero, Giulio, Italian physician, 1846–1901.
Bizzozero corpuscle—an irregularly shaped disklike cytoplasmic fragment of a megakaryocyte found in the peripheral blood where it functions in clotting. *Syn:* platelet

B

Bjerrum, Jannik P., Danish ophthalmologist, 1851–1926.
Bjerrum scotoma—a comet-shaped scotoma, occurring in glaucoma. *Syn:* sickle scotoma; Bjerrum sign
Bjerrum scotometer
Bjerrum screen—a flat, usually black surface used to measure the central 30 degrees of the field of vision. *Syn:* tangent screen
Bjerrum sign—*Syn:* Bjerrum scotoma

Bjork, V.O., 20th century Swedish cardiothoracic surgeon.
Bjork-Shiley valve—prosthetic aortic/mitral valve.

Björnstad, R., Swedish dermatologist.
Björnstad syndrome—autosomal dominant trait causing sensorineural hearing loss.

Black, Douglas A.K., Scottish physician, *1909.
Black formula—a translation of Pignet formula into British measurements.

Black, Greene V., U.S. dentist, 1836–1915.
Black classification—a classification of cavities of the teeth based upon the tooth surface(s) involved.

Black, Sir James W., joint winner of 1988 Nobel Prize for work related to drug treatment.

Blackfan, Kenneth D., U.S. physician, 1883–1941.
Diamond-Blackfan anemia—see under Diamond
Diamond-Blackfan syndrome—*Syn:* Diamond-Blackfan anemia

Blagden, Sir Charles, English physician, 1748–1820.
Blagden law—the depression of the freezing point of dilute solutions is proportional to the amount of the dissolved substance.

Blainville, Henri Marie Ducrotay de, French zoologist and anthropologist, 1777–1850.
Blainville ears—asymmetry in size or shape of the auricles.

Blair, Vilray P., U.S. surgeon, 1871–1955.
Blair ankle arthrodesis
Blair chisel

(continued)

NOTES

Blair *(continued)*
Blair elevator
Blair fusion
Blair knife
Blair saw guide
Blair technique
Blair-Brown graft—a split-thickness graft of intermediate thickness.

Blakemore, Arthur H., U.S. surgeon, 1897–1970.
Blakemore esophageal tube
Blakemore tube
Sengstaken-Blakemore tube—see under Sengstaken

Blalock, Alfred, U.S. surgeon, 1899–1965.
Blalock anastomosis
Blalock clamp
Blalock pulmonary clamp
Blalock shunt—subclavian artery to pulmonary artery shunt to increase pulmonary circulation in cyanotic heart disease with decreased pulmonary flow.
Blalock sutures
Blalock-Hanlon operation—the creation of a large atrial septal defect as a palliative procedure for complete transposition of the great arteries.
Blalock-Taussig operation—an operation for congenital malformations of the heart.
Blalock-Taussig shunt—a palliative subclavian artery to pulmonary artery anastomosis.

Bland, E.F., U.S. physician, *1901.
Bland-White-Garland syndrome—juvenile angina pectoris and myocardial infarction.

Blandin, Philippe Frédéric, French anatomist and surgeon, 1798–1849.
Blandin gland—one of the small mixed glands deeply placed near the apex of the tongue on each side of the frenulum. *SYN:* anterior lingual gland

Blasius, Gerardus, 17th century Dutch anatomist.
Blasius duct—the duct of the parotid gland opening from the cheek into the vestibule of the mouth opposite the neck of the superior second molar tooth. *SYN:* parotid duct

Blaskovics, Laszlo de, Hungarian ophthalmologist, 1869–1938.
Blaskovics operation—operation for correction of eyelid ptosis.

Blatin, Marc, French physician, 1878–1943.
Blatin syndrome—the peculiar trembling or vibratory sensation felt on palpation of a hydatid cyst. *SYN:* hydatid thrill

Blaud, P., French physician, 1774–1858.
Blaud pill—ferrous sulfate used in treatment of chlorosis. *SYN:* iron pill

Bloch, Bruno, Swiss dermatologist, 1878–1933.
Bloch-Sulzberger disease—genodermatosis that may also involve other structures. *SYN:* incontinentia pigmenti; Bloch-Sulzberger syndrome
Bloch-Sulzberger syndrome—*SYN:* Bloch-Sulzberger disease

Bloch, Konrad, joint winner of 1964 Nobel Prize for work related to cholesterol and metabolism of fatty acids.

Bloch, Marcel, French physician, 1885–1925.
  Bloch reaction—a dark staining observed in fresh tissue sections to which a solution of dopa has been applied. *Syn:* dopa reaction

Blocq, Paul O., French physician, 1860–1896.
  Blocq disease—the inability to either stand or walk in the normal manner. *Syn:* astasia-abasia

B

Bloodgood, Joseph Colt, U.S. surgeon, 1867–1935.
  Bloodgood disease
  Bloodgood operation—inguinal canal reconstruction procedure.
  blue-domed cyst of Bloodgood—breast cyst.

Bloom, David, U.S. dermatologist, *1892.
  Bloom syndrome—congenital telangiectatic erythema and dwarfism with normal body proportions except for a narrow face and dolichocephalic skull.

Blount, Walter P., U.S. orthopedist, *1900.
  Blount bent blade
  Blount blade plate
  Blount bone retractor
  Blount bone spreader
  Blount brace
  Blount disease—nonrachitic bowlegs in children. *Syn:* Blount-Barber disease
  Blount displacement osteotomy
  Blount epiphysiodesis
  Blount hip retractor
  Blount knee retractor
  Blount knife
  Blount mallet
  Blount osteotome
  Blount osteotomy
  Blount scoliosis osteotome
  Blount splint
  Blount spreader
  Blount staple
  Blount technique for osteoclasis
  Blount tibia vara
  Blount tracing technique
  Blount V-blade
  Blount-Barber disease—*Syn:* Blount disease
  Moore-Blount driver
  Moore-Blount screwdriver

Blücher, Gebhard von, Prussian field marshal, 1742–1819.
  Blücher shoe—a type of laced shoe. *Syn:* Gibson shoe

NOTES

Blum, Paul, French physician, 1878–1933.
    Gougerot and Blum disease—see under Gougerot

Blumberg, Baruch S., joint winner of 1976 Nobel Prize for work related to infectious diseases.

Blumberg, Jacob M., German surgeon and gynecologist, 1873–1955.
    Blumberg sign—pain felt upon sudden release of steadily applied pressure on a suspected area of the abdomen, indicative of peritonitis.

Blumenau, Leonid W., Russian neurologist, 1862–1932.
    Blumenau nucleus—the lateral cuneate nucleus of the medulla oblongata.

Blumenbach, Johann F., German physiologist, 1752–1840.
    Blumenbach clivus—the sloping surface from the dorsum sellae to the foramen magnum. *Syn:* clivus

Blumer, George, U.S. physician, 1858–1940.
    Blumer shelf—a shelf palpable by rectal examination, due to metastatic tumor cells gravitating from an abdominal cancer and growing in the rectovesical or rectouterine pouch. *Syn:* rectal shelf

Blythedale, Blythedale Children's Hospital, Valhalla, NY.
    Blythemobile—stretcher-wheelchair combination that can be self-propelled.

Boas, Ismar I., German gastroenterologist, 1858–1938.
    Boas sign—hyperesthesia related to acute cholecystitis.
    Boas test
    Boas-Oppler bacillus

Bobath, Berta, English physical therapist, and Karel, English neurologist.
    Bobath facilitation technique—*Syn:* Bobath method
    Bobath method—therapeutic exercise method for individuals with central nervous system lesions. *Syn:* Bobath method of exercise; Bobath proprioceptive neuromuscular facilitation; Bobath facilitation techique
    Bobath method of exercise—*Syn:* Bobath method
    Bobath proprioceptive neuromuscular facilitation—*Syn:* Bobath method
    Bobath test chart of motor ability

Bochdalek, Vincent A., Czech anatomist, 1801–1883.
    Bochdalek duct—*Syn:* duct of His; duct of Vater; thyrolingual duct
    Bochdalek foramen—a congenital defective opening through the diaphragm, connecting pleural and peritoneal cavities. *Syn:* pleuroperitoneal hiatus
    Bochdalek ganglion—a ganglion of the plexus of the dental nerve lying in the maxilla just above the root of the canine tooth.
    Bochdalek gap—a triangular area in the diaphragm devoid of muscle fibers. *Syn:* vertebrocostal trigone
    Bochdalek hernia—absence of the pleuroperitoneal membrane (usually on the left) or an enlarged Morgagni foramen which allows protrusion of abdominal viscera into the chest. *Syn:* congenital diaphragmatic hernia
    Bochdalek muscle—an occasional thin band of muscular fibers passing between the root of the tongue and the triticeal cartilage. *Syn:* musculus triticeoglossus

Bochdalek valve—a fold of mucous membrane in the lacrimal canaliculus at the lacrimal punctum. *Syn:* Foltz valvule

flower basket of Bochdalek—part of the choroid plexus of the fourth ventricle protruding through Luschka foramen and resting on the dorsal surface of the glossopharyngeal nerve.

Bock, August C., German anatomist, 1782–1833.

Bock ganglion—a small ganglionic swelling on filaments from the internal carotid plexus, lying on the undersurface of the carotid artery in the cavernous sinus. *Syn:* carotid ganglion

Bockhart, Max, German physician, 1883–1921.

Bockhart impetigo—a superficial follicular pustular eruption involving the scalp or other hairy area. *Syn:* follicular impetigo

Bodansky, Aaron, U.S. biochemist, 1887–1961.

Bodansky unit—that amount of phosphatase that liberates 1 mg of phosphorus as inorganic phosphate during the first hour of incubation with a buffered substrate containing sodium β-glycerophosphate.

Bödecker, Charles F., U.S. oral histologist, embryologist, and pathologist, *1880.

Bödecker index—a modification of the DMF caries index.

Bodian, David, U.S. anatomist, *1910.

Bodian copper-PROTARGOL stain—a stain employing a silver proteinate complex (PROTARGOL) to demonstrate axis cylinders and neurofibrils.

Bodian method

Boeck, Caesar P.M., Norwegian dermatologist, 1845–1917.

Besnier-Boeck disease—see under Besnier

Besnier-Boeck-Schaumann disease—*Syn:* Besnier-Boeck disease

Besnier-Boeck-Schaumann syndrome—*Syn:* Besnier-Boeck disease

Boeck disease—*Syn:* Besnier-Boeck disease

Boeck sarcoid—*Syn:* Besnier-Boeck disease

Boeck, Carl W., Norwegian physician, 1808–1875.

Danielssen-Boeck disease—see under Danielssen

Boehmer, F.

Boehmer hematoxylin—an alum type of hematoxylin in which natural ripening occurs in about 8 to 10 days.

Boerhaave, Hermann, Dutch physician, 1668–1738.

Boerhaave glands—*Syn:* sweat glands

Boerhaave syndrome—spontaneous rupture of the lower esophagus, a variant of Mallory-Weiss syndrome.

Bogaert, Ludo van. See under van Bogaert.

Bogorad, F.A., 20th century Russian physician.

Bogorad syndrome—in cases of facial nerve palsy, tearing occurs from one eye after eating or drinking; facial tic and taste loss may occur concurrently.

NOTES

Bogros, Antoine, 19th century French anatomist.
Bogros serous membrane—a membrane of the episcleral space (of Tenon).

Bogros, Jean-Annet, French anatomist, 1786–1823.
Bogros space—a triangular space between the peritoneum and the transversalis fascia. *Syn:* retroinguinal space

Böhler, Lorenz, Austrian orthopedic surgeon, 1885–1973.
Böhler exerciser—a device used to exercise knee extensors.
Böhler frame—orthopedic device.
Böhler iron—orthopedic device.
Böhler splint—orthopedic device.

Bohn, Heinrich, German physician, 1832–1888.
Bohn nodules—tiny multiple cysts in newborns.

Bohr, Christian, Danish physiologist, 1855–1911.
Bohr effect—the influence exerted by carbon dioxide on the oxygen dissociation curve of blood.
Bohr equation—an equation to calculate the respiratory dead space.

Bohr, Niels H.D., Danish physicist and Nobel laureate, 1885–1962.
Bohr atom—a concept or model of the atom in which the negatively charged electrons move in circular or elliptical orbits around the positively charged nucleus, energy being emitted or absorbed when electrons change from one orbit to another.
Bohr magneton—the net magnetic moment of one unpaired electron; used in electron spin resonance spectrometry for detection and estimation of free radicals. *Syn:* electron magneton
Bohr theory—that spectrum lines are produced by the quantized emission of radiant energy when electrons drop from an orbit of a higher to one of a lower energy level, or by absorption of radiation when an electron rises from a lower to a higher energy level.

Boll, Franz C., German histologist and physiologist, 1849–1879.
Boll cells—basal cells in the lacrimal gland.

Bollinger, Otto, German pathologist, 1843–1909.
Bollinger bodies—intracytoplasmic inclusion bodies observed in the infected tissues of birds with fowlpox.
Bollinger granules—irregular aggregates or colonizations of Gram-positive cocci, usually staphylococci, observed in lesions of botryomycosis.

Bollman, Jesse L., U.S. physiologist, *1896.
Mann-Bollman fistula—see under Mann, Frank C.

Bolton, Joseph S., English neurologist, 1867–1946.
Bolton plane—a roentgenographic cephalometric plane extending from the Bolton point to nasion. *Syn:* Bolton-nasion plane; Bolton-nasion line; Bolton-Broadbent plane
Bolton-Broadbent plane—*Syn:* Bolton plane
Bolton-nasion line—*Syn:* Bolton plane
Bolton-nasion plane—*Syn:* Bolton plane

Bombay, city in India
Bombay blood group—red cells resembling Group O, first seen in Bombay, India.

Bonhoeffer, Karl, German psychiatrist, 1868–1948.
Bonhoeffer sign—loss of normal muscle tone in chorea.

Bonnet, Amédée, French surgeon, 1809–1858.
Bonnet capsule—the anterior part of the vagina bulbi.

Bonnet, Charles, Swiss naturalist, 1720–1795.
Charles Bonnet syndrome—geriatric disorder marked by hallucinations.

Bonnevie, Kristine, German physician, 1872–1950.
Bonnevie-Ullrich syndrome—characteristics include hand and foot lymphedema, short stature, skin laxity.

Bonney, William F. V., English gynecologist, 1872–1953.
Bonney blue—ink for marking skin.
Bonney cervical amputation
Bonney cervical dilator
Bonney clamp
Bonney clip
Bonney forceps
Bonney hysterectomy
Bonney inflator
Bonney test—bladder test.

Bonnier, Pierre, French clinician, 1861–1918.
Bonnier syndrome—ocular disturbances, deafness, nausea, thirst, and anorexia due to a lesion of the Deiters nucleus.

Bonwill, William G.A., U.S. dentist, 1833–1899.
Bonwill triangle—an equilateral triangle formed by lines from the contact points of the lower central incisors, or the medial line of the residual ridge of the mandible, to the condyle on either side and from one condyle to the other.

Böök, Jan A., Swedish geneticist, *1915.
Böök syndrome—premolar aplasia, hyperhidrosis, and premature graying of hair.

Bordeau, Théophile de, French physician, 1722–1776.
de Bordeau theory—that each organ of the body manufactured a specific humor which it secreted into the bloodstream.

Bordet, Jules, Belgian bacteriologist and Nobel laureate, 1870–1961.
Bordet amboceptor
Bordet-Gengou bacillus—a species that causes whooping cough. *Syn: Bordetella pertussis*

(continued)

NOTES

Bordet *(continued)*

Bordet-Gengou phenomenon—the phenomenon of complement fixation.
Bordet-Gengou potato blood agar—glycerine-potato agar with 25% of blood, used for the isolation of *Bordetella pertussis*.
Bordet-Gengou reaction
Bordetella—a genus of strictly aerobic bacteria that are pathogens of the mammalian respiratory tract.

Börjeson, Mats, Swedish physician, *1922.
Börjeson-Forssman-Lehmann syndrome—a condition characterized by mental deficiency, epilepsy, hypogonadism, hypometabolism, obesity, and narrow palpebral fissures.

Born, Gustav Jacob, German embryologist, 1851–1900.
Born method of wax plate reconstruction—the making of three-dimensional models of structures from serial sections.

Bornholm, island in the Baltic Sea.
Bornholm disease—infection with Coxsackie virus causing severe abdominal and/or pleural pain.

Borrel, Amédée, French bacteriologist, 1867–1936.
Borrel blue stain—a stain for demonstrating spirochetes, treponemes, and Borrelia organisms.
Borrel bodies—particles of fowlpox virus.

Borries, T., Danish physician.
Borries syndrome—encephalitis with changes in cerebrospinal fluid suggestive of brain abscess.

Borsieri, Giovanni Battista, Italian physician, 1725–1785.
Borsieri line—*Syn:* Borsieri sign
Borsieri sign—in patients with scarlet fever, drawing the fingernail across the skin creates a white line that turns red. *Syn:* Borsieri line

Borst, Maximilian, German pathologist, 1869–1946.
Borst-Jadassohn type intraepidermal epithelioma—precancerous lesions clinically suggestive of actinic or seborrheic keratosis, with nests of immature or abnormal keratinocytes within the epidermis.

Bostock, John, English physician, 1773–1846.
Bostock catarrh—*Syn:* allergic rhinitis; hay fever
Bostock disease

Boston, Leonard N., U.S. physician, 1871–1931.
Boston exanthem
Boston sign—jerky downward movement of the upper eyelid on downward rotation of the eye, characteristic of Graves disease.

Botallo, Leonardo, Italian physician in Paris, 1530–1600.
Botallo duct—a fetal vessel connecting the left pulmonary artery with the descending aorta. *Syn:* ductus arteriosus
Botallo foramen—the orifice of communication between the two atria of the fetal heart.
Botallo ligament—the remains of the ductus arteriosus. *Syn:* ligamentum arteriosum

Böttcher, Arthur, Estonian anatomist, 1831–1889.

Böttcher canal—a duct that connects the inner aspect of the utricle with the endolymphatic duct a short distance from its origin from the saccule. *Syn:* utriculosaccular duct

Böttcher cells—cells of the basilar membrane of the cochlea.

Böttcher crystals—small crystals observed microscopically in prostatic fluid.

Böttcher ganglion—ganglion on the cochlear nerve in the internal acoustic meatus.

Böttcher space—the dilated blind extremity of the endolymphatic duct. *Syn:* endolymphatic sac

Charcot-Böttcher crystalloids—see under Charcot

Bouchard, Charles Jacques, French physician, 1837–1915.

Bouchard disease—myopathic dilation of the stomach.

Bouchard nodes—interphalangeal joint nodes, related to osteoarthritis or gout.

Bouchut, Jean A.E., French physician, 1818–1891.

Bouchut tube—a short cylindrical tube used in intubation of the larynx.

Bouillaud, Jean, French physician, 1796–1881.

Bouillaud disease—obsolete term for acute rheumatic fever with carditis.

Bouillaud sign

Bouin, Paul, French histologist, 1870–1962.

Bouin fixative—a solution of glacial acetic acid, formalin, and picric acid.

Bourdon, Eugène, French engineer and inventor, 1808–1884.

Bourdon tube—a curved tube used as a transducer to move the pointer of an aneroid manometer.

Bourgery, Marc-Jean, French anatomist and surgeon, 1797–1849.

Bourgery ligament—a fibrous band that extends across the back of the knee from its separation from the direct tendon of insertion on the medial condyle of the tibia to the lateral condyle of the femur. *Syn:* oblique popliteal ligament

Bourneville, Désiré-Magloire, French physician, 1840–1909.

Bourneville disease—phacomatosis characterized by the formation of multisystem hamartomas. *Syn:* tuberous sclerosis; Bourneville syndrome

Bourneville syndrome—*Syn:* Bourneville disease

Bourneville-Pringle disease—facial lesions with tuberous sclerosis.

Bourquin, Anne, U.S. chemist, *1897.

Sherman-Bourquin unit of vitamin B$_2$—see under Sherman

Bouveret, Leon, French physician, 1850–1926.

Bouveret disease

Bouveret syndrome—(1) paroxysmal supraventricular tachycardia; (2) gastric outlet obstruction due to gallstone passing into the duodenal bulb through a choledochoduodenal or cholecystoduodenal fistula.

NOTES

Bovero, Renaldo, 20th century Italian dermatologist.
> **Bovero muscle**—"the sucking muscle," compressor muscle of the lips. *Syn:* cutaneomucous muscle

Bovet, Daniel, Swiss-Italian pharmacologist, *1907, winner of the 1957 Nobel Prize for developing muscle relaxants and antihistamines.

Bowditch, Henry P., U.S. physiologist, 1840–1911.
> **Bowditch effect**—homeometric autoregulation of cardiac function induced by changing heart rate.
> **Bowditch law**—consistently total response to any effective stimulus. *Syn:* all or none law

Bowen, John T., U.S. dermatologist, 1857–1941.
> **Bowen disease**—a form of intraepidermal carcinoma. *Syn:* Bowen precancerous dermatosis
> **Bowen precancerous dermatosis**—*Syn:* Bowen disease
> **bowenoid cells**—cells characteristic of Bowen disease.
> **bowenoid papulosis**—a clinically benign form of intraepithelial neoplasia that microscopically resembles Bowen disease or carcinoma in situ, occurring in young individuals of both sexes on the genital or perianal skin usually as multiple well-demarcated pigmented warty papules.

Bowman, Sir William, English ophthalmologist, anatomist, and physiologist, 1816–1892.
> **Bowman capsule**—the expanded beginning of a nephron. *Syn:* glomerular capsule
> **Bowman disks**—disk resulting from transverse segmentation of striated muscular fiber treated with weak acids, certain alkaline solutions, or freezing.
> **Bowman eye knife**
> **Bowman gland**
> **Bowman iris needle**
> **Bowman iris scissors**
> **Bowman lacrimal dilator**
> **Bowman lacrimal probe**
> **Bowman membrane**—*Syn:* anterior limiting layer of cornea
> **Bowman muscle**—*Syn:* ciliary muscle
> **Bowman probe**—a double-ended probe for the lacrimal duct.
> **Bowman space**—the slitlike space between the visceral and parietal layers of the capsule of the renal corpuscle. *Syn:* capsular space
> **Bowman strabismus scissors**
> **Bowman theory**—that urine is formed by passive filtration through the glomeruli and secretion by the epithelium of the tubules.

Boyce, Frederick F., U.S. physician, *1903.
> **Boyce sign**—hand pressure on side of neck causes gurgling sound when esophageal diverticulum is present.

Boyce, William H., U.S. urologist, *1918.
> **Smith-Boyce operation**—an incision into the posterolateral renal parenchyma used for removal of renal calculi. *Syn:* anatrophic nephrotomy

Boyden, Edward A., U.S. anatomist, 1886–1977.
  Boyden meal—a meal used to test the evacuation time of the gallbladder.
  Boyden sphincter—smooth muscle sphincter that controls the flow of bile in the duodenum. *Syn:* sphincter of the common bile duct

Boyer, Baron Alexis, French surgeon, 1757–1833.
  Boyer bursa—a bursa between the posterior surface of the body of the hyoid bone and the thyrohyoid membrane. *Syn:* retrohyoid bursa
  Boyer cyst—a subhyoid cyst.

Boyle, Hon. Robert, English physicist and chemist, 1627–1691.
  Boyle law—at constant temperature, the volume of a given quantity of gas varies inversely with its absolute pressure. *Syn:* Mariotte law

Bozeman, Nathan, U.S. surgeon, 1825–1905.
  Bozeman clamp
  Bozeman curet
  Bozeman dilator
  Bozeman dressing forceps
  Bozeman forceps
  Bozeman hook
  Bozeman needle holder
  Bozeman operation—an operation for uterovaginal fistula, the cervix uteri being attached to the bladder and opening into its cavity.
  Bozeman position—knee-elbow position, the patient being strapped to supports.
  Bozeman speculum
  Bozeman sutures
  Bozeman uterine forceps
  Bozeman-Fritsch catheter—a slightly curved double-channel uterine catheter with several openings at the tip.

Bozzolo, Camillo, Italian physician, 1845–1920.
  Bozzolo sign—pulsating vessels in the nasal mucous membrane, noted occasionally in thoracic aneurysm.

Braasch, William F., U.S. urologist, 1878–1975.
  Braasch bladder specimen forceps
  Braasch bulb
  Braasch catheter—a bulb-tipped catheter used for dilation and calibration.
  Braasch cystoscope
  Braasch forceps
  Braasch ureteral catheter
  Braasch ureteral dilator

Bracht, E., 20th century German pathologist.
  Bracht-Wachter bodies—myocardial microabscesses observed in the presence of bacterial endocarditis.
  Bracht-Wachter lesion—a focal collection of lymphocytes and mononuclear cells within the myocardium in bacterial endocarditis.

NOTES

Bracht, Erich Franz, German obstetrician and gynecologist, *1882.
  Bracht maneuver—delivery of a fetus in the breech position by extension of the legs and trunk of the fetus over the symphysis pubis and abdomen of the mother.

Bradbury, Samuel, U.S. physician, 1883–1947.
  Bradbury-Eggleston syndrome—impaired peripheral vasoconstriction causing visual disturbances, dizziness, syncope, and other symptoms. *SYN:* Eggleston-Bradbury syndrome
  Eggleston-Bradbury syndrome—*SYN:* Bradbury-Eggleston syndrome

Bradford, Edward H., U.S. orthopedist, 1848–1926.
  Bradford frame—an oblong rectangular frame that permits trunk and lower extremities to move as a unit.

Bradley, W.H., 20th century English physician.
  Bradley disease—nausea and vomiting which are epidemic.

Braille, Louis, French educator, 1809–1852.
  Braille—system of raised dots placed in patterns to allow the blind to read.
  Braillophone—a combination telephone and braille system.

Brailsford, James Frederick, English radiologist, 1888–1961.
  Brailsford-Morquio disease—*SYN:* Morquio syndrome

Brain, W. Russell, Lord, English physician, 1895–1966.
  Brain reflex—extension of the arm of a hemiplegic patient when turned prone as if on all fours. *SYN:* quadripedal extensor reflex

Brandt, M.L., U.S. obstetrician, *1894.
  Brandt brassiere
  Brandt treatment

Brandt, T.E., Finnish dermatologist.
  Brandt syndrome—symptoms include fat in feces, baldness, paronychia, and pustular eruptions around the mouth and anus. *SYN:* Danbolt syndrome; Danbolt-Closs syndrome

Brandt, Thure, Swedish obstetrician and gynecologist, 1819–1895.
  Brandt massage—a gynecologic massage used to correct the faulty position of the uterus. *SYN:* Thure Brandt massage
  Brandt-Andrews maneuver—for the expression of the placenta.
  Thure Brandt massage—*SYN:* Brandt massage

Branham, H.H., 19th century U.S. surgeon.
  Branham bradycardia—*SYN:* Branham sign
  Branham sign—bradycardia following compression or excision of an arteriovenous fistula. *SYN:* Branham bradycardia

Branham, Sara Elizabeth, U.S. bacteriologist, 1888–1962.
  Branhamella—a subgenus of the genus *Moraxella*, occurring in mucous membranes of the upper respiratory tract.

Brasdor, Pierre, French surgeon, 1721–1798.
  Brasdor method—treatment of aneurysm by ligation of the artery immediately below the tumor.

Braun, Christopher Heinrich, German surgeon, 1847–1911.
Braun anastomosis—after gastroenterostomy, anastomosis between afferent and efferent loops of jejunum.

Braun-Falco, Otto, German physician.
Marghescu and Braun-Falco syndrome—see under Marghescu

Braune, Christian W., German anatomist, 1831–1892.
Braune canal—the birth canal formed by the uterine cavity, dilated cervix, vagina, and vulva.
Braune muscle—*SYN:* puborectalis muscle
Braune valve—a fold of mucous membrane at the junction of the esophagus with the stomach.

Braxton Hicks, John, English gynecologist, 1825–1897.
Braxton Hicks contraction—rhythmic myometrial activity, occurring during the course of a pregnancy, which causes no pain for the patient.
Braxton Hicks sign—irregular uterine contractions occurring after the third month of pregnancy.
Braxton Hicks version—obsolete term for internal version of the fetus, substituting the breech for the head as the leading pole.

Bray, Charles William, U.S. otologist, *1904.
Wever-Bray effect—*SYN:* Wever-Bray phenomenon
Wever-Bray phenomenon—see under Wever

Brazelton, T. Terry, U.S. pediatrician.
Brazelton Neonatal Behavioral Assessment Scale—a scale to assess the development of the neonate.

Breda, Achille, Italian dermatologist, 1850–1933.
Breda disease—a type of American leishmaniasis. *SYN:* espundia

Breen, William, U.S. physician, *1930.
Cross-McKusick-Breen syndrome

Brehmer, Hermann, German physician, 1826–1889.
Brehmer method—*SYN:* Brehmer treatment
Brehmer treatment—treatment used for pulmonary tuberculosis. *SYN:* Brehmer method

Breisky, August, Czech gynecologist, 1832–1889.
Breisky disease—eruption of papules with vulvar involvement. *SYN:* lichen sclerosus

Brenn, Lena, 20th century U.S. researcher.
Brown-Brenn stain—see under Brown, James H.

Brennemann, Joseph, U.S. pediatrician, 1872–1944.
Brennemann syndrome—lymphadenitis of the retroperitoneal and mesenteric regions as a result of throat infection.

NOTES

Brenner, Fritz, German pathologist, *1877.
Brenner tumor—a relatively infrequent benign neoplasm of the ovary.

Breschet, Gilbert, French anatomist, 1784–1845.
Breschet bones—one of the small ossicles occasionally found in the ligaments of the sternoclavicular articulation. *SYN:* os suprasternale
Breschet canals—channels in the diploë that accommodate the diploic veins. *SYN:* diploic canals
Breschet hiatus—a semilunar opening at the apex of the cochlea through which the scala vestibuli and the scala tympani of the cochlea communicate with one another. *SYN:* helicotrema
Breschet sinus—a paired dural venous sinus beginning on the parietal bone, running along the sphenoidal ridges, and emptying into the cavernous sinus. *SYN:* sphenoparietal sinus
Breschet vein—one of the veins in the diploë of the cranial bones. *SYN:* diploic vein

Brescia, Michael J., U.S. nephrologist, *1933.
Brescia-Cimino fistula—a direct, surgically created arteriovenous fistula used to facilitate chronic hemodialysis.

Breslow, Alexander, U.S. pathologist, 1928–1980.
Breslow thickness—maximal thickness of a primary cutaneous melanoma.

Bretonneau, Pierre F., French physician, 1778–1862.
Bretonneau angina—diphtheria. *SYN:* Bretonneau disease
Bretonneau disease—*SYN:* Bretonneau angina

Breuer, Josef, Austrian internist, 1842–1925.
Hering-Breuer reflex—see under Hering

Breus, Carl, Austrian obstetrician, 1852–1914.
Breus mole—an aborted ovum in which the fetal surface of the placenta presents numerous hematomata with an absence of blood vessels in the chorion.

Brewer, George E., U.S. surgeon, 1861–1939.
Brewer infarcts—dark red, wedge-shaped areas resembling infarcts, seen on section of a kidney in pyelonephritis.
Brewer operation
Brewer speculum
Brewer vaginal speculum

Bricker, Eugene M., U.S. urologist, *1908.
Bricker operation—an operation utilizing an isolated segment of ileum to collect urine from the ureters and conduct it to the skin surface.

Bright, Richard, English internist and pathologist, 1789–1858.
Bright disease—nonsuppurative nephritis with albuminuria and edema.

Brill, Nathan E., U.S. physician, 1860–1925.
Brill disease—*SYN:* Brill-Zinsser disease
Brill-Symmers disease—obsolete term for nodular lymphoma.
Brill-Zinsser disease—an endogenous reinfection associated with the "carrier state" in persons who previously had epidemic typhus fever. *SYN:* Brill disease; recrudescent typhus fever; recrudescent typhus

Brinell, Johan A., Swedish metallurgist, 1849–1925.

    Brinell hardness number—a number related to the size of the permanent impression made by a ball indenter of specified size pressed into the surface of the material under a specified load.

    Brinell scale

Brinton, William, English physician, 1823–1867.

    Brinton disease—infiltrating scirrhous carcinoma causing extensive thickening of stomach wall. *SYN:* leather-bottle stomach; linitis plastica

Briquet, Paul, French physician, 1796–1881.

    Briquet ataxia—weakening of the muscle sense and increased sensibility of the skin, in hysteria. *SYN:* hysterical ataxia

    Briquet syndrome—a chronic but fluctuating mental disorder, usually of young women, characterized by frequent complaints of physical illness involving multiple organ systems simultaneously.

Brissaud, Edouard, French physician, 1852–1909.

    Brissaud disease—habitual, repeated contraction of certain muscles, resulting in actions that can be voluntarily suppressed for only brief periods. *SYN:* tic

    Brissaud infantilism—*SYN:* infantile hypothyroidism

    Brissaud reflex—tickling the sole causes a contraction of the tensor fasciae latae muscle, even when there is no responsive movement of the toes.

    Brissaud-Marie syndrome—unilateral spasm of the tongue and lips, of hysterical nature.

Bristowe, John S., English physician, 1827–1895.

    Bristowe syndrome—symptoms caused by corpus callosum tumor.

Broadbent, Sir William H., English physician, 1835–1907.

    Bolton-Broadbent plane—*SYN:* Bolton plane

    Broadbent apoplexy—intracerebral bleeding which penetrates the lateral ventricle of the brain.

    Broadbent inverted sign—retraction of thoracic wall, synchronous with cardiac systole, visible particularly in the left posterior axillary line; sign of adherent pericardium. *SYN:* Broadbent sign

    Broadbent law—lesions of the upper segment of the motor tract cause less marked paralysis of muscles that habitually produce bilateral movements than of those that commonly act independently of the opposite side.

    Broadbent sign—*SYN:* Broadbent inverted sign

Broca, Pierre P., French surgeon, neurologist, and anthropologist, 1824–1880.

    Broca angle—the angle formed at the basion of lines drawn from the nasion and the alveolar point; the angle formed by the intersection at the biauricular axis of lines drawn from the supraorbital point and the alveolar point; the posterior superior angle of the parietal bone. *SYN:* Broca basilar angle; Broca facial angle; occipital angle of parietal bone

(continued)

NOTES

Broca *(continued)*

Broca aphasia—any of the varieties of aphasia in which the power of expression by writing, speaking, or signs is lost. *SYN:* motor aphasia

Broca area—*SYN:* Broca center

Broca basilar angle—*SYN:* Broca angle

Broca center—the posterior part of the inferior frontal gyrus of the left or dominant hemisphere, essential component of the motor mechanisms governing articulated speech. *SYN:* Broca area; motor speech center; Broca field; Brodmann area 44

Broca diagonal band—a white fiber bundle descending in the precommissural septum toward the base of the forebrain.

Broca facial angle—*SYN:* Broca angle

Broca field—*SYN:* Broca center

Broca fissure—the fissure surrounding Broca convolution.

Broca formula—a fully developed man should weigh as many kilograms as he is centimeters in height over and above 1 meter.

Broca parolfactory area—a small region of cerebral cortex on the medial surface of the frontal lobe demarcated from the subcallosal gyrus by the posterior parolfactory sulcus. *SYN:* parolfactory area

Broca pouch—a pear-shaped encapsulated collection of connective tissue and fat in each labium majus. *SYN:* pudendal sac

Broca visual plane—a plane drawn through the visual axes of each eye.

Brock, Sir Russell C., English surgeon, 1903–1980.

Brock operation—transventricular valvotomy for relief of pulmonic valvar stenosis. Obsolete procedure.

Brock syndrome—atelectasis with chronic pneumonitis of the middle lobe of the right lung, due to compression of the middle lobe bronchus, usually by enlarged lymph nodes, which may be tuberculous. *SYN:* middle lobe syndrome

Brockenbrough, E.C., U.S. surgeon, *1930.

Brockenbrough sign—a sign of idiopathic hypertrophic subaortic stenosis.

Brocq, Louis A.J., French dermatologist, 1856–1928.

Brocq disease—a variety of parapsoriasis.

Brödel, Max, German medical artist in the U.S., 1870–1941.

Brödel bloodless line—line demarcating the areas of distribution of the anterior and posterior branches of the renal artery.

Brodie, Charles Gordon, Scottish anatomist and surgeon, 1860–1933.

Brodie ligament—a fibrous band running more or less obliquely from the greater to the lesser tuberosity of the humerus, bridging over the bicipital groove. *SYN:* transverse humeral ligament

Brodie, Sir Benjamin C., English surgeon, 1783–1862.

Brodie abscess—a chronic abscess of bone surrounded by dense fibrous tissue and sclerotic bone.

Brodie bursa—(1) medial subtendinous bursa of gastrocnemius muscle; (2) *SYN:* bursa of semimembranosus muscle.

Brodie disease—(1) *SYN:* Brodie knee; (2) hysterical spinal neuralgia, simulating Pott disease.

Brodie knee—chronic hypertrophic synovitis of the knee. *SYN:* Brodie disease (1)

Brodie serocystic disease—usually benign and fast-growing postpubescent breast tumor.

Brodie-Trendelenburg test—test for varicosities in leg veins.

Brodie, Thomas Gregor, English physiologist, 1866–1916.

Brodie fluid—an aqueous salt solution used in manometers designed for testing gas evolution or uptake, as in cell respiration.

Brodmann, Korbinian, German neurologist, 1868–1918.

Brodmann area 41—*SYN:* primary auditory cortex

Brodmann area 44—*SYN:* Broca center

Brodmann areas—areas of cerebral cortex mapped out on the basis of cortical cytoarchitectural patterns.

Broesike, Gustav, German anatomist, *1853.

Broesike fossa—a peritoneal fossa. *SYN:* parajejunal fossa

Brompton, Brompton Hospital, London

Brompton cocktail—analgesic drink given to terminal cancer patients.

Brønsted, Johannes N., Danish physical chemist, 1879–1947.

Brønsted acid—an acid that is a proton donor.

Brønsted base—any molecule or ion that combines with a proton.

Brønsted theory—that an acid is a substance, charged or uncharged, liberating hydrogen ions in solution, and that a base is a substance that removes them from solution.

Brooke, Bryan N., English surgeon, *1915.

Brooke ileostomy—ileostomy in which the divided proximal ileum, brought through the abdominal wall, is evaginated and its edge is sutured to the dermis.

Brooke, Henry A.G., English dermatologist, 1854–1919.

Brooke disease—(1) *SYN:* Brooke tumor; (2) epidemic acne, possibly caused by toxic agents. *SYN:* Morrow-Brooke syndrome.

Brooke epithelioma—*SYN:* Brooke tumor

Brooke tumor—multiple small benign nodules, occurring mostly on the skin of the face, derived from basal cells of hair follicles enclosing small keratin cysts. *SYN:* trichoepithelioma; Brooke disease (1); Brooke epithelioma

Morrow-Brooke syndrome—*SYN:* Brooke disease (2)

Brophy, Truman William, U.S. oral surgeon, 1848–1928.

Brophy bistoury
Brophy bistoury knife
Brophy cleft palate knife
Brophy dressing forceps
Brophy elevator
Brophy forceps
Brophy gag
Brophy knife

(continued)

NOTES

Brophy *(continued)*
   Brophy needle
   Brophy operation—surgery to correct cleft palate.
   Brophy periosteal elevator
   Brophy periosteotome
   Brophy plate
   Brophy scissors
   Brophy tenaculum
   Brophy tenaculum retractor
   Brophy tissue forceps
   Brophy tooth elevator

Brown, George E., U.S. physician, 1885–1935.
   Hines and Brown test—see under Hines

Brown, Harold W., U.S. ophthalmologist, *1898.
   Brown syndrome—limited elevation of the eye in adduction due to fascia
   contracting the superior oblique muscle on the same side. *SYN:* tendon
   sheath syndrome
   Paterson-Brown-Kelly syndrome—see under Paterson, Donald R.

Brown, James H., U.S. microbiologist, *1884.
   Brown-Brenn stain—a method for differential staining of Gram-positive
   and Gram-negative bacteria in tissue sections.
   Brown-Brenn technique

Brown, James, U.S. plastic surgeon, 1899–1971.
   Blair-Brown graft—see under Blair
   Brown-Adson forceps—an Adson forceps with about 16 delicate teeth on
   each tip.

Brown, Michael S., joint winner of 1985 Nobel Prize for work related to
cholesterol.

Brown, Robert, English botanist, 1773–1858.
   brownian motion—*SYN:* brownian movement
   brownian movement—rapid random motion of small particles in
   suspension caused by jostling by the molecules of the suspending liquid.
   SYN: brownian motion; brownian-Zsigmondy movement; molecular
   movement; pedesis
   brownian-Zsigmondy movement—*SYN:* brownian movement

Brown-Séquard, Charles E., French physiologist and neurologist, 1817–1894.
   Brown-Séquard paralysis—*SYN:* Brown-Séquard sndrome
   Brown-Séquard syndrome—syndrome with unilateral spinal cord lesions,
   proprioception loss and weakness ipsilateral to the lesion, while pain and
   temperature loss occur contralateral. *SYN:* Brown-Séquard paralysis

Browne, Sir Denis John, English surgeon, 1892–1967.
   Denis Browne bucket
   Denis Browne forceps
   Denis Browne pouch—a common lodging site for undescended testes. *SYN:*
   superficial inguinal pouch
   Denis Browne splint—a light aluminum splint used for clubfoot.
   Denis Browne talipes hobble splint
   Denis Browne tray

Browning, William, U.S. anatomist and neurologist, 1855–1941.
  Browning vein—an inconstant vein that passes from the superficial middle cerebral vein posteriorly over the lateral aspect of the temporal lobe to enter the transverse sinus. *Syn:* inferior anastomotic vein

Bruce, Robert A., U.S. cardiologist.
  Bruce test—exercise test for individuals with coronary disease.

Bruce, Sir David, English surgeon, 1855–1931.
  Brucella abortus—infectious bacteria causing abortions in cattle, sheep, mares; causes undulant fever in man and a wasting disease in chickens. *Syn:* abortus bacillus; Bang bacillus
  Brucella—a genus of encapsulated, nonmotile bacteria (family Brucellaceae) causing infection of the genital organs, the mammary gland, and the respiratory and intestinal tracts.
  brucellosis—an infectious disease caused by *Brucella*, and transmitted by direct contact with diseased animals or through ingestion of infected meat, milk, or cheese. *Syn:* undulating fever; Malta fever; Mediterranean fever; undulant fever; febris undulans

Bruch, Carl W.L., German anatomist, 1819–1884.
  Bruch glands—lymph nodes in the palpebral conjunctiva. *Syn:* trachoma glands
  Bruch membrane—the transparent, nearly structureless inner layer of the choroid in contact with the pigmented layer of the retina. *Syn:* lamina basais choroideae

Bruck, Alfred, German physician, *1865.
  Bruck disease—a disease marked by osteogenesis imperfecta, ankylosis of the joints, and muscular atrophy.

Brücke, Ernst W. von, Austrian physiologist, 1819–1892.
  Brücke tunic—a term formerly used to designate the retina exclusive of the layer of rods and cones. *Syn:* tunica nervea
  Brücke muscle—the part of the ciliary muscle formed by the meridional fibers. *Syn:* Crampton muscle
  Brücke-Bartley phenomenon—the sensation of glare in response to successive stimuli at frequencies just below the fusion point.

Brudzinski, Josef von, Polish physician, 1874–1917.
  Brudzinski sign—neck or leg flexion tests for meningitis.

Brumpt, Emile, French parasitologist, 1877–1951.
  Brumpt white mycetoma—mycetoma caused by *Pseudallescheria boydii.*

Brunati, M., 20th century Italian physician.
  Brunati sign—corneal opacities caused by pneumonia or typhoid fever.

Brunhes, S., French physician.
  Brunhes-Chavany syndrome—*Syn:* Chavany-Brunhes syndrome
  Chavany-Brunhes syndrome—see under Chavany

NOTES

Brunn, Albert von, German anatomist, 1849–1895.
Brunn epithelial nests
Brunn membrane—the epithelium of the olfactory region of the nose.
Brunn nests—glandlike invaginations of surface transitional epithelium in the mucosa of the lower urinary tract.

Brunn, Fritz, 20th century Czech physician.
Brunn reaction—the increased absorption of water through the skin of a frog when the animal is injected with pituitrin and immersed in water.

Brunner, Johann C., Swiss anatomist, 1653–1727.
Brunner gland hamartoma
Brunner glands—small glands that secrete a substance that neutralizes gastric juice. *SYN:* duodenal glands

Brunnstrom, Signe, Swedish physical therapist.
Brunnstrom facilitation technique—*SYN:* Brunnstrom method
Brunnstrom method—exercises for individuals with central nervous system lesions. *SYN:* Brunnstrom method of exercise; Brunnstrom proprioceptive neuromuscular facilitation; Brunnstrom facilitation technique
Brunnstrom method of exercise—*SYN:* Brunnstrom method
Brunnstrom proprioceptive neuromuscular facilitation—*SYN:* Brunnstrom method

Bruns, Ludwig von, German neurologist, 1858–1916.
Bastian-Bruns law—see under Bastian
Bastian-Bruns sign—*SYN:* Bastian-Bruns law
Bruns ataxia—difficulty in moving the feet when they are in contact with the ground; a condition related to a frontal lobe lesion.
Bruns nystagmus—due to lateral brainstem compression, usually by a cerebellopontine angle mass such as an acoustic neuroma.
Bruns syndrome—lesions of cerebral fourth ventricle cause symptoms of headache, vertigo, and vomiting; if head position is altered, the patient may fall.

Brunschwig, Alexander, U.S. surgeon, 1901–1969.
Brunschwig operation—*SYN:* total pelvic exenteration

Brushfield, Thomas, English physician, 1858–1937.
Brushfield spots—light-colored condensations of the surface of the mid-iris; seen in Down syndrome.
Brushfield-Wyatt disease—a familial disorder characterized by unilateral nevus, contralateral hemiplegia, hemianopia, cerebral angioma, and mental retardation. *SYN:* nevoid amentia

Bruton, O.C., U.S. pediatrician, *1908.
Bruton agammaglobulinemia—genetic trait causing decreased quantity of gamma fraction of serum globulin; associated with increased susceptibility to pyogenic infections and observed in type III isolated growth hormone deficiency.

Bryant, Sir Thomas, English surgeon, 1828–1914.
Bryant ampulla—that portion of an artery on the proximal side of a ligature containing the clot, its upper boundary being marked by a slight constriction.

Bryant sign—in dislocation of the shoulder, an abnormal position of axillary folds occurs.

Bryant traction—traction upon the lower limb placed vertically, employed especially in fractures of the femur in children.

Bryant triangle—lines drawn on the body in fracture of the neck of the femur to determine upward displacement of the trochanter. *SYN:* iliofemoral triangle

Buchem, Francis Steven Peter van. See under van Buchem.

Büchner, Eduard, German chemist and Nobel laureate, 1860–1917.

Büchner extract—a cell-free extract of yeast.

Büchner funnel—a porcelain funnel that contains a perforated porcelain plate upon which filter paper can be laid.

Büchner, Hans E.A., German bacteriologist, 1850–1902.

Büchner extract—see under Büchner, Eduard

Buchwald, Hermann Edmund, German physician, *1903.

Buchwald atrophy—a progressive form of cutaneous atrophy.

Buck, Gurdon, U.S. surgeon, 1807–1877.

Buck extension—apparatus for applying longitudinal skin traction on the leg. *SYN:* Buck traction

Buck extension bar

Buck extension frame

Buck extension splint

Buck fascia—a deep layer which surrounds the three erectile bodies of the penis. *SYN:* fascia penis profunda

Buck femoral cement restrictor inserter

Buck fracture appliance

Buck hook

Buck knee brace

Buck method

Buck osteotome

Buck plug

Buck traction—*SYN:* Buck extension

Buck tractor

Bucky, Gustav, U.S. radiologist, 1880–1963.

Bucky diaphragm—in radiography, a diaphragm with a moving grid that avoids grid shadows. *SYN:* Potter-Bucky diaphragm

Bucky film

Bucky grid

Bucky rays

Bucky studies

Bucky technique

Bucy, Paul C., U.S. neurosurgeon, 1904–1992.

Bucy cordotomy knife

(continued)

NOTES

Bucy *(continued)*
    Bucy knife
    Bucy laminectomy rongeur
    Bucy retractor
    Bucy tube
    Klüver-Bucy syndrome—see under Klüver

Budd, George, English physician, 1808–1882.
    Budd cirrhosis—chronic enlargement of the liver without jaundice.
    Budd disease
    Budd syndrome—*SYN:* Chiari syndrome
    Budd-Chiari syndrome—*SYN:* Chiari syndrome
    Chiari-Budd syndrome—*SYN:* Chiari syndrome

Budde, E., Danish sanitary engineer, *1871.
    Budde process—a method of milk sterilization.

Budge, Julius L., German physiologist, 1811–1888.
    Budge center—the preganglionic motor neurons in the first thoracic segment of the spinal cord which give rise to the sympathetic innervation of the dilator muscle of the eye's pupil. *SYN:* ciliospinal center

Budin, Pierre C., French gynecologist, 1846–1907.
    Budin obstetrical joint—cartilaginous union between the squamous and lateral parts of the occipital bone in the newborn. *SYN:* posterior intraoccipital synchondrosis

Buecklers, M.
    Reis-Buecklers syndrome—reduction of vision with infrequent eye pain; frequent strabismus. *SYN:* corneal dystrophy

Buerger, Leo, Austrian-U.S. physician, 1879–1943.
    Buerger disease—inflammation of the entire wall and connective tissue surrounding medium-sized arteries and veins, associated with thrombotic occlusion and commonly resulting in gangrene. *SYN:* thromboangiitis obliterans; Winiwarter-Buerger disease
    Buerger exercises—exercises specifically for patients with arterial insufficiency of their lower limbs.
    Buerger-Allen exercises—exercises of the lower limbs and feet for patients with arterial insufficiency of the lower limbs.
    Winiwarter-Buerger disease—*SYN:* Buerger disease

Buhl, Ludwig Von, German physician, 1816–1880.
    Buhl disease—acute sepsis occurring in newborn infants.

Bull, Sir Graham MacGregor, South African physician.
    Bull regime—diet used in cases of acute renal failure.

Buller, Frank, Canadian ophthalmologic surgeon, 1844–1905.
    Buller bandage—*SYN:* Buller shield
    Buller shield—in eye infection, a shield used to protect the healthy eye. *SYN:* Buller bandage

Bumke, Oswald C.E., German neurologist, 1877–1950.
    Bumke pupil—dilation of the pupil in response to anxiety or other psychic stimuli.
    Bumke syndrome—*SYN:* Bumke pupil

Bunnell, Sterling, U.S. surgeon, 1882–1957.
    Bunnell atraumatic technique
    Bunnell block—a block of wood used to exercise stiffened joints.
    Bunnell dressing
    Bunnell gutter splint
    Bunnell hand drill
    Bunnell knuckle-bender splint
    Bunnell modification of Steindler flexorplasty
    Bunnell needle
    Bunnell outrigger splint
    Bunnell probe
    Bunnell pull-out wire
    Bunnell solution
    Bunnell suture—a method of tenorrhaphy using a pull-out wire affixed to buttons.
    Bunnell tendon passer
    Bunnell tendon transfer technique
    Paul-Bunnell test—see under Paul, Gustav

Bunsen, Robert W., German chemist and physicist, 1811–1899.
    Bunsen burner—a gas lamp giving a very hot but only slightly luminous flame.
    Bunsen solubility coefficient—the milliliters of gas STPD dissolved per milliliter of liquid and per atmosphere (760 mm Hg) partial pressure of the gas at any given temperature.
    Bunsen-Roscoe law—in two photochemical reactions, if the product of the intensity of illumination and the time of exposure are equal, the quantities of chemical material undergoing change will be equal. *SYN:* reciprocity law; Roscoe-Bunsen law
    Roscoe-Bunsen law—*SYN:* Bunsen-Roscoe law

Burchard, H., 19th century German chemist.
    Burchard-Liebermann reaction—a blue-green color produced by acetic anhydride with cholesterol (and other sterols) dissolved in chloroform, when a few drops of concentrated sulfuric acid are added.
    Liebermann-Burchard test—see under Liebermann

Burdach, Karl F., German anatomist and physiologist, 1776–1847.
    Burdach column—the larger lateral subdivision of the posterior funiculus. *SYN:* cuneate fasciculus; Burdach fasciculus; Burdach tract
    Burdach fasciculus—*SYN:* Burdach column
    Burdach nucleus—*SYN:* cuneate nucleus
    Burdach tract—*SYN:* Burdach column

Buren, William H. van. See under van Buren.

Bürger, Max, German physician, *1885.
    Bürger-Grütz disease—obsolete term for idiopathic hyperlipemia.
    Bürger-Grütz syndrome—an inherited disorder of lipoprotein metabolism. *SYN:* type I familial hyperlipoproteinemia

NOTES

Burghart, Hans G., German physician, 1862–1932.
    Burghart sign—*SYN:* Burghart symptom
    Burghart symptom—fine lung rales seen in early stages of pulmonary tuberculosis. *SYN:* Burghart sign

Burk, Dean, U.S. scientist, *1904.
    Lineweaver-Burk equation—see under Lineweaver
    Lineweaver-Burk plot—see under Lineweaver

Burke, Richard M., U.S. physician, *1903.
    Burke syndrome—advanced pulmonary emphysema leading to loss of pulmonary markings on x-ray. *SYN:* vanishing lung; solitary lobar atrophy; cotton candy lung; idiopathic pulmonary atrophy; De Martini-Balestra syndrome

Burkitt, Denis P., 20th century English physician in Uganda, d. 1993.
    Burkitt lymphoma—a form of malignant lymphoma reported in African children, caused by Epstein-Barr virus; a member of the family Herpesviridae.
    Burkitt tumor

Burn, J.H.
    Burn and Rand theory—that stimulation of sympathetic fibers results first in the production of acetylcholine in the postganglionic nerve endings, which then release norepinephrine to act on the active site of the effector cell.

Burnet, Sir Frank MacFarlane, joint winner of 1960 Nobel Prize for work related to immunology.

Burnett, Charles H., U.S. physician, 1901–1967.
    Burnett syndrome—a chronic disorder of the kidneys, induced by ingestion of large amounts of calcium and alkali in the therapy of peptic ulcer. *SYN:* milk-alkali syndrome

Burns, Allan, Scottish anatomist, 1781–1813.
    Burns falciform process—*SYN:* superior horn of falciform margin of saphenous opening
    Burns ligament—*SYN:* superior horn of falciform margin of saphenous opening .
    Burns space—a narrow interval between the deep and superficial layers of the cervical fascia above the manubrium of the sternum through which pass the anterior jugular veins. *SYN:* suprasternal space

Burow, Karl A. von, German surgeon, 1809–1874.
    Burow operation—an operation in which triangles of skin adjacent to a sliding flap are excised to facilitate movement of the flap.
    Burow solution—a preparation of aluminium subacetate and glacial acetic acid, used for its antiseptic and astringent action on the skin.
    Burow triangle—a triangle of skin and subcutaneous fat excised so that a pedicle flap can be advanced without buckling the adjacent tissue.
    Burow vein—one of the renal veins.

Burton, Henry, English physician, 1799–1849.
    Burton line—a bluish line on the free border of the gingiva, occurring in lead poisoning. *SYN:* lead line

Buruli, district in Uganda.
    Buruli lesion—infection with *Mycobacterium ulcerans* causing painless nodule which ulcerates on leg or forearm; common in children and first noted in Buruli.

Bury, Judson S., English dermatologist, 1852–1944.
    Bury disease—a chronic symmetrical eruption of flattened pinkish nodules. *Syn:* erythema elevatum diutinum

Buschke, Abraham, German dermatologist, 1868–1943.
    Buschke disease—obsolete eponym for cryptococcosis. *Syn:* scleredema adultorum
    Buschke-Löwenstein tumor—a large type of condyloma acuminatum found in the genitals. *Syn:* giant condyloma
    Buschke-Ollendorf syndrome—*Syn:* osteopoikilosis
    Busse-Buschke disease—see under Busse

Buselmeier, T.J., 20th century U.S. nephrologist.
    Buselmeier shunt

Busquet, G. Paul, French physician, 1866–1930.
    Busquet disease—an osteoperiostitis of the metatarsal bones, leading to exostoses on the dorsum of the foot.

Busse, Otto, German physician, 1867–1922.
    Busse saccaromyces
    Busse-Buschke disease—an acute, subacute, or chronic infection by *Cryptococcus neoformans*, causing a pulmonary, disseminated, or meningeal mycosis. *Syn:* cryptococcosis

Butcher, Richard George H., Irish surgeon, 1819–1891.
    Butcher saw—amputating saw.

Buzzard, Thomas, English physician, 1831–1919.
    Buzzard maneuver—testing the patellar reflex while the sitting patient makes firm pressure on the floor with the toes.

Buzzi, Fausto, coworker of Ernst Schweninger.
    Schweninger-Buzzi anetoderma—see under Schweninger

Byler, Amish kindred in the U.S.
    Byler disease—genetic trait in Amish children that causes fatal intrahepatic arrest of bile flow.

Bywaters, Eric G.L., English physician, *1910.
    Bywaters syndrome—lower nephron nephrosis. *Syn:* crush syndrome

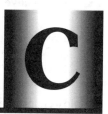

Cabot, Richard, U.S. physician, 1868–1939.
    Cabot ring bodies—ring-shaped or figure-of-eight structures found in red blood cells in severe anemias. *SYN:* Cabot rings
    Cabot rings—*SYN:* Cabot ring bodies
    Cabot-Locke murmur—an early diastolic murmur, like that of aortic insufficiency, heard best at the left lower sternal border in severe anemia.

Cacchi, Roberto, Italian physician.
    Cacchi-Ricci syndrome—*SYN:* sponge kidney; cystic disease of the renal pyramids; medullary polycystic kidney; Ricci-Cacchi syndrome
    Ricci-Cacchi syndrome—*SYN:* Cacchi-Ricci syndrome

Cacchione, Aldo, 20th century Italian psychiatrist.
    De Sanctis-Cacchione syndrome—see under Sanctis

Caffey, John Patrick, U.S. physician, radiologist, and pediatrician, the father of pediatric radiology, 1895–1978.
    Caffey disease—*SYN:* Caffey syndrome
    Caffey syndrome—neonatal subperiosteal bone formation over many bones, especially the mandible and clavicles and the shafts of long bones. *SYN:* infantile cortical hyperostosis; Caffey disease; Caffey-Silverman syndrome
    Caffey-Silverman syndrome—*SYN:* Caffey syndrome

Cajal, Santiago, Spanish histologist and Nobel laureate, 1852–1934.
    Cajal astrocyte stain—a method for demonstrating astrocytes by impregnation in a solution containing gold chloride and mercuric chloride.
    Cajal cell—*SYN:* horizontal cell of Cajal
    Cajal formol ammonium bromide solution
    Cajal gold-sublimate method
    Cajal uranium silver method
    horizontal cell of Cajal—a small fusiform cell found in the superficial layer of the cerebral cortex with its long axis placed horizontally. *SYN:* Cajal cell; astrocyte
    interstitial nucleus of Cajal—a group of neurons believed to be involved in the integration of head and eye movements. *SYN:* interstitial nucleus

Calcutta, city in India.
    Calcutta technique—a technique used in therapeutic irradiation by infrared rays; first observed in Calcutta, India.

Caldani, Leopoldo M.A., Italian anatomist, 1725–1813.
    Caldani ligament—the strong ligament that unites the clavicle to the coracoid process. *SYN:* coracoclavicular ligament

Caldwell, George W., U.S. physician, 1834–1918.
Caldwell-Luc operation—an intraoral procedure for opening into the maxillary antrum through the supradental (canine) fossa above the maxillary premolar teeth. *Syn:* intraoral antrostomy; Luc operation

Caldwell, William E., U.S. obstetrician, 1880–1943.
Caldwell-Moloy classification—a classification of the variations in the female pelvis.

Calkins, Leroy Adelbert, U.S. obstetrician-gynecologist, 1894–1960.
Calkins sign—the change of shape of the uterus from discoid to ovoid, indicating placental separation from the uterine wall.

Call, Friedrich von, Austrian physician, 1844–1917.
Call-Exner bodies—small fluid-filled spaces between granulosal cells in ovarian follicles and in ovarian tumors of granulosal origin.

Callahan, John R., U.S. endodontist, 1853–1918.
Callahan method—a method of filling the root canals of teeth by dissolving gutta-percha cones in a chloroform-rosin medium within the root canal. *Syn:* chloropercha method

Callander, Latimer, U.S. surgeon, 1892–1947.
Callander amputation—tenontoplastic amputation through the femur at the knee.
Callender derotational brace
Callender technique hip prosthesis

Calleja, Camilo, Spanish anatomist, d. 1913.
islands of Calleja—dense clusters of very small nerve cells (granule cells) characteristic of the olfactory tubercle at the base of the forebrain.

Callison, James S., U.S. physician, *1873.
Callison fluid—a diluting fluid for counting red blood cells.

Calmette, Leon A., French bacteriologist, 1863–1933.
Bacille bilié de Calmette-Guérin—an attenuated strain of *Mycobacterium bovis* used for immunization against tuberculosis and in cancer chemotherapy. *Syn:* Calmette-Guérin bacillus; Bacille Calmette-Guérin
Bacille Calmette-Guérin—*Syn:* Bacille bilié de Calmette-Guérin
bacillus Calmette-Guérin vaccine—a vaccine for tuberculosis prophylaxis. *Syn:* BCG vaccine
Calmette test—conjunctival reaction to tuberculin.
Calmette-Guérin bacillus—*Syn:* Bacille bilié de Calmette-Guérin
Calmette-Guérin vaccine—*Syn:* bacillus Calmette-Guérin vaccine

Calori, Luigi, Italian anatomist, 1807–1896.
Calori bursa—a bursa between the arch of the aorta and the trachea.

Calot, Jean-François, French surgeon, 1861–1944.
Calot node
Calot operation
Calot triangle—a triangle bounded by the cystic artery, cystic duct, and hepatic duct.

Calvé, Jacques, French orthopedic surgeon, 1875–1954.
Calvé disease—vertebral osteochondrosis.

Calvé-Perthes disease—*SYN:* Legg-Calvé-Perthes disease
Legg-Calvé-Perthes disease—see under Legg

Camera, Ugo, Italian physician.
    Camera syndrome—*SYN:* neuralgic lumbosciatic osteopathy syndrome

Camerer, Johann F.W., German pediatrician, 1842–1910.
    Camerer law—child's weight rather than age determines food
    requirement.

Cammann, George P., U.S. physician, 1804–1863.
    Cammann stethoscope

Campbell, Meredith F., 20th century U.S. pediatric urologist.
    Campbell sound—a miniature sound with a short round-tipped beak,
    especially curved for the deep urethra of the young male.

Campbell, William F., U.S. surgeon, 1867–1926.
    Campbell ligament—it maintains the characteristic hollow of the armpit.
    SYN: suspensory ligament of axilla

Camper, Pieter, Dutch physician and anatomist, 1722–1789.
    Camper chiasm—*SYN:* tendinous chiasm of the digital tendons
    Camper fascia—*SYN:* fatty layer of superficial fascia
    Camper ligament—the layer of fascia extending between the ischiopubic
    rami inferior to the sphincter urethrae and the deep transverse perineal
    muscles. *SYN:* inferior fascia of urogenital diaphragm
    Camper line—the line running from the inferior border of the ala of the
    nose to the superior border of the tragus of the ear.
    Camper plane—a plane running from the tip of the anterior nasal spine
    (acanthion) to the center of the bony external auditory meatus on the
    right and left sides.

Canada, Wilma J., 20th century U.S. radiologist.
    Cronkhite-Canada syndrome—see under Cronkhite

Canavan, Myrtelle M., U.S. pathologist, 1879–1953.
    Canavan disease—autosomal recessive degenerative disease of infancy.
    SYN: Canavan sclerosis; spongy degeneration of infancy; Canavan-van
    Bogaert-Bertrand disease
    Canavan sclerosis—*SYN:* Canavan disease
    Canavan-van Bogaert-Bertrand disease—*SYN:* Canavan disease

Cannizzaro, Stanislao, Italian chemist, 1826–1910.
    Cannizzaro reaction—formation of an acid and an alcohol by the
    simultaneous oxidation of one aldehyde molecule and reduction of
    another.

Cannon, Walter B., U.S. physiologist, 1871–1945.
    Bernard-Cannon homeostasis—see under Bernard, Claude

(continued)

NOTES

Cannon (*continued*)

    Cannon law—reaction of excessive sensitivity to chemical neurotransmitters in tissue with deficiency of autonomic supply.

    Cannon point—the location in the midtransverse colon at which innervation by superior and inferior mesenteric plexuses overlap at the junction of the primitive midgut and hindgut. *SYN:* Cannon ring

    Cannon ring—*SYN:* Cannon point

    Cannon syndrome—perspiration and palpitations due to increased secretion of adrenalin.

    Cannon theory—a theory of the emotions that animal and human organisms respond to emergency situations by increased sympathetic nervous system activity. *SYN:* emergency theory

    Cannon-Bard theory—the view that the feeling aspect of emotion and the pattern of emotional behavior are controlled by the hypothalamus.

Cantor, Meyer O., U.S. physician, *1907.

    Cantor tube—a long, single-lumen intestinal tube.

Capgras, Jean Marie Joseph, French psychiatrist, 1873–1950.

    Capgras phenomenon—*SYN:* Capgras syndrome

    Capgras syndrome—the delusional belief that a person close to the schizophrenic patient has been replaced by an impostor. *SYN:* Capgras phenomenon; illusion of doubles

Caplan, Anthony, English physician, 1907–1976.

    Caplan nodules—*SYN:* Caplan syndrome

    Caplan syndrome—intrapulmonary nodules, histologically similar to subcutaneous rheumatoid nodules, associated with rheumatoid arthritis and pneumoconiosis in coal workers. *SYN:* Caplan nodules

Capps, Joseph A., U.S. physician, 1872–1964.

    Capps reflex—obsolete eponym for vasomotor collapse at the time of crisis in pneumonia.

Capuron, Joseph, French physician, 1767–1850.

    Capuron points—the iliopubic eminences and the sacroiliac joints, constituting four fixed points in the pelvic inlet.

Carabelli, Georg (Edler von Lunkaszprie), Austrian dentist, 1787–1842.

    Carabelli tubercle—a small tubercle, resembling a supernumerary cusp, found occasionally on the lingual surface of the mesiolingual cusp of a permanent maxillary first molar. *SYN:* cusp of Carabelli

    cusp of Carabelli—*SYN:* Carabelli tubercle

Cardarelli, Antonio, Italian physician, 1831–1927.

    Cardarelli sign—laryngotracheal tube pulsation related to aortic arch dilatation and aneurysms.

Carden, Henry D., English surgeon, d. 1872.

    Carden amputation—transcondylar amputation of the leg in which the femur is sawed through the condyles just above the articular surface.

Carini, Antonino, Italian physician, 1872–1950.

    Carini syndrome—skin disease of the newborn characterized by fissures and shedding of membrane encasing the body to reveal red skin underneath. *Syn:* alligator baby; congenital icthyosiform erythroderma; lamellar desquamation of the newborn; lamellar icthyosis

Carlen, Eric, 20th century Swedish otolaryngologist.
Carlen mediastinoscope

Carmody, Thomas Edward, U.S. oral surgeon, *1875.
Carmody-Batson operation—reduction of fractures of the zygoma and zygomatic arch through an intraoral incision above the maxillary molar teeth.

Carnett, J.B., 20th century U.S. physician.
Carnett sign—pain of intra-abdominal origin with likely source in abdominal wall.

Carnoy, Jean Baptiste, French biologist, 1836–1899.
Carnoy fixative—an extremely rapid fixative used for glucogen preservation and as a nuclear fixative.

Caroli, Jacques, French physician, *1902.
Caroli disease—congenital cystic dilation of the intrahepatic bile ducts.

Carpenter, Charles J., U.S. immunologist, *1931.
Carpenter syndrome—acrocephalopolysyndactyly.

Carpenter, George Alfred, English physician, 1859–1910.
Carpenter syndrome—the association of primary hypothyroidism, primary adrenocortical insufficiency, and diabetes mellitus.

Carpentier, Alain, 20th century French cardiothoracic surgeon.
Carpentier annuloplasty
Carpentier annuloplasty ring prosthesis
Carpentier ring
Carpentier stent
Carpentier tricuspid valvuloplasty
Carpentier valve
Carpentier-Edwards aortic valve prosthesis
Carpentier-Edwards bioprosthetic valve
Carpentier-Edwards mitral annuloplasty valve
Carpentier-Edwards pericardial valve
Carpentier-Edwards porcine prosthetic valve
Carpentier-Edwards valve

Carpue, Joseph, English surgeon, 1764–1846.
Carpue method—rhinoplasty utilizing a flap from the forehead. *Syn:* Indian rhinoplasty

Carr, Francis H., English chemist, 1874–1969.
Carr-Price reaction—the basis of several quantitative techniques for the determination of vitamin A.

NOTES

Carraro, Arturo, Italian physician.
    Cararro syndrome—recessive trait causing orthopedic deformities and deaf-mutism.

Carrel, Alexis, French-U.S. surgeon and Nobel laureate, 1873–1944.
    Carrel clamp
    Carrel method
    Carrel mosquito forceps
    Carrel operation
    Carrel patch
    Carrel sutures
    Carrel treatment—treatment of wound surfaces by intermittent flushing with Dakin solution. *Syn:* Dakin-Carrel treatment
    Carrel tube
    Carrel-Lindbergh pump—a perfusion device designed for use in culture of whole organs.
    Dakin-Carrel treatment—*Syn:* Carrel treatment

Carrión, Daniel A., Peruvian medical student, 1859–1885, who inoculated himself with a disease later designated as Carri"n disease, and died thereof.
    Carrión disease—a generalized, acute, febrile, endemic, and systemic form of bartonellosis.

Carteaud, Alexandre, French physician, *1897.
    Gougerot-Carteaud syndrome—see under Gougerot, Henri

Carter, Henry V., Anglo-Indian physician, 1831–1897.
    Carter black mycetoma—mycetoma caused by *Madurella mycetomatis*.
    Carter fever—an Asiatic relapsing fever caused by *Borrelia carteri*.

Carus, Karl G., German anatomist and zoologist, 1789–1869.
    Carus circle—*Syn:* Carus curve
    Carus curve—an imaginary curved line obtained from a mathematical formula, supposed to indicate the outlet of the pelvic canal. *Syn:* Carus circle

Casal, Gasper, Spanish physician, 1691–1759.
    Casal collar—*Syn:* Casal necklace
    Casal necklace—a dermatitis partly or completely encircling the lower part of the neck in pellagra. *Syn:* Casal collar

Caslick, Edward, 20th century U.S. veterinarian.
    Caslick operation—an operation for the correction of faulty conformation of the vulva of a mare.

Casoni, Tommaro, Italian physician, 1880–1933.
    Casoni intradermal test—a test for hydatid disease. *Syn:* Casoni skin test
    Casoni skin test—*Syn:* Casoni intradermal test

Casselberry, William E., U.S. laryngologist, 1858–1916.
    Casselberry position—a prone position assumed when drinking, after intubation, in order to prevent the entrance of fluid into the tube.

Casser, Giulio, Italian anatomist, 1556–1616.
    Casser fontanel—the membranous interval on either side between the

mastoid angle of the parietal bone, the petrous portion of the temporal bone, and the occipital bone. *SYN:* mastoid fontanel

Casser perforated muscle—*SYN:* coracobrachialis muscle

Cassirer, Richard, German physician, 1868–1925.
Cassirer syndrome

Castellani, Sir Aldo, Italian physician, 1878–1971.
Castallani disease
Castallani test
Castellani bronchitis—chronic bronchitis due to infection with spirochetes and characterized by cough and bloody sputum. *SYN:* hemorrhagic bronchitis
Castellani paint—a paint used in the treatment of superficial mycotic infections. *SYN:* carbol-fuchsin paint
Castellani-Low sign—a fine tremor of the tongue observed in sleeping sickness.

Castle, William B., U.S. physician, 1897–1990.
Castle intrinsic factor—a relatively small mucoprotein required for adequate absorption of vitamin B_{12}. *SYN:* intrinsic factor

Castleman, Benjamin, U.S. pathologist, 1906–1982.
Castleman disease—solitary masses of lymphoid tissue containing concentric perivascular aggregates of lymphocytes. *SYN:* benign giant lymph node hyperplasia; Castleman tumor
Castleman tumor—*SYN:* Castleman disease

Castroviejo, Ramon, Spanish physician, *1904.
Castroviejo clip-applying forceps
Castroviejo corneal transplant marker
Castroviejo corneal transplant scissors
Castroviejo discission knife
Castroviejo electrokeratotome
Castroviejo iridocapsulotomy scissors
Castroviejo lacrimal sac probe
Castroviejo lens clamp
Castroviejo lens spoon
Castroviejo lid forceps
Castroviejo lid retractor
Castroviejo orbital aspirator
Castroviejo razor blade
Castroviejo refractor
Castroviejo scleral fold forceps
Castroviejo scleral shortening clip
Castroviejo snare enucleator
Castroviejo speculum
Castroviejo suturing forceps
Castroviejo synechia scissors
Castroviejo trephine

NOTES

Cawthorne, Terence, English physician.
Cawthorne exercises—exercises for patients with vertigo and Meniére disease.

Cayler, Glen G., U.S. physician.
Cayler syndrome—unilateral facial weakness associated with cardiac defects. *SYN:* cardiofacial syndrome

Cazenave, Pierre L. Alphée, French dermatologist, 1795–1877.
Cazenave disease
Cazenave vitiligo—obsolete term for alopecia areata.

Cecil, Arthur Bond, U.S. urologist, 1885–1967.
Cecil operation—hypospadias repair.

Ceelen, Wilhelm, 1884–1964.
Ceelen-Gellerstedt syndrome—repeated sudden attacks of dyspnea and hemoptysis leading to diffuse pulmonary hemosiderosis. *SYN:* idiopathic pulmonary hemosiderosis

Cegka, Josephus J., Czech physician, 1812–1862.
Cegka sign—cardiac dullness related to adherent pericardium.

Celestin, Felix, French physician, *1900.
Celestin tube—a plastic tube introduced through a tumor in the esophagus.

Celsius, Anders, Swedish astronomer, 1701–1744.
Celsius scale—a temperature scale that is based upon the triple point of water (defined to be 273.16 K) and assigned the value of 0.01°C.
Celsius thermometer

Celsus, Aulus (Aurelius) Cornelius, Roman physician and medical writer, *ca.* 30 B.C.–45 A.D.
Celsus 4 cardinal signs of inflammation—heat, redness, tenderness, and swelling.
Celsus alopecia—obsolete term for alopecia areata. *SYN:* Celsus vitiligo
Celsus area—obsolete term for alopecia areata.
Celsus kerion—an inflammatory fungus infection of the scalp and beard. *SYN:* tinea kerion
Celsus papules—acute papular eczema of severe type. *SYN:* lichen agrius
Celsus vitiligo—obsolete term for alopecia areata.

Cerenkov, Pavel A., Russian physicist and Nobel laureate, 1904–1990.
Cerenkov radiation—light given off by a transparent medium when a high-energy particle speeds through it at a velocity greater than that of light in that medium.

Cervenka, Jaroslav.
Cervenka syndrome—autosomal dominant trait causing facial abnormalities, joint deformity, and myopia.

Cestan, Raymond, French neurologist, 1872–1934.
Cestan-Chenais syndrome—contralateral hemiplegia, hemianesthesia, with ipsilateral hemiasynergia and lateropulsion, paralysis of the larynx and soft palate, enophthalmia, miosis, and ptosis, due to lesions of the brainstem.

Chaddock, Charles G., U.S. neurologist, 1861–1936.
    Chaddock reflex—*SYN:* Chaddock sign
    Chaddock sign—when the external malleolar skin area is irritated, extension of the great toe occurs in cases of organic disease of the corticospinal reflex paths. *SYN:* Chaddock reflex; external malleolar sign

Chadwick, James R., U.S. gynecologist, 1844–1905.
    Chadwick sign—a bluish discoloration of the cervix and vagina, a sign of pregnancy.

Chagas, Carlos, Brazilian physician, 1879–1934.
    Chagas disease—parasitic infection transmitted by certain species of reduviid (triatomine) bugs. *SYN:* South American trypanosomiasis; Chagas-Cruz disease; Cruz trypanosomiasis
    Chagas-Cruz disease—*SYN:* Chagas disease

Chailey, Chailey Heritage Craft School & Hospital, Sussex, England.
    Chailey go-cart—vehicle for children who cannot walk.

Chain, Sir Ernst Boris, 1906–1979, co-winner of 1945 Nobel Prize for work related to penicillin.

Chamberlain, W.E., U.S. radiologist, 1891–1947.
    Chamberlain line—a line drawn from the posterior margin of the hard palate to the dorsum of the foramen magnum.

Chamberlen, Peter, English obstetrician, 1560–1631.
    Chamberlen forceps—the original obstetrical forceps, without a curvature.

Champy, Christian, French physician, *1885.
    Champy fixative—cytologic fixative.

Chanarin, I., 20th century English hematologist.
    Dorfman-Chanarin syndrome—see under Dorfman

Chance, G.Q., 20th century English radiologist.
    Chance fracture—a transverse fracture, usually in the thoracic or lumbar spine, through the body of the vertebra extending posteriorly through the pedicles and the spinous process.

Chandler, Fremont A., U.S. orthopedic surgeon, 1893–1954.
    Chandler arthrodesis
    Chandler bone elevator
    Chandler felt collar splint
    Chandler forceps
    Chandler hip fusion
    Chandler laminectomy retractor
    Chandler patellar advancement
    Chandler spinal perforating forceps
    Chandler splint
    Chandler table—a table used for upper limb exercises.
    Chandler unreamed interlocking tibial nail

NOTES

Chandler, Paul A., U.S. ophthalmologist, *1896.
   Chandler iridectomy
   Chandler iris forceps
   Chandler syndrome—iris atrophy with corneal edema. *SYN:* iridocorneal
   syndrome

Changeux, Jean-Pierre, 20th century French biochemist.
   Monod-Wyman-Changeux model—see under Monod

Chantemesse, André, French bacteriologist, 1851–1919.
   Chantemesse reaction—a conjunctival reaction, especially as applied to
   typhoid.

Chaoul, Henri, Lebanese radiologist, 1887–1964.
   Chaoul therapy—x-ray therapy using low voltage.
   Chaoul tube—x-ray tube designed to allow intense but superficial
   irradiation of an area.

Chapple, Charles Culloden, U.S. pediatrician, *1903.
   Chapple syndrome—(1) unilateral facial weakness in newborn caused by
   lateral flexion of the head in utero. (2) congenital syndrome believed to
   be caused by abnormal position of the fetus in utero. *SYN:* (1)
   duosyndrome of laryngeal nerve; (2) genu recurvatum-uterine
   retroversion-dysmenorrhea syndrome

Chaput, Henri, French surgeon, 1857–1919.
   Chaput tubercle—tibial tubercle.

Charcot, Jean M., French neurologist, 1825–1893.
   Charcot arteries—any one of a variety of small cerebral arteries. *SYN:*
   lenticulostriate arteries
   Charcot arthritis
   Charcot arthropathy
   Charcot bath—for patients with arterial disorders.
   Charcot change
   Charcot disease—*SYN:* Lou Gehrig disease
   Charcot fever—*SYN:* Charcot intermittent fever
   Charcot gait—the gait of hereditary ataxia.
   Charcot intermittent fever—fever, chills, right upper quadrant pain, and
   jaundice associated with intermittently obstructing common duct stones.
   Charcot joint—a neuropathic arthropathy that occurs with tabes dorsalis
   (tabetic neurosyphilis). *SYN:* tabetic arthropathy
   Charcot laryngeal vertigo—fainting as a result of a coughing spell, most
   often occurring in heavy-set male smokers with chronic bronchitis. *SYN:*
   Charcot vertigo; tussive syncope
   Charcot spine
   Charcot syndrome—a condition caused by ischemia of the muscles. *SYN:*
   intermittent claudication
   Charcot triad—(1) in multiple (disseminated) sclerosis, the three
   symptoms: nystagmus, tremor, and scanning speech; (2) combination of
   jaundice, fever, and upper abdominal pain that occurs as a result of
   cholangitis.
   Charcot vertigo—*SYN:* Charcot laryngeal vertigo
   Charcot-Böttcher crystalloids—spindle-shaped crystalloids found in human
   Sertoli cells.

Charcot-Leyden crystals—crystals found in the sputum in bronchial asthma. *Syn:* asthma crystals; Charcot-Neumann crystals; Leyden crystals; Charcot-Robin crystals

Charcot-Marie-Tooth disease—a group of three familial peripheral neuromuscular disorders, sharing the common feature of marked wasting of the more distal extremities. *Syn:* peroneal muscular atrophy

Charcot-Neumann crystals—*Syn:* Charcot-Leyden crystals

Charcot-Robin crystals—*Syn:* Charcot-Leyden crystals

Charcot-Weiss-Baker syndrome—stimulation of a hyperactive carotid sinus, causing a marked fall in blood pressure. *Syn:* carotid sinus syndrome

Charcot-Wilbrand syndrome—inability to recognize objects by sight, usually caused by bilateral parieto-occipital lesions.

Erb-Charcot disease—see under Erb

Chargaff, Erwin, Austrian-U.S. biochemist, *1905.

Chargaff rule—in double-stranded DNA the content of adenine residues equals the number of thymine and the number of cytosine equals the number of guanine.

Charles, Jacques, French physicist, 1746–1823.

Charles law—all gases expand equally on heating. *Syn:* Gay-Lussac law

Charlin, C. Carlos, Chilean ophthalmologist, 1886–1945.

Charlin syndrome—multiple symptoms of the nose resulting from neuralgia of the nasociliary nerve. *Syn:* nasociliary neuralgia

Charlouis, M., 19th century Dutch army surgeon in Java.

Charlouis disease—an infectious tropical disease caused by *Treponema pertenue* and characterized by the development of crusted granulomatous ulcers on the extremities. *Syn:* yaws

Charlton, Willy, German physician, *1889.

Schultz-Charlton phenomenon—*Syn:* Schultz-Charlton reaction

Schultz-Charlton reaction—see under Schultz, Werner

Charnley, Sir John, English surgeon, 1911–1988.

Charnley acetabular cup prosthesis
Charnley arthrodesis
Charnley arthrodesis clamp
Charnley bone clamp
Charnley bone clasp
Charnley brace handle
Charnley cemented hip prosthesis
Charnley centering drill
Charnley compression arthrodesis
Charnley compression fusion
Charnley device
Charnley femoral broach

(continued)

NOTES

Charnley *(continued)*
    Charnley femoral condyle drill
    Charnley femoral prosthesis pusher
    Charnley hip arthroplasty—a form of total hip replacement consisting of the application of an acetabular cup and a femoral head prosthesis.
    Charnley hip prosthesis
    Charnley implant
    Charnley incision
    Charnley knee prosthesis
    Charnley narrow stem component
    Charnley pilot drill
    Charnley pin
    Charnley pin clamp
    Charnley pin retractor
    Charnley rasp
    Charnley reamer
    Charnley self-retaining retractor
    Charnley standard stem retractor
    Charnley towel

Charrière, Joseph F.B., French instrument maker, 1803–1876.
    Charrière scale—a scale for grading sizes of sounds, tubules, and catheters. *SYN:* French scale

Charters, W.J., U.S. dentist.
    Charters method—a method of tooth brushing utilizing a restricted circular motion with the bristles inclined coronally at a 45-degree angle.

Chaslin, Philippe, French physician, *1857.
    Chaslin gliosis—sclerosis of glial fibers in brain tissue of epileptics causing pathological changes.

Chassaignac, Edouard P.M., French surgeon, 1804–1879.
    Chassaignac space—potential space between the pectoralis major and the mammary gland.
    Chassaignac tubercle—the anterior tubercle of the transverse process of the sixth cervical vertebra, against which the carotid artery may be compressed by the finger. *SYN:* carotid tubercle

Chastek, S.J., U.S. breeder of foxes.
    Chastek paralysis—disease of foxes and mink caused by eating certain types of raw fish which contain a thiamin-destroying enzyme with resultant loss of appetite, emaciation, paralysis, and death.

Chaudhry, Anand P.
    Gorlin-Chaudhry-Moss syndrome—see under Gorlin, Robert

Chauffard, Anatole M.E., French physician, 1855–1932.
    Chauffard syndrome—the symptoms of Still disease in one suffering from bovine or other nonhuman form of tuberculosis. *SYN:* Still-Chauffard syndrome
    Minkowski-Chauffard syndrome—see under Minkowski
    Still-Chauffard syndrome—*SYN:* Chauffard syndrome

Chaussier, François, French physician, 1746–1828.
  Chaussier areola—a ring of indurated tissue surrounding the lesion of cutaneous anthrax.
  Chaussier line—the anteroposterior line of the corpus callosum as appearing on median section of the brain.
  Chaussier sign—severe pain in the epigastrium, a prodrome of eclampsia.

Chauveau, J.-B. Auguste, French veterinarian, physiologist, and microbiologist, 1827–1917.
  Chauveau bacterium—former name for *Clostridium chauvoei.*

Chavany, Jean A.E., French physician, 1892–1959.
  Brunhes-Chavany syndrome—*SYN:* Chavany-Brunhes syndrome
  Chavany-Brunhes syndrome—persistent headaches and various mental disorders caused by calcification of the falx cerebri. *SYN:* Brunhes-Chavany syndrome

Chayes, Herman E.S., U.S. prosthodontist, 1880–1933.
  Chayes method—a method of replacing lost teeth.

Cheadle, Walter B., English pediatrician, 1835–1910.
  Cheadle disease—a cachectic condition in infants, resulting from malnutrition. *SYN:* infantile scurvy

Cheatle, Sir George L., English surgeon, 1865–1951.
  Cheatle slit—a longitudinal incision into the antimesenteric border of the small intestine.

Chédiak, Moisés, 20th century Cuban physician.
  Chédiak test
  Chédiak-Higashi anomaly—*SYN:* Chédiak-Steinbrink-Higashi syndrome
  Chédiak-Higashi disease—*SYN:* Chédiak-Steinbrinck-Higashi syndrome
  Chédiak-Steinbrinck-Higashi anomaly—*SYN:* Chédiak-Steinbrinck-Higashi syndrome
  Chédiak-Steinbrinck-Higashi syndrome—hereditary, fatal disorder of granulation and nuclear structure of all types of leukocytes. *SYN:* Chédiak-Steinbrinck-Higashi anomaly; Béguez César disease; Chédiak-Higashi disease

Chenais, Louis J., French physician, 1872–1950.
  Cestan-Chenais syndrome—see under Cestan

Cheney, William D., U.S. radiologist, *1918.
  Cheney syndrome—acro-osteolysis with osteoporosis and changes in the skull and mandible.
  Cheney-Hajdu syndrome—*SYN:* Hajdu-Cheney syndrome
  Hajdu-Cheney syndrome—see under Hajdu

Cherenkov, var. of Cerenkov

NOTES

Cheyne, John, Scottish physician, 1777–1836.
    Cheyne nystagmus
    Cheyne-Stokes breathing—*Syn:* Cheyne-Stokes respiration
    Cheyne-Stokes psychosis—a mental state characterized by anxiety and
    restlessness, accompanying Cheyne-Stokes respiration.
    Cheyne-Stokes respiration—the pattern of breathing characteristically seen
    in coma. *Syn:* Cheyne-Stokes breathing

Chiari, Hans, German pathologist, 1851–1916.
    Arnold-Chiari deformity—*Syn:* Arnold-Chiari malformation
    Arnold-Chiari malformation—see under Arnold, Julius
    Arnold-Chiari syndrome—*Syn:* Arnold-Chiari malformation
    Budd-Chiari syndrome—*Syn:* Chiari syndrome
    Chiari disease—*Syn:* Chiari syndrome
    Chiari II syndrome—elongation of medulla and cerebellar tonsils and
    vermis with displacement through the foramen magnum into the upper
    spinal canal.
    Chiari net—abnormal fibrous or lacelike strands in the right atrium.
    Chiari syndrome—thrombosis of the hepatic vein with great enlargement
    of the liver and extensive development of collateral vessels, intractable
    ascites, and severe portal hypertension. *Syn:* Budd-Chiari syndrome;
    Chiari-Budd syndrome; Chiari disease; Rokitansky disease (2); Budd
    syndrome
    Chiari-Budd syndrome—*Syn:* Chiari syndrome

Chiari, Johann B., German obstetrician, 1817–1854.
    Chiari-Frommel syndrome—unphysiological lactation and amenorrhea
    following pregnancy, but not caused by infant's nursing. *Syn:* Frommel-
    Chiari syndrome
    Frommel-Chiari syndrome—*Syn:* Chiari-Frommel syndrome

Chido, first patient in whom this specific antigen was first seen.
    Chido blood group—found in red cells and plasma in 98% of population.

Chievitz, Johan H., Danish anatomist, 1850–1901.
    Chievitz layer—in the developing retina of an embryo, a transitory zone
    between the inner and outer neuroblastic layers that is devoid of nuclei.
    Chievitz organ—a normal epithelial structure, possibly a neurotransmitter,
    found at the angle of the mandible with branches of the buccal nerve.

Chilaiditi, Demetrius, Austrian radiologist, *1883.
    Chilaiditi syndrome—interposition of the colon between the liver and the
    diaphragm.

Chinese restaurant, a dining establishment that serves Chinese food.
    Chinese restaurant syndrome—chest pain, facial pressure, and burning
    sensation that develops after persons sensitive to monosodium glutamate
    ingest this food additive. *Syn:* Kwok quease

Cholewa, Erasmus R., German physician, 1845–1931.
    Cholewa-Itard sign—*Syn:* Itard-Cholewa sign
    Itard-Cholewa sign—see under Itard

Chopart, François, French surgeon, 1743–1795.
    Chopart amputation—amputation through the midtarsal joint. *Syn:*
    mediotarsal amputation

Chopart ankle dislocation
Chopart articulation
Chopart brace
Chopart fracture
Chopart joint—the synovial joints which act as a unit in allowing the front of the foot to pivot relative to the back of the foot about the longitudinal axis of the foot. *SYN:* transverse tarsal joint
Chopart osseous joint injury
Chopart partial foot prosthesis

Chotzen, F., 20th century German physician.
 Chotzen syndrome—syndactyly, mild mental retardation, hypertelorism, and occasional ptosis.

Christ, J., German dermatologist, 1871–1948.
 Christ-Siemens-Touraine syndrome—congenitally defective or absent sweat glands, smooth, finely wrinkled skin, sunken nose, malformed and missing teeth, sparse fragile hair, and associated with deformed nails, absent breast tissue, mental retardation, or syndactyly. *SYN:* anhidrotic ectodermal dysplasia

Christensen, Erna, Danish pathologist, 1906–1967.
 Christensen-Krabbe disease—familial progressive spastic paresis of extremities with destruction and disorganization of nerve cells of the cerebral cortex. *SYN:* poliodystrophia cerebri progressiva infantalis

Christian, Henry A., U.S. internist, 1876–1951.
 Christian disease—(1) *SYN:* Hand-Schüller-Christian disease; (2) *SYN:* Weber-Christian disease.
 Christian syndrome—*SYN:* Hand-Schüller-Christian disease
 Hand-Schüller-Christian disease—see under Hand, Alfred
 Weber-Christian disease—see under Weber, Frederick

Christison, Sir Robert, Scottish physician, 1797–1882.
 Christison formula—*SYN:* Häser formula

Christmas, Stephen, patient with disease.
 Christmas disease—a clotting disorder caused by hereditary deficiency of factor IX. *SYN:* hemophilia B
 Christmas factor—*SYN:* factor IX coagulation factor

Churchill, E.D., U.S. thoracic surgeon, *1895.
 Churchill-Cope reflex—distention of pulmonary vascular bed results in increase in respiratory rate.

Churg, Jacob, U.S. pathologist, *1910.
 Churg-Strauss syndrome—asthma, fever, eosinophilia, and varied symptoms and signs of vasculitis, primarily affecting small arteries, with vascular and extravascular granulomas. *SYN:* allergic granulomatous angiitis; allergic granulomatosis

NOTES

Chvostek, Franz, Austrian surgeon, 1834–1884.
    Chvostek sign—facial irritability in tetany, unilateral spasm of the orbicularis oculi or oris muscle being excited by a slight tap over the facial nerve just anterior to the external auditory meatus. *Syn:* Weiss sign; Chvostek tremor
    Chvostek tremor—*Syn:* Chvostek sign

Ciaccio, Carmelo, Italian pathologist, 1877–1956.
    Ciaccio fluid
    Ciaccio method
    Ciaccio stain—a method for demonstrating complex insoluble intracellular lipids.

Ciaccio, Giuseppe V., Italian anatomist, 1824–1901.
    Ciaccio glands—*Syn:* accessory lacrimal glands

Cimino, James E., U.S. nephrologist, *1928.
    Brescia-Cimino fistula—see under Brescia

Citelli, Salvatore, Italian laryngologist, 1875–1947.
    Citelli syndrome—nasopharyngeal obstruction caused by adenoid tissue and associated with mental retardation, sinus infection, and inability to concentrate.

Civatte, Achille, French dermatologist, 1877–1956.
    Civatte bodies—eosinophilic hyaline spherical bodies seen in or just beneath the epidermis, particularly in lichen planus, formed by necrosis of individual basal cells. *Syn:* colloid bodies
    Civatte disease—*Syn:* poikiloderma of Civatte
    poikiloderma of Civatte—reticulated pigmentation and telangiectasia of the sides of the cheeks and neck; common in middle-aged women. *Syn:* Civatte disease

Civinini, Filippo, Italian anatomist, 1805–1844.
    Civinini canal—a canal in the petrotympanic or glaserian fissure near its posterior edge through which the chorda tympani nerve issues from the skull. *Syn:* anterior canaliculus of chorda tympani
    Civinini ligament—a membranous ligament extending from the spine of the sphenoid to the upper part of the posterior border of the lateral pterygoid lamina. *Syn:* pterygospinous ligament
    Civinini process—a sharp projection from the posterior edge of the lateral pterygoid plate of the sphenoid bone. *Syn:* pterygospinous process

Clado, Spiro, French gynecologist, 1856–1905.
    Clado anastomosis—anastomosis in the right suspensory ligament of the ovary between the appendicular and ovarian arteries.
    Clado band—the suspensory ligament of the ovary.
    Clado ligament—a mesenteric fold running from the broad ligament on the right side to the appendix.
    Clado point—a point at the lateral border of the rectus abdominis muscle where marked tenderness on pressure is felt in some cases of appendicitis.

Clapton, Edward, English physician, 1830–1909.
    Clapton line—a greenish discoloration of the marginal gingiva in cases of chronic copper poisoning.

Clara, Max, Austrian anatomist, *1899.
 Clara cell—a rounded, club-shaped, nonciliated cell protruding between ciliated cells in bronchiolar epithelium; believed to be secretory in function. *Syn:* bronchiolar exocrine cell
 Clara hematoxylin

Clark, Alonzo, U.S. pharmacologist, 1807–1887.
 Clark sign—absence of liver dullness in the presence of peritonitis.
 Clark weight rule—an obsolete rule for an approximate child's dose.

Clark, Earl Perry, U.S. biochemist, *1892.
 Clark-Collip method—method for detecting calcium and urea in serum and blood.

Clark, Eliot R., U.S. anatomist, 1881–1963.
 Sandison-Clark chamber—see under Sandison

Clark, Leland, Jr., U.S. biochemist, *1918.
 Clark electrode—used to measure oxygen pressure in arterial blood samples.

Clark, Wallace H., Jr., U.S. dermatopathologist, *1924.
 Clark level—the level of invasion of primary malignant melanoma of the skin, recorded by Roman numerals I, II, III, IV, V.

Clarke, Cecil, 20th century English physician.
 Clarke-Hadfield syndrome—a congenital metabolic disorder in which secretions of exocrine glands are abnormal. *Syn:* cystic fibrosis

Clarke, Jacob A.L., English anatomist, 1817–1880.
 Clarke column—a column of large neurons that gives rise to the dorsal spinocerebellar tract. *Syn:* thoracic nucleus

Clauberg, Karl W., German bacteriologist, *1893.
 Clauberg test—a test for progestational activity.
 Clauberg unit

Claude, Albert, *1879, co-winner of the 1974 Nobel Prize for work related to cell structure and organization.

Claude, Henri, French psychiatrist, 1869–1945.
 Claude syndrome—midbrain syndrome with oculomotor palsy on the side of the lesion and incoordination on the opposite side.

Claudius, Friedrich M., German anatomist, 1822–1869.
 Claudius cells—columnar cells on the floor of the ductus cochlearis external to the organ of Corti.
 Claudius fossa—a depression in the parietal peritoneum of the pelvis that lodges the ovary. *Syn:* ovarian fossa

Claybrook, Edwin B., U.S. surgeon, 1871–1931.
 Claybrook sign—in rupture of abdominal viscus, transmission of breath and heart sounds through the abdominal wall.

NOTES

Cleemann, Richard Alsop, U.S. physician, 1840–1912.
   Cleemann sign—in fracture of the femur with overriding of the fragments, wrinkling of the skin occurs directly above the patella.

Cleland, John, Scottish anatomist, 1835–1925.
   Cleland ligaments—digital ligaments.

Cleland, W. Wallace, U.S. biochemist, *1930.
   Cleland reagent—a substance used to reduce disulfide bonds in proteins. *Syn:* dithiothreitol

Clérambault, C. G. See under de Clérambault.

Cléret, M., 20th century French physician.
   Launois-Cléret syndrome—*Syn:* Fröhlich syndrome

Clevenger, Shobal V., U.S. neurologist, 1843–1920.
   Clevenger fissure—the sulcus on the basal aspect of the temporal lobe that separates the fusiform gyrus from the inferior temporal gyrus on its lateral side. *Syn:* inferior temporal sulcus

Clias, Phokion Heinrich, U.S. therapist, 1780–1854.
   Clias exercises—basic exercises for younger individuals. *Syn:* Clias method
   Clias method—*Syn:* Clias exercises

Cloquet, Hippolyte, French anatomist, 1787–1840.
   Cloquet space—a space between the ciliary zonule and the vitreous body.

Cloquet, Jules G., French anatomist, 1790–1883.
   Cloquet canal—a minute canal running through the vitreous from the discus nervi optici to the lens. *Syn:* hyaloid canal
   Cloquet canal remnants
   Cloquet hernia—a femoral hernia perforating the aponeurosis of the pectineus and insinuating itself between this aponeurosis and the muscle, therefore lying behind the femoral vessels.
   Cloquet septum—the delicate fibrous membrane that closes the femoral ring at the base of the femoral canal. *Syn:* femoral septum
   node of Cloquet—one of the deep inguinal lymph nodes located in or adjacent to the femoral canal. *Syn:* Rosenmüller node; Rosenmüller gland

Closs, K., Finnish dermatologist.
   Danbolt-Closs syndrome—*Syn:* Brandt syndrome

Cloudman, Arthur M., U.S. zoologist and pathologist, *1901.
   Cloudman melanoma—a transplantable melanoma that arose spontaneously in a mouse of DBA strain and which grows and metastasizes in mice of related strains.

Clouston, H.R., 20th century Canadian physician.
   Clouston syndrome—autosomal dominant trait resulting in congenital dystrophy of hair and nails. *Syn:* hidrotic ectodermal dysplasia

Clutton, Henry H., English surgeon, 1850–1909.
   Clutton joints—symmetrical arthrosis, especially of the knee joints, in cases of congenital syphilis.

Coats, George, English ophthalmologist, 1876–1915.

    Coats disease—a chronic abnormality characterized by deposition of cholesterol in outer retinal layers and subretinal space. *SYN:* exudative retinitis

Cobb, Stanley, U.S. neuropathologist, *1887.

    Cobb chisel

    Cobb curet

    Cobb gouge

    Cobb method

    Cobb osteotome

    Cobb periosteal elevator

    Cobb retractor

    Cobb spinal elevator

    Cobb syndrome—cutaneous angiomas, usually in a dermatomal distribution on the trunk, associated with vascular abnormality of the spinal cord and resulting neurologic symptoms. *SYN:* cutaneomeningospinal angiomatosis

    Cobb technique

Cock, E., English surgeon, 1805–1892.

    Cock tumor—*SYN:* infected sebaceous cyst

Cockayne, Edward A., English physician, 1880–1956.

    Cockayne disease—*SYN:* Cockayne syndrome

    Cockayne syndrome—dwarfism, senile appearance, pigmentary degeneration of the retina, optic atrophy, deafness, sensitivity to sunlight, and mental retardation. *SYN:* Cockayne disease

    Weber-Cockayne syndrome—see under Weber, Frederick

Cockett, Frank Bernard, English surgeon.

    Cockett and Dodd operation—varicose vein surgery.

Codman, Ernest Amory, U.S. surgeon, 1869–1940.

    Codman angle

    Codman cartilage clamp

    Codman classification

    Codman drill

    Codman exercises

    Codman incision

    Codman saber-cut shoulder approach

    Codman shunt

    Codman sign—in the absence of rotator cuff function, hunching of the shoulder occurs when the deltoid muscle contracts.

    Codman sponge

    Codman triangle—in radiology, the interface between growing bone tumor and normal bone, presenting as an incomplete triangle formed by periosteum.

    Codman tumor—chondroblastoma of the proximal humerus.

(continued)

NOTES

Codman *(continued)*
> **Codman vein stripper**
> **Codman wire-passing drill**

Coffey, Robert, U.S. surgeon, 1869–1933.
> **Coffey incision**
> **Coffey suspension**—an operative technique following partial excision of the cornu, as in salpingectomy, whereby the broad and the round ligaments are sutured over the cornual wound to restore continuity of the peritoneum and to suspend the uterus on the operated side.
> **Coffey ureterointestinal anastomosis**

Coffin, Grange S., U.S. pediatrician, *1923.
> **Coffin-Lowry syndrome**—*Syn:* Coffin-Siris syndrome
> **Coffin-Siris syndrome**—mental retardation with wide bulbous (pugilistic) nose, low nasal bridge, moderate hirsutism, and digital anomalies. *Syn:* Coffin-Lowry syndrome

Cogan, David G., U.S. ophthalmologist, 1908–1993.
> **Cogan syndrome**—a nonsyphilitic interstitial keratitis with vertigo and tinnitus, followed by deafness. *Syn:* oculovestibulo-auditory syndrome
> **Cogan-Reese syndrome**—syndrome of glaucoma, iris atrophy, decreased corneal endothelium, anterior peripheral synechia, and multiple iris nodules. *Syn:* iridocorneal endothelial syndrome

Cohen, Stanley, *1922, co-winner of 1986 Nobel Prize for work related to growth factors.

Cohnheim, Julius F., German histologist, pathologist, and physiologist, 1839–1884.
> **Cohnheim area**—a shrinkage artifact of fixation. *Syn:* Cohnheim field
> **Cohnheim field**—*Syn:* Cohnheim area
> **Cohnheim theory**—that neoplasms originate from various cell rests. *Syn:* emigration theory

Coiter, Volcher, Dutch surgeon and anatomist, 1534–1600.
> **Coiter muscle**—draws medial end of eyebrow downward and wrinkles forehead vertically. *Syn:* corrugator supercilii muscle

Cole, Laurent, French pathologist, *1903.
> **Benedict-Hopkins-Cole reagent**—see under Benedict, Stanley

Coley, W.B., U.S. surgeon, 1862–1936.
> **Coley fluid**—*Syn:* Coley toxin
> **Coley toxin**—injection with this bacterial toxin causes a febrile reaction and reduction in size of tumor mass. *Syn:* Coley fluid

Colles, Abraham, Irish surgeon, 1773–1843.
> **Colles fascia**—*Syn:* superficial fascia of perineum
> **Colles fracture**—a fracture of the lower end of the radius with displacement of the distal fragment dorsally.
> **Colles ligament**—a triangular fibrous band extending from the aponeurosis of the external oblique to the pubic tubercle of the opposite side. *Syn:* reflected inguinal ligament
> **Colles operation**
> **Colles sling**

Colles space—*Syn:* superficial perineal space
Colles splint

Collet, Frédric-Justin, French otolaryngologist, *1870.
    Collet-Sicard syndrome—unilateral lesions of cranial nerves IX, X, XI, and XII, producing Vernet syndrome and paralysis of the tongue on the same side.

Collier, James S., English physician, 1870–1935.
    Collier sign—unilateral or bilateral lid retraction due to midbrain lesion. *Syn:* Collier tucked lid sign
    Collier tract—a longitudinal bundle of fibers extending from the upper border of the mesencephalon into the cervical segments of the spinal cord. *Syn:* medial longitudinal fasciculus
    Collier tucked lid sign—*Syn:* Collier sign

Collins, Edward Treacher, English ophthalmologist, 1862–1919.
    Treacher Collins syndrome—mandibulofacial dysostosis, when limited to the orbit and malar region. *Syn:* Nager-Reynier syndrome

Collip, James B., Canadian endocrinologist, 1892–1965.
    Anderson-Collip test—see under Anderson, Evelyn
    Clark-Collip method—see under Clark, Earl Perry
    Collip unit—dosage of parathyroid extract.
    Noble-Collip procedure—see under Noble

Collis, John Leighton, English thoracic surgeon, *1911.
    Collis antireflux operation
    Collis forceps
    Collis gastroplasty—a technique for lengthening the esophagus.
    Collis mouth gag
    Collis repair
    Collis spirometer
    Collis technique

Colonna, Paul Crenshaw, U.S. surgeon, 1892–1966.
    Colonna arthroplasty
    Colonna hip fracture classification
    Colonna operation—procedure for correction of congenital hip dislocation.
    Colonna reconstruction

Comby, Jules, French pediatrician, 1853–1947.
    Comby sign—an early sign of measles, consisting of thin whitish patches on the gums and buccal mucous membrane, formed of desquamating epithelial cells.

Comolli, Antonio, Italian pathologist, *1879.
    Comolli sign—in cases of fracture of the scapula, a typical triangular cushion-like swelling appears, corresponding to the outline of the scapula.

NOTES

Compton, Arthur H., U.S. physicist and Nobel laureate in 1927 for his work in physics, 1892–1962.

    Compton effect—in electromagnetic radiations of medium energy, a decrease in energy of the bombarding photon with the dislodgement of an orbital electron, usually from an outer shell. *Syn:* Compton scattering

    Compton scattering—*Syn:* Compton effect

Concato, Luigi M., Italian physician, 1825–1882.

    Concato disease—chronic inflammation with effusions in several serous cavities resulting in fibrous thickening of the serosa and constrictive pericarditis. *Syn:* polyserositis

Conn, Harold J., U.S. microbiologist, 1886–1975.

    Hucker-Conn stain—a crystal violet-ammonium oxalate mixture used in Gram stain.

Conn, Jerome, U.S. physician, *1907.

    Conn syndrome—an adrenocortical disorder caused by excessive secretion of aldosterone. *Syn:* primary aldosteronism

Connell, F. Gregory, U.S. surgeon, 1875–1968.

    Connell airway

    Connell breathing tube

    Connell ether vapor tube

    Connell incision

    Connell operation

    Connell suture—a continuous suture used for inverting the gastric or intestinal walls in performing an anastomosis.

Conradi, Andrew, Norwegian physician, 1809–1869.

    Conradi line—a line corresponding approximately to the lower edge of the cardiac area.

Conradi, Erich, 20th century German physician.

    Conradi disease—congenital shortening of the humerus and femur, with stippled epiphyses, high-arched palate, cataracts, erythroderma in the newborn, and scaling followed by follicular atrophoderma. *Syn:* chondrodystrophia congenita punctata; Conradi syndrome; Conradi-Hunermann disease

    Conradi syndrome—*Syn:* Conradi disease

    Conradi-Hunermann disease—*Syn:* Conradi disease

Conradi, Heinrich, German bacteriologist, *1876.

    Conradi-Drigalski agar—a selective, nutrient medium for isolation of *Salmonella typhi* and other intestinal pathogens from fecal specimens. *Syn:* Drigalski-Conradi agar

    Drigalski-Conradi agar—*Syn:* Conradi-Drigalski agar

Contino, Antonino, Italian ophthalmologist, 1878–1951.

    Contino epithelioma—papilloma of the eye.

    Contino glaucoma

Converse, John M., U.S. plastic surgeon, 1909–1981.

    Converse alar elevator

    Converse alar retractor

    Converse bistoury

Converse curet
Converse hinged skin hook
Converse knife
Converse method—earlobe reconstruction procedure.
Converse nasal chisel
Converse nasal retractor
Converse nasal rongeur
Converse nasal root rongeur
Converse nasal saw
Converse nasal speculum
Converse nasal tip scissors
Converse needle holder
Converse operation
Converse osteotome
Converse rasp
Converse raspatory
Converse splint

Cooke, A. Bennett, U.S. physician, *1869.
Cooke speculum—a three-pronged speculum for rectal examinations and operations.

Cooley, Denton, 20th century U.S. surgeon.
Cooley anastomosis
Cooley anastomosis clamp
Cooley anastomosis forceps
Cooley aortic aneurysm clamp
Cooley aortic clamp
Cooley aortic retractor
Cooley aortic vent needle
Cooley arterial occlusion forceps
Cooley arteriotomy scissors
Cooley atrial retractor
Cooley auricular appendage forceps
Cooley bronchial clamp
Cooley bulldog clamp
Cooley cardiac tucker
Cooley cardiovascular forceps
Cooley cardiovascular scissors
Cooley cardiovascular suction tube
Cooley caval occlusion clamp
Cooley chisel
Cooley coarctation clamp
Cooley coarctation forceps
Cooley coronary dilator
Cooley curved forceps
Cooley dilator

(continued)

NOTES

Cooley (*continued*)
    Cooley double-angled jaw forceps
    Cooley first-rib shears
    Cooley graft clamp
    Cooley graft forceps
    Cooley iliac clamp
    Cooley iliac forceps
    Cooley intrapericardial anastomosis
    Cooley microvascular needle holder
    Cooley neonatal retractor
    Cooley neonatal vascular clamp
    Cooley partial occlusion clamp
    Cooley patent ductus clamp
    Cooley patent ductus forceps
    Cooley pediatric aortic forceps
    Cooley pediatric clamp
    Cooley pediatric dilator
    Cooley peripheral vascular forceps
    Cooley probe-point scissors
    Cooley renal clamp
    Cooley reverse-cut scissors
    Cooley rib contractor
    Cooley rib retractor
    Cooley sternotomy retractor
    Cooley suction tube
    Cooley sump tube
    Cooley tangential pediatric forceps
    Cooley tissue forceps
    Cooley U-sutures
    Cooley valve dilator
    Cooley vascular forceps
    Cooley vascular tissue forceps
    Cooley vena cava catheter clamp
    Cooley vena cava clamp

Cooley, Thomas B., U.S. pediatrician, 1871–1945.
    Cooley anemia—the syndrome of severe anemia with multiple organ disorders. *SYN:* thalassemia major
    Cooley trait—*SYN:* thalassemia minor

Coolidge, William D., U.S. physicist, 1873–1974.
    Coolidge tube—a kind of x-ray tube.

Coombs, Carey F., English physician, 1879–1932.
    Coombs murmur—a blubbering apical mid-diastolic murmur occurring in the acute stage of rheumatic mitral valvulitis and disappearing as the valvulitis subsides. *SYN:* Carey Coombs murmur

Coombs, Robin R.A., English veterinarian and immunologist, *1921.
    Coombs serum—serum from a rabbit or other animal previously immunized with purified human globulin to prepare antibodies directed against IgG and complement. *SYN:* antihuman globulin
    Coombs test—a test for antibodies, the so-called anti-human globulin test using either the direct or indirect Coombs tests. *SYN:* antiglobulin test

direct Coombs test—a test for detecting sensitized erythrocytes in erythroblastosis fetalis and in cases of acquired immune hemolytic anemia.

Gell and Coombs reactions—see under Gell

indirect Coombs test—a test routinely performed in cross-matching blood or in the investigation of transfusion reaction.

Coons, A.H., U.S. immunologist, *1912.

Coons fluorescent antibody method—method used to localize cell antigens.

Cooper, Sir Astley Paston, English anatomist and surgeon, 1768–1841.

Cooper fascia—one of the coverings of the spermatic cord, formed of delicate connective tissue and of muscular fibers derived from the internal oblique muscle (cremaster muscle). *SYN:* cremasteric fascia

Cooper hernia—a femoral hernia with two sacs. *SYN:* bilocular femoral hernia; Hey hernia

Cooper herniotome—a slender bistoury with short cutting edge for dividing the constricting tissues at the neck of a hernial sac.

Cooper ligament repair

Cooper ligaments—(1) *SYN:* suspensory ligaments of breast; (2) *SYN:* pectineal ligament; (3) *SYN:* transverse ligament of elbow.

Cooper neuralgia—*SYN:* mastodynia

Cooper testis—neuralgia of the testicles.

suspensory ligaments of Cooper—*SYN:* Cooper ligaments (1)

Cooperman, H.N., U.S. dentist.

Cooperman-Miura syndrome—retrusion of the mandible causing tongue-uvula impingement; symptoms include respiratory disorders, headache, temporomandibular joint dysfunction. *SYN:* uvula-tongue malposture; Miura-Cooperman syndrome

Miura-Cooperman syndrome—*SYN:* Cooperman-Miura syndrome

Coopernail, George P., U.S. surgeon, 1876–1962.

Coopernail sign—in fracture of the pelvis, occurrence of ecchymosis of the perineum and scrotum, or labia.

Cope, O.J., U.S. surgeon, *1902.

Churchill-Cope reflex—see under Churchill

Cope, Sir Vincent Z., English surgeon, 1881–1974.

Cope biopsy needle

Cope clamp—a clamp used in excision of colon and rectum.

Cope double-ended retractor

Coplin, W.M.I., U.S. physician, 1864–1928.

Coplin jar—glass jar used to hold staining slides.

Coppet, Louis de, French physicist, 1841–1911.

Coppet law—solutions having the same freezing point have equal concentrations of dissolved substances.

NOTES

Corbus, Budd Clarke, U.S. urologist, 1876–1954.
 Corbus disease—spirochete causing infection that erodes the glans penis.
 SYN: balanitis gangrenosa

Cords, Richard, German ophthalmologist, *1861.
 Cords angiopathy—thrombosis of a retinal vein that can eventually lead to
 visual field reduction; occurs in children.

Corey, R.B., U.S. chemist, 1897–1971.
 Pauling-Corey helix—see under Pauling

Cori, Carl F., Czech-U.S. biochemist and Nobel laureate, 1896–1984.
 Cori cycle—the phases in the metabolism of carbohydrate.
 Cori ester—an important intermediate in glycogenesis and glycogenolysis.
 SYN: D-glucose 1-phosphate

Cori, Gerty Theresa, Czech-U.S. biochemist and Nobel laureate, 1896–1957.
 Cori disease—glycogenosis due to amylo-1,6-glucosidase deficiency,
 resulting in accumulation of abnormal glycogen with short outer chains in
 liver and muscle. *SYN:* type 3 glycogenosis
 Cori syndrome—*SYN:* McArdle syndrome

Cormack, Alan M., joint winner of 1979 Nobel Prize for work related to CT
 scan.

Cornell, William Mason, U.S. psychiatrist, 1802–1895.
 Cornell Medical Index—psychological test designed to screen for potential
 instability in World War II soldiers.
 Cornell Word Form—word-association test.

Corner, Edred M., English surgeon, 1873–1950.
 Corner tampon—a plug of omentum stuffed into a wound of the stomach
 or intestine as a temporary tampon.

Corner, George W., U.S. anatomist, 1889–1981.
 Corner-Allen test—a test for progestational activity.
 Corner-Allen unit—a unit of progestational activity, measured in rabbits.

Cornet, Georg, German bacteriologist, 1858–1915.
 Cornet forceps

Cornil, L.
 Roussy-Cornil syndrome—see under Roussy

Coroli, J., French gastroenterologist.
 Coroli syndrome—intrahepatic biliary tract cystic dilatation often
 accompanied by bile stones and increased incidence of adenocarcinoma
 in the intrahepatic bile ducts.

Corrigan, Sir Dominic J., Irish pathologist and clinician, 1802–1880.
 Corrigan disease—reflux of blood through an incompetent aortic valve
 into the left ventricle during ventricular diastole. *SYN:* aortic regurgitation
 Corrigan pulse—the collapsing or water-hammer-type pulse in aortic
 regurgitation or peripheral arterial dilation, characterized by an abrupt
 rise and rapid fall away.

Corti, Marquis Alfonso, Italian anatomist, 1822–1888.
 Corti arch—the arch formed by the junction of the heads of Corti inner
 and outer pillar cells.

Corti auditory teeth—tooth-shaped formations or ridges occurring on the vestibular lip of the limbus lamina spiralis of the cochlear duct. *SYN:* auditory teeth

Corti canal—*SYN:* Corti tunnel

Corti cells—sensory cells in the organ of Corti in synaptic contact with sensory as well as efferent fibers of the cochlear (auditory) nerve. *SYN:* cochlear hair cells

Corti ganglion—an elongated ganglion of bipolar sensory nerve cell bodies on the cochlear part of the vestibulocochlear nerve in the spiral canal of the modiolus. *SYN:* spiral ganglion of cochlea

Corti membrane—a gelatinous membrane that overlies the spiral organ (Corti) in the inner ear. *SYN:* tectorial membrane of cochlear duct

Corti organ—a prominent ridge of highly specialized epithelium in the floor of the cochlear duct. *SYN:* spiral organ

Corti pillars—cells forming the outer and inner walls of the tunnel in the organ of Corti. *SYN:* pillar cells; Corti rods; pillar cells of Corti

Corti rods—*SYN:* Corti pillars

Corti tunnel—the spiral canal in the organ of Corti, filled with fluid and occasionally crossed by nonmedullated nerve fibers. *SYN:* Corti canal

pillar cells of Corti—*SYN:* Corti pillars

Corvisart des Marets, Baron Jean N., French clinician, 1755–1821.
Corvisart disease
Corvisart facies—the characteristic facies seen in cardiac insufficiency or aortic regurgitation.

Costen, James B., U.S. otolaryngologist, 1895–1962.
Costen syndrome—a symptom complex of loss of hearing, otalgia, tinnitus, dizziness, headache, and burning sensation of the throat, tongue, and side of the nose.

Cotard, Jules, French neurologist, 1840–1887.
Cotard syndrome—psychotic depression involving delusion of the existence of one's body, along with ideas of negation and suicidal impulses.

Cotte, Gaston, French surgeon, 1879–1951.
Cotte operation—cutting of the presacral nerve to relieve severe dysmenorrhea. *SYN:* presacral neurectomy

Cotting, Benjamin E., U.S. surgeon, 1812–1898.
Cotting operation—repair of ingrown toenail.

Cotton, Frank A., U.S. chemist, *1930.
Cotton effect—a change in the sign of optical rotation of a specimen as the wavelength of observation is changed.

Cotton, Frederick J., U.S. physician, 1869–1938.
Cotton fracture—tibial fracture.

NOTES

Cotugno, var. of Cotunnius
    Cotugno disease—*SYN:* sciatica

Cotunnius, Domenico, Italian anatomist, 1736–1822.
    aqueductus cotunnii—a bony canal of the petrous portion of the temporal bone, giving passage to the endolymphatic duct and a small vein. *SYN:* aqueduct of vestibule; Cotunnius aqueduct; Cotunnius canal
    Cotunnius aqueduct—*SYN:* aqueductus cotunnii
    Cotunnius canal—*SYN:* aqueductus cotunnii
    Cotunnius disease—pain in the lower back and hip radiating down the back of the thigh into the leg now known to usually be due to herniated lumbar disk compromising the L5 or S1 root. *SYN:* sciatica
    Cotunnius liquid—the fluid contained within the osseus labyrinth. *SYN:* perilymph; liquor cotunnii
    Cotunnius space—the dilated blind extremity of the endolymphatic duct. *SYN:* endolymphatic sac
    liquor cotunnii—*SYN:* Cotunnius liquid

Councilman, William T., U.S. pathologist, 1854–1933.
    Councilman body—an eosinophilic globule seen in the liver in yellow fever, derived from necrosis of a single hepatic cell. *SYN:* Councilman lesion; Councilman cell
    Councilman cell—*SYN:* Councilman body
    Councilman lesion—*SYN:* Councilman body

Cournand, André, F., French-U.S. physiologist, *1895, joint winner of 1956 Nobel Prize for work related to circulation and cardiac catheterization.
    Cournand arterial needle
    Cournand catheter
    Cournand needle

Courvoisier, Ludwig G., French surgeon, 1843–1918.
    Courvoisier gallbladder—an enlarged, often palpable, gallbladder in a patient with carcinoma of the head of the pancreas.
    Courvoisier law—enlargement of the gallbladder with jaundice is likely to result from carcinoma of the head of the pancreas and not from a stone in the common duct. *SYN:* Courvoisier sign
    Courvoisier sign—*SYN:* Courvoisier law

Couto, Miguel, South American physician, 1864–1934.
    Couto disease—visceral organ fatty degeneration.

Couvelaire, Alexandre, French obstetrician, 1873–1948.
    Couvelaire uterus—extravasation of blood into the uterine musculature and beneath the uterine peritoneum in association with severe forms of abruptio placentae. *SYN:* uteroplacental apoplexy

Cowdry, Edmund Vincent, U.S. cytologist, 1888–1975.
    Cowdry type A inclusion bodies—droplet-like masses of acidophilic material surrounded by clear halos within nuclei, with margination of chromatin on the nuclear membrane.
    Cowdry type B inclusion bodies—droplet-like masses of acidophilic material surrounded by clear halos within nuclei, without other nuclear changes during early stages of development of the inclusion.

Cowen, J.P., 20th century U.S. ophthalmologist.
    Cowen sign—sign of Graves disease.

Cowper, William, English anatomist, 1666–1709.
    Cowper cyst—a retention cyst of a bulbourethral gland.
    Cowper gland—*SYN:* bulbourethral gland
    Cowper ligament—the part of the fascia lata which is anterior to and provides origin for fibers of the pectineus muscle.
    cowperitis—inflammation of Cowper gland.

Coxsackie, city in New York where virus was first isolated.
    Coxsackie disease—*SYN:* Coxsackie virus
    Coxsackie virus—*SYN:* Coxsackie disease

Crabtree, Herbert G., 20th century English physician and biochemist.
    Crabtree effect—inhibition of cellular respiration of isolated systems by high concentrations of glucose.

Crafoord, Clarence, Swedish surgeon, *1899.
    Crafoord aortic clamp
    Crafoord bronchial forceps
    Crafoord clamp—a clamp used in heart, lung, and vascular operations.
    Crafoord coarctation clamp
    Crafoord coarctation forceps
    Crafoord forceps
    Crafoord hemostat
    Crafoord lobectomy scissors
    Crafoord operation
    Crafoord pulmonary forceps
    Crafoord thoracic scissors

Crafts, Leo M., U.S. neurologist, 1863–1938.
    Crafts test—test related to organic disease of pyramidal tract.

Cramer, Friedrich, German surgeon, 1847–1903.
    Cramer wire splint—a flexible splint consisting of two stout parallel wires with finer cross wires. *SYN:* ladder splint

Crampton, Charles Ward, U.S. physician, *1877.
    Crampton test—a test for physical condition and resistance.

Crampton, Sir Philip, Irish surgeon, 1777–1858.
    Crampton line—a guide to the common iliac artery.
    Crampton muscle—*SYN:* Brücke muscle

Crandall, Barbara F., U.S. physician.
    Crandall syndrome—recessive trait causing deafness, baldness, and hypogonadism.

Crawford, Brian H., English physicist, *1906.
    Stiles-Crawford effect—see under Stiles

NOTES

Credé, Karl S.F., German obstetrician and gynecologist, 1819–1892.
  Credé maneuver—*SYN:* Credé method (3)
  Credé method—(1) instillation of 0.1% silver nitrate in eyes of neonates; (2) resting the hand on the fundus uteri from the moment of the expulsion of the fetus; (3) use of manual pressure on a bladder to express urine. *SYN:* Credé maneuver

Creutzfeldt, Hans Gerhard, German neuropsychiatrist, 1885–1964.
  Creutzfeldt-Jakob disease—a form of subacute spongiform encephalopathy caused by a transmissible agent that has not been completely defined. *SYN:* transmissible dementia; Jakob-Creutzfeldt disease; mad cow disease
  Jakob-Creutzfeldt disease—*SYN:* Creutzfeldt-Jakob disease

Creveld, S. van. See under van Creveld.

Crichton-Browne, Sir James, English physician, 1840–1938.
  Crichton-Browne sign—a slight tremor at the angles of the mouth and at the outer canthus of each eye in general paresis.

Crick, Francis H.C., English biochemist and Nobel laureate, *1916.
  Watson-Crick helix—see under Watson, James

Crigler, John F., U.S. physician, *1919.
  Crigler-Najjar disease—*SYN:* Crigler-Najjar syndrome
  Crigler-Najjar syndrome—a rare defect in ability to form bilirubin glucuronide due to deficiency of bilirubin-glucuronide glucuronosyltransferase. *SYN:* Crigler-Najjar disease

Crile, George W., U.S. surgeon, 1864–1943.
  Crile appendiceal clamp
  Crile arterial forceps
  Crile blade
  Crile clamp—a clamp for temporary stoppage of blood flow.
  Crile dissector
  Crile gall duct forceps
  Crile gall hemostats
  Crile needle holder
  Crile single hook
  Crile spatula
  Crile vagotomy stripper

Crocq, Jean, Belgian physician, 1868–1925.
  Crocq disease—a circulatory disorder. *SYN:* acrocyanosis

Crohn, Burrill, B., U.S. gastroenterologist, 1884–1983.
  Crohn disease—a subacute chronic enteritis. *SYN:* regional enteritis

Cronin, Thomas D., U.S. plastic surgeon, *1906.
  Cronin cheiloplasty
  Cronin cleft palate elevator
  Cronin implant
  Cronin mammary implant
  Cronin method—nasal tip operation.
  Cronin palate elevator

Cronin palate knife
Cronin Silastic mammary prosthesis

Cronkhite, Leonard W., Jr., U.S. physician, *1919.
    Cronkhite-Canada syndrome—a sporadically occurring syndrome of gastrointestinal polyps with diffuse alopecia and nail dystrophy.

Crooke, Arthur, English pathologist, *1905.
    Crooke granules—lumpy masses of basophilic material in the pituitary associated with Cushing disease or following the administration of ACTH.
    Crooke hyaline change—replacement of cytoplasmic granules of basophil cells of the anterior pituitary by homogenous hyaline material. *Syn:* Crooke hyaline degeneration
    Crooke hyaline degeneration—*Syn:* Crooke hyaline change

Crookes, Sir William, English physicist and chemist, 1832–1919.
    Crookes glass—a spectacle lens combined with metallic oxides to absorb ultraviolet or infrared rays.

Crosby, William Holmes, Jr., U.S. physician, *1914.
    Crosby capsule—an attachment to the end of a flexible tube used for peroral biopsy of the small intestine.
    Crosby syndrome—recessive trait causing hemolytic anemia.

Cross, Harold E., U.S. physician, *1937.
    Cross syndrome—autosomal recessive trait resulting in corneal opacity and albinism, mental retardation.
    Cross-McKusick-Breen syndrome
    McKusick-Cross syndrome—*Syn:* McKusick syndrome

Crosti, A., 20th century Italian dermatologist.
    Gianotti-Crosti syndrome—see under Gianotti

Crouzon, Octave, French physician, 1874–1938.
    Crouzon disease—craniostosis with widening of the skull and high forehead, ocular hypertelorism, exophthalmos, beaked nose, and hypoplasia of the maxilla. *Syn:* craniofacial dysostosis
    Crouzon-Apert disease—*Syn:* Apert syndrome

Crowe, Samuel J., U.S. physician, 1883–1955.
    Crowe sign—in the presence of lateral sinus thrombosis, internal jugular vein compression resulting in engorgement of retinal vessels.
    Crowe-Davis mouth gag—*Syn:* Davis-Crowe mouth gag
    Davis-Crowe mouth gag—see under Davis, John

Crozat, George B., U.S. dentist, *1876.
    Crozat appliance—orthodontic appliance.
    Crozat clasp—dental appliance clasp.
    Crozat dental orthopedics
    Crozat philosophy

(continued)

NOTES

Crozat *(continued)*
    Crozat removable orthodontic appliance
    Crozat therapy

Cruchet, Jean R., French physician.
    Cruchet disease—*Syn:* torticollis.

Crutchfield, William G., U.S. neurosurgeon, *1900.
    Crutchfield clamp
    Crutchfield drill
    Crutchfield operation
    Crutchfield reduction technique
    Crutchfield skeletal traction
    Crutchfield skull-tip pin
    Crutchfield tongs
    Crutchfield tongs prosthesis
    Crutchfield traction
    Crutchfield traction bow
    Crutchfield traction tongs

Cruveilhier, Jean, French pathologist and anatomist, 1791–1874.
    Cruveilhier atrophy
    Cruveilhier disease—*Syn:* Lou Gehrig disease
    Cruveilhier fascia—*Syn:* superficial fascia of perineum
    Cruveilhier fossa—a longitudinal hollow on the posterior surface of the superior portion (root) of the medial pterygoid plate. *Syn:* scaphoid fossa; fossa navicularis cruveilhier
    Cruveilhier joint—a pivot synovial joint between the dens of the axis and the ring formed by the anterior arch and the transverse ligament of the atlas. *Syn:* median atlantoaxial joint
    Cruveilhier ligaments—the counterparts in the foot of the palmar ligaments in the hand. *Syn:* plantar ligaments
    Cruveilhier nodules
    Cruveilhier palsy—*Syn:* Lou Gehrig disease
    Cruveilhier plexus—a nerve plexus formed by communications between the dorsal primary rami of the first three cervical nerves.
    Cruveilhier sign—palpable groin swelling noted when patient coughs.
    Cruveilhier tumor
    Cruveilhier ulcer
    Cruveilhier-Baumgarten disease—*Syn:* Cruveilhier-Baumgarten syndrome
    Cruveilhier-Baumgarten murmur—a venous murmur heard over collateral veins, connecting portal and caval venous systems, on the abdominal wall.
    Cruveilhier-Baumgarten sign—a murmur over the umbilicus often in the presence of caput medusae.
    Cruveilhier-Baumgarten syndrome—cirrhosis of the liver with patent umbilical or paraumbilical veins and varicose periumbilical veins (caput medusae). *Syn:* Cruveilhier-Baumgarten disease
    fossa navicularis cruveilhier—*Syn:* Cruveilhier fossa

Cruz, G. Oswaldo, Brazilian physician, 1872–1917.
    Chagas-Cruz disease—*Syn:* Chagas disease
    Cruz phenomenon—*Syn:* Kernohan-Woltman syndrome

Cruz trypanosomiasis—*SYN:* Chagas disease
Oswaldocruzia—genus of parasite which reside in the intestines and lungs of amphibians and reptiles.

Cryer, Matthew H., U.S. surgeon, 1840–1921.
    Cryer elevator—dental elevator.

Csillag, J.
    Csillag disease—chronic atrophic and lichenoid dermatitis.

Cuignet, Ferdinand L.J., 19th century French ophthalmologist.
    Cuignet method—skiascopy. *SYN:* retinoscopy

Cullen, Thomas S., U.S. gynecologist, 1868–1953.
    Cullen sign—periumbilical darkening of the skin from blood, a sign of intraperitoneal hemorrhage, especially in ruptured ectopic pregnancy.

Culp, Ormond S., U.S. urologist, 1910–1977.
    Culp biopsy needle
    Culp pyeloplasty—a reconstructive technique for correction of uteropelvic obstruction.
    Culp ureteropelvioplasty

Cummer, William E., Canadian dentist, 1879–1942.
    Cummer classification—a listing of several types of removable partial dentures in accordance with the distribution of direct retainers.
    Cummer guideline—a line which serves as a guide in the proper location of various parts of a clasp assembly for a removable partial denture. *SYN:* survey line

Cureton, Thomas Kirk, U.S. physical educator, 1901–1976.
    Cureton exercises—a physical education system.

Curie, Marie, French physicist, 1867–1934.
    curie—a unit of measurement of radioactivity.

Curie, P., French physicist, 1859–1906.
    curie—a unit of measurement of radioactivity.

Curling, Thomas B., English surgeon, 1811–1888.
    Curling ulcer—an ulcer of the duodenum in a patient with extensive superficial burns, intracranial lesions, or severe bodily injury. *SYN:* stress ulcers

Curschmann, Heinrich, German physician, 1846–1910.
    Curschmann disease—hyaloserositis of the liver. *SYN:* frosted liver
    Curschmann spirals—spirally twisted masses of mucus occurring in the sputum in bronchial asthma.
    Curschmann-Batten-Steinhert syndrome—rare hereditary condition resulting in atrophy of testicles in addition to muscle membrane abnormality which causes myotonia. *SYN:* myotonia dystrophia

NOTES

Curtis, Arthur H., U.S. gynecologist, 1881–1955.
    Fitz-Hugh and Curtis syndrome—see under Fitz-Hugh, T.

Curtius, Friedrich, German physician, 1896–1975.
    Curtius syndrome—(1) hypertrophy of a part or system of the body with various associated disorders. *SYN:* hemihypertrophy; (2) ovarian insuffiency with various associated disorders.

Cushing, Harvey W., U.S. neurosurgeon, 1869–1939.
    Cushing basophilism—*SYN:* Cushing syndrome
    Cushing bone rongeur
    Cushing brain depressor
    Cushing brain forceps
    Cushing brain spatula
    Cushing cranial bur
    Cushing cranial rongeur forceps
    Cushing disease—adrenal hyperplasia (Cushing syndrome) caused by an ACTH-secreting basophil adenoma of the pituitary. *SYN:* Cushing pituitary basophilism
    Cushing dressing forceps
    Cushing dural hook
    Cushing dural hook knife
    Cushing effect—*SYN:* Cushing phenomenon
    Cushing Gigli-saw guide
    Cushing nerve retractor
    Cushing perforator
    Cushing perforator drill
    Cushing periosteal elevator
    Cushing phenomenon—a rise in systemic blood pressure when the intracranial pressure acutely increases. *SYN:* Cushing effect; Cushing response
    Cushing pituitary basophilism—*SYN:* Cushing disease
    Cushing response—*SYN:* Cushing phenomenon
    Cushing self-retaining retractor
    Cushing straight retractor
    Cushing syndrome—a disorder resulting from increased adrenocortical secretion of cortisol. *SYN:* Cushing basophilism; Gallais syndrome; Itsenko-Cushing syndrome; adrenalism
    Cushing syndrome medicamentosus—a variable number of the signs and symptoms of Cushing syndrome.
    Cushing ulcer
    Itsenko-Cushing syndrome—*SYN:* Cushing syndrome

Cushing, Hayward W., U.S. surgeon, 1854–1934.
    Cushing suture—a running horizontal mattress suture used to approximate two adjacent surfaces.

Cuvier, Baron Georges L.C.F.D. de la, French scientist, 1769–1832.
    Cuvier ducts—obsolete term for the common cardinal veins.
    Cuvier veins—the common cardinal vein of the embryo.

Cyon, Elie de, Russian physiologist, 1843–1912.
    Cyon nerve—a branch of the vagus which ends in the aortic arch and base of the heart. *SYN:* aortic nerve

Cyriax, Edward F., 20th century English orthopedic surgeon.

    Cyriax syndrome—costal cartilage lesions cause a "slipping" sensation of the ribs; pain radiates to shoulder and arm and is often confused with angina pectoris.

Czapek, Friedrich J.F., Czech botanist, 1868–1921.

    Czapek solution agar—a culture medium used for the cultivation of fungus species and for identification of *Aspergillus* and *Penicillium* species. *SYN:* Czapek-Dox medium

    Czapek-Dox medium—*SYN:* Czapek solution agar

Czerny, Vincenz, German surgeon, 1842–1916.

    Czerny herniorrhaphy

    Czerny incision

    Czerny operation

    Czerny rectal speculum

    Czerny suture—the first row of the Czerny-Lembert intestinal suture.

    Czerny-Lembert suture—an intestinal suture in two rows combining the Czerny suture (first) and the Lembert suture (second).

C

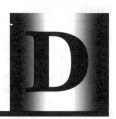

d'Arcet, Jean, French chemist, 1725–1801.
    d'Arcet metal—an alloy of lead, bismuth, and tin used in dentistry.

d'Arsonval, Jacques Arsène, French biophysicist, 1851–1940.
    d'Arsonval current—an alternating electric current having a frequency of 10,000 or more per second. *SYN:* high-frequency current
    d'Arsonval galvanometer—a sensitive galvanometer consisting of a moving coil suspended in a permanent magnetic field between delicate metallic wires.

D'Éspine, Jean H.A., French physician, 1846–1930.
    D'Éspine sign—bronchophony over the spinous processes heard at a lower level than in health, in pulmonary tuberculosis.

d'Herelle, Felix H., Canadian physician and bacteriologist, 1873–1949.
    d'Herelle phenomenon—*SYN:* Twort-d'Herelle phenomenon
    Twort-d'Herelle phenomenon—see under Twort

d'Ocagne, Philbert M., French mathematician, 1862–1938.
    d'Ocagne nomogram—an alignment chart.

Da Fano, Corrado D., Italian-U.S. anatomist, 1879–1927.
    Da Fano stain—a silver stain that produces a blackening of Golgi elements after tissues are fixed in a mixture of nitrate and formalin.

Daae, Anders, Norwegian physician, 1838–1910.
    Daae disease—an acute infectious disease usually occurring in epidemic form, characterized by paroxysms of pain and associated with strains of *Enterovirus* coxsackievirus type B. *SYN:* epidemic pleurodynia

Dacie, Sir John V., English physician.
    Dacie syndrome—massive splenomegaly, etiology unknown.

DaCosta, Jacob M., U.S. surgeon, 1833–1900.
    DaCosta disease
    DaCosta syndrome—a syndrome of functional nervous and circulatory irregularities. *SYN:* neurocirculatory asthenia

Dagnini, G., Italian physician, *1905.
    Scaglietti-Dagnini syndrome—*SYN:* Erdheim syndrome

Dagnini, Giuseppe, Italian physician, 1866–1928.
    Aschner-Dagnini reflex—*SYN:* Aschner phenomenon

Dakin, Henry, U.S. chemist, 1880–1952.
    Dakin catheter
    Dakin dressing
    Dakin fluid—*SYN:* Dakin solution
    Dakin solution—a bactericidal wound irrigant. *SYN:* Dakin fluid
    Dakin tube
    Dakin-Carrel treatment—*SYN:* Carrel treatment

Dalcroze, Emile-Jacques, Swiss composer and educator, 1865–1950.
    Dalcroze eurhythmics—a method of musical education used in therapy.

Dale, Sir Henry Hallett, English physiologist and Nobel laureate, 1875–1968.
    Dale reaction—*SYN:* Schultz-Dale reaction
    Dale-Feldberg law—an identical chemical transmitter is liberated at all the functional terminals of a single neuron.
    Schultz-Dale reaction—see under Schultz

Dalen, Johan A., Swedish ophthalmologist, 1866–1940.
    Dalen-Fuchs nodules—collections of epithelial cells lying between the Bruch membrane and the retinal pigment epithelium in sympathetic ophthalmia and rarely in other granulomatous intraocular inflammations.

Dalldorf, G.J., U.S. pathologist, *1900.
    Dalldorf test—test for capillary fragility.

Dalrymple, John, English oculist, 1804–1852.
    Dalrymple disease
    Dalrymple sign—retraction of the upper eyelid in Graves disease, causing abnormal wideness of the palpebral fissure.

Dalton, John, English chemist, mathematician, and natural philosopher, 1766–1844.
    Dalton law—each gas in a mixture of gases exerts a pressure proportionate to the percentage of the gas and independent of the presence of the other gases present. *SYN:* law of partial pressures
    Dalton-Henry law—in dissolving a mixture of gases, a liquid will absorb as much of each gas in the mixture as if that were the only gas dissolved.

Dam, Carl P. Henrik, Danish biochemist and 1943 Nobel laureate for discovery of vitamin K, 1895–1976.
    Dam unit—a unit of activity of vitamin K.

Dana, Charles L., U.S. neurologist, 1852–1935.
    Dana operation—section of posterior spinal root. *SYN:* posterior rhizotomy
    Dana syndrome—degenerative disease of the spinal cord associated with pernicious anemia.
    Putnam-Dana syndrome—see under Putnam

Danbolt, Niels Christian, Norwegian dermatologist, *1900.
    Danbolt syndrome—*SYN:* Brandt syndrome
    Danbolt-Closs syndrome—*SYN:* Brandt syndrome

Dance, Jean B.H., French physician, 1797–1832.
    Dance sign—*SYN:* signe de Dance
    signe de Dance—slight retraction in area of right iliac fossa sometimes seen in presence of intussusception. *SYN:* Dance sign

Dandy, Walter E., U.S. surgeon, 1886–1946.
  Dandy ventriculostomy
  Dandy clamp
  Dandy forceps
  Dandy hemostat
  Dandy nerve hook
  Dandy neurosurgical scissors
  Dandy operation
  Dandy suction tube
  Dandy-Walker syndrome—developmental anomaly of the fourth ventricle associated with atresia of the foramina of Luschka and Magendie that results in cerebellar hypoplasia, hydrocephalus, and posterior fossa cyst formation.

Dane, David S., 20th century English virologist.
  Dane method
  Dane particles—the larger spherical forms of hepatitis-associated antigens.

Danforth, William Clark, U.S. obstetrician-gynecologist, 1878–1949.
  Danforth sign—shoulder pain on inspiration, due to irritation of the diaphragm by a hemoperitoneum in ruptured ectopic pregnancy.

Danielli, J.F., English biologist, *1911.
  Davson-Danielli model—see under Davson

Danielssen, Daniel C., Norwegian physician, 1815–1894.
  Danielssen disease—*SYN:* anesthetic leprosy
  Danielssen-Boeck disease—*SYN:* anesthetic leprosy

Danlos, Henri A., French dermatologist, 1844–1912.
  Danlos phenomenon
  Danlos syndrome
  Ehlers-Danlos syndrome—see under Ehlers

Danysz, Jean, Polish pathologist in France, 1860–1928.
  Danysz phenomenon—reduction of the neutralizing effect of an antitoxin when toxin is mixed with it in divided portions.

Darier, Jean F., French dermatologist, 1856–1938.
  Darier disease—a familial, autosomal dominant eruption of pruritic keratotic papules on the trunk, face, scalp, and axillae. *SYN:* keratosis follicularis
  Darier sign—urtication on stroking of cutaneous lesions of urticaria pigmentosa (mastocytosis).

Darkschewitsch, Liverij Osipovich, Russian neurologist, 1858–1925.
  nucleus of Darkschewitsch—an ovoid cell group in the ventral central gray substance rostral to the oculomotor nucleus.

Darkshevich, var. of Darkschewitsch

D

NOTES

Darling, Samuel Taylor, U.S. physician in Panama, 1872–1925.
> **Darling disease**—a widely distributed infectious disease caused by *Histoplasma capsulatum* and manifested by a primary benign pneumonitis. *SYN:* histoplasmosis

Darrow, D.C., U.S. pediatrician, 1895–1965.
> **Darrow solution**—potassium-containing electrolyte solution.

Darwin, Charles R., English biologist and evolutionist, 1809–1882.
> **darwinian ear**—an auricle in which the upper border is not rolled over to form the helix, but projects upward as a flat, sharp edge.
> **darwinian reflex**—the tendency of young infants to grasp a bar and hang suspended.
> **darwinian theory**—the theory of the origin of species and of the development of higher organisms from lower forms through natural selection.
> **darwinian tubercle**—a small projection from the upper end of the posterior portion of the incurved free margin of the helix. *SYN:* auricular tubercle

Daubenton, Louis J.M., French physician, 1716–1799.
> **Daubenton angle**—an angle formed by the junction of lines coming from the basion and from the projection in the median plane of the lower border of the orbits. *SYN:* angulus occipitalis ossis parietalis; occipital angle of parietal bone
> **Daubenton line**—the line passing between the opisthion and the basion.
> **Daubenton plane**—the plane of the foramen magnum.

Dausset, Jean, joint winner of 1980 Nobel Prize for work related to cell structures and regulation of immunological reactions.

David, W. Walter, German physician, *1908.
> **David disease**—hemorrhage of gingivae and mucous membranes due to ovarian hormone deficiency.

Davidoff, M. von, German histologist, d. 1904.
> **Davidoff cells**—*SYN:* Paneth granular cells

Davidson, Edward C., U.S. surgeon, 1894–1933.
> **Davidson bur**
> **Davidson clamp**
> **Davidson collector**
> **Davidson forceps**
> **Davidson muscle clamp**
> **Davidson periosteal elevator**
> **Davidson retractor**
> **Davidson syringe**—a rubber tube intersected with a compressible bulb designed to take up fluid.
> **Davidson trocar**

Daviel, Jacques, French oculist, 1696–1762.
> **Daviel cataract extraction**
> **Daviel chalazion knife**
> **Daviel knife**
> **Daviel lens loupe**
> **Daviel lens spoon**

Daviel operation—extracapsular cataract extraction.

Daviel scoop

Daviel spoon—a small oval-shaped instrument for removing the remains of a cataract after discission.

Davies, J.N.P., U.S. pathologist, *1915.

Davies disease—thickening of the ventricular endocardium by fibrosis leading to progressive right and left ventricular failure with mitral and tricuspid insufficiency. *SYN:* endomyocardial fibrosis

Davis, John Staige, U.S. surgeon, 1872–1946.

Crowe-Davis mouth gag—*SYN:* Davis-Crowe mouth gag

Davis graft—small pieces (2 to 3 mm) of full-thickness skin. *SYN:* pinch graft

Davis-Crowe mouth gag—instrument used for opening the mouth, depressing the tongue, maintaining the airway, and transmitting volatile anesthetics during tonsillectomy or other oropharyngeal surgery.

Davson, H., English physiologist.

Davson-Danielli model—model of cell membrane.

Dawbarn, Robert Hugh Mackay, U.S. surgeon, 1860–1915.

Dawbarn sign—pain of subacromial bursitis disappears when the arm is abducted.

Dawson, James R., U.S. pathologist, *1908.

Dawson encephalitis—a rare chronic, progressive encephalitis caused by the measles virus. *SYN:* subacute sclerosing panencephalitis

Day, Richard H., U.S. physician, 1813–1892.

Day test—a test for blood.

Day, Richard L., U.S. pediatrician, *1905.

Riley-Day syndrome—see under Riley

de Bordeau, Théophile. See under Bordeau.

de Clérambault, G.G. de, French psychiatrist, 1872–1934.

Clérambault syndrome—psychosis primarily affecting females in which patient believes she is loved by someone of high status. *SYN:* de Clérambault syndrome

Clérambault-Kandinsky complex—psychosis in which patient believes his mind is controlled by a source outside himself. *SYN:* Clérambault-Kandinsky syndrome

Clérambault-Kandinsky syndrome—*SYN:* Clérambault-Kandinsky complex

de Clérambault syndrome—*SYN:* Clérambault syndrome

De Duve, Christian, joint winner of 1974 Nobel Prize for work related to cell structure and organization.

de Lange, Cornelia, Dutch pediatrician, 1871–1950.

Cornelia de Lange syndrome—*SYN:* de Lange syndrome

(continued)

NOTES

de Lange *(continued)*

 de Lange syndrome—a congenital anomaly characterized by impaired development, mental retardation, characteristic facies with synophrys and hairline well down on forehead, depressed bridge of nose with uptilted tip of nose, small head with low-set ears, and flat spadelike hands with simian crease and short tapering fingers. *Syn:* Amsterdam syndrome; Cornelia de Lange syndrome

De Martini, A., Italian physician

 De Martini-Balestra syndrome—*Syn:* Burke syndrome

De Morgan, Campbell, English physician, 1811–1876.

 Campbell De Morgan spots—congenital anomaly in which proliferation of blood vessels leads to a mass resembling a neoplasm; primarily seen on skin and in subcutaneous tissue; incidence increases with age. *Syn:* cherry angioma

 De Morgan spots—a red papule due to weakening of the capillary wall. *Syn:* senile hemangioma

de Morsier, G., 20th century Swiss neurologist.

 de Morsier syndrome—congenital optic nerve hypoplasia associated with midline cerebral anomalies. *Syn:* septo-optic dysplasia

de Musset, L.C. Alfred. See under Musset.

de Pezzer, Oscar M.B., French surgeon, 1853–1917.

 de Pezzer catheter—a self-retaining catheter with a bulbous extremity.
 de Pezzer mushroom-tipped catheter
 de Pezzer self-retaining catheter
 Pezzer catheter
 Pezzer drain

de Quervain, Fritz, Swiss surgeon, 1868–1940.

 de Quervain disease—fibrosis of the sheath of a tendon of the thumb. *Syn:* radial styloid tendovaginitis
 de Quervain fracture—fracture of navicular bone with dislocation of lunar bone.
 de Quervain incision
 de Quervain release
 de Quervain tenolysis
 de Quervain tenosynovitis
 de Quervain thyroiditis—thyroiditis with round cell infiltration, destruction of thyroid cells, epithelial giant cell proliferation, and evidence of regeneration. *Syn:* subacute granulomatous thyroiditis
 Quervain abdominal retractor
 Quervain cranial forceps
 Quervain elevator
 Quervain forceps
 Quervain incision
 Quervain release
 Quervain rongeur

De Sanctis, Carlo, Italian psychiatrist, *1888.

 De Sanctis-Cacchione syndrome—xeroderma pigmentosum with mental deficiency, dwarfism, and gonadal hypoplasia.

De Toni, Giovanni, Italian pediatrician, 1895–1973.
   De Toni-Fanconi syndrome—the most common of a group of diseases
   with characteristic renal tubular dysfunction disorders. *SYN:* cystinosis
   Debré-De Toni-Fanconi syndrome—*SYN:* Fanconi syndrome (2)

De Vries, Andre, Israeli physician.
   De Vries syndrome—congenital disorder associated with bleeding
   tendency and syndactyly.

de Wecker, Louis H., French physician, 1832–1906.
   de Wecker cannula
   de Wecker eye implant
   de Wecker forceps
   de Wecker iridectomy scissors
   de Wecker iris scissors
   de Wecker iris spatula
   de Wecker operation
   de Wecker scissors—a small scissors with sharp points for intraocular
   cutting of the iris and lens capsule.
   de Wecker sclerotomy
   de Wecker syringe cannula

Dean, Henry Trendley, U.S. dentist and epidemiologist, 1893–1962.
   Dean fluorosis index—an index that measures the degree of mottled
   enamel (fluorosis) in teeth.
   Dean periosteal elevator

Deaver, George G., U.S. physiatrist, 1890–1973.
   Deaver method—a method of motor reeducation.

Deaver, John B., U.S. surgeon, 1855–1931.
   Deaver blade
   Deaver clamp
   Deaver hemostat
   Deaver incision—an incision in the right lower abdominal quadrant, with
   medial displacement of the rectus muscle.
   Deaver operating scissors
   Deaver retractor
   Deaver skin incision
   Deaver T-tube

DeBakey, Michael Ellis, U.S. heart surgeon, *1908.
   DeBakey aortic aneurysm clamp
   DeBakey arterial clamp
   DeBakey Autraugrip forceps
   DeBakey ball-valve prosthesis
   DeBakey Beaver blade
   DeBakey bulldog clamp

(continued)

D

NOTES

DeBakey *(continued)*
    DeBakey chest retractor
    DeBakey classification—three types of dissections of the aorta: type I, type II, type III, type IIIA.
    DeBakey coarctation clamp
    DeBakey dissecting forceps
    DeBakey endarterectomy scissors
    DeBakey forceps—nontraumatic forceps used to pick up blood vessels.
    DeBakey graft
    DeBakey heart valve
    DeBakey implant
    DeBakey needle
    DeBakey patent ductus clamp
    DeBakey scissors
    DeBakey stripper
    DeBakey tangential occlusion clamp
    DeBakey tunneler
    DeBakey valve prosthesis
    DeBakey vascular dilator
    DeBakey Vasculour-II vascular prosthesis

Debler, K., German physician.
    Debler anemia—inherited form of hemolytic anemia.

Debove, George M., French physician, 1845–1920.
    Debove disease—splenomegaly.

Debré, Robert, French pediatrician and bacteriologist, 1882–1978.
    Debré phenomenon—in measles, the failure of the rash to develop at the site of immune serum injection.
    Debré-De Toni-Fanconi syndrome—*Syn:* Fanconi syndrome (2)
    Debré-Fibiger syndrome—pyloric pseudospasm causing vomiting and dehydration and which can lead to death. *Syn:* Pirie syndrome; Fibiger-Debré-Von Gierke syndrome
    Debré-Marie syndrome—(1) infectious edematous polyneuropathy; (2) dwarfism and underdevelopment of sexual organs.
    Debré-Semelaigne syndrome—*Syn:* Kocher-Debré-Semelaigne syndrome
    Fibiger-Debré-von Gierke syndrome—*Syn:* Debré-Fibiger syndrome
    Kocher-Debré-Semelaigne syndrome—see under Kocher
    Pirie syndrome—*Syn:* Debré-Fibiger syndrome

Deen, Izaak A. van. See under van Deen.

Deetjen, Hermann, German physician, 1867–1915.
    Deetjen bodies—a disklike cytoplasmic fragment found in the peripheral blood where it functions in clotting. *Syn:* platelet

Degos, R., French dermatologist, *1904.
    Degos acanthoma—obsolete term for clear cell acanthoma.
    Degos disease—a cutaneovisceral syndrome characterized by pathognomonic umbilicated porcelain-white papules followed by peritonitis, progressive neurological disability, and death. *Syn:* malignant atrophic papulosis; Degos syndrome
    Degos syndrome—*Syn:* Degos disease

Kohlmeier-Degos syndrome—vascular occlusive disorder predominantly involving the small arteries of the skin and bowel.

Dehio, Karl K., Russian physician, 1851–1927.
Dehio test—a test to determine the cause of bradycardia. *Syn:* atropine test

Deiters, Otto F.K., German anatomist, 1834–1863.
Deiters cells—the supporting cells of the organ of Corti; one of the large neuroglia cells of nervous tissue. *Syn:* phalangeal cell; astrocyte
Deiters nucleus—lateral vestibular nucleus.
Deiters terminal frames—platelike structures in the organ of Corti uniting the outer phalangeal cells with Hensen cells.

Dejerine, Joseph J., Paris neurologist, 1849–1917.
Dejerine anterior bulbar syndrome—occlusion of anterior spinal arteries with involvement of cortical spinal tract, hypoglossal nerves, and medial lemnisci.
Dejerine cortical sensory syndrome—(1) radiculitis; (2) bulbar syndrome caused by medullar lesion and resulting in cranial nerve paralysis in the area; (3) polyneuropathy resulting in depression of deep sensation; tactile sensation remains normal.
Dejerine disease—*Syn:* Dejerine-Sottas disease
Dejerine hand phenomenon—clonic contractions of the flexors of the hand (wrist) on tapping the dorsum of the hand or the volar side of the forearm near the wrist, exaggerated in pyramidal tract lesions. *Syn:* Dejerine reflex
Dejerine reflex—*Syn:* Dejerine hand phenomenon
Dejerine sign—aggravation of symptoms of radiculitis by the acts of coughing, sneezing, or straining to defecate.
Dejerine-Landouzy dystrophy—*Syn:* Landouzy-Dejerine dystrophy
Dejerine-Landouzy myopathy—*Syn:* Landouzy-Dejerine dystrophy
Dejerine-Lichtheim phenomenon—*Syn:* Lichtheim sign
Dejerine-Roussy syndrome—infraction of posteroinferior thalamus causing transient hemiparesis, severe loss of superficial and deep sensation with preservation of crude pain in the limbs with decreased sensation; the limbs frequently have vasomotor or trophic disturbances. *Syn:* thalamic syndrome
Dejerine-Sottas disease—a familial type of demyelinating sensorimotor polyneuropathy that begins in early childhood and is slowly progressive. *Syn:* Dejerine disease; progressive hypertrophic polyneuropathy; Dejerine-Sottas neuropathy
Dejerine-Sottas neuropathy—*Syn:* Dejerine-Sottas disease
Landouzy-Dejerine dystrophy—see under Landouzy

Dejerine-Klumpke, Augusta, French neurologist, 1859–1927.
Dejerine-Klumpke palsy—*Syn:* Klumpke palsy
Dejerine-Klumpke syndrome—*Syn:* Klumpke palsy

(continued)

NOTES

Dejerine-Klumpke *(continued)*
    Klumpke palsy—a type of brachial birth palsy in which there is paralysis of the muscles of the distal forearm and hand. *Syn:* Dejerine-Klumpke palsy; Klumpke paralysis; Dejerine-Klumpke syndrome
    Klumpke paralysis—*Syn:* Klumpke palsy

del Castillo, E.B., 20th century Argentinian physician.
    Ahumada-del Castillo syndrome—see under Ahumada
    Argonz-del Castillo syndrome—*Syn:* Ahumada-del Castillo syndrome
    del Castillo syndrome—*Syn:* Sertoli-cell-only syndrome

Delafield, Francis, U.S. physician and pathologist, 1841–1915.
    Delafield hematoxylin—an alum type of hematoxylin used in histology.

Delbet, Pierre, French surgeon, 1861–1925.
    Delbet sign—in a case of aneurysm of a main artery, efficient collateral circulation if the nutrition of the part below is well maintained, despite the fact that the pulse has disappeared.
    Delbet splint for heel fracture

Delbrück, Max, joint winner of 1969 Nobel Prize for work related to viruses.

DeLee, Joseph B., U.S. obstetrician and gynecologist, 1869–1942.
    DeLee trap meconium aspirator
    DeLee catheter
    DeLee forceps
    DeLee infant catheter
    DeLee maneuver—a method by which obstetrical forceps are used to rotate the fetal head. *Syn:* key-in-lock maneuver
    DeLee obstetrical forceps
    DeLee ovum forceps
    DeLee pelvimeter
    DeLee uterine packing forceps
    DeLee-Hillis stethoscope

Delmege, Jean A., 20th century French physician.
    Delmege sign—early tuberculosis sign.

DeLorme, Thomas L., U.S. orthopedic surgeon.
    DeLorme exercises—progressive resistance exercise system.
    DeLorme table—an exercise table with adjustable parts.

Delsarte, Francois-Alexandre-Nicolas, 1811–1871.
    Delsarte exercises—*Syn:* Delsarte system
    Delsarte system—a method of breathing, speaking, posture, etc. *Syn:* Delsarte exercises; delsartism

Demarquay, Jean N., French surgeon, 1811–1875.
    Demarquay symptom—absence of elevation of the larynx during deglutition, said to indicate syphilitic induration of the trachea.

Demoivre, Abraham, English mathematician, 1667–1754.
    Demoivre formula—an obsolete formula for calculating life expectancy.

Denis Browne, See under Browne, Sir Denis John.

Denman, Thomas, English obstetrician, 1733–1815.
Denman spontaneous evolution—a mechanism of spontaneous molding of the fetus and impaction of the shoulder with prolapse of the arm noted in some cases of transverse lie.

Dennie, C.C., U.S. dermatologist, 1883–1971.
Dennie-Marfan syndrome—juvenile spastic paraplegia and mental retardation due to congenital syphilis.

Denny-Brown, Derek E., New Zealand neurologist in England and U.S., 1901–1981.
Denny-Brown syndrome—bronchogenic carcinoma.

Denonvilliers, Charles P., French surgeon, 1808–1872.
Denonvilliers aponeurosis—a fascial layer that extends superiorly from the central tendon of the perineum to the peritoneum between the prostate and rectum. *Syn:* rectovesical septum
Denonvilliers blepharoplasty
Denonvilliers fascia
Denonvilliers ligament—the localized thickening of the superior fascia of the pelvic diaphragm anteriorly that anchors the prostate and neck of the bladder to the pubis on each side. *Syn:* puboprostatic ligament
Denonvilliers space

Denucé, Jean L.P., French surgeon, 1824–1889.
Denucé ligament—fibers that pass from the distal margin of the radial notch of the ulna to the neck of the radius. *Syn:* quadrate ligament

Denys, Joseph, Belgian bacteriologist, 1857–1932.
Denys-Leclef phenomenon—enhanced phagocytosis by leukocytes of microorganisms in the presence of immune serum.

Dercum, Francis X., U.S. neurologist, 1856–1931.
Dercum disease—a condition characterized by a deposit of symmetrical nodular or pendulous masses of fat in various regions of the body, with discomfort or pain. *Syn:* adiposis dolorosa

Desault, Pierre J., French surgeon, 1744–1795.
Desault bandage—a bandage for fracture of the clavicle.
Desault ligature—a ligature of the femoral artery in the adductor muscle, for treatment of popliteal aneurysm.
Desault sign
Desault wrist bandage
Desault wrist dislocation

Descartes, René, French philosopher, mathematician, physiologist, 1596–1650.
cartesian—relating to Cartesius, latinized form of Descartes.
Descartes law—for two given media, the sine of the angle of incidence bears a constant relation to the sine of the angle of refraction. *Syn:* law of refraction

D

NOTES

Descemet, Jean, French physician, 1732–1810.
> **Descemet membrane**—a transparent homogeneous acellular layer between the substantia propria and the endothelial layer of the cornea. *SYN:* posterior limiting layer of cornea

Deschamps, Joseph F., French surgeon, 1740–1824.
> **Deschamps needle**—a needle with a long shaft for passing sutures in the deep tissues.

Desmarres, Louis A., French ophthalmologist, 1810–1882.
> **Desmarres dacryoliths**—*SYN: Nocardia* dacryoliths
> **Desmarres fixation pick**
> **Desmarres lid elevator**
> **Desmarres marker**
> **Desmarres refractor**

Deutschländer, Carl E. W., German surgeon, 1872–1942.
> **Deutschländer disease**—tumor of one of the metatarsal bones; a fatigue fracture of one of the metatarsals. *SYN:* march fracture

Deventer, Hendrik van, Dutch obstetrician, 1651–1724.
> **Deventer pelvis**—a pelvis with shortened anteroposterior diameter.

Devic, Eugène, French physician, 1869–1930.
> **Devic disease**—a demyelinating disorder consisting of a transverse myelopathy and optic neuritis. *SYN:* neuromyelitis optica

Devine, Sir Hugh B., Australian surgeon, 1878–1959.
> **Devine exclusion**—exclusion of the lower part of the stomach, followed by gastrojejunostomy, for treatment of duodenal ulcer.

Dewar, Sir James, English chemist, 1842–1923.
> **Dewar flask**—a glass vessel with two walls, the space between which is evacuated. *SYN:* vacuum flask

Di Guglielmo, Giovanni, Italian physician, 1886–1961.
> **Di Guglielmo anemia**—*SYN:* Di Guglielmo disease
> **Di Guglielmo disease**—*SYN:* Di Guglielmo syndrome
> **Di Guglielmo syndrome**—acute form of erythremic myelosis. *SYN:* Di Guglielmo disease; Mortensen syndrome

Diamond, Louis K., U.S. physician, *1902.
> **Diamond-Blackfan anemia**—autosomal recessive normocytic normochromic anemia. *SYN:* congenital hypoplastic anemia; Diamond-Blackfan syndrome
> **Diamond-Blackfan syndrome**—*SYN:* Diamond-Blackfan anemia
> **Gardner-Diamond syndrome**—see under Gardner

Dick, George Frederick, U.S. internist, 1881–1967.
> **Dick method**—*SYN:* Dick test
> **Dick test**—an intracutaneous test of susceptibility to the erythrogenic toxin of *Streptococcus pyogenes* responsible for the rash and other manifestations of scarlet fever. *SYN:* Dick method
> **Dick test toxin**—a test for scarlet fever antibodies. *SYN:* streptococcus erythrogenic toxin

Dick, Gladys R.H., U.S. internist, 1881–1963.
  Dick method—*SYN:* Dick test
  Dick test—see under Dick, George

Dickens, Frank, English biochemist, *1899.
  Dickens shunt—a secondary pathway for the oxidation of *d*-glucose (not occurring in skeletal muscle), generating reducing power in the cytoplasm outside the mitochondria and synthesizing pentoses and a few other sugars. *SYN:* Warburg-Lipmann-Dickens-Horecker shunt; pentose phosphate pathway
  Warburg-Lipmann-Dickens-Horecker shunt—*SYN:* Dickens shunt

Dieffenbach, Johann F., German surgeon, 1792–1847.
  Dieffenbach method—plastic surgery for covering a defect by sliding a flap with broad pedicle.

Diego, Venezuelan patient in whom a blood group antigen was originally found.
  Diego antigen—dominant inherited blood group antigen presumably of Mongolian origin.

Dieker, H., U.S. physician.
  Miller-Dieker syndrome—see under Miller, James

Diels, Otto, German chemist and Nobel laureate, 1876–1954.
  Diels hydrocarbon—a phenanthrene derivative obtained by the dehydrogenation of various steroids.

Dietl, Józef, Polish physician, 1804–1878.
  Dietl crisis—paroxysmal attacks of lumbar and abdominal pain with nausea and vomiting, resulting from kinking of the ureter in persons with floating kidney. *SYN:* incarceration symptom

Dieulafoy, Georges, French physician, 1839–1911.
  Dieulafoy disease—*SYN:* Dieulafoy erosion
  Dieulafoy erosion—acute ulcerative gastroenteritis complicating pneumonia, possibly caused by overproduction of adrenal steroid hormones. *SYN:* Dieulafoy disease
  Dieulafoy lesion
  Dieulafoy theory—an obsolete theory that appendicitis is always the result of the transformation of the appendicular canal into a closed cavity.
  Dieulafoy vascular malformation of the stomach

DiGeorge, Angelo M., U.S. pediatrician, *1921.
  DiGeorge syndrome—a condition arising from developmental failure of the third and fourth pharyngeal pouches, associated with facial deformity, hypoparathyroidism, and deficiency in cellular (T-lymphocyte) immunity. *SYN:* congenital aplasia of thymus; immunodeficiency with hypoparathyroidism; pharyngeal pouch syndrome; third and fourth pharyngeal pouch syndrome

NOTES

D

123

Dighton, C.A.C., English otolaryngologist, *1885.
   Dighton syndrome—genetic trait causing abnormal fragility and plasticity of bone and deafness.

Dimmer, Friedrich, Austrian ophthalmologist, 1855–1926.
   Dimmer keratitis—coin-shaped or round, discrete, grayish areas 0.5 to 1.5 mm in diameter scattered throughout the various layers of the cornea. *Syn:* keratitis nummularis

Diogenes, of Sinope, Greek philosopher, 412–323 B.C.
   Diogenes cup—the palm of the hand when contracted and deepened by the action of the muscles on either side. *Syn:* poculum diogenis
   Diogenes syndrome—condition of self-neglect generally observed in older individuals, associated with deficiencies in nutrition.
   poculum diogenis—*Syn:* Diogenes cup

Dische, Zacharias, 20th century Austrian-U.S. biochemist, *1895.
   Dische reaction—the assay of DNA by means of the blue color formed with diphenylamine in acid (Dische reagent).
   Dische reagent—acid used in assay of DNA.
   Dische-Schwarz reagent—reagent used in the colorimetric detection of RNA.

Disse, Josef, German anatomist, 1852–1912.
   Disse space—the potential extravascular space between the liver sinusoids and liver parenchymal cells. *Syn:* perisinusoidal space

Dittrich, Franz, German pathologist, 1815–1859.
   Dittrich plugs—minute, dirty-grayish, foul-smelling masses of bacteria and fatty acid crystals in the sputum in pulmonary gangrene and fetid bronchitis. *Syn:* Traube plugs
   Dittrich stenosis—narrowing of the outflow tract of the right ventricle below the pulmonic valve. *Syn:* infundibular stenosis

Divry, P., Belgian neurologist.
   Divry-van Bogaert disease—multiple angiomas of skin and cerebral meninges with progressive loss of myelin in white matter.

Dodd, Harold C., English surgeon.
   Cockett and Dodd operation—see under Cockett

Döderlein, Albert, S.G., German obstetrician, 1860–1941.
   Döderlein bacillus—a large, Gram-positive bacterium occurring in normal vaginal secretions.

Doehle, var. of Döhle
   Doerfler, Leo, U.S. audiologist, *1919.
   Doerfler-Stewart test—used in differentiating between functional and organic hearing loss. *Syn:* D-S test

Dogiel, Alexander S., Russian histologist, 1852–1922.
   Dogiel corpuscle—an encapsulated sensory nerve ending.

Dogiel, Jan von, Russian anatomist and physiologist, 1830–1905.
   Dogiel cells—the different cell types in cerebrospinal ganglia.

Doherty, Peter C., joint winner of 1996 Nobel Prize for work related to immunity.

Döhle, Karl G.P., German histologist and pathologist, 1855–1928.

Döhle bodies—found in neutrophils of patients with infections, burns, trauma, pregnancy, or cancer. *Syn:* Döhle inclusions; leukocyte inclusions

Döhle inclusions—*Syn:* Döhle bodies

Döhle-Heller aortitis—a common manifestation of tertiary syphilis, involving the thoracic aorta, where destruction of elastic tissue in the media results in dilation and aneurysm formation. *Syn:* syphilitis aortitis

Doisy, Edward A., U.S. biochemist and Nobel laureate, 1893–1986.

Allen-Doisy test—see under Allen, Edgar

Allen-Doisy unit—see under Allen, Edgar

Dollinger, Albert, German physician, *1888.

Bielschowsky-Dollinger syndrome—*Syn:* Dollinger-Bielschowsky syndrome

Dollinger-Bielschowsky syndrome—genetic disorder with onset between three and four years of age, resulting in mental deterioration, hearing and visual disorders. *Syn:* Bielschowsky syndrome; Bielschowsky-Dollinger syndrome

Domagk, Gerhard, winner of 1939 Nobel Prize for work related to prontosil.

Donaldson, Susanne W., U.S. nurse.

Donaldson scale—a scale used to score a patient's activities of daily living.

Donath, Julius, German physician, 1870–1950.

Donath-Landsteiner cold autoantibody—an autoantibody of the IgG class responsible for paroxysmal cold hemoglobinuria. *Syn:* cold hemolysin

Donath-Landsteiner phenomenon—the hemolysis which results in a sample of blood of a subject of paroxysmal hemoglobinuria when the sample is cooled to around 5°C and then warmed again.

Landsteiner-Donath test

Donders, Franz C., Dutch ophthalmologist, 1818–1889.

Donders glaucoma—obsolete term for open-angle glaucoma.

Donders law—rotation of the eyeball is determined by the distance of an object from the median plane and the line of the horizon.

Donders pressure—an increase of about 6 mm Hg shown by a manometer connected with the trachea when the thorax of the corpse is opened, caused by the collapse of the lungs when air is admitted to the thorax.

Donders rings—an obsolete term for the iridescent rings or halos observed by a cloudy cornea due to acute glaucoma.

space of Donders—the space between the dorsum of the tongue and the hard palate when the mandible is in rest position following the expiratory cycle of respiration.

Donnan, Frederick G., English physical chemist, 1870–1956.

Donnan equilibrium—the equilibrium of small ions between a solution with charged macromolecules, and one without. *Syn:* Gibbs-Donnan equilibrium

Gibbs-Donnan equilibrium—*Syn:* Donnan equilibrium

NOTES

Donné, Alfred, French physician, 1801–1878.
   Donné corpuscle—one of numerous bodies present in the colostrum, supposed to be modified leukocytes containing fat droplets. *Syn:* colostrum corpuscle

Donohue, William L., Canadian pathologist, *1906.
   Donohue disease—a congenital form of dwarfism. *Syn:* leprechaunism

Donovan, Charles, Irish surgeon, 1863–1951.
   Donovan bodies—clusters of blue or black staining, bipolar chromatin condensations in large mononuclear cells in granulation tissue infected with *Calymmatobacterium granulomatis.*
   Leishman-Donovan body—see under Leishman

Doose, H., 20th century German pediatrician and epileptologist.
   Doose syndrome—a rare familial type of primary generalized myoclonic astatic epilepsy.

Doppler, Christian J., Austrian mathematician and physicist in U.S., 1803–1853.
   Doppler bidirectional test
   Doppler echocardiography—use of Doppler ultrasonography techniques to augment two-dimensional echocardiography by allowing velocities to be registered within the echocardiographic image. *Syn:* duplex echocardiography
   Doppler effect—a change in frequency is observed when the sound and observer are in relative motion away from or toward each other. *Syn:* Doppler phenomenon; Doppler principle
   Doppler flow test
   Doppler measurement
   Doppler phenomenon—*Syn:* Doppler effect
   Doppler principle—*Syn:* Doppler effect
   Doppler probe
   Doppler pulse evaluation
   Doppler scope
   Doppler shift—the magnitude of the frequency change in hertz when sound and observer are in relative motion away from or toward each other.
   Doppler ultrasonography—application of the Doppler effect in ultrasound to detect movement of scatterers (usually red blood cells) by the analysis of the change in frequency of the returning echoes.
   Doppler ultrasound flowmeter
   Doppler ultrasound segmental blood pressure testing

Dorello, Primo, Italian anatomist, *1872.
   Dorello canal—a bony canal sometimes found at the tip of the temporal bone enclosing the abducens nerve and inferior petrosal sinus.

Dorendorf, Hans, German physician, 1866–1953.
   Dorendorf sign—fullness of one supraclavicular groove in an aneurysm of the aortic arch.

Dorfman, Maurice L., 20th century Israeli dermatologist.
   Dorfman-Chanarin syndrome—congenital ichthyosis, leukocyte vacuoles, and variable involvement of other organ systems. *Syn:* neutral lipid storage disease

Döring, G., German neurologist.
Pette-Döring disease—see under Pette

Dormia, Enrico, Italian professor of urology.
Dormia basket—device used to remove calculi from ureter.
Dormia biliary stone basket
Dormia dislodger
Dormia extracorporeal shockwave lithotripsy system
Dormia gallstone lithotriptor
Dormia lithotriptor
Dormia stone basket
Dormia stone basket catheter
Dormia stone dislodger
Dormia ureteral basket
Dormia ureteral stone dislodger
Dormia waterbath lithotriptor

Dorno, Carl, Swiss climatologist, 1865–1942.
Dorno rays—the biologically active ultraviolet rays.

Dorset, Marion, U.S. bacteriologist, 1872–1935.
Dorset culture egg medium—a medium for cultivating *Mycobacterium tuberculosis.*

Douglas, Beverly, U.S. surgeon, *1891.
Douglas graft—obsolete term for sieve graft.

Douglas, Claude G., English physiologist, 1882–1963.
Douglas bag—a large bag in which expired gas is collected for several minutes to determine oxygen consumption in humans under conditions of actual work.

Douglas, James, Scottish anatomist in London, 1675–1742.
cavum douglasi—*SYN:* Douglas cul-de-sac
Douglas abscess—suppuration in Douglas pouch.
Douglas cul-de-sac—a pocket formed by the deflection of the peritoneum from the rectum to the uterus. *SYN:* rectouterine pouch; cavum douglasi; Douglas pouch
Douglas fold—a fold of peritoneum, containing the rectouterine muscle, forming the lateral boundary of the rectouterine (Douglas) pouch. *SYN:* sacrouterine fold
Douglas line—a crescentic line that marks the lower limit of the posterior layer of the sheath of the rectus abdominis muscle. *SYN:* arcuate line of rectus sheath
Douglas pouch—*SYN:* Douglas cul-de-sac

Douglas, John C., Irish obstetrician, 1777–1850.
Douglas mechanism—mechanism of spontaneous evolution in transverse lie.

(continued)

NOTES

Douglas (*continued*)

Douglas spontaneous evolution—a mechanism whereby molding of the fetus and impaction of the shoulder and prolapsed arm occurs in transverse lie, allowing vaginal delivery with the lateral aspect of the thorax following the prolapsed shoulder.

Dover, Thomas, English physician, 1660–1742.
Dover powder—a sedative.

Down, John Langdon H., English physician, 1828–1896.
Down syndrome—a chromosomal dysgenesis syndrome consisting of a variable constellation of abnormalities, caused by triplication or translocation of chromosome 21. *Syn:* trisomy 21 syndrome; Langdon Down syndrome
Langdon Down syndrome—*Syn:* Down syndrome

Downey, H., U.S. hematologist, 1877–1959.
Downey cell—the atypical lymphocyte of infectious mononucleosis.

Downey, June Etta, U.S. psychologist, 1875–1932.
Downey Will-Temperament Tests—use of handwriting tasks to measure differences in temperament and/or personality.

Downs, William B., U.S. orthodontist, 1899–1966.
Downs analysis—a series of cephalometric criteria used as an aid in orthodontic diagnosis.

Dox, Arthur W., U.S. chemist, *1882.
Czapek-Dox medium—*Syn:* Czapek solution agar

Doyère, Louis, French physiologist, 1811–1863.
Doyère eminence—the slightly elevated area of the striated muscle fiber surface that corresponds to the site of the motor end plate.

Doyle, J.B., U.S. gynecologist, *1907.
Doyle operation—paracervical uterine denervation.

Doyne, Robert Walter, English ophthalmologist, 1857–1916.
Doyne choroiditis—genetic trait resulting in retinal degeneration and retinal drusen.
Doyne honeycomb choroidopathy—obsolete term for macular drusen.
Doyne iritis—grey precipitate found on iris.

Dragendorff, Georg J.N., German physician and pharmaceutical chemist, 1836–1898.
Dragendorff solution
Dragendorff test—a qualitative test for bile.

Drager, Glenn A., U.S. neurologist, *1917.
Shy-Drager syndrome—see under Shy

Dräger, Heinrich, German manufacturer of industrial and diving respiratory apparatus, *1898.
Dräger respirometer—an inferential meter to measure tidal and minute volume.

Dragstedt, L.R., U.S. surgeon, 1893–1975.
Dragstedt operation—procedure for repair duodenal ulcer.

Draper, John W., English chemist, 1811–1882.
    Draper law—a chemical change is produced in a photochemical substance only by those light rays that are absorbed by that substance.

Drash, Allan, U.S. physician, *1931.
    Drash syndrome—pseudohermaphroditism.

Dresbach, Melvin, U.S. physician, 1874–1946.
    Dresbach anemia—inherited blood disorder resulting in elliptical red cells.
    Dresbach syndrome

Dressler, William, U.S. physician, 1890–1969.
    Dressler beat—presence of Dressler beats strongly supporting the diagnosis of ventricular tachycardia by interruption of it.
    Dressler syndrome—*Syn:* pericarditis

Dreyer, Georges, English pathologist, 1873–1934.
    Dreyer formula—an obsolete formula indicating relationship between vital capacity and body surface area.

Driesch, H.A.E., German biologist, 1867–1941.
    Driesch law of constant volume—number of cells determines total mass of an organ.

D

Drigalski, Wilhelm von, German bacteriologist, 1871–1950.
    Conradi-Drigalski agar—see under Conradi
    Drigalski-Conradi agar—*Syn:* Conradi-Drigalski agar

Drinker, Philip, U.S. industrial hygienist, 1894–1972.
    Drinker respirator—a mechanical respirator in which the body except the head is encased within a metal tank, which is sealed at the neck with an airtight gasket. *Syn:* iron lung; tank respirator

Drummond, Sir David, English physician, 1852–1932.
    artery of Drummond—artery formed by anastomoses between the right and left colic arteries. *Syn:* marginal artery of colon
    Drummond sign—in certain cases of aortic aneurysm, a puffing sound synchronous with cardiac systole, heard from the nostrils when the mouth is closed.

Du Bois-Reymond, Emil H., German physiologist, 1818–1896.
    Du Bois-Reymond law—a motor nerve responds, not to the absolute value, but to the alteration of value from moment to moment, of the electric current. *Syn:* law of excitation

Duane, Alexander, U.S. ophthalmologist, 1858–1926.
    Duane syndrome—a retraction of the globe and pseudoptosis on attempted adduction. *Syn:* retraction syndrome

Dubin, I. Nathan, U.S. pathologist, 1913–1980.
    Dubin-Johnson syndrome—*Syn:* chronic idiopathic jaundice

NOTES

Dubini, Angelo, Italian physician, 1813–1902.
   Dubini disease—infection of the central nervous system resulting in usually fatal form of chorea. *SYN:* electrolepsy

DuBois, Eugene F., U.S. physiologist, 1882–1959.
   Aub-DuBois table—see under Aub, Joseph
   DuBois formula—a formula for predicting a person's surface area from weight and height.
   Meeh-DuBois formula—see under Meeh

Dubois, Paul, French obstetrician, 1795–1871.
   Dubois abscesses—small cysts of the thymus reported in congenital syphilis but also found in the absence of syphilis. *SYN:* thymic abscesses; Dubois disease
   Dubois disease—*SYN:* Dubois abscesses

Duboscq, Jules, French optician, 1817–1886.
   Duboscq colorimeter—an apparatus for measuring the depth of tint in a fluid.

Dubowitz, Victor, South African-English pediatrician, *1931.
   Dubowitz score—a method of clinical assessment of gestational age in the newborn.
   Dubowitz syndrome—congenital dwarfism.

Dubreuil-Chambardel, Louis, French dentist, 1879–1927.
   Dubreuil-Chambardel syndrome—simultaneous caries of the upper incisor teeth occurring in either sex between the ages of 14 and 17.

Dubreuilh, M.W., 20th century French dermatologist.
   precancerous melanosis of Dubreuilh—obsolete term for lentigo maligna.

Duchenne, Guillaume B.A., French neurologist, 1806–1875.
   Aran-Duchenne disease—*SYN:* Lou Gehrig disease
   Duchenne attitude—paralysis of trapezius resulting in shoulder lowering on external rotation.
   Duchenne disease—(1) *SYN:* Duchenne dystrophy; (2) progressive bulbar paralysis.
   Duchenne dystrophy—the most common childhood muscular dystrophy, with onset usually before age 6. *SYN:* pseudohypertrophic muscular dystrophy; Duchenne disease (1); childhood muscular dystrophy
   Duchenne paralysis—brachial birth palsy in which there is paralysis of upper arm and shoulder girdle muscles due to lesion of upper trunk of brachial plexus or roots of fifth and sixth cervical roots.
   Duchenne sign—falling in of the epigastrium during inspiration in paralysis of the diaphragm.
   Duchenne syndrome—subacute or chronic anterior spinal paralysis combined with multiple neuritis.
   Duchenne-Aran disease—*SYN:* Lou Gehrig disease
   Duchenne-Erb paralysis—*SYN:* Erb palsy
   Duchenne-Erb syndrome—*SYN:* Erb palsy
   Duchenne-Griesinger disease—*SYN:* Duchenne muscular atrophy; Duchenne muscular dystrophy
   Erb-Duchenne paralysis—*SYN:* Erb palsy

Duckworth, Sir Dyce, English physician, 1840–1928.
  Duckworth phenomenon—respiratory arrest before cardiac arrest as a result of intracranial disease.

Ducrey, Augusto, Italian dermatologist, 1860–1940.
  Ducrey bacillus—a species which causes soft chancre (chancroid). *Syn: Haemophilus ducreyi*
  Ducrey test—an intradermal test, using inactivated *Haemophilus ducreyi*, for diagnosis of chancroid. *Syn:* Ito-Reenstierna test

Duddell, Benedict, 18th century English oculist.
  Duddell membrane—considered to be a highly developed basement membrane. *Syn:* posterior limiting layer of cornea

Duffy, patient in whom this antigen was first found in 1950.
  Duffy antigen—may be related to resistance to malarial infection.
  Duffy blood group

Dugas, Louis A., U.S. physician, 1806–1884.
  Dugas test—in the case of an injured shoulder, if the elbow cannot be made to touch the chest while the hand rests on the opposite shoulder, the injury is a dislocation and not a fracture of the humerus.

Duhot, Robert, 19th century Belgian urologist and dermatologist.
  Duhot line—line from the superior iliac spine to the sacral apex.

D

Duhring, Louis A., U.S. dermatologist, 1845–1913.
  Duhring disease—a chronic skin disease marked by a symmetric itching eruption of vesicles and papules that occur in groups. *Syn:* dermatitis herpetiformis

Dührssen, Alfred, German obstetrician-gynecologist, 1862–1933.
  Dührssen incisions—three surgical incisions of an incompletely dilated cervix used as a means of effecting immediate delivery of the fetus.
  Dührssen operation
  Dührssen tampon
  Dührssen vaginal fixation

Duke, William Waddell Duke, U.S. pathologist, 1883–1945.
  Duke bleeding time test—a bleeding time test in which an incision is made in the earlobe and the time until bleeding stops is measured.

Dukes, Clement, English physician, 1845–1925.
  Dukes disease—*Syn:* Filatov-Dukes disease
  Filatov-Dukes disease—see under Filatov, Nil

Dukes, Cuthbert E., English pathologist, 1890–1977.
  Dukes classification—a classification of the extent of operable adenocarcinoma of the colon or rectum: Dukes A, Dukes B, Dukes B_2, Dukes C_1, Dukes C_2.

Dulbecco, Renato, joint winner of 1975 Nobel Prize for work related to tumor viruses and cell material.

NOTES

Dulong, Pierre L., French chemist, 1785–1838.
Dulong-Petit law—the specific heats of many solid elements are inversely proportional to their atomic weights.

Dumontpallier, Alphonse, French physician, 1827–1899.
Dumontpallier pessary—*SYN:* Mayer pessary

Duncan, David Beattie, Australian-U.S. statistician, 1916*.
Duncan multiple-range test—a test designed to compare various means.

Duncan, James M., Scottish gynecologist, 1826–1890.
Duncan curet
Duncan endometrial biopsy curet
Duncan endometrial curet
Duncan fold
Duncan folds—the folds on the peritoneal surface of the uterus immediately after delivery.
Duncan mechanism—passage of the placenta from the uterus with the rough side foremost.
Duncan position
Duncan ventricle—a slitlike, fluid-filled space of variable width between the left and right transparent septum, which may communicate with the third ventricle. *SYN:* cavity of septum pellucidum

Duncan, one of the first individuals to carry recessive trait that causes propensity to malignant B-cell lymphoproliferative disease.
Duncan disease—immunodeficiency disease with propensity to B-cell malignant lymphoproliferative disease in the presence of Epstein-Barr virus, leading to death. *SYN:* Duncan syndrome
Duncan syndrome—*SYN:* Duncan disease

Dunlop, John, U.S. orthopedic surgeon, *1876.
Dunlop elbow traction
Dunlop sleeve
Dunlop stripper
Dunlop thrombus stripper
Dunlop traction

Dunn, R.L.
Lison-Dunn stain—see under Lison

Duplay, Emanuel Simon, French surgeon, 1836–1924.
Duplay disease—*SYN:* subacromial bursitis
Duplay syndrome

Dupré, 17th century Paris surgeon and anatomist.
Dupré muscle—*SYN:* articularis genu muscle

Dupuy-Dutemps, Louis, French ophthalmologist, 1871–1946.
Dupuy-Dutemps operation—a modified dacryocystorhinostomy for stenosis of the lacrimal duct.

Dupuytren, Baron Guillaume, French surgeon and surgical pathologist, 1777–1835.
Dupuytren amputation—amputation of the arm at the shoulder joint.
Dupuytren canal—one of the veins in the diploë of the cranial bones. *SYN:* diploic vein

Dupuytren contracture—a disease of the palmar fascia resulting in thickening and shortening of fibrous bands on the palmar surface of the hand and fingers.
Dupuytren diathesis
Dupuytren disease of the foot—nodular fibroblastic proliferation in plantar fascia of one or both feet. *Syn:* plantar fibromatosis
Dupuytren enterotome
Dupuytren exostosis
Dupuytren fascia—the thickened, central portion of the fascia ensheathing the hand. *Syn:* palmar aponeurosis
Dupuytren fracture—fracture of lower part of fibula, with dislocation of ankle. *Syn:* Pott I syndrome
Dupuytren hydrocele—bilocular hydrocele in which the sac fills the scrotum and also extends into the abdominal cavity beneath the peritoneum.
Dupuytren knife
Dupuytren operation
Dupuytren sign—(1) in congenital dislocation, free up and down movement of the head of the femur occuring upon intermittent traction; (2) a crackling sensation on pressure over the bone in certain cases of sarcoma.
Dupuytren splint
Dupuytren suture—a continuous Lembert suture.
Dupuytren tourniquet—an instrument for compression of the abdominal aorta.

Duran-Reynals, Francisco, U.S. bacteriologist, 1899–1958.
   Duran-Reynals permeability factor—a soluble enzyme product prepared from mammalian testes. *Syn:* hyaluronidase

Durante, Gustave, French physician, 1865–1934.
   Durante disease—abnormal fragility and plasticity of bone. *Syn:* osteogenesis imperfecta

Dürck, Hermann, German pathologist, 1869–1941.
   Dürck nodes—perivascular chronic inflammatory infiltrates in the brain, occurring in human trypanosomiasis.

Duret, Henri, French neurosurgeon, 1849–1921.
   Duret hemorrhage—small brainstem hemorrhage resulting from brainstem distortion secondary to transtentorial herniation.
   Duret lesion—small hemorrhage(s) in the floor of the fourth ventricle or beneath the aqueduct of Sylvius.

Durham, Arthur E., English surgeon, 1834–1895.
   Durham needle
   Durham operation
   Durham tracheostomy tube
   Durham tracheotomy trocar

(continued)

NOTES

Durham *(continued)*
Durham trocar
Durham tube—a jointed tracheotomy tube.

Duroziez, Paul L., French physician, 1826–1897.
Duroziez disease—congenital stenosis of the mitral valve.
Duroziez murmur—a two-phase murmur over peripheral arteries, especially the femoral artery, due to rapid ebb and flow of blood during aortic insufficiency. *SYN:* Duroziez sign
Duroziez sign—*SYN:* Duroziez murmur

Dusard, surname of individuals in which syndrome was discovered.
Dusard syndrome—autosomal dominant disorder of qualitatively abnormal fibrinogens; causes inadequate lysis of fibrin with probable thrombotic tendency.

Dutcher, Thomas F., U.S. pathologist, *1923.
Dutcher body—a type of cytoplasm found in benign and malignant conditions.

Dutton, Joseph Everett, English physician, 1877–1905.
Dutton disease—African tick-borne relapsing fever caused by *Borrelia duttonii* and spread by the soft tick, *Ornithodoros moubata*. *SYN:* Dutton relapsing fever
Dutton relapsing fever—*SYN:* Dutton disease

Duverney, Joseph G., French anatomist, 1648–1730.
Duverney fissures—(usually) two vertical fissures in the anterior portion of the cartilage of the external auditory meatus, filled by fibrous tissue. *SYN:* notches in cartilage of external acoustic meatus
Duverney foramen—the passage, below and behind the portal hepatis, connecting the two sacs of the peritoneum. *SYN:* epiploic foramen
Duverney gland—one of two mucoid-secreting tubuloalveolar glands on either side of the lower part of the vagina, the equivalent of the bulbourethral glands in the male. *SYN:* greater vestibular gland
Duverney muscle—*SYN:* lacrimal part of orbicularis oculi muscle

Dwyer, Allan Frederick, Australian orthopedic surgeon, 1920–1975.
Dwyer fusion—method of spinal fusion.
Dwyer instrumentation

Dwyer, Frederick Charles, English orthopedic surgeon.
Dwyer osteotomy—a procedure for club foot.

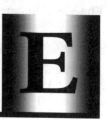

Eagle, Harry, U.S. physician and cell biologist, 1905–1992.

    Eagle basal medium—a solution of various salts used as a tissue culture medium.

    Eagle minimum essential medium—a tissue culture medium similar to Eagle basal medium but with different amounts and a few exclusions (e.g., antibiotics and phenol red).

Eagle, W., 20th century U.S. otolaryngologist.

    Eagle syndrome—facial pain due to an elongated styloid process.

Eales, Henry, English ophthalmologist, 1852–1913.

    Eales disease—peripheral retinal periphlebitis causing recurrent retinal or intravitreous hemorrhages in young adults.

Earle, Wilton R., U.S. pathologist, 1902–1962.

    Earle L fibrosarcoma—a transplantable fibrosarcoma derived from subcutaneous tissue of a mouse of C3H strain, grown in tissue culture to which 20-methylcholanthrene had been added.

    Earle medium

    Earle solution

Eaton, Lee M., U.S. neurologist, 1905–1958.

    Eaton-Lambert syndrome—*Syn:* Lambert-Eaton syndrome

    Lambert-Eaton syndrome—see under Lambert, Edward H.

Eaton, Monroe D., U.S. microbiologist, 1904–1958.

    Eaton agent—a species causing primary atypical pneumonia. *Syn: Mycoplasma pneumoniae*; Eaton virus

    Eaton agent pneumonia—an acute systemic disease with involvement of the lungs, caused by *Mycoplasma pneumoniae*. *Syn:* primary atypical pneumonia

    Eaton virus—*Syn:* Eaton agent

Ebbinghaus, Hermann, German, 1850–1909.

    Ebbinghaus test—a psychological test in which the patient is asked to complete certain sentences from which several words have been left out.

Eberth, Karl J., German physician, 1835–1926.

    Eberth bacillus—a species that causes typhoid fever and is transmitted in contaminated water and food. *Syn: Salmonella typhi*; typhoid bacillus

    Eberth lines—lines appearing between the cells of the myocardium when stained with silver nitrate.

    Eberth perithelium—an incomplete layer of connective tissue cells encasing the blood capillaries.

Ebner, Victor von. See under von Ebner.

Ebstein, Wilhelm, German physician, 1836–1912.
    Armanni-Ebstein change—see under Armanni
    Armanni-Ebstein kidney—*SYN:* Armanni-Ebstein change
    Armanni-Ebstein nephropathy—see under Armanni
    Ebstein anomaly—congenital downward displacement of the tricuspid valve into the right ventricle. *SYN:* Ebstein disease; Ebstein malformation
    Ebstein disease—*SYN:* Ebstein anomaly
    Ebstein malformation—*SYN:* Ebstein anomaly
    Ebstein sign—in pericardial effusion, obtuseness of the cardiohepatic angle on percussion.
    Murchison-Pel-Ebstein syndrome—see under Murchison
    Pel-Ebstein disease—*SYN:* Pel-Ebstein fever
    Pel-Ebstein fever—see under Pel

Eccles, Sir John Carew, joint winner of 1963 Nobel Prize for work related to nerve cell membrane.

Eck, Nikolai V., Russian physiologist, 1849–1917.
    Eck fistula—transposition of the portal circulation to the systemic by making an anastomosis between the vena cava and portal vein.
    reverse Eck fistula—side-to-side anastomosis of the portal vein with the inferior vena cava and ligation of the latter above the anastomosis but below the hepatic veins.

Ecker, Alexander, German anatomist, 1816–1887.
    Ecker fissure—a fissure between the petrous part of the temporal bone and the basilar part of the occipital bone that extends anteromedially from the jugular foramen. *SYN:* petro-occipital fissure

Ecker, Enrique E., U.S. bacteriologist, 1887–1966.
    Ecker fluid—dilating fluid.
    Rees-Ecker fluid—see under Rees

Ecklin, Theophil, Swiss physician.
    Ecklin anemia—a generally fatal form of anemia of the newborn.

Economo, Constantin von. See under von Economo.

Eddowes, A., English dermatologist, 1850–1946.
    Eddowes disease—osteogenesis imperfecta *SYN:* Eddowes syndrome
    Eddowes syndrome—*SYN:* Eddowes disease

Edelman, Gerald M., U.S. biochemist, *1929, co-winner of the 1972 Nobel Prize for his work in identifying and separating heavy and light chains in antibody molecules.

Edelmann, Adolf, Polish physician, 1885–1939.
    Edelmann syndrome—(1) chronic infectious anemia; (2) chronic pancreatitis.

Edinburgh University, institution of higher learning in Edinburgh, Scotland.
    Edinburgh University solution—antiseptic wound irrigation solution. *SYN:* Eusol
    Eusol—*SYN:* Edinburgh University solution

Edinger, Ludwig, German anatomist, 1855–1918.
    Edinger-Westphal nucleus—a small group of preganglionic parasympathetic motor neurons in the midline near the rostral pole of the oculomotor nucleus of the midbrain.

Edlefsen, Gustav J.F., German physician, 1842–1910.
    Edlefsen reagent—an alkaline permanganate solution used in the determination of sugar in the urine.

Edman, Pehr, Australian scientist, 1916–1977.
    Edman method
    Edman reagent—a method of identifying N-terminal amino acids. *Syn:* phenylisothiocyanate

Edridge-Green, Frederick W., English ophthalmologist, 1863–1953.
    Edridge-Green lamp—a test for color blindness now seldom used.

Edsall, David L., U.S. physician, 1869–1945.
    Edsall disease—heat cramp. *Syn:* myalgia thermica

Edwards, James Hilton, English physician and medical geneticist, *1928.
    Edwards Personal Preferences Schedule—personality inventory test.
    Edwards syndrome—characterized by mental retardation, abnormal skull shape, lowset and malformed ears, small mandible, cardiac defects, short sternum, diaphragmatic or inguinal hernia, Meckel diverticulum, abnormal flexion of fingers, and dermatoglyphic anomalies. *Syn:* trisomy 18 syndrome

Edwards, M.L., U.S. physician, *1906.
    Carpentier-Edwards aortic valve prosthesis
    Carpentier-Edwards bioprosthesis
    Carpentier-Edwards bioprosthetic valve
    Carpentier-Edwards mitral annuloplasty valve
    Carpentier-Edwards pericardial valve
    Carpentier-Edwards porcine prosthetic valve
    Carpentier-Edwards valve
    Starr-Edwards aortic valve prosthesis—see under Starr
    Starr-Edwards ball valve prosthesis—see under Starr
    Starr-Edwards ball-cage valve—see under Starr
    Starr-Edwards disk valve prosthesis—see under Starr
    Starr-Edwards heart valve—see under Starr
    Starr-Edwards hermetically sealed pacemaker—see under Starr
    Starr-Edwards mitral prosthesis—see under Starr
    Starr-Edwards pacemaker—see under Starr
    Starr-Edwards prosthesis—see under Starr
    Starr-Edwards prosthetic aortic valve—see under Starr
    Starr-Edwards prosthetic mitral valve—see under Starr
    Starr-Edwards Silastic valve—see under Starr
    Starr-Edwards silicone rubber ball valve—see under Starr
    Starr-Edwards valve—see under Starr

E

NOTES

Efron, M.L.
    Paine-Efron syndrome—see under Paine

Egger, Fritz, Swiss internist, 1863–1938.
    Egger line—seldom-used term for the circular line of adhesion between the vitreous and posterior lens.

Eggers, George William Nordholtz, U.S. orthopedic surgeon, 1896–1963.
    Eggers bone plate
    Eggers contact splint
    Eggers neurectomy
    Eggers plate—orthopedic fixation plate.
    Eggers screw
    Eggers tendon transfer
    Eggers tenodesis

Eggleston, Cary, U.S. physician, 1884–1966.
    Bradbury-Eggleston syndrome—see under Bradbury
    Eggleston method—obsolete term for rapid digitalization by means of large doses of digitalis leaf or tincture frequently repeated.
    Eggleston-Bradbury syndrome—*Syn:* Bradbury-Eggleston syndrome

Ehlers, Edward L., Danish dermatologist, 1863–1937.
    Ehlers-Danlos syndrome—a group of inherited generalized connective tissue diseases.

Ehrenritter, Johann, Austrian anatomist, d. 1790.
    Ehrenritter ganglion—the upper and smaller of two ganglia on the glossopharyngeal nerve as it traverses the jugular foramen. *Syn:* superior ganglion of glossopharyngeal nerve

Ehret, Heinrich, German physician, *1870.
    Ehret phenomenon—a sudden throb felt by the finger on the brachial artery, said to indicate fairly accurately the diastolic pressure.
    Ehret syndrome—efforts to compensate for pain by assuming the least painful posture resulting in contractures and muscle atrophy.

Ehrlich, Paul, German bacteriologist, immunologist, and Nobel laureate, 1854–1915.
    Ehrlichia—a genus of small, often pleomorphic, coccoid to ellipsoidal, nonmotile, Gram-negative bacteria (order Rickettsiales) that are the etiologic agents of ehrlichiosis and are transmitted by ticks.
    Ehrlich anemia—anemia resulting from hypoplastic or aplastic bone marrow. *Syn:* aplastic anemia
    Ehrlich diazo reagent—two solutions, one of sodium nitrite, the other of acidified sulfanilic acid, used in bringing about diazotization. *Syn:* diazo reagent
    Ehrlich inner body—a round oxyphil body found in the red blood cell in case of hemocytolysis due to a specific blood poison. *Syn:* Heinz-Ehrlich body
    Ehrlich phenomenon—the difference between the amount of diphtheria toxin that will exactly neutralize one unit of antitoxin.
    Ehrlich postulate—that cells contain surface extensions or side chains (haptophores) that bind to the antigenic determinants of a toxin (toxophores). *Syn:* side-chain theory

Ehrlich side-chain theory

Ehrlich test—urobilinogen test using Ehrlich reagent.

Ehrlich theory—*Syn:* side-chain theory

Ehrlich tumor—solid or ascitic transplantable tumor derived from breast carcinoma in mice.

Ehrlich unit

Ehrlich-Türk line—seldom-used term for the thin vertical deposition of material on the posterior surface of the cornea seen in uveitis.

Heinz-Ehrlich body—*Syn:* Ehrlich inner body

Eichhorst, Hermann L., Swiss physician, 1849–1921.

Eichhorst corpuscles—the globular forms sometimes occurring in the poikilocytosis of pernicious anemia.

Eichhorst neuritis—inflammation of the connective tissue framework of a nerve. *Syn:* interstitial neuritis

Eicken, Karl von, German laryngologist, 1873–1960.

Eicken method—facilitation of hypopharyngoscopy by means of forward traction on the cricoid cartilage by a laryngeal probe.

Eijkman, Christiaan, Dutch physiologist, 1858–1930, co-winner of the 1929 Nobel Prize for the discovery of thiamine, an antineuritic vitamin.

Eimer, Gustav Heinrich Theodor, German zoologist, 1843–1898.

Eimeria—the largest, most economically important, and most widespread genus of the coccidial protozoa (family Eimeriidae, class Sporozoea).

Einthoven, Willem, Dutch physiologist and Nobel laureate, 1860–1927.

Einthoven equation—*Syn:* Einthoven law

Einthoven law—in the electrocardiogram the potential of any wave or complex in lead II is equal to the sum of its potentials of leads I and III. *Syn:* Einthoven equation

Einthoven string galvanometer—the original instrument on which Einthoven developed the first electrocardiogram.

Einthoven triangle—an imaginary equilateral triangle with the heart at its center, its equal sides representing the three standard limb leads of the electrocardiogram.

Eisenlohr, Carl, German physician, 1847–1896.

Eisenlohr syndrome—numbness and weakness in the extremities; paralysis of the lips, tongue, and palate; and dysarthria.

Eisenmenger, Victor, German physician, 1864–1932.

Eisenmenger complex—the combination of ventricular septal defect with pulmonary hypertension and consequent right-to-left shunt through the defect, with or without an associated overriding aorta. *Syn:* Eisenmenger disease; Eisenmenger tetralogy; Eisenmenger defect

Eisenmenger defect—*Syn:* Eisenmenger complex

Eisenmenger disease—*Syn:* Eisenmenger complex

(continued)

NOTES

Eisenmenger *(continued)*
　　Eisenmenger syndrome—cardiac failure usually due to the Eisenmenger complex, a ventricular septal defect.
　　Eisenmenger tetralogy—*SYN:* Eisenmenger complex

Eisenson, Jon, U.S. speech pathologist.
　　Eisenson test—a test for aphasia.

Ejrup, Erick, 20th century Swedish internist.
　　Ejrup maneuver—demonstration of collateral circulation by reduction in the prominence of activity of the greater arteries and reduced pulse volume following muscular activity.

Ekbom, K.A., Swedish neurologist, *1907.
　　Ekbom syndrome—*SYN:* restless legs syndrome

Ekman, Olof J., Swedish physician, 1764–1839.
　　Ekman syndrome—abnormal fragility and plasticity of bone. *SYN:* osteogenesis imperfecta.

Elaut, Leon J.S., 20th century Belgian pathologist.
　　Elaut triangle—triangle formed by the iliac arteries and the promontory of the sacrum.

Elion, Gertrude B., joint winner of 1988 Nobel Prize for work related to drug treatment.

Ellenberg, Max, U.S. physician.
　　Ellenberg syndrome—peripheral neuropathy associated with diabetes mellitus; spontaneous recovery has been noted.

Ellik, Milo, U.S. urologist, *1905.
　　Ellik bladder evacuator
　　Ellik evacuator—an instrument used to evacuate tissue fragments, blood clots, or calculi from the urinary bladder.
　　Ellik kidney stone basket
　　Ellik loop stone dislodger
　　Ellik meatotome
　　Ellik sound

Elliot, John W., U.S. surgeon, 1852–1925.
　　Elliot position—a supine position used to facilitate abdominal section.

Elliot, Robert H., English ophthalmologist, 1864–1936.
　　Elliot corneal trephination
　　Elliot operation—trephining of the eyeball at the corneoscleral margin to relieve tension caused by glaucoma.

Elliott, Thomas R., English physician, 1877–1961.
　　Elliott law—adrenaline acts upon those structures innervated by sympathetic nerve fibers.
　　Elliott treatment regulator—a regulator used to control heat, circulation, and pressure of water through Elliott applicators.

Ellis, Calvin, U.S. physician, 1826–1883.
　　Ellis sign—line of dullness related to pleuritic exudate resorption.

Ellis, Richard W.B., English physician, 1902–1966.

    Ellis-van Creveld syndrome—triad of chondrodysplasia, ectodermal dysplasia, and polydactyly, with congenital heart defects in over half of patients. *Syn:* chondroectodermal dysplasia

Ellison, Edwin H., U.S. physician, 1918–1970.

    Zollinger-Ellison syndrome—see under Zollinger

    Zollinger-Ellison tumor—see under Zollinger

Ellsworth, Read McLane, U.S. physician, 1899–1970.

    Ellsworth-Howard test—used in the diagnosis of pseudohypoparathyroidism.

Eloesser, Leo, U.S. thoracic surgeon, 1881–1976.

    Eloesser flap

    Eloesser procedure—transposition of a tonguelike skin flap pedicle from the chest wall into the depths of an incision that communicates with an empyema or peripheral lung abscess.

Elsberg, C.A., U.S. physician.

    Elsberg syndrome—acute urinary retention in women, often associated with genital herpes.

Elschnig, Anton, German ophthalmologist, 1863–1939.

    Elschnig blepharorrhaphy

    Elschnig bodies

    Elschnig canthorrhaphy

    Elschnig capsular forceps

    Elschnig cataract knife

    Elschnig corneal knife

    Elschnig cyclodialysis spatula

    Elschnig extrusion needle

    Elschnig eye spoon

    Elschnig iridectomy

    Elschnig lens scoop

    Elschnig lid retractor

    Elschnig pearls—the proliferated anterior capsule of the lens of the eye after surgical capsulotomy or injury.

    Elschnig pterygium knife

    Elschnig refractor

    Elschnig spots—isolated choroidal bright yellow or red spots with black pigment flecks at their borders, seen by ophthalmoscope in advanced hypertensive retinopathy.

    Elschnig syndrome—ocular deformities often associated with cleft palate.

    Elschnig trephine

    Koerber-Salus-Elschnig syndrome—*Syn:* Parinaud I syndrome

Elsner, Christoph F., German physician, 1749–1820.

    Elsner asthma—chest pain caused by oxygen deficiency in the heart muscle, often precipitated by stress, associated with pathological heart conditions.

E

NOTES

Ely, L.W., U.S. orthopedic surgeon, 1868–1944.
    Ely sign—discomfort indicative of hip lesion or psoas muscle irritation on testing.
    Ely test—a test for hip extension.

Embden, Gustav G., German biochemist, 1874–1933.
    Embden ester—significant in the understanding of sugar metabolism.
    Embden-Meyerhof pathway—the anaerobic glycolytic pathway by which D-glucose is converted to lactic acid. *SYN:* Embden-Meyerhof-Parnas pathway
    Embden-Meyerhof-Parnas pathway—*SYN:* Embden-Meyerhof pathway
    Robison-Embden ester—see under Robison

Emmet, Thomas A., U.S. gynecologist, 1828–1919.
    Emmet forceps
    Emmet hemostatic bag
    Emmet needle—a needle that is used to pass a ligature around an undissected structure.
    Emmet operation—suture repair of a cervix uteri laceration. *SYN:* trachelorrhaphy
    Emmet ovarian trocar
    Emmet probe
    Emmet tenaculum
    Emmet uterine probe
    Emmet uterine scissors

Enders, John F., U.S. microbiologist, 1897–1985, co-winner of the 1954 Nobel Prize for the discovery that some viruses can be grown, studied, and isolated, making vaccine production possible.

Endo, Shigeru, Japanese bacteriologist, 1869–1937.
    Endo agar—a medium useful in the bacteriological examination of water. *SYN:* Endo medium
    Endo fuchsin agar—nutrient agar used as a culture medium to differentiate *Salmonella typhi* from coliform bacteria. *SYN:* fuchsin agar
    Endo medium—*SYN:* Endo agar

Engelmann, Guido, German surgeon, *1876.
    Camurata-Engelmann syndrome—*SYN:* Engelmann disease
    Engelmann disease—progressive, symmetrical fusiform enlargement of the shafts of long bones. *SYN:* Camurata-Engelmann syndrome; diaphysial dysplasia

Engelmann, Theodor W., German physiologist, 1843–1909.
    Engelmann basal knobs—obsolete term for blepharoplast.

Englisch, Josef, Austrian physician, 1835–1915.
    Englisch sinus—a paired dural venous sinus running in the groove on the petrooccipital fissure connecting the cavernous sinus with the superior bulb of the internal jugular vein. *SYN:* inferior petrosal sinus

Enroth, Emil, Finnish ophthalmologist, 1879–1953.
    Enroth sign—in Graves disease, edema of the eyelids, especially of the upper eyelid near the supraorbital margin.

Epple, associate of Leonard S. Fosdick.
    Fosdick-Hansen-Epple test—see under Fosdick

Epstein, A.A., U.S. physician, 1880–1965.
    Epstein syndrome—symptoms include edema, protein concentration in urine, low concentration of albumin in the blood, and hyperlipidemia. *Syn:* nephrotic syndrome

Epstein, Alois, German pediatrician, 1849–1918.
    Epstein disease—one of a group of local infections suggesting diphtheria, but caused by microorganisms other than *Corynebacterium diphtheriae.* *Syn:* diphtheroid
    Epstein pearls—multiple small white epithelial inclusion cysts found in the midline of the palate in newborn infants.
    Epstein sign—lid retraction in an infant, giving it a frightened expression and a wild glance.
    Epstein symptom

Epstein, E., German physician.
    Epstein-Goedel syndrome—hematological disorder resulting in prolonged bleeding time despite increased platelets; accompanied by splenomegaly, hematemesis, and thrombosis.

Epstein, Michael Anthony, English virologist, *1921.
    Epstein-Barr virus—a herpesvirus that causes infectious mononucleosis. *Syn:* EB virus

Eranko, Eino, Finnish anatomist, *1924.
    Eranko fluorescence stain—exposure of frozen sections to formaldehyde, which produces a strong yellow-green fluorescence from cells containing norepinephrine.

Erasmus, L.D., South African physician.
    Erasmus syndrome—scleroderma with silicosis, associated with pulmonary symptoms.

Erb, Wilhelm H., German neurologist, 1840–1921.
    Duchenne-Erb paralysis—*Syn:* Erb palsy
    Duchenne-Erb syndrome—*Syn:* Erb palsy
    Erb atrophy—a form of progressive muscular atrophy in which the disease begins in the muscle and not in the spinal centers. *Syn:* progressive muscular dystrophy
    Erb disease—progressive weakness and atrophy of the muscles of the tongue, lips, palate, pharynx, and larynx, most often caused by motor neuron disease. *Syn:* progressive bulbar paralysis
    Erb formula—the portion of the brachial plexus that can be stimulated through intact skin.
    Erb palsy—a type of brachial birth palsy in which there is paralysis of the muscles of the upper arm and shoulder girdle. *Syn:* Erb paralysis;

(continued)

NOTES

E

Erb *(continued)*

Duchenne-Erb paralysis; Duchenne-Erb syndrome; Erb-Duchenne paralysis

Erb paralysis—*Syn:* Erb palsy

Erb sign—*Syn:* Erb-Westphal sign

Erb spinal paralysis—chronic myelitis of syphilitic origin.

Erb-Charcot disease—a type of cerebral palsy. *Syn:* spastic diplegia; spastic paraplegia

Erb-Duchenne paralysis—*Syn:* Erb palsy

Erb-Goldflam disease—*Syn:* Goldflam disease

Erb-Westphal sign—abolition of the patellar tendon reflex in certain diseases of the spinal cord and occasionally in brain disease. *Syn:* Westphal phenomenon; Erb sign; Westphal sign; Westphal-Erb sign

Goldflam-Erb disease

Nievergelt-Erb syndrome—*Syn:* Nievergelt syndrome

Westphal-Erb sign—*Syn:* Erb-Westphal sign

Erben, Siegmund, Austrian neurologist, *1863.

Erben phenomenon—vagal stimulation slowing of the pulse when head and trunk are flexed. *Syn:* Erben reflex; Erben sign

Erben reflex—*Syn:* Erben phenomenon

Erben sign—*Syn:* Erben phenomenon

Erdheim, Jakob, Austrian physician, 1874–1937.

Erdheim disease—a disease of unknown cause that may be inherited and that predisposes to dissecting aneurysms. *Syn:* cystic medial necrosis

Erdheim syndrome—acromegaly causing cervical stiffening and often associated with clavicular hypertrophy. *Syn:* Scaglietti-Dagnini syndrome

Erdheim tumor—a suprasellar neoplasm, usually cystic, that develops from the nests of epithelium derived from Rathke pouch. *Syn:* craniopharyngioma

Erdmann, Hugo, German chemist, 1862–1910.

Erdmann reagent—a mixture of sulfuric and nitric acids, used in testing alkaloids.

Erichsen, Sir John, English surgeon, 1818–1896.

Erichsen disease—neurosis following spinal injury. *Syn:* railway spine

Erichsen sign—in sacroiliac disease, pain when sudden pressure approximates the iliac bones.

Erlanger, Joseph, U.S. physiologist, 1874–1965, joint winner of 1944 Nobel Prize for work related to nerve fibers.

Erlenmeyer, Emil, German chemist, 1825–1909.

Erlenmeyer flask—shaped so that its liquid content can be shaken laterally without spilling.

Erlenmeyer flask deformity—a deformity at the distal end of the femur with the result that the bone is wide for a much longer distance up the shaft than normal.

Ernst, Paul, German pathologist, 1859–1937.

Babès-Ernst bodies—see under Babès

Babès-Ernst granules—*Syn:* Babès-Ernst bodies

Ernst-Babès granules—*Syn:* Babès-Ernst bodies

Esbach, Georges H., French physician, 1843–1890.
  Esbach reagent—picric acid, citric acid, and water (in the proportions 1, 2, and 97) used for the detection of albumin in the urine.

Escamilla, Roberto Francisco, Mexican-U.S. physician, *1905.
  Escamilla-Lisser syndrome—adult hypothyroidism.
  Escamilla-Lisser-Shepardson syndrome

Escat, Etienne, French physician, 1865–1948.
  Escat phlegmon—abscess of connective tissue in the region of tonsils.

Escherich, Theodor, German physician, 1857–1911.
  Escherichia coli—a species that occurs normally in the intestines of humans and is a frequent cause of infections of the urogenital tract and of diarrhea in infants. *Syn:* colibacillus; colon bacillus
  Escherich sign—in hypoparathyroidism (latent tetany) tapping the skin at the angle of the mouth causes protrusion of the lips.

Escobar, Victor, 20th century U.S. physician.
  Escobar syndrome—syndrome manifested by orthopedic and cranial anomalies due to recessive trait. *Syn:* multiple pterygium syndrome

Esmarch, Johann F.A. von, German surgeon, 1823–1908.
  Esmarch bandage—*Syn:* Esmarch tourniquet
  Esmarch operation
  Esmarch probe
  Esmarch roll dressing
  Esmarch scissors
  Esmarch shears
  Esmarch tin bullet probe
  Esmarch tourniquet—a narrow hard rubber tourniquet with a chain fastener. *Syn:* Esmarch bandage
  Esmarch tube

Esser, Johannes F.S., Dutch surgeon, 1877–1946.
  Esser eyelid operation
  Esser graft—a skin graft wrapped (raw side out) around a bolus of dental compound and inserted into a prepared surgical pocket. *Syn:* inlay graft
  Esser implant
  Esser operation
  Esser prosthesis

Essick, C., 20th century U.S. anatomist.
  Essick cell bands—groups of cells in the developing rhombencephalon which migrate in two bands, one of which eventually forms the inferior olivary nucleus and the arcuate nucleus, and the other the pontine nuclei.

Estes, William L., Jr., U.S. surgeon, 1885–1940.
  Estes operation—an operation for sterility in which a portion of an ovary is implanted on one uterine cornu.

E

NOTES

Estlander, Jakob A., Finnish surgeon, 1831–1881.
    Abbe-Estlander cheiloplasty
    Estlander cheiloplasty
    Estlander flap—a full-thickness flap of the lip, transferred from the side of one lip to the same side of the other lip.
    Estlander operation—use of an Estlander flap in plastic surgery of the lips.

Eulenburg, Albert, German neurologist, 1840–1917.
    Eulenburg disease—a nonprogressive myotonia induced by exposure of muscles to cold. *SYN:* congenital paramyotonia

Euler, Ulf Von, Swedish physiologist, 1905–1983, joint winner of 1970 Nobel Prize for work related to neural transmittors.

Eustachio, Bartolommeo E., Italian anatomist, 1524–1574.
    eustachian catheter—a catheter used for catheterization of the middle ear through the eustachian tube.
    eustachian cushion—a ridge in the nasopharyngeal wall posterior to the opening of the eustachian tube. *SYN:* torus tubarius
    eustachian tonsil—a collection of lymphoid nodules near the pharyngeal opening of the auditory tube. *SYN:* tubal tonsil
    eustachian tube—a tube leading from the tympanic cavity to the nasopharynx. *SYN:* auditory tube; tuba eustachiana; tuba eustachii
    eustachian tuber—a slight projection from the labyrinthine wall of the middle ear below the fenestra vestibuli (ovalis).
    eustachian valve—an endocardial fold extending from the anterior inferior margin of the inferior vena cava to the anterior part of the limbus fossa ovalis. *SYN:* valve of inferior vena cava
    tuba eustachiana—*SYN:* eustachian tube
    tuba eustachii—*SYN:* eustachian tube

Evans, Dillwyn, Welsh orthopedic surgeon, 1910–1974.
    Dillwyn Evans procedure—procedure related to club foot.

Evans, H.M., U.S. anatomist and physiologist, 1882–1971.
    Evans blue—a diazo dye used as a vital stain for following diffusion through blood vessel walls. *SYN:* azovan blue

Evans, Robert S., U.S. physician, *1912.
    Evans syndrome—acquired hemolytic anemia and thrombocytopenia.

Everett, Charles E., a patient at the Georgia Warm Springs Foundation for whom the crutch was made.
    Everett crutch—aluminum variety of crutch. *SYN:* Warm Springs crutch; metal triceps crutch

Eversbusch, Oskar, German ophthalmologist, 1853–1912.
    Eversbusch operation—correction of upper eyelid ptosis.

Ewart, William, English physician, 1848–1929.
    Ewart procedure—elevation of the larynx between the thumb and forefinger to elicit tracheal tugging.
    Ewart sign—in large pericardial effusions, an area of dullness with bronchial breathing and bronchophony below the angle of the left scapula. *SYN:* Pins sign

Ewing, James H., pathologist, 1798–1827.

    Ewing sign—dullness on percussion to the inner side of the angle of the left scapula, denoting an accumulation of fluid in the pericardium behind the heart.

Ewing, James, U.S. pathologist, 1866–1943.

    Ewing sarcoma—*Syn:* Ewing tumor

    Ewing tumor—a malignant neoplasm that involves bones of the extremities, including the shoulder girdle, with a predilection for the metaphysis. *Syn:* endothelial myeloma; Ewing sarcoma

Exner, Siegmund, Austrian physiologist, 1846–1926.

    Call-Exner bodies—see under Call

    Exner plexus—a plexus formed by tangential nerve fibers in the superficial plexiform or molecular layer of the cerebral cortex.

Exton, William G., U.S. physician, 1876–1943.

    Exton reagent—a test for albumin.

Eysenck, Hans J., German-English psychologist, *1916.

    Eysenck Personality Inventory

E

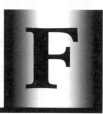

Faber, Knud H., Danish physician, 1862–1956.
    Faber anemia—a form of chronic hypochromic microcytic anemia associated with achlorhydria or achylia gastrica. *Syn:* achlorhydric anemia; Faber syndrome
    Faber syndrome—*Syn:* Faber anemia

Fabricius, Girolamo (Hieronymus ab Aquapendente), Italian anatomist and embryologist, 1537–1619.
    bursa fabricii—in poultry, a blind saclike structure located on the posterodorsal wall of the cloaca. *Syn:* bursa of Fabricius
    bursa of Fabricius—*Syn:* bursa fabricii
    Fabricius ship—the outlines of the sphenoid, occipital, and frontal bones, from their fancied resemblance to the hull of a ship.

Fabry, Johannes, German dermatologist, 1860–1930.
    Anderson-Fabry disease—*Syn:* Fabry disease
    Fabry disease—an X-linked recessive disorder of glycosphingolipid metabolism. *Syn:* diffuse angiokeratoma; glycolipid lipidosis; Anderson-Fabry disease

Faget, Jean C., French physician, 1818–1884.
    Faget sign—a slow pulse with an elevated temperature, often seen in yellow fever.

Fahr, Theodore, German physician, 1877–1945.
    Fahr disease—progressive calcific deposition in the walls of blood vessels of the basal ganglia, occasionally associated with mental retardation and extrapyramidal symptoms.

Fahraeus, Robert (Robin) Sanno, Swedish pathologist, 1888–1968.
    Fahraeus method
    Fahraeus-Lindqvist effect—decrease in apparent viscosity that occurs when a suspension, such as blood, is made to flow through a tube of smaller diameter.

Fahrenheit, Gabriel D., German-Dutch physicist, 1686–1736.
    Fahrenheit scale—a thermometer scale in which the freezing point of water is 32°F and the boiling point of water 212°F.

Fairbank disease—*Syn:* hyperostosis generalisata

Fairley, K.F., Australian physician, *1927.
    Fairley test—test to identify site of infection within the bladder.

Fallopius, Gabriele, Italian anatomist, 1523–1562.

 fallopian aqueduct—the bony passage in the temporal bone through which the facial nerve passes. *Syn:* facial canal; fallopian canal

 fallopian arch—*Syn:* fallopian ligament

 fallopian artery

 fallopian canal—*Syn:* fallopian aqueduct

 fallopian cannula

 fallopian catheter

 fallopian hiatus—the opening on the anterior aspect of the petrous part of the temporal bone which leads to the facial canal and gives passage to the greater petrosal nerve. *Syn:* hiatus of facial canal

 fallopian ligament—forms the floor of the inguinal canal and gives origin to lowermost fibers of internal oblique and transversus abdominis muscles. *Syn:* fallopian arch; inguinal ligament

 fallopian neuritis—*Syn:* facial paralysis

 fallopian pregnancy—*Syn:* tubal pregnancy

 fallopian tube—one of the tubes leading on either side from the upper or outer extremity of the ovary to the fundus of the uterus. *Syn:* uterine tube; tuba fallopiana

 tuba fallopiana—*Syn:* fallopian tube

 tuba fallopii

Fallot, Étienne-Louis A., French physician, 1850–1911.

 Fallot tetrad—*Syn:* tetralogy of Fallot

 Fallot tetralogy—*Syn:* tetralogy of Fallot

 Fallot triad—*Syn:* trilogy of Fallot

 pentalogy of Fallot—Fallot tetralogy with, in addition, a patent foramen ovale or atrial septal defect.

 tetralogy of Fallot—a set of congenital cardiac defects. *Syn:* Fallot tetrad; Fallot tetralogy

 trilogy of Fallot—atrial septal defect associated with pulmonic stenosis and right ventricular hypertrophy. *Syn:* Fallot triad

Falls, H.F., U.S. internist, *1911.

 Rundles-Falls syndrome—see under Rundles

Falret, Jean-Pierre, French psychiatrist, 1794–1870.

 Falret disease—manic-depressive psychosis. *Syn:* circular insanity; cyclic insanity

Falta, Wilhelm, Austrian physician, 1875–1950.

 Falta syndrome—insuffiency of the pituitary and other glands.

Fañanás, J., Spanish physician.

 Fañanás cell—a specialized astrocyte found in the cerebellar cortex.

Fanconi, Guido, Swiss pediatrician, 1892–1979.

 De Toni-Fanconi syndrome—see under De Toni

 Debré-De Toni-Fanconi syndrome—*Syn:* Fanconi syndrome (2)

 Fanconi anemia—a type of idiopathic refractory anemia characterized by pancytopenia, hypoplasia of the bone marrow, and congenital anomalies. *Syn:* congenital pancytopenia; congenital aplastic anemia; Fanconi syndrome (1)

 Fanconi pancytopenia—*Syn:* congenital pancytopenia

Fanconi syndrome—(1) *SYN:* Fanconi anemia; (2) a group of conditions with characteristic disorders of renal tubular function.
Lignac-Fanconi syndrome—see under Lignac
Wissler-Fanconi syndrome—see under Wissler

Farabeuf, Louis H., French surgeon, 1841–1910.
Farabeuf amputation—amputation of the leg or of the foot.
Farabeuf bone-holding forceps
Farabeuf double-ended retractor
Farabeuf elevator
Farabeuf forceps
Farabeuf raspatory
Farabeuf retractor
Farabeuf saw
Farabeuf triangle—the triangle formed by the internal jugular and facial veins and the hypoglossal nerve.

Faraday, Michael, English physicist and chemist, 1791–1867.
farad—a practical unit of electrical capacity.
faraday—96,485.309 Coulombs per mole, the amount of electricity required to reduce one equivalent of silver ion.
Faraday cage—cage designed to enclose and protect an electric instrument from outside electric interference.
Faraday constant
Faraday laws—the amount of an electrolyte decomposed by an electric current is proportional to the amount of the current.
faradic bath—water bath in which there is faradic current.
faradic current—current that stimulates muscle through its nerve.
faradism—*SYN:* faradization
faradization—use of the faradic current. *SYN:* faradism

Farber, Sidney, U.S. pediatric pathologist, 1903–1973.
Farber disease—a form of mucolipodosis, developing soon after birth because of deficiency of ceramidase. *SYN:* disseminated lipogranulomatosis; Farber syndrome
Farber syndrome—*SYN:* Farber disease

Farnsworth, Dean, U.S. naval officer, 1902–1959.
Farnsworth-Munsell color test—a test for color perception.

Farr, William, English medical statistician, 1807–1883.
Farr law—the curve of cases of an epidemic rises rapidly at first, then climbs slowly to a peak from which the fall is steeper than the previous rise.

Farre, Arthur, English obstetrician and gynecologist, 1811–1887.
Farre line—a whitish line marking the insertion of the mesovarium at the hilum of the ovary.

NOTES

Farre, John R., English physician, 1775–1862.
Farre tubercles—masses beneath the liver capsule, sometimes associated with hepatic carcinoma.

Fauchard, Pierre, French dentist, 1678–1761.
Fauchard disease—marginal periodontitis.

Faught, Francis A., 20th century U.S. chemist.
Faught sphygmomanometer

Favre, Maurice, French physician, 1876–1954.
Favre disease—(1) lymphogranuloma venereum; (2) venous insufficiency resulting in angiodermatitis of lower limbs.
Gamna-Favre bodies—see under Gamna
Nicolas-Favre disease—see under Nicolas

Fay, Temple S., U.S. neurosurgeon, 1895–1963.
Fay exercises—*Syn:* Fay reflex therapy
Fay method—*Syn:* Fay reflex therapy
Fay reflex therapy—exercise used for patients with neuromuscular disorders. *Syn:* Fay exercises; Fay method
Fay suction elevator
Fay suction tube

Fazio, E., Italian physician, 1849–1902.
Fazio-Londe atrophy—hereditary trait leading to muscular atrophy. *Syn:* Fazio-Londe disease
Fazio-Londe disease—*Syn:* Fazio-Londe atrophy

Fechner, Gustav T., German physicist, 1801–1887.
Fechner paradox—refers to apparent increase in brightness of a figure when viewed with one eye after first viewing with both eyes.
Fechner-Weber law—*Syn:* Weber-Fechner law
Weber-Fechner law—see under Weber

Fede, Francesco, Italian physician, 1832–1913.
Fede-Riga disease—*Syn:* Riga-Fede disease
Riga-Fede disease—see under Riga

Federici, Cesare, Italian physician, 1838–1892.
Federici sign—intestinal perforation causing cardiac sounds to be heard on auscultation of abdomen.

Feer, Emil, Swiss pediatrician, 1864–1955.
Feer disease—pain in peripheral or acral parts of the body; caused almost exclusively by mercury poisoning in children. *Syn:* acrodynia; pink disease; Swift disease

Fegeler, F., German dermatologist.
Fegeler syndrome—neck injury causing capillary nevus.

Fehling, Hermann von, German chemist, 1812–1885.
Fehling reagent—*Syn:* Fehling solution
Fehling solution—an alkaline copper tartrate solution formerly used for detection of reducing sugars. *Syn:* Fehling reagent
Fehling test—test used to reduce substances in urine.

Feil, André, French physician, *1884.
　　Feil-Klippel syndrome—*SYN:* Klippel-Feil syndrome
　　Klippel-Feil syndrome—see under Klippel

Feingold, M.
　　Palant-Feingold-Berkman syndrome—see under Palant

Feiss, Henry O., 20th century U.S. orthopedic surgeon.
　　Feiss line—a line running from the medial malleolus to the plantar aspect
　　of the first metatarsophalangeal joint.

Feldberg, Wilhelm, English physiologist, *1900.
　　Dale-Feldberg law—see under Dale, Sir Henry

Feldenkrais, Moshe, Israeli physicist, 1904–1979.
　　Feldenkrais exercises—system used to improve posture, movement, and
　　body awareness.

Feldman, Harry Alfred, U.S. epidemiologist, *1914.
　　Sabin-Feldman dye test—see under Sabin

Felix, Arthur, Polish bacteriologist, 1887–1956.
　　Weil-Felix reaction—*SYN:* Weil-Felix test
　　Weil-Felix test—see under Weil

Felton, Lloyd D., U.S. physician, 1885–1953.
　　Felton phenomenon—in laboratory animals, immunologic
　　unresponsiveness or tolerance to pneumococcal polysaccharide on
　　administration of large doses of antigen.

Felty, Augustus R., U.S. physician, 1895–1964.
　　Felty syndrome—rheumatoid arthritis with splenomegaly and leukopenia.

Fendt, H., 19th century Austrian dermatologist.
　　Spiegler-Fendt pseudolymphoma—see under Spiegler
　　Spiegler-Fendt sarcoid—*SYN:* Spiegler-Fendt pseudolymphoma

Fenn, Wallace Osgood, U.S. physiologist, 1893–1971.
　　Fenn effect—the increased liberation of heat in a stimulated muscle when
　　it is allowed to do mechanical work.

F

Fenwick, Edwin Hurry, English urologist, 1856–1944.
　　Fenwick-Hunner ulcer—*SYN:* Hunner ulcer

Fenwick, Samuel, English physician, 1821–1902.
　　Fenwick disease—idiopathic gastric atrophy.

Féréol, Louis H.F., French physician, 1825–1891.
　　Féréol node—subcutaneous nodes seen around joints in the presence of
　　acute rheumatism.

Ferguson Smith, John, English physician, 1888–1978.
　　Ferguson Smith epithelioma—squamous epithelioma, self-healing.

NOTES

Fergusson, Sir William, Scottish surgeon, 1808–1877.
> **Fergusson incision**—an incision used in maxillectomy, along the junction of cheek and nose, to bisect the upper lip.

Fernbach, Auguste, French microbiologist, 1860–1939.
> **Fernbach flask**—a flask used in microbial fermentations where a large surface area of the liquid substrate is required.

Ferrata, Adolfo, Italian physician, 1880–1946.
> **Ferrata cell**—primitive cell believed to be capable of developing into all types of blood cells. *Syn:* hemohistioblast

Ferrein, Antoine, French anatomist, 1693–1769.
> **Ferrein canal**—a space between the closed lids and the eyeball through which the tears flow to the punctum lacrimale. *Syn:* rivus lacrimalis
> **Ferrein cords**
> **Ferrein foramen**—the opening on the anterior aspect of the petrous part of the temporal bone which leads to the facial canal and gives passage to the greater petrosal nerve. *Syn:* hiatus of facial canal
> **Ferrein ligament**—the capsular ligament that passes obliquely down and backward across the lateral surface of temporomandibular joint. *Syn:* lateral temporomandibular ligament
> **Ferrein pyramid**—the center of the renal lobule, which has the shape of a small, steep pyramid, consisting of straight tubular parts. *Syn:* medullary ray; processus ferreini
> **Ferrein tube**—*Syn:* convoluted tubule of kidney
> **Ferrein vasa aberrantia**—biliary canaliculi that are not connected with hepatic lobules.
> **processus ferreini**—*Syn:* Ferrein pyramid

Ferry, Erwin S., U.S. physicist, 1868–1956.
> **Ferry-Porter law**—the critical fusion is directly proportional to the logarithm of the light intensity.

Feulgen, Robert, German nucleic acid biochemist and cytochemist, 1884–1955. First to detect DNA in cells by a specific cytochemical test.
> **Feulgen reaction**—DNA staining reaction.
> **Feulgen test**

Fevold, Harry Leonard, U.S. biochemist, *1902.
> **Fevold test**—a test to determine the chemical nature of a substance by means of reagents.

Fèvre, Marcel Paul Luis Edmond, French orthopedic surgeon, *1897.
> **Fèvre-Lanquepin syndrome**—popliteal webbing associated with multiple anomalies. *Syn:* popliteal pterygium

Fiamberti, Adamo Mario, Italian psychiatrist, *1894.
> **Fiamberti hypothesis**—theory that schizophrenia results from acetylcholine deficiency due to infection or toxicity.

Fibiger, Johannes A.G., Danish pathologist, 1867–1928.
> **Fibiger tumor**—gastric squamous cell carcinoma in rats caused by larvae of Spiroptera neoplastica nematode.
> **Fibiger-Debré-von Gierke syndrome**—*Syn:* Debré-Fibiger syndrome

Fick, Adolf, German physician, 1829–1901.
   Fick method—cardiac output can be calculated as the quotient of total body oxygen consumption divided by the difference in oxygen content of arterial blood and mixed venous blood. *Syn:* Fick principle
   Fick principle—*Syn:* Fick method

Fiedler, Carl L.A., German physician, 1835–1921.
   Fiedler disease
   Fiedler myocarditis—an acute interstitial myocarditis of unknown cause, the endocardium and pericardium being unaffected. *Syn:* acute isolated myocarditis

Fielding, George H., English anatomist, 1801–1871.
   Fielding membrane—in neuroanatomy, a thin sheet of fibers in the lateral wall of the temporal and occipital horns of the lateral ventricle, continuous with the corpus callosum. *Syn:* tapetum

Fiessinger, Noël Armand, French physician, 1881–1946.
   Fiessinger-Leroy-Reiter syndrome—*Syn:* Reiter syndrome

Figueira, Fernandes, Brazilian pediatrician, d. 1928.
   Figueira syndrome—weakness of the neck muscles with slight spasticity of the muscles of the lower extremities and increased tendon reflexes.

Filatov, Nil, Russian pediatrician, 1847–1902.
   Filatov disease—*Syn:* Filatov-Dukes disease
   Filatov spots—*Syn:* Koplik spots
   Filatov-Dukes disease—exanthem-producing infectious disease of childhood, etiology unknown. *Syn:* Dukes disease; Filatov disease; parascarlatina; fourth disease; scarlatinella

Filatov, Vladimir P., Russian ophthalmologist, 1875–1956.
   Filatov flap—a flap in which the sides of the pedicle are sutured together to create a tube, with the entire surface covered by skin. *Syn:* tubed flap
   Filatov operation—obsolete term for penetrating keratoplasty.
   Filatov-Gillies flap—*Syn:* tubed flap
   Filatov-Gillies tubed pedicle—*Syn:* tubed flap

Filatow, var. of Filatov

Fildes, Sir Paul Gordon, English bacteriologist, *1882.
   Fildes enrichment agar
   McIntosh-Fildes jar

Filipovitch, Casimir, 19th century Polish physician.
   Filipovitch sign—yellow discoloration of palms of hands and soles of feet due to typhoid.

Filmer, David L., U.S. biochemist, *1932.
   Adair-Koshland-Némethy-Filmer model—*Syn:* Koshland-Némethy-Filmer model
   Koshland-Némethy-Filmer model—see under Koshland

NOTES

Finckh, Johann, German psychiatrist, *1873.
    Finckh test—a psychological test.

Fink, R.P., 20th century U.S. anatomist.
    Fink-Heimer stain—a method used for histologic demonstration of degenerating nerve fibers and terminals of the central nervous system.

Finkeldey, Wilhelm, 20th century German pathologist.
    Finkeldey cells—*Syn:* Warthin-Finkeldey cells
    Warthin-Finkeldey cells—see under Warthin

Finkelstein, Harry, U.S. surgeon, 1865–1939.
    Finkelstein maneuver
    Finkelstein test—test indicative of de Quervain tenosynovitis.

Finkelstein, Heinrich, German pediatrician, 1865–1942.
    Finkelstein feeding—form of infant feeding based on decrease in milk sugar.

Finney, John M.T., U.S. surgeon, 1863–1942.
    Finney gastroduodenostomy
    Finney gastroenterostomy
    Finney operation—gastroduodenostomy which creates, by the technique of closure, a large opening to ensure free emptying from the stomach.
    Finney pyloroplasty—operation to provide a wider opening between stomach and duodenum.

Finochietto, Enrique, Argentinian surgeon, 1881–1948.
    Finochietto artery clamp
    Finochietto clamp carrier
    Finochietto forceps
    Finochietto laminectomy retractor
    Finochietto needle
    Finochietto needle holder
    Finochietto operation
    Finochietto retractor
    Finochietto rib retractor
    Finochietto rib spreader
    Finochietto scissors
    Finochietto spreader
    Finochietto stirrup—used for traction in leg fractures.
    Finochietto thoracic forceps
    Finochietto thoracic scissors

Finsen, Niels Ryberg, Danish physician, 1860–1904, 1903 Nobel Prize winner for work related to disease treatment, particularly lupus vulgaris.
    finsen—*Syn:* finsen unit
    Finsen bath—ultraviolet irradiation.
    Finsen carbon arc light
    Finsen lamp—carbon-arc lamp.
    Finsen method—to treat by using concentrated ultraviolet rays. *Syn:* Finsen therapy
    Finsen retractor
    Finsen therapy—*Syn:* Finsen method
    finsen unit—erythemal flux density of irradiation. *Syn:* finsen

Fisch, L., English physician.
    Fisch-Renwick syndrome—disorder resulting in congenital deafness, abnormal distance between paired organs, and white forelock. *Syn:* Renwick-Fisch syndrome
    Renwick-Fisch syndrome—*Syn:* Fisch-Renwick syndrome

Fischer, Emil, German chemist and Nobel laureate, 1852–1919.
    Fischer projection formulas of sugars—representations, by projection, of cyclic sugars, or derivatives thereof, in which the carbon chain is depicted vertically.
    Kiliani-Fischer reaction
    Kiliani-Fischer synthesis—see under Kiliani

Fischer, Louis, U.S. pediatrician, 1864–1944.
    Fischer sign—an obsolete sign of tuberculosis. *Syn:* Fischer symptom
    Fischer symptom—*Syn:* Fischer sign
    Fishberg

Fishberg, Arthur M., U.S. physician, 1898–1992.
    Fishberg concentration test—a test of renal water conservation.

Fisher, Miller, U.S. neurologist, *1910.
    Fisher syndrome—a syndrome characterized by ophthalmoplegia, ataxia, and areflexia; a form of polyneuroradiculitis.

Fisher, Ronald A., English statistician, 1890–1962.
    Fisher exact test—a statistical hypothesis test.

Fitz, Reginald Heber, U.S. physician, 1843–1913.
    Fitz syndrome—*Syn:* acute pancreatitis

Fitz-Hugh, Thomas, Jr., U.S. physician, 1894–1963.
    Fitz-Hugh and Curtis syndrome—perihepatitis in women with a history of gonococcal or chlamydial salpingitis.

Fitzgerald, (origin unknown).
    Fitzgerald trait—defect resulting in prolongation of clotting tests but seldom causing hemostatic symptoms. *Syn:* Flaujeauc and Williams trait; kalikrein deficiency
    Fitzgerald-Gardner syndrome—genetic trait resulting in multiple tumors, osteomas of the skull, epidermoid cysts, fibromas, and multiple polyposis predisposing to carcinoma of the colon.

Fitzsimmons, J.S., English physician.
    Fitzsimmons syndrome—hereditary syndrome resulting in limb spasticity, mental retardation, and foot deformities.

Flack, Martin, English physiologist, 1882–1931.
    Flack node—*Syn:* Keith and Flack node
    Flack test—a cardiopulmonary test.
    Keith and Flack node—see under Keith

F

NOTES

Flatau, Edward, Polish neurologist, 1869–1932.
    Flatau law—a law concerning the eccentric position of the long spinal tracts.
    Flatau syndrome—recessive trait resulting in bizarre movements brought on by physical activity. *Syn:* torsion dystonia
    Flatau-Schilder disease—*Syn:* Schilder disease

Flaujeauc, one of two patients in whom Flaujeauc and Williams trait was detected.
    Flaujeauc and Williams trait—*Syn:* Fitzgerald trait

Flechsig, Paul E., German neurologist, 1847–1929.
    Flechsig areas—three divisions (anterior, lateral, posterior) of each lateral half of the medulla as seen on transverse section, marked off by the root fibers of the hypoglossal and vagus nerves.
    Flechsig fasciculi—fasciculus anterior proprius and fasciculus lateralis proprius. *Syn:* Flechsig ground bundles
    Flechsig ground bundles—Flechsig fasciculi
    Flechsig tract—a compact bundle of heavily myelinated, thick fibers at the periphery of the dorsal half of the lateral funiculus of the spinal cord. *Syn:* posterior spinocerebellar tract
    oval area of Flechsig
    semilunar nucleus of Flechsig—the small ventral region of the ventral posteromedial nucleus of thalamus in which the fibers of the gustatory lemniscus and secondary trigeminal tracts terminate. *Syn:* arcuate nucleus of thalamus

Flegel, Heinz, German dermatologist, *1923.
    Flegel disease—small keratotic papules on the dorsa of the feet and legs, and occasionally elsewhere, with pinpoint keratotic papules of the palms and soles. *Syn:* hyperkeratosis lenticularis perstans

Fleisch, Alfred, Swiss physician and physiologist, *1892.
    Fleisch pneumotachograph—a pneumotachograph that measures flow in terms of the proportional pressure drop across a resistance consisting of numerous capillary tubes in parallel.

Fleischer, Bruno, German ophthalmologist, 1874–1965.
    Fleischer corneal ring
    Fleischer lines
    Fleischer ring—an incomplete ring often present at the base of the keratoconus cone.
    Fleischer vortex—congenital whorl-like opacities in the cornea. *Syn:* cornea verticillata
    Fleischer-Strümpell ring—*Syn:* Kayser-Fleischer ring
    Kayser-Fleischer ring—see under Kayser

Fleischmann, Friedrich Ludwig, 19th century German anatomist.
    Fleischmann bursa—an inconstant serous bursa at the level of the frenulum linguae, between the surface of the genioglossus muscle and the mucous membrane of the floor of the mouth. *Syn:* sublingual bursa; bursa sublingualis

Fleischner, Felix, Austrian-U.S. radiologist, 1893–1969.
    Fleischner lines—coarse linear shadows on chest x-ray, indicating bands of subsegmental atelectasis.

Fleisher, Thomas A., U.S. physician.
    Fleisher syndrome—genetically transmitted syndrome related to growth
    hormone deficiency and immune system deficiencies.

Fleitmann, Theodore, 19th century German chemist.
    Fleitmann test—a test for arsenic.

Fleming, Sir Alexander, Scottish bacteriologist, 1881–1955, co-winner of the 1945
Nobel Prize for the discovery of penicillin.

Flemming, Walther, German anatomist, 1843–1905.
    Flemming fixative—a cytoplasmic and chromosomal fixative.
    Flemming triple stain—a stain comprised of safranin, methyl violet, and
    orange G.
    germinal center of Flemming—the lightly staining center in a lymphatic
    nodule in which the predominant cells are large lymphocytes and
    macrophages. *SYN:* reaction center
    intermediate body of Flemming—a dense stalk of residual interzonal
    spindle fibers (microtubules) and actin-containing filaments that is
    formed during anaphase of mitosis. *SYN:* midbody

Flesch, Rudolf, Austrian educator, *1911.
    Flesch formula—a method of determining the difficulty of a written
    passage used in determining patient comprehension of hospital consent
    forms.

Fletcher, patient in whom Fletcher defect was first noted.
    Fletcher defect—slow contact activation in coagulation of the blood.
    Fletcher factor—factor found in coagulation studies, revealing a slow
    contact activation but not associated with bleeding abnormalities. *SYN:*
    prekallikrein

Flexner, Simon, U.S. pathologist, 1863–1946.
    Flexner bacillus—the most common cause of dysentery epidemics and
    sometimes of infantile gastroenteritis. *SYN: Shigella flexneri*

Flieringa, Henri J., Dutch ophthalmologist, *1891.
    Flieringa fixation ring
    Flieringa ring—a stainless steel ring sutured to the sclera to prevent
    collapse of the globe in difficult intraocular operations.
    Flieringa scleral ring

F

Flindt, N., Danish physician, 1843–1913.
    Flindt spots—*SYN:* Koplik spots

Flint, Austin, Jr., U.S. physiologist, 1836–1915.
    Flint arcade—a series of vascular arches at the bases of the pyramids of
    the kidney.

Flint, Austin, U.S. physician, 1812–1886.
    Austin Flint murmur—*SYN:* Flint murmur

(continued)

NOTES

Flint *(continued)*
> **Austin Flint phenomenon**—*SYN:* Flint murmur
> **Austin Flint respiration**
> **Flint murmur**—a diastolic murmur, similar to that of mitral stenosis, heard best at the cardiac apex in some cases of free aortic insufficiency. *SYN:* Austin Flint phenomenon; Austin Flint murmur

Flocks, Milton, U.S. ophthalmologist, *1914.
> **Harrington-Flocks test**—see under Harrington

Flood, Valentine, Irish anatomist and surgeon, 1800–1847.
> **Flood ligament**—a band of the coracohumeral ligament, attached to the lower part of the lesser tuberosity of the humerus.

Florence, Albert, French physician, 1851–1927.
> **Florence crystals**—brown rhombic crystals formed at the interface between a drop of Lugol solution and a drop of fluid that contains semen.

Florey, Sir Howard W., Australian-English pathologist and Nobel laureate, 1898–1968.
> **Florey unit**—1 unit equals 0.6 μg of crystalline sodium salt of penicillin. *SYN:* Oxford unit

Florschütz, Georg, German physician, *1859.
> **Florschütz formula**—the correct relation of height to the abdominal circumference.

Flourens, Marie J.P., French physiologist, 1794–1867.
> **Flourens theory**—that thought is a process depending upon the action of the entire cerebrum.

Flower, Sir William H., English surgeon and anatomist, 1831–1899.
> **Flower bone**—a sutural bone occasionally present at the pterion or junction of the parietal, frontal, greater wing of the sphenoid, and squamous portion of the temporal bones. *SYN:* epipteric bone
> **Flower dental index**—a system of numbers for indicating comparative size of the teeth. *SYN:* dental index

Flynn, P., 20th century U.S. physician.
> **Flynn phenomenon**—a pupillary response to light, the reverse of that expected. *SYN:* paradoxical pupillary reflex
> **Flynn-Aird syndrome**—a familial syndrome characterized by muscle wasting, ataxia, dementia, skin atrophy, and ocular anomalies.

Fogarty, Thomas J., U.S. thoracic surgeon, *1934.
> **Fogarty arterial embolectomy**
> **Fogarty biliary probe**
> **Fogarty catheter**—a catheter used to remove arterial emboli and thrombi from major veins. *SYN:* balloon-tip catheter
> **Fogarty clamp**—a clamp with rubber-shod blades having serrated surfaces, to provide an atraumatic grip on tissues.
> **Fogarty forceps**
> **Fogarty irrigation catheter**
> **Fogarty venous thrombectomy catheter**

Foix, Charles, French neurologist, 1882–1927.

    Foix syndrome—paralysis of cranial nerves III through VI resulting in proptosis and eyelid edema; trigeminal neuralgia may also be present.

    Foix-Alajouanine myelitis—a disorder of the lower spinal cord in adult males resulting in progressive paraplegia. *SYN:* subacute necrotizing myelitis

    Foix-Alajouanine syndrome—thrombophlebitis of spinal veins resulting in a subacute ascending painful flaccid paralysis from necrotic myelitis.

    Foix-Cavany-Marie syndrome—constellation of faciopharyngoglossomasticatory diplegia, usually caused by bilateral large artery infarcts of the opercular cortex.

Foley, Frederic E.B., U.S. urologist, 1891–1966.

    Foley acorn-bulb catheter

    Foley bag

    Foley balloon catheter

    Foley catheter—a catheter with a retaining balloon.

    Foley cone-tip catheter

    Foley forceps

    Foley hemostatic bag

    Foley operation—*SYN:* Foley Y-plasty pyeloplasty

    Foley plate

    Foley pyeloplasty

    Foley three-way catheter

    Foley ureteropelvioplasty

    Foley vas isolation forceps

    Foley Y-plasty pyeloplasty—a reconstructive procedure for correction of ureteropelvic obstruction. *SYN:* Foley operation

    Foley Y-type ureteropelvioplasty

    Foley Y-V pyeloplasty

Folin, Otto K.O., U.S. biochemist, 1867–1934.

    Folin reaction—the reaction of amino acids in alkaline solution with 1,2-naphthoquinone-4-sulfonate (Folin reagent) to yield a red color. *SYN:* Folin reagent

    Folin reagent—*SYN:* Folin reaction

    Folin test—a quantitative test for urea.

    Folin-Looney test—a test for tyrosine that gives a blue color in alkaline solution with a reagent consisting of sodium tungstate, phosphomolybdic acid, and phosphoric acid.

    Lowry-Folin assay—*SYN:* Lowry protein assay

Folling, Ivar A., Norwegian physician, 1888–1973.

    Folling disease—congenital deficiency of phenylalanine 4-monooxygenase or occasionally of dihydropherine reductase or of dihydrobiopterin synthetase that can cause brain damage and other neurologic abnormalities. *SYN:* phenylketonuria

F

NOTES

Foltz, Jean C.E., French anatomist and ophthalmologist, 1822–1876.
   Foltz valvule—*Syn:* Bochdalek valve

Fones, Alfred Civilion, U.S. dentist, 1869–1938.
   Fones method of tooth brushing
   Fones technique

Fong, E.E., U.S. radiologist, *1912.
   Fong lesion—genetic trait resulting in abnormality of thumb and great toe nails; may result in iliac bone abnormalities and abnormalities of the renal system. *Syn:* Fong syndrome; nail-patella syndrome
   Fong syndrome—*Syn:* Fong lesion

Fonio, Anton, Swiss physician, *1889.
   Fonio solution—a diluent with magnesium sulfate, used for stained smears of blood platelets.

Fontan, Francois, French thoracic surgeon, *1929.
   Fontan operation—*Syn:* Fontan procedure
   Fontan procedure—placement of a conduit (usually valved) from the right atrium to the main pulmonary artery as a bypass to a hypoplastic right ventricle, as in tricuspid atresia. *Syn:* Fontan operation

Fontana, Arturo, Italian dermatologist, 1873–1950.
   Fontana stain—a traditional method for silver-impregnation of treponemes and other spirochetal forms.
   Fontana-Masson silver stain—*Syn:* Masson-Fontana ammoniacal silver stain
   Masson-Fontana ammoniacal silver stain—see under Masson

Fontana, Felice, Italian physiologist, 1730–1805.
   Fontana canal—the vascular structure encircling the anterior chamber of the eye and through which the aqueous is returned to the blood circulation. *Syn:* sinus venosus sclerae
   Fontana spaces—irregularly shaped endothelium-lined spaces within the trabecular reticulum, through which the aqueous filters to reach the sinus venosus sclerae. *Syn:* spaces of iridocorneal angle

Foot, N.C., 20th century U.S. pathologist.
   Foot reticulin impregnation stain—a silver stain.

Forbes, Anne P., 20th century U.S. physician.
   Forbes-Albright syndrome—pituitary tumor in a patient without acromegaly, which secretes excessive amounts of prolactin and produces persistent lactation.

Forbes, Gilbert B., U.S. pediatrician, *1915.
   Forbes disease—(1) storage of excess amounts of glycogen. *Syn:* type 11 Cori; (2) glycogenosis due to amylo-1,6-glucosidase deficiency, resulting in accumulation of abnormal glycogen with short outer chains in liver and muscle. *Syn:* type 3 glycogenosis.

Forbes, Thomas R.
   Hooker-Forbes test—see under Hooker

Forchheimer, Frederick, U.S. physician, 1853–1913.
   Forchheimer sign—the presence in German measles of a reddish maculopapular eruption on the soft palate.

Fordyce, John A., U.S. dermatologist, 1858–1925.

    Fordyce angiokeratoma—asymptomatic vascular papules of the scrotum.

    Fordyce disease—*Syn:* Fordyce spots

    Fordyce granules—*Syn:* Fordyce spots

    Fordyce lesion—scrotal angiomas of no significance.

    Fordyce spots—a condition marked by the presence of numerous small, yellowish-white bodies or granules on the inner surface and vermilion border of the lips. *Syn:* pseudocolloid of lips; Fordyce disease; Fordyce granules

    Fox-Fordyce disease—see under Fox

Forel, Auguste H., Swiss neurologist, 1848–1931.

    fields of Forel—three circumscript, myelin-rich regions of the subthalamus. *Syn:* campi foreli; tegmental fields of Forel

    Forel commissure

    Forel decussation

    Forel field

    Forel space

    tegmental fields of Forel—*Syn:* fields of Forel

Forestier, Jacques, French rheumatologist, *1890.

    Forestier disease—a generalized spinal and extraspinal articular disorder characterized by calcification and ossification of ligaments. *Syn:* diffuse idiopathic skeletal hyperostosis

Formad, Henry, U.S. physician, 1847–1892.

    Formad kidney—an enlarged and deformed kidney, sometimes seen in chronic alcoholism.

Forssell, Gösta, Swedish radiologist, 1876–1950.

    Forssell sinus—mucosal folds surround this smooth space in the stomach wall.

Forssell, Jarl, Finnish physician, 1912–1964.

    Forssell syndrome—polycythemia.

Forssman, Hans, Swedish physician, *1912.

    Börjeson-Forssman-Lehmann syndrome—see under Börjeson

Forssman, John, Swedish bacteriologist and pathologist, 1868–1947.

    Forssman antibody—a heterogenetic antibody specific for the Forssman group of heterogenetic antigens. *Syn:* heterophile antibody; heterophil antibody

    Forssman antigen—the antibody that develops in infectious mononucleosis reacts specifically with the Forssman antigen.

    Forssman antigen-antibody reaction—the combination of Forssman antibody with heterogenetic antigen of the Forssman type. *Syn:* Forssman reaction

    Forssman reaction—*Syn:* Forssman antigen-antibody reaction

Forssmann, Werner Theodor Otto, German surgeon, 1904–1979, and co-winner of 1956 Nobel Prize for work related to circulation and heart catheterization.

F

NOTES

Förster, Richard, German ophthalmologist, 1825–1902.
Förster eye forceps
Förster iris forceps
Förster photometer
Förster uveitis—syphilitic inflammation, with diffuse nodules involving the choroid and retinal vasculitis.

Fosdick, Leonard S., U.S. chemist, *1903.
Fosdick-Hansen-Epple test—a test for determining dental caries activity based on a solution of powdered human enamel in a saliva-glucose-enamel mixture.

Foshay, Lee, U.S. bacteriologist, 1896–1961.
Foshay test—an intradermal test for cat-scratch disease or tularemia, using material prepared from suppurative lymph nodes of persons known to have had the disease.

Fothergill, John, English physician, 1712–1780.
Fothergill disease—severe, paroxysmal bursts of pain in one or more branches of the trigeminal nerve. *Syn:* trigeminal neuralgia; anginose scarlatina; Fothergill neuralgia
Fothergill neuralgia—*Syn:* Fothergill disease
Fothergill sign—in rectus sheath hematoma, the hematoma produces a mass that does not cross the midline and remains palpable when the rectus muscle is tense.

Fothergill, William E., English gynecologist, 1865–1926.
Fothergill operation—*Syn:* Manchester operation
Fothergill suture

Fouchet, André, French physician, *1894.
Fouchet reagent—a test for bilirubin.
Fouchet stain—Fouchet reagent employed to demonstrate bile pigments.

Fountain, R.B., English physician.
Fountain syndrome—recessive trait related to mental retardation, bone abnormalities, and tissue swelling.

Fourier, J.B.J., French mathematician and administrator, 1768–1830.
Fourier analysis—used in reconstruction of images in computed tomography and magnetic resonance imaging in radiology and in analysis of any kind of signal for its frequency content. *Syn:* Fourier transform; Fourier law
Fourier law—*Syn:* Fourier analysis
Fourier transform—*Syn:* Fourier analysis

Fourneau, Ernest F.A., French chemist and pharmacologist, 1872–1949.
Fourneau 693—a synthetic organic compound of antimony used in the treatment of several protozoal diseases and for the relief of pain in multiple myeloma. *Syn:* ethylstibamine
Fourneau 710—a synthetic antimalarial agent.
Fourneau 933—used as a diagnostic test for pheochromocytoma. *Syn:* piperoxan hydrochloride

Fournier, Jean A., French syphilographer, 1832–1914.
Fournier disease—infective gangrene involving the scrotum. *Syn:* Fournier gangrene; syphiloma of Fournier

Fournier gangrene—*Syn:* Fournier disease
syphiloma of Fournier—*Syn:* Fournier disease

Foville, Achille L., French neurologist, 1799–1878.
    Foville fasciculus—a slender, compact fiber bundle that connects the amygdala with the hypothalamus and other basal forebrain regions. *Syn:* terminal stria
    Foville paralysis—*Syn:* Foville syndrome
    Foville syndrome—a form of alternating hemiplegia characterized by abducens paralysis on one side, paralysis of the extremities on the other. *Syn:* Foville paralysis

Fowler, Edson Brady, U.S. surgeon, 1865–1942.
    Fowler procedure—orthopedic procedure performed on metatarsal heads.

Fowler, George R., U.S. surgeon, 1848–1906.
    Fowler position—an inclined position obtained by raising the head of the bed about 60–90 cm to promote better dependent drainage after an abdominal operation.

Fowler, Thomas, English physician, 1736–1801.
    Fowler solution—solution of potassium arsenate used in treatment of leukemia.

Fox, George H., U.S. dermatologist, 1846–1937.
    Fox-Fordyce disease—a rare chronic pruritic eruption of dry papules and distended ruptured apocrine glands, with follicular hyperkeratosis of the nipples, axillae, and pubic and sternal regions. *Syn:* apocrine miliaria

Fox, Lewis, U.S. periodontist, *1903.
    Goldman-Fox knives—see under Goldman, Henry

Fraccaro, M., Italian physician.
    Schmid-Fraccaro syndrome—see under Schmid

Fraenkel, Albert, German physician, 1848–1916.
    Fraenkel pneumococcus—normal inhabitants of the respiratory tract and perhaps the most common cause of lobar pneumonia, they are relatively common causative agents of meningitis, sinusitis, and other infections. *Syn: Streptococcus pneumoniae*; Fraenkel-Weichselbaum pneumococcus
    Fraenkel-Weichselbaum pneumococcus—*Syn:* Fraenkel pneumococcus

F

Fraley, Elwin E., U.S. urologist, *1934.
    Fraley syndrome—dilation of the upper pole renal calices due to stenosis of the upper infundibulum.

Franceschetti, Adolphe, Swiss ophthalmologist, 1896–1968.
    Franceschetti syndrome—mandibulofacial dysostosis, when complete or nearly complete.
    Franceschetti-Jadassohn syndrome—*Syn:* Naegeli syndrome

NOTES

Francis, C.A., English otolaryngologist, 1898–1951.
Francis triad—aspirin sensitivity in conjunction with asthma and nasal polyps.

Francis, Edward, U.S. physician, 1872–1957.
Francis disease—tularemia.

Francke, Karl E., German physician, 1859–1920.
Francke needle—a small lancet-shaped, spring-activated needle, used to evacuate a small effusion of blood.

Franco, Pierre, French surgeon, 1500–1561.
Franco operation—cystotomy.

François, Jules, Belgian ophthalmologist, *1907.
François syndrome—*Syn:* Hallermann-Streif syndrome

Frank, A.E., German physician, 1884–1957.
Frank capillary toxicosis—purpura without any platelet count decrease. *Syn:* nonthrombocytopenic purpura

Frank, Otto, German physiologist, 1865–1944.
Frank-Starling curve—*Syn:* Starling curve

Frank, Rudolf, Austrian surgeon, 1862–1913.
Ssabanejew-Frank operation—see under Ssabanejew

Frank, Sanders T., U.S. thoracic physician, *1938.
Frank sign—oblique earlobe fissure associated with hypertension, heart disease, and diabetes; acquired as opposed to congenital.

Franke, Gustav, German physician, *1878.
Franke syndrome—abnormalities of the palate, septal deviation, and enlarged adenoids leading to infections and breathing through the mouth rather than the nose. *Syn:* Franke triad
Franke triad—*Syn:* Franke syndrome

Fränkel, var. of Fraenkel

Frankenhäuser, Ferdinand, German gynecologist, 1832–1894.
Frankenhäuser ganglion—a gangliated autonomic plexus on each side of the cervix of the uterus, derived from the inferior hypogastric plexus. *Syn:* uterovaginal plexus

Franklin, Benjamin, U.S. physicist and statesman, 1706–1790.
Franklin spectacles—an early form of bifocal spectacles in which the lower half of the lens is for near vision, the upper half for distant vision. *Syn:* divided spectacles
franklinic—denoting static or frictional electricity.

Franklin, Edward C., U.S. physician, *1928.
Franklin disease—common features include anemia, lymphocytosis, eosinophilia, thrombocytopenia, hyperuricemia, lymphadenopathy, and hepatosplenomegaly. *Syn:* γ-heavy-chain disease

Fraser, Alexander, Canadian pathologist, 1869–1939.
Fraser-Lendrum stain for fibrin—a multistaining procedure after Zenker fixative in which fibrin, keratin, and some cytoplasmic granules appear red, erythrocytes appear orange, and collagen appears green.

Fraser, George R., English geneticist, *1932.
　　Fraser syndrome—an association of cryptophthalmus with multiple anomalies. *Syn:* cryptophthalmus syndrome

Fraumeni, Joseph F., Jr., 20th century epidemiologist.
　　Li-Fraumeni cancer syndrome—see under Li

Fraunhofer, Joseph von, German optician, 1787–1826.
　　Fraunhofer lines—a number of the most prominent of the absorption lines of the solar spectrum.

Frazier, Charles H., U.S. surgeon, 1870–1936.
　　Frazier dural guide
　　Frazier incision
　　Frazier needle—a needle for draining lateral ventricles of brain.
　　Frazier stylet
　　Frazier suction tip
　　Frazier suction tube
　　Frazier-Spiller operation—division or section of a sensory root of the fifth cranial nerve, accomplished through a subtemporal approach.

Frederick, Maurice Hugh, joint winner of 1963 Nobel Prize for work related to nuclear acids.

Fredet, Pierre, French surgeon, 1870–1946.
　　Fredet-Ramstedt operation—*Syn:* Ramstedt operation

Freeman, Charles.
　　Freeman rule—a person is not responsible for crimes committed if that person has a condition which prevents him/her from knowing what s/he is doing.

Freeman, Ernest A., English orthopedic surgeon, 1900–1975.
　　Freeman-Sheldon syndrome—*Syn:* craniocarpotarsal dystrophy

Frei, Wilhelm S., German dermatologist, 1885–1943.
　　Frei disease—lymphogranuloma venereum.
　　Frei test—an intracutaneous diagnostic test for lymphogranuloma venereum. *Syn:* Frei-Hoffmann reaction
　　Frei-Hoffmann reaction—*Syn:* Frei test

F

Freiberg, Albert Henry, U.S. surgeon, 1869–1940.
　　Freiberg cartilage knife
　　Freiberg disease—epiphysial ischemic (aseptic) necrosis of the second metatarsal head.
　　Freiberg hip retractor
　　Freiberg infraction
　　Freiberg meniscectomy knife
　　Freiberg traction
　　Freiberg tractor

NOTES

Frejka, B., Czech orthopedist, *1890.
    Frejka cast
    Frejka hip pillow
    Frejka jacket
    Frejka orthosis
    Frejka pillow splint—a pillow splint used for abduction and flexion of the femurs in treatment of congenital hip dysplasia or dislocation in infants.
    Frejka splint
    Frejka traction

Frenkel, Heinrich S., Swiss neurologist, 1860–1931.
    Frenkel exercises—exercises designed for reeducating those with incoordination problems. *SYN:* Frenkel method
    Frenkel method—*SYN:* Frenkel exercises
    Frenkel symptom—diminished
    Frenkel tracks—a method of painting footprints or other marks on a floor to use as a guide for patients with ataxia in walking reeducation.

Frenkel, Henri, French ophthalmologist, 1864–1934.
    Frenkel anterior ocular traumatic syndrome—an obsolete term for traumatic iridoplegia.

Frerichs, Friedrich T. von, German pathologist and clinician, 1819–1885.
    Frerichs theory—that uremia represents a toxic condition caused by ammonium carbonate, which is formed as the result of the action of a plasma enzyme on the increased amounts of urea.

Fresnel, Augustin Jean, French physicist, 1788–1827.
    Fresnel lens—a lens with a surface consisting of a concentric series of zones that duplicate the power of a lens or prism but with less thickness. *SYN:* lighthouse lens; Fresnel prism
    Fresnel prism—*SYN:* Fresnel lens

Freud, Sigmund, Austrian neurologist and psychiatrist, 1856–1939, founder of psychoanalysis.
    Freud theory—a comprehensive theory of how personality is formed and develops in normal and emotionally disturbed individuals.
    freudian—relating to or described by Freud.
    freudian fixation
    freudian psychoanalysis—the theory and practice of psychoanalysis and psychotherapy as developed by Freud.
    freudian slip—a mistake in speech or deed which presumably suggests some underlying motive, often sexual or aggressive in nature.

Freud, Emanuel, Austrian physician, *1869.
    Freud dermatitis—application of cosmetics causes erythema at application site and later brown pigmentation when that area of skin is exposed to sunlight. *SYN:* bergamot dermatitis

Freund, Jules, U.S. bacteriologist, 1891–1960.
    Freund complete adjuvant—water-in-oil emulsion of antigen, to which killed mycobacteria or tuberculosis bacteria are added.
    Freund incomplete adjuvant—water-in-oil emulsion of antigen, without mycobacteria.

Freund, Wilhelm A., German gynecologist, 1833–1918.
Freund anomaly—a narrowing of the upper aperture of the thorax by shortening of the first rib and its cartilage.
Freund operation—(1) total abdominal hysterectomy for uterine cancer; (2) chondrotomy to relieve Freund anomaly.

Frey, Lucie, Polish physician, 1852–1932.
Frey syndrome—localized flushing and sweating of the ear and cheek in response to eating. *SYN:* auriculotemporal nerve syndrome

Frey, Max von, German physician, 1852–1932.
Frey hairs—short hairs of varying degrees of stiffness, set into a light wooden handle and used for assessing sensation.

Freyer, Sir Peter J., English surgeon, 1851–1921.
Freyer drain
Freyer operation—prostate enucleation.
Freyer suprapubic drain

Frias, Jaime L., 20th century Chilean pediatrician.
Opitz-Frias syndrome—see under Opitz

Fridenberg, Percy H., U.S. ophthalmologist, 1868–1960.
Fridenberg stigometric card test—an obsolete test of vision and accommodation for illiterates.

Friderichsen, Carl, Danish physician, *1886.
Friderichsen syndrome—*SYN:* Waterhouse-Friderichsen syndrome
Friderichsen-Waterhouse syndrome—*SYN:* Waterhouse-Friderichsen syndrome
Waterhouse-Friderichsen syndrome—see under Waterhouse

Friedlander, var. of Friedländer.

Friedländer, Carl, German pathologist, 1847–1887.
Friedländer bacillus—capsular types 1, 2, and 3 of this organism may be causative agents in pneumonia. *SYN: Klebsiella pneumoniae*
Friedländer disease
Friedländer pneumobacillus
Friedländer pneumonia—a form of pneumonia caused by infection with *Klebsiella pneumoniae.*
Friedländer stain for capsules—an obsolete stain employing gentian violet.

Friedman, Arnold Phineas, U.S. physician, *1909.
Friedman-Roy syndrome—familial syndrome resulting in mental deficiency, strabismus, clubfoot, and other abnormalities.

Friedman, Emanuel A., U.S. obstetrician, *1926.
Friedman curve—a graph on which hours of labor are plotted against cervical dilation in centimeters.

Friedman, M., U.S. physiologist and physician, *1903.
Friedman test—modified Asheim-Zondek test for pregnancy.

F

NOTES

169

Friedmann, Max, German physician, 1858–1925.
    Friedmann syndrome—(1) juvenile epilepsy, petit mal type; (2) juvenile spastic paralysis due to congenital syphilis; (3) progressive form of encephalitis related to cerebral vasomotor disorder. *SYN:* postconcussion syndrome

Friedreich, Nikolaus, German neurologist, 1825–1882.
    Friedreich ataxia—sclerosis of the posterior and lateral columns of the spinal cord, occurring in children and marked by ataxia in the lower extremities, extending to the upper, followed by paralysis and contractures. *SYN:* hereditary spinal ataxia; Biemond ataxia
    Friedreich disease—*SYN:* Friedreich spasms; paramyoclonus multiplex
    Friedreich phenomenon—the tympanitic percussion sound over a pulmonary cavity is slightly raised in pitch on deep inspiration.
    Friedreich sign—in adherent pericardium, sudden collapse of the previously distended veins of the neck at each diastole of the heart.
    Friedreich spasms—*SYN:* Friedreich disease

Friend, Charlotte, U.S. microbiologist, *1921.
    Friend disease—mouse leukemia caused by the Friend leukemia virus.
    Friend leukemia virus—*SYN:* Friend virus
    Friend virus—a strain of the splenic group of mouse leukemia viruses, related to Moloney and Rauscher viruses. *SYN:* Swiss mouse leukemia virus; Friend leukemia virus

Fritsch, Heinrich, German gynecologist, 1844–1915.
    Bozeman-Fritsch catheter—see under Bozeman

Froehde, A., 19th century German chemist.
    Froehde reagent—sodium molybdate 1, in strong sulfuric acid 1000.

Froehlich, var. of Fröhlich

Fröhlich, Alfred, Austrian neurologist and pharmacologist, 1871–1953.
    Fröhlich dwarfism—dwarfism with Fröhlich syndrome.
    Fröhlich syndrome—dystrophia adiposogenitalis, originally involving an adenohypophysial tumor. *SYN:* Launois-Cléret syndrome

Frohn, Damianus, German physician, *1843.
    Frohn reagent—used to test for alkaloids and sugar.

Froin, Georges, French physician, 1874–1932.
    Froin syndrome—an alteration in cerebrospinal fluid noted in loculated portions of the subarachnoid space isolated from spinal fluid circulation by an inflammatory or neoplastic obstruction. *SYN:* loculation syndrome

Froment, Jules, Lyon physician, 1878–1946.
    Froment sign—flexion of the distal phalanx of the thumb when a sheet of paper is held between the thumb and index finger in ulnar nerve palsy.

Frommann, Carl, German anatomist, 1831–1892.
    Frommann lines—transverse marks on nerve fibers.

Frommel, Richard, German gynecologist, 1854–1912.
    Chiari-Frommel syndrome—see under Chiari
    Frommel disease—prolonged lactation causing uterine involution.

Frommel operation
Frommel-Chiari syndrome—*SYN:* Chiari-Frommel syndrome

Froriep, August von, German anatomist, 1849–1917.
Froriep ganglion—a temporary collection of nerve cells on the dorsal aspect of the hypoglossal nerve in the embryo.
Froriep induration—induration of a muscle through an interstitial growth of fibrous tissue. *SYN:* myositis fibrosa

Frost, Albert D., U.S. ophthalmologist, 1889–1945.
Frost operation
Frost suture—intermarginal suture between the eyelids to protect the cornea.

Frostig, Marianne B., Austrian-U.S. psychologist, *1906.
Frostig Developmental Test of Visual Perception—designed for use with children who are learning-disabled.
Frostig Movement Skills Test Battery—a test designed to determine learning problems by evaluating juvenile sensorimotor skills.

Frugoni, Cesare, Italian physician, *1881.
Frugoni disease—proliferation of eosinophils causing arthralgias, respiratory and gastrointestinal problems. *SYN:* infectious eosinophilia
Frugoni syndrome—splenomegaly due to splenic vein thrombosis.

Fryns, J.P., Belgian physician.
Fryns syndrome—genetic disorder resulting in limb abnormalities and pulmonary defects.

Fuchs, Ernst, Austrian ophthalmologist, 1851–1930.
angle of Fuchs—a crevice between the ciliary and pupillary zones of the iris, formed by atrophy of superficial layers of the iris in the pupillary zone.
Dalen-Fuchs nodules—see under Dalen
Fuchs adenoma—a benign epithelial tumor of the nonpigmented epithelium of the ciliary body, rarely exceeding 1 mm in diameter.
Fuchs atrophy—optic nerve peripheral atrophy.
Fuchs black spot—an area of pigment proliferation in the macular region in degenerative myopia.
Fuchs capsule forceps
Fuchs capsulotomy forceps
Fuchs coloboma—a congenital inferior crescent on the choroid at the edge of the optic disk. *SYN:* congenital conus
Fuchs crypt
Fuchs dystrophy—congenital degenerative eye disease.
Fuchs epithelial dystrophy—epithelial edema secondary to endothelial dystrophy of the cornea.
Fuchs heterochromic cyclitis—*SYN:* Fuchs syndrome

(continued)

F

NOTES

Fuchs *(continued)*
    Fuchs keratome
    Fuchs phenomenon—degeneration of third cranial nerve resulting in paradoxical retraction of lid in association with eye movements.
    Fuchs spur—part of the insertion of the dilator muscle onto the iris sphincter.
    Fuchs stoma—small depression on the surface of the iris near the margin of the pupil.
    Fuchs syndrome—syndrome characterized by heterochromia of the iris, iridocyclitis, keratic precipitates, and cataract. *Syn:* Fuchs heterochromic cyclitis
    Fuchs two-way eye syringe
    Fuchs uveitis—anterior uveitis and depigmentation of the iris. *Syn:* heterochromic uveitis

Fukala, Vincenz, Austrian ophthalmologist, 1847–1911.
    Fukala operation—eye lens removal.

Fukuyama, Yukio, 20th century Japanese physician.
    Fukuyama dystrophy—*Syn:* Fukuyama syndrome
    Fukuyama syndrome—recessive genetic trait resulting in progressive muscular dystrophy and brain disorders. *Syn:* Fukuyama dystrophy

Fürbringer, Paul W., German physician, 1849–1930.
    Fürbringer sign—sign related to subphrenic abscess.

Fürmaier, A.
    Fürmaier syndrome—lumbar rigidity causing difficulty in forward flexion of lumbar spine, caused by nerve root compression due to tumor or formation of posttraumatic cicatrix.

Futcher, Palmer Howard, U.S.-Canadian physician, *1910.
    Futcher line—a dorsoventral line of pigmentation occurring symmetrically and bilaterally for about 10 cm along the lateral edge of the biceps muscle. *Syn:* Voigt lines

G

Gabriel, William Bashall, English surgeon, *1893.
Gabriel proctoscope
Gabriel syringe—used for injection of hemorrhoids.

Gaddum, John H., English biochemist, *1900.
Gaddum and Schild test—a sensitive method for identification of
epinephrine in tissue or other material.

Gaenslen, Frederick J., U.S. surgeon, 1877–1937.
Gaenslen fracture
Gaenslen incision
Gaenslen osteomyelitis
Gaenslen sign—pain on hyperextension of the hip with pelvis fixed by
flexion of opposite hip.
Gaenslen split-heel incision
Gaenslen technique
Gaenslen test

Gaertner, Hermann Treschow, Danish surgeon, 1785–1827.
Gaetner duct—mesonephric duct.

Gaffky, Georg T.A., German hygienist, 1850–1918.
Gaffky scale—*Syn:* Gaffky table
Gaffky table—a numerical rating for the classification of tuberculosis. *Syn:*
Gaffky scale

Gairdner, Sir William T., Scottish physician, 1824–1907.
Gairdner disease—attacks of cardiac distress accompanied by
apprehension. *Syn:* angina pectoris sine dolore; angor pectoris

Gaisbock, var. of Gaisböck

Gaisböck, Felix, German physician, 1868–1955.
Gaisböck disease—polycythemia associated with hypertension but without
splenomegaly. *Syn:* Gaisböck syndrome; polycythemia hypertonica
Gaisböck syndrome—*Syn:* Gaisböck disease

Gajdusek, D. Carleton, U.S. pediatrician, *1923, joint winner of 1976 Nobel
Prize for work related to infectious diseases.

Galant, Nikolay Fedorovich, Russian hygienist, *1893.
Galant abdominal response
Galant hip guide
Galant hip prosthesis

(continued)

Galant *(continued)*

Galant reflex—a deep abdominal reflex in which there is a contraction of the abdominal muscles on tapping the anterior superior iliac spine. *SYN:* lower abdominal periosteal reflex

Galeati, Domenico, Italian physician, 1686–1775.

Galeati glands—the tubular glands in the mucous membrane of the small and large intestines. *SYN:* intestinal glands

Galeazzi, Riccardo, Italian surgeon, 1886–1952.

Galeazzi fracture—fracture of the shaft of the radius with dislocation of the distal radioulnar joint.
Galeazzi patellar operation
Galeazzi realignment
Galeazzi sign
Galeazzi test

Galen, Claudius, Greek physician and medical scientist in Rome, *c.* 130–201 A.D.

Galen anastomosis—*SYN:* communicating branch of superior laryngeal nerve with recurrent laryngeal nerve
Galen bandage
Galen dressing
Galen foramen
Galen nerve—*SYN:* communicating branch of superior laryngeal nerve with recurrent laryngeal nerve
Galen ventricle
galenical—referring to medicine prepared from plants rather than chemicals.
great cerebral vein of Galen—a large, unpaired vein formed by the junction of the two internal cerebral veins. *SYN:* great vein of Galen
great vein of Galen—*SYN:* great cerebral vein of Galen
veins of Galen—*SYN:* internal cerebral veins

Gall, Franz J., German-Austrian anatomist, 1758–1828.

Gall craniology—an obsolete doctrine. *SYN:* phrenology

Gallais, Alfred, French physician.

Gallais syndrome—*SYN:* Cushing syndrome

Gallavardin, Louis, French physician, 1875–1957.

Gallavardin phenomenon—dissociation between the noisy and musical elements of the murmur of aortic stenosis.

Gallie, William E., Canadian surgeon, 1882–1959.

Gallie arthrodesis
Gallie atlantoaxial fusion technique
Gallie fascia needle
Gallie herniorrhaphy
Gallie procedure
Gallie spinal fusion
Gallie subtalar ankle fusion
Gallie technique

Gallie tendon passer

Gallie transplant—narrow strips of the femoral fascia lata used for suture material.

Galton, Sir Francis, English scientist, 1822–1911.

Galton delta—a more or less well-marked triangle in a fingerprint; in dermatoglyphics, the figure at the base of each finger in the palm. *Syn:* triradius

Galton law—in a population mating at random, the progeny of a parent with an extreme value for a measurable phenotype will tend to have values nearer the population mean than in the extreme parent. *Syn:* law of regression to mean

Galton system of classification of fingerprints—a system of classification based on the variations in the patterns of the ridges, which are grouped into arches, loops, and whorls.

Galton whistle—a cylindrical whistle attached to a compressible bulb used to test hearing.

Galvani, Luigi, Italian physician and anatomist, 1737–1798.

galvanic bath—water bath that is charged with galvanic current.

galvanic current—continuous one-direction electric current.

galvanic skin response—skin's response to electric stimulation. *Syn:* electrodermal response

galvanic-faradic test—an electrodiagnostic test of muscles.

galvanism—oral manifestations of direct current electricity occurring when dental restorations with dissimilar electric potentials (such as silver and gold) are placed in the mouth. *Syn:* voltaism

galvanometer—an instrument used to measure current.

Gamgee, Joseph Sampson, English surgeon, 1828–1886.

Gamgee tissue—a thick layer of absorbent cotton between two layers of absorbent gauze, used in surgical dressings.

Gammel, John A., U.S. physician.

Gammel syndrome—paraneoplastic disorder resulting in erythematous lesions associated with neoplasms of internal organs. *Syn:* erythema gyratum repens

Gamna, Carlos, Italian physician, 1896–1950.

Gamna disease—a form of chronic splenomegaly.

Gamna-Favre bodies—characteristic, relatively large, intracytoplasmic basophilic inclusion bodies observed in lymphogranuloma venereum.

Gamna-Gandy bodies—small firm spheroidal or irregular foci occurring chiefly in the spleen in such conditions as congestive splenomegaly and sickle cell disease. *Syn:* siderotic nodules; Gandy-Gamna bodies

Gandy-Gamna bodies—*Syn:* Gamna-Gandy bodies

Gamper, E., Austrian neurologist, 1887–1938.

Gamper bowing reflex—when holding the sacrum of severely brain-

(continued)

G

NOTES

Gamper (*continued*)

> damaged children and sometimes normal but premature infants, the hips are extended and head and trunk elevate in bowlike fashion from supine position.

Gamstorp, Ingrid, Swedish pediatric neurologist, *1924.

> **Gamstorp disease**—dominant trait resulting in periodic paralysis and usually accompanied by hyperkalemia.
>
> **Gamstorp-Wohlfart syndrome**—genetic trait resulting in muscle wasting, increased muscle contractility, and increased perspiration.

Gandy, Charles, French physician, *1872.

> **Gamna-Gandy bodies**—see under Gamna
>
> **Gandy-Gamna bodies**—*SYN:* Gamna-Gandy bodies
>
> **Gandy-Nanta disease**—siderotic splenomegaly.

Ganong, William F., U.S. physiologist, *1924.

> **Lown-Ganong-Levine syndrome**—see under Lown

Ganser, Siegbert J.M., German psychiatrist, 1853–1931.

> **basal nucleus of Ganser**—a group of large cells in the innominate substance, ventral to the lentiform nucleus. *SYN:* nucleus basalis of Ganser
>
> **Ganser commissures**—the commissural fibers that lie above and behind the optic chiasm. *SYN:* commissurae supraopticae
>
> **Ganser syndrome**—a psychotic-like condition, without the symptoms and signs of a traditional psychosis, occurring typically in prisoners who feign insanity. *SYN:* syndrome of approximate relevant answers; syndrome of deviously relevant answers; nonsense syndrome
>
> **nucleus basalis of Ganser**—*SYN:* basal nucleus of Ganser

Gant, Samuel, U.S. surgeon, 1870–1944.

> **Gant clamp**—a right-angled clamp used in hemorrhoidectomy.

Gantzer, Carol F.L., 17th century German anatomist.

> **Gantzer accessory bundle**
>
> **Gantzer muscle**—an accessory muscle extending from the superficial flexor of the digits to the deep flexor of the digits.

Ganz, William, U.S. cardiologist, *1919.

> **Ganz-Edwards coronary infusion catheter**
>
> **Swan-Ganz balloon flotation catheter**
>
> **Swan-Ganz bipolar pacing catheter**
>
> **Swan-Ganz catheter**—see under Swan
>
> **Swan-Ganz flow-directed catheter**
>
> **Swan-Ganz pacing TD catheter**

Garbe, William, Canadian dermatologist, *1908.

> **Sulzberger-Garbe disease**—see under Sulzberger
>
> **Sulzberger-Garbe syndrome**—*SYN:* Sulzberger-Garbe disease

Garceau, George J., U.S. orthopedic surgeon, 1896–1977.

> **Garceau approach**
>
> **Garceau bougie**
>
> **Garceau catheter**
>
> **Garceau cheilectomy**

Garceau clubfoot procedure
Garceau method—a method used to treat fractures of the surgical neck of the humerus.
Garceau tendon technique

Garcin, Raymond, French physician, 1897–1971.
Garcin syndrome—tumors of the nasopharynx involving all or most unilateral cranial nerves without involving the brain.

Garden, Robert Symon, English orthopedic surgeon.
Garden alignment index
Garden classification
Garden femoral neck fracture
Garden grades—classification system for femoral neck fractures (I-IV).
Garden procedure

Gardner, Eldon J., U.S. geneticist, *1909.
Fitzgerald-Gardner syndrome—see under Fitzgerald
Gardner syndrome—multiple polyposis predisposing to carcinoma of the colon.

Gardner, F.H.
Gardner-Diamond syndrome—a condition usually occurring in women in which the individual bruises easily. *Syn:* autoerythrocyte sensitization syndrome

Gareis, Frank J., U.S. physician.
Gareis syndrome—mental retardation, X-linked, associated with missing extensor pollicis brevis tendons causing bilateral thumb clasping.

Gariel, Maurice, French physician, 1812–1878.
Gariel pessary—a hollow, inflatable, rubber pessary made in the form of a ring or a pear.

Garland, George M., U.S. physician, 1848–1926.
Garland triangle—a triangular area of relative resonance in the lower back, found in the same side as a pleural effusion.

Garland, Hugh, English neurologist.
Marinesco-Sjögren-Garland syndrome—see under Marinesco

Garré, Carl, Swiss surgeon, 1857–1928.
Garré disease—fusiform thickening or increased density of bones. *Syn:* sclerosing osteitis
Garré osteomyelitis—chronic osteomyelitis with proliferative periostitis; a focal gross thickening of the periosteum with peripheral reactive bone formation resulting from mild infection.

G

Garrod, A.E., English physician, 1857–1936.
Garrod hypothesis—one enzyme defect per gene.
Garrod pads—pads on the dorsum of proximal interphalangeal joints, may be painful on flexion.

NOTES

Gartner, Herman T., Danish anatomist and surgeon, 1785–1827.

    Gartner canal—a rudimentary vestige of the mesonephric duct in the female into which the tubules of the epoöphoron open. *SYN:* longitudinal duct of epoöphoron; Gartner duct

    Gartner cyst—a cyst of the principal duct in the vestigial structures of the paroöphoron in the cervix or anterolateral vaginal wall.

    Gartner duct—*SYN:* Gartner canal

Gärtner, August, German physician, 1848–1934.

    Gärtner bacillus—a widely distributed species that occurs in humans and in domestic and wild animals, especially rodents. *SYN: Salmonella enteritidis*

    Gärtner method—a method of measuring venous pressure.

    Gärtner tonometer—an apparatus for estimating blood pressure.

    Gärtner vein phenomenon—fullness of the veins of the arm and hand held below heart level and collapsed at a certain variable distance above that level.

Gaskell, Walter H., English physiologist, 1847–1914.

    Gaskell bridge—a bundle of modified cardiac muscle fibers. *SYN:* atrioventricular bundle

    Gaskell clamp—an instrument for crushing the atrioventricular bundle in experimental animals and thus producing heart block.

Gass, J. Donald M., U.S. ophthalmologist, *1928.

    Gass cannula

    Gass cataract-aspirating cannula

    Gass corneoscleral punch

    Gass muscle hook

    Gass scleral marker

    Gass scleral punch

    Irvine-Gass syndrome—see under Irvine

Gasser, Johann L., Austrian anatomist, 1723–1765.

    gasserian ganglion—the large flattened sensory ganglion of the trigeminal nerve. *SYN:* trigeminal ganglion

Gasser, Konrad J., Swiss pediatrician, *1912.

    Gasser cells—cytoplasmic inclusions that stain dark red-purple.

    Gasser syndrome—(1) acute transient erythropoietic tissue aplasia, in children; no known cause; (2) acute renal failure, hemolytic anemia, and other disorders occurring in children under the age of 4; often associated *Escherichia coli* infection-induced diarrhea.

Gastaut, Henri, French biologist, *1915.

    Gastaut syndrome—juvenile hemiplegic epilepsy with ipsilateral signs.

    Lennox-Gastaut syndrome—see under Lennox

Gatch, Willis Dew, U.S. surgeon, 1878–1961.

    Gatch bed—a bed with 3 sections for independent elevation of a patient's head and knees.

Gaucher, Philippe C.E., French physician, 1854–1918.

    Gaucher cells—large, finely and uniformly vacuolated cells derived from the reticuloendothelial system and found especially in the spleen, lymph nodes, liver, and bone marrow of patients with Gaucher disease.

Gaucher disease—a lysosomal storage disease. *SYN:* familial splenic anemia; cerebroside lipidosis

Gaucher type of histiocyte

pseudo-Gaucher cell—a plasma cell, microscopically resembling a Gaucher cell, found in the bone marrow in some cases of multiple myeloma.

Gauer, Otto Hans, German physiologist, 1909–1979.
  Henry-Gauer response—see under Henry, James

Gauss, Johann K.F., German physicist, 1777–1855.
  gauss—a unit of magnetic field intensity.
  gaussian curve—a specific bell-shaped frequency distribution. *SYN:* normal distribution; gaussian distribution
  gaussian distribution—*SYN:* gaussian curve

Gauss, Karl J., German gynecologist, 1875–1957.
  Gauss sign—marked mobility of the uterus in the early weeks of pregnancy.

Gaussel, A., French physician, 1871–1937.
  Grasset-Gaussel phenomenon—*SYN:* Grasset phenomenon

Gavard, Hyacinthe, French anatomist, 1753–1802.
  Gavard muscle—oblique fibers in the muscular coat of the stomach.

Gay, Alexander H., Russian anatomist, 1842–1907.
  Gay glands—large apocrine sweat glands surrounding the anus. *SYN:* circumanal glands

Gay-Lussac, Joseph L., French naturalist, 1778–1850.
  Gay-Lussac equation—the overall chemical equation for alcoholic fermentation.
  Gay-Lussac law—*SYN:* Charles law

Gayet, Charles Jules Alphonse, French physician, 1833–1904.
  Gayet disease—*SYN:* Wernicke syndrome
  Gayet-Wernicke syndrome—*SYN:* Wernicke syndrome

Gee, Samuel J., English pediatrician and physician, 1839–1911.
  Gee disease—malabsorption syndrome in infants. *SYN:* Gee-Herter disease; Gee-Thaysen disease; Heubner-Herter disease
  Gee-Herter disease—*SYN:* Gee disease
  Gee-Herter-Heubner disease
  Gee-Thaysen disease—*SYN:* Gee disease

Gegenbaur, Carl, German anatomist, 1826–1903.
  Gegenbaur cell—bone-producing cell.

Gehrig, Henry Louis, U.S. baseball player, New York Yankees; 1903–1941, victim of Lou Gehrig disease.
  Lou Gehrig disease—a disease of the motor tracts of the lateral columns and anterior horns of the spinal cord, causing progressive muscular

G

(continued)

NOTES

Gehrig *(continued)*
 atrophy. *Syn:* amyotrophic lateral sclerosis; Aran-Duchenne disease; Aran-Duchenne dystrophy; Duchenne-Aran disease; Cruveilhier disease; Cruveilhier palsy; Charcot disease

Geigel, Richard, German physician, 1859–1930.
 Geigel reflex—in the female, a contraction of the muscular fibers at the upper edge of Poupart ligament on gently stroking the inner side of the thigh.

Geiger, Hans, German physicist, 1882–1945.
 Geiger-Müller counter—an instrument for measuring radioactivity by counting the emission of radioactive particles.
 Geiger-Müller tube

Gélineau, Jean Baptiste Edouard, French physician, 1859–1906.
 Gélineau disease—*Syn:* Gélineau syndrome
 Gélineau syndrome—a sleep disorder that usually appears in young adulthood. *Syn:* narcolepsy; Gélineau disease; Gélineau-Redlich syndrome
 Gélineau-Redlich syndrome—*Syn:* Gélineau syndrome

Gell, Philip G., English immunologist, *1914.
 Gell and Coombs reactions—allergic reaction.

Gellé, Marie-Ernst, French otologist, 1834–1923.
 Gellé test—a test of the mobility of the ossicles using a vibrating tuning fork.

Gellerstedt, Nils, *1896.
 Ceelen-Gellerstedt syndrome—see under Ceelen

Gély, Jules A., French surgeon, 1806–1861.
 Gély suture—a cobbler's suture used in closing intestinal wounds.

Gengou, Octave, French bacteriologist, 1875–1957.
 Bordet-Gengou bacillus—see under Bordet
 Bordet-Gengou phenomenon—see under Bordet
 Bordet-Gengou potato blood agar—see under Bordet
 Bordet-Gengou reaction
 Gengou phenomenon—noncellular antigens.

Gennari, Francesco, Italian anatomist, 1750–1795.
 Gennari band—*Syn:* line of Gennari
 Gennari stria—*Syn:* line of Gennari
 line of Gennari—a prominent white line appearing in perpendicular sections of the visual cortex. *Syn:* Gennari band; Gennari stria; stripe of Gennari
 stripe of Gennari—*Syn:* line of Gennari

Georgi, Walter, German bacteriologist, 1889–1920.
 Sachs-Georgi test—see under Sachs

Geraghty, John T., U.S. physician, 1876–1924.
 Geraghty test—obsolete test for renal function. *Syn:* phenolsulfonphthalein test
 Rowntree and Geraghty test—see under Rowntree

Gerbode, Frank

Gerbode annuloplasty
Gerbode cardiovascular tissue forceps
Gerbode defect—a defect in the interventricular portion of the membranous septum, associated with a communication between the right ventricle and the right atrium through an abnormality in the tricuspid valve.
Gerbode dilator
Gerbode mitral dilator
Gerbode mitral valvulotome
Gerbode mitral valvulotomy dilator
Gerbode patent ductus clamp
Gerbode rib spreader
Gerbode sternal retractor
Gerbode valve dilator

Gerdy, Pierre N., French surgeon, 1797–1856.

Gerdy fibers—a thickening of the deep fascia in the most distal part of the base of the triangular palmar aponeurosis. *SYN:* superficial transverse metacarpal ligament
Gerdy fontanel—an occasional fontanel-like defect in the sagittal suture in the newborn. *SYN:* sagittal fontanel
Gerdy hyoid fossa—a space that contains the bifurcation of the common carotid artery. *SYN:* carotid triangle
Gerdy interatrial loop—a muscular fasciculus in the interatrial septum of the heart, passing backward from the atrioventricular groove.
Gerdy ligament—the continuation of the clavipectoral fascia downward to attach to the axillary fascia. *SYN:* suspensory ligament of axilla
Gerdy tubercle—a tubercle on the lateral side of the upper end of the tibia giving attachment to the iliotibial tract and some fibers of the tibialis anterior muscle.

Gerhardt, Carl J., German physician, 1833–1902.

Gerhardt disease—*SYN:* Gerhardt-Mitchell disease
Gerhardt reaction—*SYN:* Gerhardt test for acetoacetic acid
Gerhardt sign—complete bilateral paralysis of the adductor muscles of the larynx with severe inspiratory dyspnea. *SYN:* Biermer sign
Gerhardt syndrome—bilateral laryngeal abductor paralysis.
Gerhardt test for acetoacetic acid—*SYN:* Gerhardt reaction
Gerhardt-Mitchell disease—paroxysmal throbbing and burning pain in the skin affecting the hands and feet, accompanied by a dusky mottled redness of the parts with increased skin temperature. *SYN:* erythromelalgia; Weir Mitchell disease; Mitchell disease; Gerhardt disease
Gerhardt-Semon law—obsolete law formerly used to account for the position of affected vocal cords after injury to the recurrent laryngeal nerve(s).

G

NOTES

Gerhardt, Charles F., French chemist, 1816–1856.
Gerhardt test for urobilin in the urine—the urobilin is extracted with chloroform and then treated with iodine and potassium hydrate.

Gerlach, Joseph, German anatomist, 1820–1896.
Gerlach annular tendon—the thickened portion of the circumference of the tympanic membrane that is fixed in the tympanic sulcus. *SYN:* fibrocartilaginous ring of tympanic membrane
Gerlach tonsil—a collection of lymphoid nodules near the pharyngeal opening of the auditory tube. *SYN:* tubal tonsil
Gerlach valve—a fold of mucous membrane, simulating a valve, sometimes found at the origin of the vermiform appendix. *SYN:* valve of vermiform appendix; valvula processus vermiformis
Gerlach valvula—the network of fibers at the iridocorneal angle between the anterior chamber of the eye and the venous sinus of the sclera. *SYN:* trabecular reticulum

Gerlier, Felix, Swiss physician, 1840–1914.
Gerlier disease—a paroxysmal attack of severe vertigo, not accompanied by deafness or tinnitus, due to unilateral vestibular dysfunction. *SYN:* vestibular neuronitis; Gerlier syndrome
Gerlier syndrome—*SYN:* Gerlier disease

Gerold, M., German physician.
Baller-Gerold syndrome—see under Baller
Gerold-Baller syndrome—*SYN:* Baller-Gerold syndrome

Gerota, Dimitru, Romanian anatomist and surgeon, 1867–1939.
Gerota capsule—*SYN:* Gerota fascia
Gerota fascia—the condensation of the fibroareolar tissue and fat surrounding the kidney to form a sheath for the organ. *SYN:* renal fascia; Gerota capsule
Gerota method—injection of the lymphatics with a dye that is soluble in chloroform or ether but not in water.

Gersh, Isidore, U.S. histologist, *1907.
Altmann-Gersh method—see under Altmann

Gerstmann, Josef, Austrian neurologist, 1887–1969.
Gerstmann syndrome—finger agnosia, agraphia, confusion of laterality of body, and acalculia caused by lesions between the occipital area and the angular gyrus.
Gerstmann-Sträussler syndrome—a more chronic cerebellar form of spongiform encephalopathy.

Geschickter, Charles F., U.S. physician.
Geschickter tumor—a bone tumor, often malignant, occurring most frequently in adults between the ages of 20 and 40; found on the femur or humerus.

Gesell, Arnold L., U.S. psychologist, 1880–1961.
Gesell Development Scales—designed to test the development of infants and preschoolers. *SYN:* Gesell test
Gesell test—*SYN:* Gesell Development Scales

Gey, George O., U.S. physician and researcher, *1899.
   Gey solution—a salt solution used for culturing animal cells.

Ghilarducci, Francesco, Italian physician, 1857–1924.
   Ghilarducci reaction

Ghon, Anton, Czech pathologist, 1866–1936.
   Ghon complex—*SYN:* Ghon tubercle
   Ghon focus—*SYN:* Ghon tubercle
   Ghon lesion
   Ghon node
   Ghon primary lesion—*SYN:* Ghon tubercle
   Ghon tubercle—calcification seen in pulmonary parenchyma and hilar
     nodes resulting from earlier infection with tuberculosis. *SYN:* Ghon
     complex; Ghon focus; Ghon primary lesion
   Ghon-Sachs bacillus—*SYN:* Sachs bacillus

Giacomini, Carlo, Italian anatomist, 1841–1898.
   band of Giacomini—*SYN:* uncus band of Giacomini
   frenulum of Giacomini—*SYN:* uncus band of Giacomini
   uncus band of Giacomini—a slender whitish band crossing transversally
     the surface of the recurved part of the uncus gyri parahippocampalis.
     SYN: band of Giacomini; frenulum of Giacomini; cauda fasciae dentatae;
     tail of dentate gyrus

Gianelli, Giuseppe, Italian physician, 1799–1871.
   Gianelli sign—*SYN:* Tournay phenomenon

Giannuzzi, Guiseppe, Italian anatomist, 1839–1876.
   Giannuzzi crescents—the serous cells at the distal end of a mucous,
     tubuloalveolar secretory unit of certain salivary glands. *SYN:* serous
     demilunes; Giannuzzi demilunes
   Giannuzzi demilunes—*SYN:* Giannuzzi crescents

Gianotti, Fernando, Italian dermatologist, *1920.
   Gianotti-Crosti syndrome—a cutaneous manifestation of hepatitis B
     infection occurring in young children. *SYN:* papular acrodermatitis of
     childhood

Giard, Alfred, French biologist, 1846–1908.
   Giardia lamblia—protozoa which causes diarrhea and adominal
     discomfort.
   giardiasis—infection with Giardia.

Gibbon, John H., U.S. surgeon, 1903–1973.
   Landis-Gibbon test—see under Landis
   Mayo-Gibbon heart-lung machine—see under Mayo, Charles

Gibbon, Norman Otway Knight, English urologist.
   Gibbon catheter—urinary catheter.
   Gibbon hydrocele
   Gibbon ureteral stent

G

NOTES

Gibbs, J. Willard, U.S. mathematician and physicist, 1839–1903.
Gibbs energy of activation—energy that must be added to that already possessed by a molecule(s) in order to initiate a reaction.
Gibbs free energy
Gibbs theorem—substances that lower the surface tension of the pure dispersion medium tend to collect in its surface, whereas substances that raise the surface tension tend to remain out of the surface film.
Gibbs-Donnan equilibrium—*SYN:* Donnan equilibrium
Gibbs-Helmholtz equation—an equation expressing the relationship in a galvanic cell between the chemical energy transformed and the maximal electromotive force obtainable. *SYN:* Helmholtz-Gibbs theory
Helmholtz-Gibbs theory—*SYN:* Gibbs-Helmholtz equation

Gibert, Camille Melchior, French physician, 1797–1866.
Gibert disease—inflammatory skin disease causing macules over trunk and extremities.

Gibney, Virgil P., U.S. orthopedist, 1847–1927.
Gibney bandage
Gibney boot—adhesive tape treatment of a sprained ankle.
Gibney disease
Gibney dressing
Gibney fixation bandage—herring bone strapping of the foot and leg for sprain of the ankle.
Gibney perispondylitis
Gibney strapping

Gibson, George A., Scottish physician, 1854–1913.
Gibson murmur—the typical continuous murmur of patent ductus arteriosus.

Gibson, Kasson C., U.S. dentist, 1849–1925.
Gibson bandage—a bandage for stabilizing a fracture of the mandible.

Gibson, Quentin Howieson, English physician.
Gibson disease—recessive trait which renders hemoglobin unable to bind with oxygen, causing dyspnea and fatigue after physical exertion.

Giedion, Andreas, Swiss physician.
Giedion syndrome—genetic recessive or dominant trait causing orofacial defects and abnormalities of the phalanges. *SYN:* trichorhinophalangeal syndrome

Giemsa, Gustav, German bacteriologist, 1867–1948.
Giemsa chromosome banding stain—a unique chromosome staining technique used in human cytogenetics to identify individual chromosomes. *SYN:* G-banding stain
Giemsa stain—compound used for demonstrating Negri bodies, *Tunga* species, spirochetes and protozoans, and differential staining of blood smears.

Gierke, Edgar von, German pathologist, 1877–1945.
Gierke disease—glycogenosis due to glucose 6-phosphatase deficiency, resulting in accumulation of excessive amounts of glycogen of normal chemical structure, particularly in liver and kidney. *SYN:* type 1 glycogenosis; von Gierke disease; von Gierke syndrome

von Gierke disease—*SYN:* Gierke disease
von Gierke syndrome—*SYN:* Gierke disease

Gierke, Hans P.B., German anatomist, 1847–1886.
    Gierke corpuscles—*SYN:* thymic corpuscles
    Gierke respiratory bundle—primary sensory fibers that enter with the vagus, glossopharyngeal, and facial nerves, and in part convey information from stretch receptors and chemoreceptors in the walls of the cardiovascular, respiratory, and intestinal tracts. *SYN:* solitary tract

Gieson, Ira van. See under van Gieson.

Gifford, Harold, U.S. ophthalmologist, 1858–1929.
    Gifford applicator
    Gifford corneal applicator
    Gifford corneal curet
    Gifford fixation forceps
    Gifford holder
    Gifford iris forceps
    Gifford keratotomy
    Gifford needle holder
    Gifford reflex—constriction of both pupils when an effort is made to close eyelids forcibly held apart. *SYN:* eye-closure pupil reaction
    Gifford sign—difficulty in everting the upper eyelid in Graves disease.

Gigli, Leonardo, Italian gynecologist, 1863–1908.
    Gigli operation—severance of the pubic bone a few centimeters lateral to the symphysis to permit the passage of a living child. *SYN:* pubiotomy
    Gigli pubiotomy
    Gigli saw—a hand-held wire saw for use in craniotomy or pubiotomy.
    Gigli-saw blade
    Gigli-saw conductor
    Gigli-saw guide
    Gigli-saw handle
    Gigli-saw wire

Gil-Vernet, Jose Maria Vila, Spanish urologist, *1922.
    Gil-Vernet dissection
    Gil-Vernet operation—extension of a standard pyelotomy into the lower pole infundibulum through the avascular plane between the posterior and basilar segmental renal arteries. *SYN:* extended pyelotomy
    Gil-Vernet pyelolithotomy
    Gil-Vernet renal sinus retractor
    Gil-Vernet retractor

Gilbert, Nicholas A., French physician, 1858–1927.
    Gilbert disease—*SYN:* familial nonhemolytic jaundice
    Gilbert syndrome—*SYN:* familial nonhemolytic jaundice

Gilbert, Walter, U.S. microbiologist and Nobel laureate, *1932.
    Maxim-Gilbert sequencing—see under Maxim

G

NOTES

Gilchrist, Thomas C., U.S. physician, 1862–1927.
    Gilchrist disease—a chronic granulomatous and suppurative disease caused by *Blastomyces dermatitidis*. *SYN:* blastomycosis
    Gilchrist mycosis—obsolete term for blastomycosis.

Gilford, Hastings, English physician, 1861–1941.
    Hutchinson-Gilford disease—see under Hutchinson
    Hutchinson-Gilford syndrome—*SYN:* Hutchinson-Gilford disease

Gilles de la Tourette, Georges, French physician, 1857–1904.
    Gilles de la Tourette disease—*SYN:* Tourette syndrome
    Gilles de la Tourette syndrome—*SYN:* Tourette syndrome
    Tourette disease—*SYN:* Tourette syndrome
    Tourette syndrome—a disorder characterized by multiple motor and vocal tics. *SYN:* Gilles de la Tourette disease; Tourette disease; Gilles de la Tourette syndrome

Gillespie, Frank D., U.S. ophthalmologist, *1927.
    Gillespie syndrome—hereditary syndrome resulting in absence of the iris and other abnormalities.

Gillette, Eugène P., French surgeon, 1836–1886.
    Gillette suspensory ligament—longitudinal fiber of the esophagus that attaches to the posterior aspect of the cricoid cartilage of the larynx. *SYN:* cricoesophageal tendon

Gilliam, David Tod, U.S. gynecologist, 1844–1923.
    Gilliam operation—an operation for retroversion of the uterus by suturing round ligaments to abdominal wall fascia.
    Gilliam suspension of uterus

Gillies, Sir Harold D., English plastic surgeon, 1882–1960.
    Filatov-Gillies flap—see under Filatov, Vladimir
    Filatov-Gillies tubed pedicle—see under Filatov, Vladimir
    Gillies approach
    Gillies construction of replacement thumb
    Gillies ectropion graft
    Gillies elevation procedure
    Gillies flap
    Gillies graft
    Gillies hook
    Gillies horizontal dermal suture
    Gillies implant
    Gillies incision
    Gillies needle holder
    Gillies operation—a technique for reducing fractures of the zygoma and the zygomatic arch through an incision in the temporal region above the hairline.
    Gillies prosthesis
    Gillies scissors
    Gillies skin hook
    Gillies tissue forceps
    Gillies up-and-down flap
    Gillies zygomatic hook

Gilman, Alfred G., joint winner of 1994 Nobel Prize for work related to G-proteins.

Gilmer, Thomas L., U.S. oral surgeon, 1849–1931.
    Gilmer intermaxillary fixation—*Syn:* Gilmer wiring
    Gilmer tooth splint
    Gilmer wiring—a method of intermaxillary fixation in which single opposing teeth are wired circumferentially, and the wires are twisted together. *Syn:* Gilmer intermaxillary fixation

Gimbernat, Don Manuel L.A. de, Spanish anatomist and surgeon, 1734–1816.
    Gimbernat ligament—a curved fibrous band that forms the medial boundary of the femoral ring. *Syn:* lacunar ligament

Girard, A., Swiss-born U.S. surgeon, 1841–1914.
    Girard reagent—the hydrazine of betaine chloride, used to extract ketonic steroids by forming water-soluble hydrazones with them.

Girdlestone, Gathorne Robert, English orthopaedist, 1881–1950.
    Girdlestone procedure—complete resection or excision of the head and neck of the femur.
    Girdlestone resection
    Girdlestone resection arthroplasty

Giroux, Jean Marie, Canadian physician.
    Giroux-Barbeau syndrome—dominant trait causing plaques in the neonate with development of neurologic disorders in adulthood.

Givens, Maurice H., U.S. biochemist, *1888.
    Givens method—measurement of digestion.

Gjessing, Leiv Rolvssoen, Norwegian physician, *1918.
    Gjessing syndrome—nitrogen retention resulting in periodic catatonia which responds to thyroid therapy.

Glanzmann, Eduard, Swiss clinician, 1887–1959.
    Glanzmann and Riniker lymphocytophthisis—agammaglobulinemia, absent thymus, severe cytopenia, recurring infections, and inability to form antibodies.
    Glanzmann disease—*Syn:* Glanzmann thrombasthenia
    Glanzmann thrombasthenia—a hemorrhagic diathesis due to defect in platelet membrane glycoprotein IIb-IIIa complex. *Syn:* Glanzmann disease; hereditary hemorrhagic thrombasthenia; constitutional thrombopathy

Glaser, Johann H., Swiss anatomist, 1629–1675.
    glaserian artery—*Syn:* anterior tympanic artery
    glaserian fissure—*Syn:* petrotympanic fissure

Glasgow, William C., U.S. physician, 1845–1907.
    Glasgow sign—a systolic murmur heard over the brachial artery in aortic aneurysm.

G

NOTES

Glauber, Johann R., German chemist, 1604–1668.
  Glauber salt—an ingredient of many of the natural laxative waters, and also used as a hydragogue cathartic. *SYN:* sodium sulfate

Gleason, Donald F., U.S. pathologist, *1920.
  Gleason score
  Gleason tumor grade—a classification of adenocarcinoma of the prostate.

Glénard, F., French physician, 1848–1920.
  Glénard disease—intraabdominal organ ptosis.

Glenner, George B., U.S. pathologist and histologist, *1927.
  Glenner-Lillie stain for pituitary—a modification of Mann methyl blue-eosin stain.

Gley, Marcel E.E., French physiologist, 1857–1930.
  Gley cells—testicular interstitial cells.
  Gley glands

Glisson, Francis, English physician, anatomist, physiologist and pathologist, 1597–1677.
  Glisson capsule—a layer of connective tissue ensheathing the liver, hepatic artery, portal vein, and bile ducts. *SYN:* fibrous capsule of liver
  Glisson cirrhosis—chronic perihepatitis with thickening and subsequent contraction, resulting in atrophy and deformity of the liver. *SYN:* capsular cirrhosis of liver
  Glisson disease
  Glisson sling—used in cervical traction to support the head.
  Glisson sphincter—the smooth muscle sphincter of the hepatopancreatic ampulla within the duodenal papilla. *SYN:* sphincter of hepatopancreatic ampulla

Gluge, Gottlieb, German histologist, 1812–1898.
  Gluge corpuscles—large pus cells containing fat droplets.

Gmelin, Leopold, German physiologist and chemist, 1788–1853.
  Gmelin test—a test for bile in body fluid. *SYN:* Rosenbach-Gmelin test
  Rosenbach-Gmelin test—*SYN:* Gmelin test

Godélier, Charles P., French physician, 1813–1877.
  Godélier law—tuberculosis of the peritoneum is always associated with tuberculosis of the pleura on one or both sides.

Godman, John D., U.S. anatomist, 1794–1830.
  Godman fascia—an extension of the pretracheal fascia into the thorax and onto the pericardium.

Godtfredsen, E., English ophthalmologist.
  Godtfredsen syndrome—invasive tumor of the cavernous sinus causing ipsilateral blindness, trigeminal neuralgia, paralysis of 12th cranial nerve, and ophthalmoplegia.

Godwin, John T., U.S. pathologist, *1917.
  Godwin tumor—benign tumorlike masses of lymphoid tissue in the parotid gland, containing scattered small islands of epithelial cells. *SYN:* benign lymphoepithelial lesion

Goeckerman, William H., U.S. dermatologist, 1884–1954.
    Goeckerman light therapy
    Goeckerman treatment—a treatment for psoriasis.

Goedel, A., German physician.
    Epstein-Goedel syndrome—see under Epstein

Goeminne, Luc, Belgian physician.
    Goeminne syndrome—congenital disorder resulting in torticollis, facial
    asymmetry, renal problems, pigmented nevi, varicose veins of lower
    extremities, hyperpigmentation.

Gofman, Moses, German physician, *1887.
    Gofman test—a test for various serum lipoproteins that contain
    cholesterol, as an index of the tendency to the development of
    atheromatous lesions and arteriosclerosis.

Goggia, Carlo P., Italian physician, 1871–1948.
    Goggia sign—fibrillation of the biceps muscle, when pinched and tapped,
    is confined to a limited area in cases of debilitating disease, whereas in
    health it is general.

Goldberg, Morton F., U.S. physician, *1937.
    Goldberg syndrome—galactosialidosis.

Goldblatt, Harry, U.S. pathologist, 1891–1977.
    Goldblatt clamp
    Goldblatt hypertension—increased blood pressure following obstruction of
    blood flow to one kidney. *SYN:* Goldblatt phenomenon
    Goldblatt kidney—a kidney whose arterial blood supply has been
    compromised, as a consequence of which arterial hypertension develops.
    Goldblatt phenomenon—*SYN:* Goldblatt hypertension

Goldenhar, M., 20th century French physician.
    Goldenhar syndrome—a syndrome characterized by epibulbar dermoids,
    preauricular appendages, micrognathia, and vertebral and other
    anomalies. *SYN:* oculoauriculovertebral dysplasia

Goldflam, Samuel V., Polish neurologist, 1852–1932.
    Erb-Goldflam disease—*SYN:* Goldflam disease
    Goldflam disease—disorder of neuromuscular transmission, marked by
    fluctuating weakness, of oculofacial and proximal limb muscles. *SYN:*
    myasthenia gravis; Erb-Goldflam disease; Goldflam symptom complex;
    Hoppe-Goldflam disease
    Goldflam symptom complex—*SYN:* Goldflam disease
    Hoppe-Goldflam disease—*SYN:* Goldflam disease

G

Goldman, David E., U.S. physiologist, *1911.
    Goldman equation—an equation derived to predict membrane potentials
    in terms of the membrane's permeability to ions and their concentrations
    (continued)

NOTES

Goldman *(continued)*
on either side. *Syn:* constant field equation; Goldman-Hodgkin-Katz equation

Goldman-Hodgkin-Katz equation—*Syn:* Goldman equation

Goldman, Henry M., U.S. periodontist, *1911.
Goldman-Fox knives—a set of knives used in periodontal surgery.

Goldmann, Hans, Swiss ophthalmologist, *1899.
Goldmann applanation tonometer—an applanation tonometer that flattens only 3 sq mm of cornea, used with a slit-lamp.
Goldmann contact lens
Goldmann contact lens prism
Goldmann expressor
Goldmann goniolens
Goldmann implant
Goldmann lens
Goldmann macular contact lens
Goldmann multimirror lens implant
Goldmann perimeter—a projection perimeter that adds further precision by controlling the surrounding illumination.
Goldmann serrated knife
Goldmann tonometer

Goldscheider, J.K.A.E. Alfred, German neurologist, 1858–1935.
Goldscheider disease—loosening of the epidermis with formation of bullae. *Syn:* epidermolysis bullosa
Goldscheider test—determination of the temperature sense by touching the skin with a sharp-pointed metallic rod, heated to varying degrees.

Goldstein, Hyman I., U.S. physician, 1887–1954.
Goldstein toe sign—increased space between the great toe and the second toe, seen in mongolism and occasionally in cretinism.

Goldstein, Joseph L., U.S. physician, *1940, joint winner of 1985 Nobel Prize for work related to cholesterol.

Goldstein, K., U.S. neurologist, 1878–1965.
Goldstein catastrophic reaction—when trying to perform a cognitive skill which has been lost, patients are seen to exhibit extreme agitation and anger.

Goldthwait, Joel E., U.S. surgeon, 1866–1961.
Goldthwait sign—in sprain of sacroiliac ligaments, flexion of the hip with extended knee elicits pain in the sacroiliac region.

Golgi, Camillo, Italian histologist and Nobel laureate, 1843–1926.
Golgi apparatus—a membranous system of cisternae and vesicles concerned with intracellular transport of membrane-bounded secretory proteins. *Syn:* dictyosome; Holmgrén-Golgi canals; Golgi complex; Golgi body; Golgi internal reticulum
Golgi body—*Syn:* Golgi apparatus
Golgi cells
Golgi complex—*Syn:* Golgi apparatus
Golgi corpuscle
Golgi internal reticulum—*Syn:* Golgi apparatus

Golgi osmiobichromate fixative—an osmic-bichromate mixture used to demonstrate nerve cells and their processes.

Golgi stain—any of several methods for staining nerve cells, nerve fibers, and neuroglia.

Golgi tendon organ—a proprioceptive sensory nerve ending embedded among the fibers of a tendon. *SYN:* neurotendinous organ; neurotendinous spindle

Golgi zone—part of the cytoplasm occupied by the Golgi apparatus.

Golgi-Mazzoni corpuscle—an encapsulated sensory nerve ending.

Holmgrén-Golgi canals—*SYN:* Golgi apparatus

Goll, Friedrich, Swiss anatomist, 1829–1903.

Goll column—*SYN:* fasciculus gracilis

nucleus of Goll—the medial one of the three nuclei of the dorsal column. *SYN:* gracile nucleus

tract of Goll—*SYN:* fasciculus graclis

Goltz, Robert W., U.S. dermatologist, *1923.

Goltz syndrome—*SYN:* focal dermal hypoplasia

Gombault, François A.A., French neurologist and pathologist, 1844–1904.

Gombault triangle

Gomori, George, Hungarian histochemist in the U.S., 1904–1957.

Gomori chrome alum hematoxylin-phloxine stain—a technique used to demonstrate cytoplasmic granules.

Gomori method for chromaffin

Gomori nonspecific alkaline phosphatase stain—for histological demonstration of enzymes.

Gomori one-step trichrome stain—a connective tissue stain.

Gomori silver impregnation stain—a reliable method for reticulin, as an aid in the diagnosis of neoplasm and early cirrhosis of the liver.

Grocott-Gomori methenamine-silver stain—a modification of Gomori methenamine-silver stain for fungi.

Gompertz, Benjamin, English actuary, 1779–1865.

Gompertz hypothesis—a theory that the force of mortality increases in geometrical progression.

Gompertz law—after age 35–40, the increase in mortality with age tends to be logarithmic.

Gonin, Jules, Swiss ophthalmic surgeon, 1870–1935.

Gonin cautery

Gonin marker

Gonin operation—retinal detachment repair.

Good, Robert A., U.S. pediatrician, *1922.

Good syndrome—agammaglobulinemia resulting in recurrent infections.

NOTES

Goodell, William, U.S. gynecologist, 1829–1894.
 Goodell dilator—obsolete term for a uterine dilator.
 Goodell sign—softening of the cervix and vagina as being usually indicative of pregnancy.

Goodenough, Florence L., U.S. psychologist, *1886.
 Goodenough Draw-a-Man Test—an intelligence test.

Goodpasture, Ernest W., U.S. pathologist, 1886–1960.
 Goodpasture disease
 Goodpasture epitope
 Goodpasture reactivity
 Goodpasture stain—a stain for Gram-negative bacteria, using aniline fuchsin.
 Goodpasture syndrome—glomerulonephritis that usually progresses rapidly to produce death from renal failure, and the lungs at autopsy show extensive hemosiderosis or recent hemorrhage.

Goodsall, David H., English surgeon, 1843–1906.
 Goodsall rule—a guide for classifying anal fistulas.

Goormaghtigh, Norbert, Belgian physician, 1890–1960.
 Goormaghtigh cells—modified smooth muscle cells primarily of the afferent arteriole of the renal glomerulus. *Syn:* juxtaglomerular cells

Gopalan, C., Indian biochemist, *1918.
 Gopalan syndrome—severe discomfort of the feet associated with elevated skin temperature and excessive sweating.

Gordon, Alfred, U.S. neurologist, 1874–1953.
 Gordon reflex—dorsal flexion of the great toe produced by firm lateral pressure on the calf muscles. *Syn:* paradoxical flexor reflex
 Gordon sign—a sign of organic hemiplegia. *Syn:* finger phenomenon
 Gordon symptom—the occurrence of an appreciable interval after the production of a reflex before relaxation. *Syn:* tonic reflex

Gordon, Mervyn H., English physician, 1872–1953.
 Gordon test—a spinal fluid test for proteins.

Gordon, Richard D., Australian endocrinologist, *1934.
 Gordon test—a test formerly used for Hodgkin disease.

Gorham, Lemuel W., U.S. physician, 1885–1968.
 Gorham disease—extensive decalcification of a single bone. *Syn:* disappearing bone disease

Gorlin, Richard, U.S. physiologist and cardiologist, *1926.
 Gorlin formula—a formula for calculating the area of the orifice of a cardiac valve.

Gorlin, Robert J., U.S. oral pathologist, *1923.
 Gorlin sign—unusual ease in touching the tip of the nose with the tongue.
 Gorlin syndrome—a syndrome of myriad basal cell nevi with development of basal cell carcinomas in adult life. *Syn:* basal cell nevus syndrome
 Gorlin-Chaudhry-Moss syndrome—craniofacial dysostosis, patent ductus arteriosus, hypertrichosis, hypoplasia of the labia majora, and dental and ocular abnormalities.

Gorman, P.
    Paget-Gorman sign language—*Syn:* Paget sign language

Goslee, Hart J., U.S. dentist, 1871–1930.
    Goslee tooth—metal-based artificial tooth.

Gosselin, Léon Athanese, French surgeon, 1815–1887.
    Gosselin fracture—V-shaped fracture of distal end of tibia.

Göthlin, Gustaf F., Swedish physiologist, 1874–1949.
    Göthlin test—a capillary fragility test to determine the presence or absence of scurvy.

Gottlieb, Bernhard, Viennese dentist, 1885–1950.
    Gottlieb epithelial attachment—a band of epithelium that forms a protective barrier between periodontal tissue and materials in the oral cavity.

Gottron, Heinrich A., German physician, 1890–1974.
    Arndt-Gottron syndrome—see under Arndt, G.

Gottschaldt, Kurt, German psychologist, *1902.
    Gottschaldt figures—geometric figures used to test perception of forms.

Gottstein, Jacob, German otologist, 1832–1895.
    Gottstein fibers—fibers related to auditory nerve.

Gougerot, Claude, French physician.
    Beuermann-Gougerot disease—*Syn:* Schenck disease

Gougerot, Henri, French physician, 1881–1955.
    Gougerot and Blum disease—an eruption of lichenoid papules on the legs. *Syn:* pigmented purpuric lichenoid dermatosis
    Gougerot disease—dermatologic disorder resulting in papular lesions, macules and dermal/dermohypodermal nodularity. *Syn:* Gougerot trilogy
    Gougerot trilogy—*Syn:* Gougerot disease
    Gougerot-Carteaud syndrome—discrete and confluent gray-brown papules of the anterior and posterior mid-chest. *Syn:* confluent and reticulate papillomatosis
    Gougerot-Sjögren disease—*Syn:* Sjögren syndrome

Gould, Sir Alfred P., English surgeon, 1852–1922.
    Gould electromagnetic flowmeter
    Gould suture—an intestinal mattress suture.

Gouley, John W.S., U.S. urologist, 1832–1920.
    Gouley catheter
    Gouley dilator
    Gouley guide
    Gouley tunneled urethral sound
    Gouley urethral sound

NOTES

Gowers, Sir William R., English neurologist, 1845–1915.

Gowers column—a bundle of fibers that conveys proprioceptive and exteroceptive information largely from the opposite lower extremity. *Syn:* anterior spinocerebellar tract; Gowers tract

Gowers contraction—contraction of the calf muscles when the anterior surface of the leg is struck. *Syn:* front-tap contraction

Gowers disease—a distal type of progressive muscular dystrophy. *Syn:* saltatory spasm

Gowers solution—solution used to count red blood cells.

Gowers syndrome—syndrome consisting of palpitation, chest pain, respiratory difficulties, and disturbances in gastric motility, now considered psychogenic. *Syn:* vagal attack; vasovagal attack

Gowers tract—*Syn:* Gowers column

Graaf, Reijnier de, Dutch physiologist and histologist, 1641–1673.

graafian follicle—a follicle in which the oocyte attains its full size. *Syn:* vesicular ovarian follicle

Gradenigo, Giuseppe, Italian physician, 1859–1926.

Gradenigo syndrome—petrositis with abducens paralysis and pain in the temporal region, due to localized meningitis involving the fifth and sixth nerves.

Graefe, Albrecht von, German ophthalmologist, 1828–1870.

Graefe cataract knife

Graefe disease—chronic progressive ophthalmoplegia.

Graefe eye speculum

Graefe forceps—a small thumb forceps with one horizontal row of six or eight delicate teeth across each tip.

Graefe iris forceps

Graefe knife—a narrow-bladed knife used in making a section of the cornea.

Graefe operation—(1) cataract removal by a limbal incision with capsulotomy and iridectomy; both operations were landmarks in the field of ophthalmic surgery; (2) iridectomy for glaucoma.

Graefe sign—in Graves disease, lag of the upper eyelid as it follows the rotation of the eyeball downward. *Syn:* von Graefe sign

Graefe spots—small areas over the vertebrae or near the supraorbital foramen, pressure upon which causes relaxation of blepharofacial spasm.

pseudo-Graefe phenomenon—retraction of the upper eyelid on downward movement of the eyes.

von Graefe cautery

von Graefe cystitome

von Graefe electrocautery

von Graefe knife needle

von Graefe sign—*Syn:* Graefe sign

von Graefe strabismus hook

Graefenberg, Ernst, German gynecologist in America, 1881–1957.

Graefenberg ring—obsolete term for a silver or silkworm gut ring designed for insertion into the uterine cavity as a means of contraception.

Gräfe, var. of Graefe

Gräfenberg, var. of Graefenberg
   Graffe, var. of Graefe

Graffi, Arnold, German pathologist, *1910.
   Graffi virus—a mouse myeloleukemia virus from filtrates of transplantable tumors.

Graham, Evarts Ambrose, U.S. surgeon, 1883–1957.
   Graham-Cole test—a radiographic study of the gallbladder. *SYN:* cholecystography

Graham, Thomas, English chemist, 1805–1869.
   Graham law—the relative rapidity of diffusion of two gases varies inversely as the square root of their densities, i.e., their molecular weights.

Graham Little, Sir Ernest Gordon, English physician, 1867–1950.
   Graham Little syndrome—follicular hyperkeratosis of the scalp with lymphocytic perifolliculitis and lichen planus elsewhere. *SYN:* lichen planopilaris

Graham Steell, see under Steell.

Gram, Hans C.J., Danish bacteriologist, 1853–1938.
   Gram iodine—a solution containing iodine and potassium iodide, used in Gram stain.
   Gram stain—a method for differential staining of bacteria.
   Weigert-Gram stain—see under Weigert

Grancher, Jacques Joseph, French physician, 1843–1907.
   Grancher disease—pneumonia with lung splenization.

Grandry, M., 19th century French anatomist.
   Grandry corpuscles—general sensory endings in the beak, mouth, and tongue of birds.

Granger, Amedee, U.S. radiologist, 1879–1939.
   Granger line—on lateral skull x-ray, the line produced by the groove of the optic chiasm or sulcus prechiasmatis.

Granit, Ragnar A., Finnish-Swedish neurophysiologist and Nobel laureate, 1900–1991.
   Granit loop—the reflex arc consisting of small anterior horn cells and neuroma which initiates the afferent impulses that pass through the posterior root to the anterior horn cells. *SYN:* gamma loop

Grasbeck, Ralph, Finnish physician, *1930.
   Grasbeck-Imerslund syndrome—*SYN:* Imerslund-Grasbeck syndrome
   Imerslund-Grasbeck syndrome—see under Imerslund

Graser, Ernst, German physician, 1860–1929.
   Graser diverticulum—*SYN:* sigmoid diverticulum

NOTES

Grasset, Joseph, French physician, 1849–1918.
    Grasset law—*Syn:* Landouzy-Grasset law
    Grasset phenomenon—in organic paralysis of the lower extremity, the patient, lying on his back, can raise either limb separately but not both together. *Syn:* Grasset-Gaussel phenomenon
    Grasset sign—normal contraction of the sternocleidomastoid muscle on the paralyzed side in cases of hemiplegia.
    Grasset-Gaussel phenomenon—*Syn:* Grasset phenomenon
    Landouzy-Grasset law—see under Landouzy

Gratiolet, Louis P., French anatomist, physiologist, and physician, 1815–1865.
    Gratiolet fibers—the massive fanlike fiber system passing from the lateral geniculate body of the thalamus to the visual cortex. *Syn:* optic radiation; Gratiolet radiation
    Gratiolet radiation—*Syn:* Gratiolet fibers

Gräupner, Sigurd C., German physician, 1861–1916.
    Gräupner method—obsolete term for a test of the sufficiency of the heart muscle.

Graves, Robert James, Irish physician, 1796–1853.
    Graves disease—thyroid dysfunction and all or any of its clinical associations. *Syn:* Basedow disease; ophthalmic hyperthyroidism; Parry disease
    Graves ophthalmopathy—exophthalmos associated with thyroid disease. *Syn:* endocrine ophthalmopathy; Graves orbitopathy
    Graves orbitopathy—*Syn:* Graves ophthalmopathy

Grawitz, Paul, German pathologist, 1850–1932.
    Grawitz basophilia—a condition in which basophilic erythrocytes are found in circulating blood, as in certain instances of leukemia, advanced anemia, malaria, and plumbism. *Syn:* basophilia
    Grawitz tumor—obsolete term for renal adenocarcinoma.

Grebe, Hans, German physician.
    Grebe syndrome—genetic trait resulting in dwarfism with extremely short limbs, legs being more severely affected than arms.

Greeff, C. Richard, German ophthalmologist, 1862–1938.
    Prowazek-Greeff bodies—see under Prowazek

Greene, Charles L., U.S. physician, 1862–1929.
    Greene sign—cardiac border displacement due to pleural effusion.

Greenfield, Joseph G., English neuropathologist, 1884–1958.
    Greenfield disease—metabolic disorder.

Greenhow, Edward H., English physician, 1814–1888.
    Greenhow disease—excoriations and melanoderma caused by scratching the bites of the body louse, *Pediculus corporis*. *Syn:* parasitic melanoderma

Gregg, Sir Norman, Australian ophthalmologist, 1902–1966.
    Gregg triad—deafness, cataracts, and heart defects found in children whose mothers contracted rubella while pregnant.

Greig, David M., Scottish physician, 1864–1936.
 Greig syndrome—increased width between the eyes due to an enlarged sphenoid bone. *Syn:* ocular hypertelorism

Greissinger, Georg, German prosthetist, 1903–1972.
 Greissinger foot—prosthetic foot that has ankle motion in all directions.

Grey Turner, see under Turner.

Gridley, Mary F., U.S. medical technologist, 1908–1954.
 Gridley stain—a silver staining method for reticulum.
 Gridley stain for fungi—a method for fixed tissue sections.

Griesinger, Wilhelm, German neurologist, 1817–1868.
 bilious typhoid of Griesinger—*Syn:* Griesinger disease
 Duchenne-Griesinger disease—see under Duchenne
 Griesinger disease—a severe form of louse-borne relapsing fever caused by *Borrelia recurrentis*. *Syn:* bilious typhoid of Griesinger
 Griesinger symptom—edema of the superficial tissues at the tip of the mastoid process in cases of thrombosis of the sigmoid sinus.

Griffiths, Ruth, English psychologist, *1909.
 Griffiths Mental Development Scale—designed to determine developmental level of infants and children up to age two.

Grignolo, Antonio, Italian ophthalmologist.
 Grignolo syndrome—anterior chamber pus accumulation, inflammation of the iris, uveal inflammation, exudative erythema, frequently exacerbated.

Grindon, Joseph, U.S. physician.
 Grindon disease—inflammation of hair follicles resulting in reversible baldness.

Grinspan, D., Argentinian physician.
 Grinspan syndrome—lichen planus, hypertension, and diabetes mellitus.

Griscelli, Claude, French physician.
 Griscelli syndrome—genetic trait causing partial albinism and frequent episodes of fever, decrease in blood platelets, and neutropenia.

Grisel, P., French physician.
 Grisel syndrome—torticollis resulting from subluxation of atlantoaxial joint.

Gritti, Rocco, Italian surgeon, 1828–1920.
 Gritti operation—*Syn:* Gritti-Stokes amputation
 Gritti-Stokes amputation—supracondylar amputation of the femur. *Syn:* Gritti operation

Grocco, Pietro, Italian physician, 1857–1916.
 Grocco sign—acute dilation of the heart following a muscular effort.

(continued)

G

NOTES

Grocco *(continued)*
Grocco triangle—a triangular patch of dullness at the base of the chest near the spinal column, on the side opposite a pleural effusion. *Syn:* paravertebral triangle
Orsi-Grocco method—see under Orsi

Groenouw, Arthur, German ophthalmologist, 1862–1945.
Groenouw corneal dystrophy—a granular type of corneal dystrophy.

Groffith, Joseph, English physician.
Groffith degeneration—degeneration of undescended testicles.

Grönblad, Ester E., Swedish ophthalmologist, 1898–1942.
Grönblad-Strandberg syndrome—angioid streaks of the retina together with pseudoxanthoma elasticum of the skin.

Gross, Ludwik, 20th century U.S. oncologist.
Gross leukemia virus—*Syn:* Gross virus
Gross virus—a strain of mouse leukemia virus. *Syn:* Gross leukemia virus

Gross, Samuel David, U.S. physician, 1805–1884.
Gross disease—disease in which the walls of the anus develop large pouches which may contain hardened feces.

Grover, Ralph W., U.S. dermatologist, *1920.
Grover disease—a pruritic papular eruption. *Syn:* transient acantholytic dermatosis

Groves, Ernest William Hey, English surgeon, 1872–1944.
Hey Groves clamp—orthopedic clamp

Gruber, George B., German physician, 1884–1977.
Martin-Gruber anastomosis—see under Martin, August
Meckel-Gruber syndrome—see under Meckel, Johann F., the younger

Gruber, Josef, Austrian otologist, 1827–1900.
Gruber method—a modification of the Politzer method in which the patient does not swallow, but says "hoc" at the instant of compression of the bag.

Gruber, Max von, German hygienist, 1853–1927.
Gruber reaction—*Syn:* Widal reaction
Gruber-Widal reaction—*Syn:* Widal reaction

Gruber, Wenzel (Wenaslaus) L., Russian anatomist, 1814–1890.
Gruber cul-de-sac—a lateral diverticulum in the suprasternal space.
Gruber-Landzert fossa—the variable peritoneal recess which lies behind the inferior duodenal fold and along the ascending part of the duodenum. *Syn:* inferior duodenal recess

Gruby, David, French physician, 1810–1898.
Gruby disease—*Syn:* tinea tonsurans

Grutz, var. of Grütz

Grütz, O., German dermatologist, *1886.
Bürger-Grütz disease—see under Bürger, Max
Bürger-Grütz syndrome—see under Bürger, Max

Grynfeltt, Joseph C., French surgeon, 1840–1913.
    Grynfeltt triangle—lumbar hernia occurs in this space. *Syn:* Lesshaft triangle

Guarnieri, Giuseppi, Italian physician, 1856–1918.
    Guarnieri bodies—intracytoplasmic acidophilic inclusion bodies observed in epithelial cells in smallpox and vaccinia infections, and which include aggregations of Paschen bodies or virus particles.
    Guarnieri gelatin agar—a type of agar, similar to Stoddart gelatin agar, used for the cultivation of *Streptococcus pneumoniae.*

Gubler, Adolphe, French physician, 1821–1879.
    Gubler line—the level of the superficial origin of the trigeminus on the pons, a lesion below which causes Gubler paralysis.
    Gubler paralysis—*Syn:* Gubler syndrome
    Gubler syndrome—a form of alternating hemiplegia characterized by contralateral hemiplegia and ipsilateral facial paralysis. *Syn:* Millard-Gubler syndrome; Gubler paralysis
    Gubler tumor—a fusiform swelling on the wrist in lead palsy.
    Millard-Gubler syndrome—*Syn:* Gubler paralysis

Gudden, Bernhard A. von, German neurologist, 1824–1886.
    Gudden commissures—the commissural fibers that lie above and behind the optic chiasm. *Syn:* commissurae supraopticae
    Gudden ganglion—a median, unpaired, ovoid cell group at the base of the midbrain tegmentum between the cerebral peduncles. *Syn:* interpeduncular nucleus
    Gudden tegmental nuclei—collective term for two small round cell groups in the caudal part of the midbrain associated with the mamillary body by way of the mamillary peduncle and mamillotegmental tract. *Syn:* tegmental nuclei

Guedel, Arthur Ernest, U.S. anesthetist, *1883.
    Guedel airway—rubber oropharyngeal airway.

Guéneau de Mussy, Noël F.O., French physician, 1813–1885.
    de Mussy point—in the presence of diaphragmatic pleurisy, a point on the left sternal border at the end of the tenth rib which is exceedingly painful when pressure is applied. *Syn:* Guéneau de Mussy point
    Guéneau de Mussy point—*Syn:* de Mussy point

Guérin, Alphonse F.M., French surgeon, 1816–1895.
    Guérin fold—*Syn:* Guérin valve
    Guérin fracture—a fracture of the facial bones. *Syn:* LeFort I fracture; horizontal fracture
    Guérin glands—*Syn:* glands of the female urethra
    Guérin sinus—a cul-de-sac or diverticulum behind the valve of the navicular fossa.

G

(continued)

NOTES

Guérin *(continued)*

Guérin valve—a fold of mucous membrane sometimes found in the root of the navicular fossa of the urethra. *SYN:* valve of navicular fossa; Guérin fold

Guérin, Camille, French bacteriologist, 1872–1961.

Bacille bilié de Calmette-Guérin—see under Calmette

bacillus Calmette-Guérin vaccine—see under Calmette

Calmette-Guérin bacillus—*SYN:* Bacille bilié de Calmette-Guérin

Calmette-Guérin vaccine—*SYN:* bacillus Calmette-Guérin vaccine

Guidi, Guido, Italian physician, 1508–1569.

Guidi canal—*SYN:* pterygoid canal

Guillain, Georges, French neurologist, 1876–1961.

Guillain-Barré reflex—plantar flexion of the foot and toes elicited by tapping the sole near its outer edge. *SYN:* aponeurotic reflex

Guillain-Barré syndrome—a syndrome marked by paresthesia of the limbs, muscular weakness or a flaccid paralysis, and increased protein in the cerebrospinal fluid without increase in cell count. *SYN:* acute idiopathic polyneuritis

Landry-Guillain-Barré syndrome—*SYN:* Landry syndrome

Guillemin, Roger, French-American physician, *1924, joint winner of 1977 Nobel Prize for work related to production of peptide hormone.

Guldberg, C., Norwegian chemist, 1862–1902.

Guldberg-Waage law—the rate of a chemical reaction is proportional to the concentrations of the reacting substances. *SYN:* law of mass action

Gull, Sir William, English physician, 1816–1890.

Gull disease—hypothyroidism.

Gullstrand, Allvar, Swedish ophthalmologist and Nobel laureate, 1862–1930.

Gullstrand slitlamp—in ophthalmology, an instrument consisting of a microscope combined with a rectangular light source that can be narrowed into a slit. *SYN:* slitlamp

Gumprecht, Ferdinand, German physician, *1864.

Gumprecht shadows—immature leukocytes that have undergone partial breakdown. *SYN:* smudge cells

Klein-Gumprecht shadow nuclei—see under Klein

Gunn, Robert Marcus, English ophthalmologist, 1850–1909.

Gunn dots—minute, highly glistening, white or yellowish specks usually seen in the posterior part of the fundus.

Gunn phenomenon—an increase in the width of the eyelids during chewing. *SYN:* jaw-winking syndrome; Gunn syndrome; Marcus Gunn syndrome

Gunn pupil—*SYN:* Marcus Gunn pupil

Gunn sign—compression of the underlying vein at arteriovenous crossings seen ophthalmoscopically in arteriolar sclerosis. *SYN:* Marcus Gunn sign

Gunn syndrome—*SYN:* Gunn phenomenon

Marcus Gunn pupil—relative afferent pupillary defect. *SYN:* Gunn pupil; Marcus Gunn syndrome

Marcus Gunn sign—*SYN:* Gunn sign
Marcus Gunn syndrome—*SYN:* Gunn phenomenon

Gunning, var. of Günning

Gunning, Thomas B., U.S. dentist, 1813–1889.
    Gunning splint—a prosthesis fabricated from models of endentulous maxillary and mandibular arches in order to aid in reduction and fixation of a fracture.

Günning, Jan W., Dutch chemist, 1827–1901.
    Günning reaction—the formation of iodoform from acetone by iodine and ammonia in alcohol.
    Günning test—test for urine acetone.

Günz, Justus, German anatomist, 1714–1751.
    Günz ligament—a portion of the superficial layer of the obturator membrane.

Günzberg, Alfred, German physician, 1861–1937.
    Günzberg reagent—phloroglucin and vanillin used as a reagent in Günzberg test.
    Günzberg test—a test for hydrochloric acid utilizing phloroglucin vanillin (Günzberg reagent), with which a bright red color is produced in the presence of the acid.

Gurdjieff, Georg Ivanovich, Armenian philosopher, 1877–1949.
    Gurdjieff exercises—rhythmic exercises used for self-development.

Gussenbauer, Carl, German surgeon, 1842–1903.
    Gussenbauer suture—a figure-of-eight suture for the intestine, resembling the Czerny-Lembert suture but not including the mucous membrane.

Guthrie, George J., English ophthalmologist, 1785–1856.
    Guthrie muscle—constricts membranous urethra. *SYN:* sphincter urethrae

Guthrie, Robert, U.S. pediatrician, *1916.
    Guthrie test—bacterial inhibition assay for detection of phenylketonuria in the newborn.

Guthrie-Smith, Olive F., English physical therapist, 1883–1956.
    Guthrie-Smith apparatus—*SYN:* Guthrie-Smith bed
    Guthrie-Smith bed—*SYN:* Guthrie-Smith apparatus
    Guthrie-Smith suspension exercises—*SYN:* weightless exercises

Gutierrez, Robert, U.S. physician, *1895.
    Gutierrez syndrome—*SYN:* horseshoe kidney

Gutmann, Carl, German physician, *1872.
    Michaelis-Gutmann body—see under Michaelis

Guttman, Louis, Israeli psychologist, *1906.
    Guttman scale—attitude scale. *SYN:* cumulative scale

G

NOTES

Guttmann, Paul, German physician, 1834–1893.

> **Guttmann sign**—thyroid gland bruit heard in patients with thyrotoxicosis.

Gutzeit, Max A.G., German chemist, 1847–1915.

> **Gutzeit test**—a test for arsenic.

Guyon, Felix J.C., French surgeon, 1831–1920.

> **Guyon amputation**—amputation above the malleoli, a modification of Syme amputation.
>
> **Guyon bougie**
>
> **Guyon canal**
>
> **Guyon catheter guide**
>
> **Guyon clamp**
>
> **Guyon curettage**
>
> **Guyon dilator**
>
> **Guyon exploratory bougie**
>
> **Guyon isthmus**—an elongated constriction at the junction of the body and cervix of the uterus. *SYN:* isthmus of uterus
>
> **Guyon sign**—ballottement of the kidney in cases of nephroptosis, especially when there is also a renal tumor.
>
> **Guyon sound**
>
> **Guyon ureteral sound**
>
> **Guyon vessel clamp**

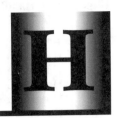

Haab, Otto, Swiss ophthalmologist, 1850–1931.
Haab degeneration
Haab eye knife
Haab magnet—a magnet that is used to extract metallic foreign bodies from the eye.
Haab needle
Haab reflex—a pupillary reflex. *Syn:* cerebral cortex reflex
Haab scleral resection knife

Haber, Henry, 20th century English dermatologist.
Haber syndrome—a permanent flushing and telangiectasia of the face with prominent follicular openings, small papules with scaling, and minute pitted areas.

Habermann, Rudolf, German dermatologist, 1884–1941.
Habermann disease
Mucha-Habermann disease—see under Mucha
Mucha-Habermann syndrome—*Syn:* Mucha-Habermann disease

Hadfield, Geoffrey, English physician, 1889–1968.
Clarke-Hadfield syndrome—see under Clarke, Cecil

Hadorn, W., Swiss physician.
Albright-Hadorn syndrome—see under Albright

Haeckel, Ernst, German naturalist, 1834–1919.
Haeckel gastrea theory—that the two-layered gastrula is the ancestral form of all multicellular animals. *Syn:* gastrea theory
Haeckel law—the theory that ontogeny is an abbreviated recapitulation of phylogeny. *Syn:* recapitulation theory

Haenel, Hans G., German neurologist, 1874–1942.
Haenel symptom—absence of sensation on pressure of the eyeball in the tabes.

Haenszel, William, U.S. epidemiologist and statistician, *1910.
Mantel-Haenszel test—see under Mantel

Haferkamp, Otto, German physician, *1929.
Haferkamp syndrome—syndrome resulting in anemia, arteriosclerosis of renal arteries, fat metabolism disorders.

Haffkine, Waldemar M.W., Russian physician, 1860–1930.
Haffkine vaccine—a killed culture of *Vibrio cholerae*; a killed plague bacillus (*Yersinia pestis*) vaccine.

Hagedorn, Werner, German surgeon, 1831–1894.
   Hagedorn cheiloplasty
   Hagedorn needle—a curved surgical needle that is flattened on the sides.
   Hagedorn needle holder
   Hagedorn operation
   Hagedorn suture needle

Haglund, S.E. Patrick, Swedish orthopedist, 1870–1937.
   Haglund deformity—*SYN:* Haglund disease
   Haglund disease—an abnormal prominence of the posterior superior lateral aspect of the os calcis, caused by a gait disorder. *SYN:* Haglund deformity

Hagner, Francis R., U.S. surgeon, 1873–1940.
   Hagner bag—bag used to prevent postprostatectomy hemorrhage.
   Hagner bag catheter
   Hagner hemostatic bag
   Hagner operation
   Hagner urethral bag

Hahn, Eugen H., German physician, 1841–1902.
   Hahn sign—side-to-side head rotation seen in childhood cerebellar disease.

Haidinger, Wilhelm von, Austrian mineralogist, 1795–1871.
   Haidinger brushes—the perception of two dark yellowish brushes when an evenly illuminated surface is viewed through a polarizing lens.

Hailey, Hugh E., U.S. dermatologist, *1909.
   Hailey-Hailey disease—recurrent eruption of vesicles and bullae. *SYN:* benign familial chronic pemphigus

Hailey, W. Howard, U.S. dermatologist, 1898–1967.
   Hailey-Hailey disease—recurrent eruption of vesicles and bullae. *SYN:* benign familial chronic pemphigus

Hajdu, Nicholas, Czech physician, *1908.
   Cheney-Hajdu syndrome—*SYN:* Hajdu-Cheney syndrome
   Hajdu-Cheney syndrome—missing terminal phalanges on extremities giving appearance of clubbing; may be accompanied by scoliosis, tooth loss, and other defects. *SYN:* Cheney-Hajdu syndrome

Hakim, S., 20th century U.S. neurologist.
   Hakim catheter
   Hakim reservoir
   Hakim shunt
   Hakim syndrome—in the presence of normal pressure hydrocephalus, the patient experiences urinary incontinence, dementia, gait apraxia. *SYN:* Hakim-Adams syndrome; HA syndrome
   Hakim tube
   Hakim valve
   Hakim-Adams syndrome—*SYN:* Hakim syndrome

Hakola, H. P. A., Finnish physician.
   Hakola syndrome—genetic trait resulting in progressive dementia and cystic changes in bones.

Halbeisen, William A., U.S. physician, *1915.
    Stryker-Halbeisen syndrome—see under Stryker

Halberstaedter, Ludwig, German physician, 1876–1949.
    Halberstaedter-Prowazek bodies—*SYN:* Prowazek-Greef bodies

Halbrecht, J., U.S. physician.
    Halbrecht syndrome—jaundice appearing in newborns within 24 hours of birth and related to ABO blood type incompatibility between mother and infant.

Haldane, John S., Scottish physiologist at Oxford, 1860–1936.
    Haldane apparatus—a device used for analyzing respiratory gases.
    Haldane chamber—an obsolete chamber for metabolic studies on animals.
    Haldane effect—the promotion of carbon dioxide dissociation by oxygenation of hemoglobin.
    Haldane relationship—a mathematical relationship between the equilibrium constant of an enzyme-catalyzed reaction and all of that enzyme's kinetic parameters.
    Haldane transformation—multiplication of inspired oxygen concentration by the ratio of expired to inspired nitrogen concentrations in the calculation of oxygen consumption or respiratory quotient by the open circuit method.
    Haldane tube—a tube for securing human alveolar air samples.
    Haldane-Priestley sample—an approximation of alveolar gas obtained from the end of a sudden maximal expiration into a Haldane tube.

Hales, Stephen, English physiologist, 1677–1761.
    Hales piesimeter—a glass tube inserted into an artery at right angles to its axis to measure pressure.

Hallauer, Otto, 19th century Swiss ophthalmologist.
    Hallauer glasses—glasses which prohibit blue and ultraviolet rays from passing through them.

Hallberg, Josef H., 20th century U.S. electrician.
    Hallberg effect—peaks and troughs in wave fields have opposite electrical signs.

Hallé, Adrien J.M.N., French physician, 1859–1947.
    Hallé point—a point where the ureter can be most readily palpated.

Haller, Albrecht von, Swiss physiologist, 1708–1777.
    Haller annulus—*SYN:* Haller insula
    Haller ansa—*SYN:* communicating branch of facial nerve with glossopharyngeal nerve
    Haller arches
    Haller circle—(1) a network of branches of the short ciliary arteries on the sclera around the point of entrance of the optic nerve. *SYN:* vascular

(continued)

H

NOTES

Haller *(continued)*
circle of optic nerve; (2) a venous plexus in the areola surrounding the nipple. *Syn:* areolar venous plexus.
Haller cones—the coiled portion of the efferent ductules that constitute the head of the epididymis. *Syn:* lobules of epididymis
Haller habenula—rarely used term for the cordlike remains of the vaginal process of the peritoneum. *Syn:* Scarpa habenula
Haller insula—a doubling of the thoracic duct for part of its course through the thorax. *Syn:* Haller annulus
Haller line—a thickened band of pia mater along the midline of the anterior surface of the spinal cord. *Syn:* linea splendens
Haller plexus—a nervous plexus of sympathetic filaments and branches of the external laryngeal nerve on the surface of the inferior constrictor muscle of the pharynx.
Haller rete—the network of canals at the termination of the straight tubules in the mediastinum testis. *Syn:* rete testis
Haller tripod—abdominal artery. *Syn:* celiac trunk
Haller tunica vasculosa—the vascular, pigmentary, or middle coat of the eye, comprising the choroid, ciliary body, and iris. *Syn:* vascular tunic of eye
Haller unguis—the lower of two elevations on the medial wall of the posterior horn of the lateral ventricle of the brain. *Syn:* calcar avis
Haller vas aberrans—a narrow, coiled tubule frequently connected to the first part of the ductus deferens or to the lower part of the ductus epididymitis. *Syn:* inferior aberrant ductule
Haller vascular tissue—the outer portion of the choroid of the eye containing the largest blood vessels. *Syn:* vascular lamina of choroid

Hallermann, Wilhelm, German ophthalmologist, *1901.
Hallermann-Streiff syndrome—a syndrome of bony anomalies of the calvaria, face, and jaw, with curved nose and multiple ocular defects. *Syn:* dyscephalia mandibulo-oculofacialis; François syndrome; Hallermann-Streiff-François syndrome
Hallermann-Streiff-François syndrome—*Syn:* Hallermann-Streiff syndrome

Hallervorden, Julius, German neurologist, 1882–1965.
Hallervorden syndrome—*Syn:* Hallervorden-Spatz syndrome
Hallervorden-Spatz disease—*Syn:* Hallervorden-Spatz syndrome
Hallervorden-Spatz syndrome—a disorder characterized by dystonia with other extrapyramidal dysfunctions. *Syn:* status dysmyelinisatus; Hallervorden syndrome; Hallervorden-Spatz disease

Hallgren, Bertil, 20th century Swedish geneticist.
Hallgren syndrome—vestibulocerebellar ataxia, pigmentary retinal dystrophy, congenital deafness, and cataract.

Hallion, Louis, French physiologist, 1862–1940.
Hallion test—a test of collateral circulation. *Syn:* Tuffier test

Hallopeau, François H., French dermatologist, 1842–1919.
Hallopeau disease—a sterile pustular eruption of the fingers and toes. *Syn:* pustulosis palmaris et plantaris; pemphigus vegetans
Hallopeau-Siemens syndrome

Hallwachs, Wilhelm L.F., German physiologist, 1859–1922.
  Hallwachs effect—electronic or electric effects produced by action of light.

Halstead, Ward C., U.S. psychologist, 1908–1968.
  Halstead-Reitan battery—a battery of neuropsychological tests used to study brain-behavior functions. *SYN:* Tactual Performance Test

Halsted, William Stewart, U.S. surgeon, 1852–1922.
  Halsted clamp
  Halsted curved mosquito forceps
  Halsted hemostat
  Halsted incision
  Halsted law—transplanted tissue will grow only if there is a lack of that tissue in the host.
  Halsted mattress sutures
  Halsted operation—excision of the breast as well as the pectoral muscles, lymphatic-bearing tissue in the axilla, and various other tissues. *SYN:* radical mastectomy
  Halsted suture—a suture used for exact skin approximation.

Ham, Thomas Hale, U.S. physician, *1905.
  Ham test—lysis of the patient's red cells in acidified fresh serum. *SYN:* acidified serum test

Hamburger, Hartog J., Dutch physiologist, 1859–1924.
  Hamburger law—albumins and phosphates pass from red corpuscles to serum, and chlorides pass from serum to cells when blood is acid; the reverse occurs when blood is alkaline.
  Hamburger phenomenon—movement of chloride from plasma to erythrocyte interior, or vice versa. *SYN:* chloride shift

Hamilton, Frank Hastings, U.S. surgeon, 1813–1886.
  Hamilton pseudophlegmon—a trophic affection of the subcutaneous connective tissue, marked by a circumscribed swelling which may become indurated and red, but never suppurates.

Hamman, Louis, U.S. physician, 1877–1946.
  Hamman crunch
  Hamman disease—*SYN:* Hamman syndrome
  Hamman murmur—*SYN:* Hamman sign
  Hamman sign—a crunching, rasping sound, synchronous with heartbeat, heard over the precordium and sometimes at a distance from the chest in mediastinal emphysema. *SYN:* Hamman murmur
  Hamman syndrome—spontaneous mediastinal emphysema, resulting from rupture of alveoli. *SYN:* Hamman disease
  Hamman-Rich syndrome—*SYN:* usual interstitial pneumonia of Liebow

Hammarsten, Olof, Swedish physiological chemist, 1841–1932.
  Hammarsten reagent—a mixture of hydrochloric acid and alcohol to test for bile.

H

NOTES

Hammerschlag, Albert, Austrian physician, 1863–1935.
  Hammerschlag method—a hydrometric method of determining the specific gravity of the blood.

Hammond, William A., U.S. neurologist, 1828–1900.
  Hammond disease—a condition in which there is a constant succession of involuntary movements of the fingers and hands, and sometimes of the toes and feet. *SYN:* athetosis

Hampton, Aubrey Otis, U.S. radiologist, 1900–1955.
  Hampton hump—a juxtapleural pulmonary soft tissue density on a chest x-ray, described as a manifestation of pulmonary infarction.
  Hampton line—a thin radiolucent band across the neck of a contrast-filled benign gastric ulcer, indicating mucosal edema.
  Hampton maneuver—rolling a supine patient to the right and then left side to obtain an air contrast x-ray in gastrointestinal fluoroscopy.
  Hampton technique—obsolete term for atraumatic, nonpalpation, fluoroscopic examination of the upper gastrointestinal tract in peptic ulcer disease with acute hemorrhage.

Hancock, Henry, English surgeon, 1809–1880.
  Hancock amputation—amputation of the foot through the astragalus.

Hand, Alfred, U.S. pediatrician, 1868–1949.
  Hand-Schüller-Christian disease—the chronic disseminated form of Langerhans cell histiocytosis. *SYN:* Christian disease (1); Schüller disease; Christian syndrome; Schüller syndrome; normal cholesteremic xanthomatosis

Hanflig, Samuel S., U.S. orthopedic surgeon, 1901–1966.
  Hanflig technique of neck traction—a method of cervical traction.

Hanfmann, Eugenia, Russian-U.S. psychologist, *1905.
  Hanfmann-Kasanin Concept Formation Test—a test to assess conceptual thinking.

Hanhart, Ernst, Swiss internist, 1891–1973.
  Hanhart syndrome—hypoplasia of the mandible with malformed and missing teeth, birdlike face, and severe deformities of the hands and forearms and sometimes of feet and legs. *SYN:* micrognathia with peromelia

Hanks, Horace Tracy, U.S. surgeon, 1837–1900.
  Hanks dilators—uterine dilators of solid metal construction.

Hanlon, C. Rollins, U.S. cardiovascular and thoracic surgeon, *1915.
  Blalock-Hanlon operation—see under Blalock

Hannover, Adolph, Danish anatomist, 1814–1894.
  Hannover canal—the potential space between the ciliary zonule and the vitreous body.

Hanot, Victor C., French physician, 1844–1896.
  Hanot cirrhosis—a condition characterized by obstructive jaundice with hyperlipemia, pruritus, and hyperpigmentation of the skin. *SYN:* primary biliary cirrhosis

Hansemann, D.P. von. See under von Hansemann.

Hansen, Gerhard A., Norwegian physician, 1841–1912.
    Fosdick-Hansen-Epple test—see under Fosdick
    Hansen bacillus—a species that causes Hansen disease. *SYN:*
    Mycobacterium leprae
    Hansen disease—*SYN:* leprosy

Harada, Einosuke, Japanese surgeon, 1892–1947.
    Harada disease—*SYN:* Harada syndrome
    Harada syndrome—bilateral retinal edema, uveitis, choroiditis, and retinal
    detachment, with deafness, graying of the hair, and alopecia. *SYN:* Harada
    disease; uveomeningitis syndrome; uveoencephalitis

Harden, Sir Arthur, English biochemist and Nobel laureate, 1865–1940.
    Harden-Young ester—important intermediate in sugar metabolism.

Harder, Johann J., Swiss anatomist, 1656–1711.
    Harder gland—the deep gland of the semilunar conjunctival fold found in
    animals such as pig and deer.

Harding, Harold E., 20th century English pathologist.
    Harding-Passey melanoma—a melanin-forming tumor that is
    transplantable to mice of many strains.

Hardy, Godfrey H., English mathematician, 1877–1947.
    Hardy-Weinberg equilibrium—the state in which the genetic structure of
    the population conforms to the prediction of the Hardy-Weinberg law.
    SYN: random mating equilibrium
    Hardy-Weinberg law—if mating occurs at random with respect to any one
    autosomal locus in a population in which the gene frequencies are equal
    in the two sexes, and the factors tending to change gene frequencies are
    absent or negligible, then in one generation the probabilities of all
    possible genotypes will on average equal the same proportions as if the
    genes were assembled at random.

Hardy, LeGrand, U.S. ophthalmologist, 1895–1954.
    Hardy enucleator
    Hardy-Rand-Ritter test—a test for color vision deficiency.

Hare, Edward S., English surgeon, 1812–1838.
    Hare syndrome—lower trunk brachial plexopathy and Horner syndrome
    due to malignant tumor in region of superior pulmonary sulcus. *SYN:*
    Pancoast syndrome

Harkavy, Joseph, U.S. physician, *1890.
    Harkavy syndrome—probable allergic reaction causing pleurisy,
    pericarditis, and neurologic symptoms.

Harken, Dwight, U.S. Army surgeon.
    Harken cardiovascular forceps
    Harken clamp
    Harken needle

(continued)

NOTES

Harken *(continued)*
    Harken prosthetic valve
    Harken retractor
    Harken rib spreader
    Harken valve
    Harken-Cooley forceps

Harley, George, Scottish physician, 1829–1896.
    Harley disease—hemoglobin in the urine. *Syn:* Dressler syndrome

Harnasch, Hans M. E., German physician, *1907.
    Harnasch disease—loss of bone tissue in hands and feet.

Harrington, David O., U.S. ophthalmologist, *1904.
    Harrington-Flocks test—an obsolete rapid screening test for visual field defects.

Harrington, Paul R., U.S. orthopedic surgeon, *1911.
    Harrington clamp
    Harrington deep surgical scissors
    Harrington flat wrench
    Harrington hook driver
    Harrington instrumention
    Harrington operation
    Harrington retractor
    Harrington rod instrumentation
    Harrington scissors
    Harrington spinal elevator
    Harrington spinal fusion
    Harrington spinal instrumentation
    Harrington strut
    Harrington thoracic forceps
    Harrington tonometer

Harris, Henry A., English anatomist, 1886–1968.
    Harris lines—dense lines parallel to the growth plates of long bones on x-rays. *Syn:* growth arrest lines

Harris, Henry F., U.S. physician, 1867–1926.
    Harris hematoxylin—an alum type of hematoxylin.

Harris, R.I., 20th century Canadian orthopedist.
    Harris anterolateral approach
    Harris brace-type reamer
    Harris broach
    Harris cement gun
    Harris cemented hip prosthesis
    Harris center-cutting acetabular reamer
    Harris condylocephalic nailing
    Harris condylocephalic rod
    Harris femoral component removal
    Harris growth arrest line
    Harris hip scale
    Harris hip status system
    Harris lateral approach

Harris medullary nail
Harris plate
Harris prosthesis
Harris splint sling
Harris superior acetabular graft
Harris view
Harris wire tier
Salter-Harris classification of epiphysial plate injuries—see under Salter

Harris, Robert L., Canadian surgeon
Harris footprint mat—a rubber mat that is used for taking footprints.

Harris, Seale, U.S. physician, 1870–1957.
Harris syndrome—hypoglycemia due to pancreatic disorders.

Harris, Wilfred, English physician, 1869–1960.
Harris migraine—recurrent facial pain and headache, more common in men than in women. *SYN:* periodic migrainous neuralgia

Harrison, Edward, English physician, 1766–1838.
Harrison groove—a deformity of the ribs.

Hartel, Fritz, 20th century German surgeon.
Hartel technique—a method of reaching the gasserian ganglion for the relief of trigeminal neuralgia.

Hartline, Haldan Keffer, U.S. physician and physiologist, joint winner of 1967 Nobel Prize for work related to the eye.

Hartman, Alexis F., U.S. pediatrician, 1898–1964.

Hartman, LeRoy L., U.S. dentist, 1893–1951.
Hartman solution—a solution used to desensitize dentin in dental operations.

Hartmann, Alexis F., U.S. pediatrician, 1898–1964.
Hartmann solution—*SYN:* lactated Ringer solution
Shaffer-Hartmann method—see under Shaffer

Hartmann, Arthur, German laryngologist, 1849–1931.
Hartmann adenoidal curet
Hartmann curet—a curet for the removal of adenoids.
Hartmann ear forceps
Hartmann ear rongeur
Hartmann eustachian catheter
Hartmann mastoid rongeur
Hartmann nasal dressing forceps
Hartmann nasal speculum
Hartmann punch
Hartmann tonsillar punch
Hartmann tuning fork

NOTES

Hartmann, Henri A.C.A., French surgeon, 1860–1952.
Hartmann colostomy
Hartmann knife
Hartmann mosquito forceps
Hartmann operation—resection of the rectosigmoid colon beginning at or just above the peritoneal reflexion and extending proximally, with closure of the rectal stump and end-colostomy.
Hartmann pouch—a spheroid or conical pouch at the junction of the neck of the gallbladder and the cystic duct. *Syn:* pelvis of gallbladder; fossa provesicalis; ampulla of gallbladder
Hartmann resection
Hartmann speculum

Harvey, William, English physician, 1578–1657.
Harvey sign—related to venous refill.

Häser, Heinrich, German physician, 1811–1884.
Häser formula—a formula to determine the number of grams of urinary solids per liter. *Syn:* Trapp-Häser formula; Christison formula; Trapp formula
Trapp-Häser formula—*Syn:* Häser formula

Hashimoto, Japanese surgeon, 1881–1934.
Hashimoto disease—*Syn:* Hashimoto thyroiditis
Hashimoto struma—*Syn:* Hashimoto thyroiditis
Hashimoto thyroiditis—diffuse infiltration of the thyroid gland with lymphocytes. *Syn:* Hashimoto disease; lymphadenoid goiter; Hashimoto struma; struma lymphomatosa; autoimmune thyroiditis

Haslam, John, English physician, 1764–1844.
Haslam-Pinel syndrome—a type of schizophrenia. *Syn:* Pinel-Haslam syndrome
Pinel-Haslam syndrome—*Syn:* Haslam-Pinel syndrome

Hasner, Joseph Ritter von, Czech ophthalmologist, 1819–1892.
Hasner fold—a fold of mucous membrane guarding the lower opening of the nasolacrimal duct. *Syn:* lacrimal fold; Hasner valve
Hasner lid
Hasner operation
Hasner valve—*Syn:* Hasner fold

Hassall, Arthur, English physician, 1817–1894.
Hassall bodies—small spherical bodies of keratinized and usually squamous epithelial cells found in the medulla of the lobules of the thymus. *Syn:* thymic corpuscle; Virchow-Hassall bodies; Hassall concentric corpuscle
Hassall concentric corpuscle—*Syn:* Hassall bodies
Hassall-Henle bodies—hyaline bodies on the posterior surface of Descemet membrane at the periphery of the cornea. *Syn:* Henle warts
Virchow-Hassall bodies—*Syn:* Hassall bodies

Hasselbalch, Karl, Danish biochemist and physician, 1874–1962.
Henderson-Hasselbalch equation—see under Henderson

Haudek, Martin, Austrian radiologist, 1880–1931.
Haudek niche—an obsolete term for the radiographic appearance in

profile of contrast material filling a gastric ulcer in the wall of the stomach.

Hauser, G.A., 20th century German gynecologist.
Mayer-Rokitansky-Küster-Hauser syndrome—see under Mayer
Rokitansky-Küster-Hauser syndrome—*Syn:* Mayer-Rokitansky-Küster-Hauser syndrome

Havers, Clopton, English anatomist, 1650–1702.
Havers glands—collections of adipose tissue in the hip, knee, and other joints, covered by synovial membrane. *Syn:* synovial glands
haversian canals—vascular canals that run longitudinally in the center of haversian systems of compact osseous tissue. *Syn:* Leeuwenhoek canals
haversian lamella—one of the concentric tubular layers of bone surrounding the central canal in an osteon. *Syn:* concentric lamella
haversian spaces—spaces in bone formed by the enlargement of haversian canals.
haversian system—a central canal containing capillaries and the concentric osseous lamellae around it occurring in compact bone. *Syn:* osteon

Hawley, C.A., 20th century U.S. orthodontist.
Hawley appliance—*Syn:* Hawley retainer
Hawley bite plate
Hawley chart
Hawley retainer—a removable wire and acrylic palatal appliance used to stabilize teeth following orthodontic tooth movement. *Syn:* Hawley appliance

Hawley, George Waller, U.S. surgeon, 1875–1940.
Hawley table—operating table for orthopedic procedures.

Haworth, Sir Walter Norman, English chemist and Nobel laureate, 1883–1950.
Haworth conformational formulas of cyclic sugars—for the pyranoses, these depict those shapes on which 0 to 2 ring-atoms lie outside the plane of the ring.
Haworth perspective formulas of cyclic sugars—these formulas depict the planar conformation, a situation not usually met.

Hayem, Georges, French physician, 1841–1933.
Hayem hematoblast—an irregularly shaped, disklike cytoplasmic fragment of a megakaryocyte found in the peripheral blood where it functions in clotting. *Syn:* platelet
Hayem solution—a blood diluent used prior to counting red blood cells.
Hayem-Widal syndrome—obsolete term for acquired hemolytic icterus. *Syn:* Widal syndrome

Hayflick, Leonard, U.S. microbiologist, *1928.
Hayflick limit—the limit of human cell division in subcultures.

NOTES

H

Haygarth, John, English physician, 1740–1827.
  Haygarth nodes—exostoses associated with lateral deflection of the fingers toward the ulnar side, occurring in rheumatoid arthritis. *Syn:* Haygarth nodosities
  Haygarth nodosities—*Syn:* Haygarth nodes

Head, Sir Henry, English neurologist, 1861–1940.
  Head areas—areas of skin exhibiting reflex hyperesthesia and hyperalgesia due to visceral disease.
  Head lines—bands of cutaneous hyperesthesia associated with acute or chronic inflammation of the viscera. *Syn:* Head zones; tender zones; tender lines
  Head zones—*Syn:* Head lines

Heaf, Frederick R.G., English physician, 1894–1973.
  Heaf gun—inoculation gun.

Heaney, Noble Sproat, U.S. gynecological surgeon and obstetrician, 1880–1955.
  Heaney clamp
  Heaney curet
  Heaney hysterectomy forceps
  Heaney needle holder
  Heaney operation—technique for vaginal hysterectomy.
  Heaney retractor
  Heaney suture
  Heaney uterine curet
  Heaney vaginal hysterectomy

Heath, Christopher, English surgeon, 1835–1905.
  Heath clip
  Heath curet
  Heath dilator
  Heath dissector
  Heath forceps
  Heath operation—division of mandibular ascending rami.
  Heath scissors
  Heath trephiine flap dissector
  Parker-Heath anterior chamber syringe
  Parker-Heath cautery
  Parker-Heath electrocautery
  Parker-Heath piggyback

Hebb, Donald O., Canadian psychologist, *1904.
  Hebb learning theory

Heberden, William, English physician, 1710–1801.
  Heberden angina—severe constricting pain in the chest. *Syn:* angina pectoris; Rougnon-Heberden disease
  Heberden anomaly
  Heberden asthma
  Heberden disease—small joint rheumatism, with distal interphalangeal joint nodules and angina.
  Heberden nodes—small exostoses found on the terminal phalanges of the fingers in osteoarthritis. *Syn:* Heberden nodosities; Rosenbach disease (1); tuberculum arthriticum

Heberden nodosities—*Syn:* Heberden nodes
Heberden rheumatism
Rougnon-Heberden disease—*Syn:* Heberden angina

Hebra, Ferdinand von, Austrian dermatologist, 1816–1880.
  Hebra disease—an acute eruption of macules, papules, or subdermal vesicles presenting a multiform appearance. *Syn:* erythema multiforme; familial nonhemolytic jaundice
  Hebra prurigo—a severe form of chronic dermatitis with secondary infection. *Syn:* prurigo agria; prurigo ferox

Hecht, Victor, early 20th century Austrian pathologist.
  Hecht pneumonia—a rare complication of measles, with the postmortem finding of multinucleated giant cells lining the alveoli. *Syn:* giant cell pneumonia

Heck, John W., U.S. dentist, *1923.
  Heck disease—multiple soft nodular lesions of the lips, buccal mucosa, tongue, and other oral sites in children and adolescents. *Syn:* focal epithelial hyperplasia

Hedblom, Carl Arthur, U.S. physician, 1879–1934.
  Hedblom syndrome—inflammation of the diaphragm.

Hedström, Gustav, Swedish endodontist.
  Hedström file—a coarse root canal file similar to a rasp.

Heerfordt, Christian Frederick, Danish ophthalmologist, *1871.
  Heerfordt disease—chronic enlargement of the parotid glands and inflammation of the uveal tract accompanied by a long-continued fever of low degree. *Syn:* uveoparotid fever
  Heerfordt syndrome

Hefke, Hans William, U.S. radiologist, *1871.
  Hefke-Turner sign—inflammatory hip disease found in children. *Syn:* Turner-Hefke sign
  Turner-Hefke sign—*Syn:* Hefke-Turner sign

Hegar, Alfred, German gynecologist, 1830–1914.
  Hegar bougie
  Hegar dilators—a series of cylindrical bougies of graduated sizes used to dilate the cervical canal.
  Hegar needle holder
  Hegar operation
  Hegar sign—softening and compressibility of the lower segment of the uterus in early pregnancy.

Hegglin, Robert M.P., 20th century Swiss physician.
  Hegglin anomaly—a disorder in which neutrophils and eosinophils contain Döhle bodies and in which there is faulty maturation of platelets, with thrombocytopenia. *Syn:* May-Hegglin anomaly

(continued)

H

NOTES

Hegglin (*continued*)

Hegglin syndrome—an energy-dynamic cardiac insufficiency during diabetic coma and other metabolic disorders. *SYN:* May-Hegglin syndrome

May-Hegglin anomaly—*SYN:* Hegglin anomaly

May-Hegglin syndrome—*SYN:* Hegglin syndrome

Hehner, Otto, English chemist, 1853–1924.

Hehner number—the weight or percentage of the nonvolatile fatty acids yielded by 5 g of a saponified fat or oil. *SYN:* Hehner value

Hehner value—*SYN:* Hehner number

Heidbreder, Edna, U.S. psychologist, *1890.

Heidbreder test—*SYN:* Minnesota Mechanical Ability Test

Heidelberg, city in Germany.

Heidelberg arm—a pneumatic prosthesis with a hand. Created at the University Clinic in Heidelberg, Germany.

Heidenhain, Adolf, German neurologist, *1893.

Heidenhain syndrome—dementia of presenile type, associated with limb rigidity, ataxia, and blindness due to lesions of neurons.

Heidenhain, Rudolph P., German histologist and physiologist, 1834–1897.

Biondi-Heidenhain stain—see under Biondi

Heidenhain azan stain—a technique to stain nuclei and erythrocytes red, muscle orange, glia fibrils reddish, mucin blue, and collagen and reticulum dark blue.

Heidenhain crescents—the serous cells at the distal end of a mucous, tubuloalveolar secretory unit of certain salivary glands. *SYN:* serous demilunes; Heidenhain demilunes

Heidenhain demilunes—*SYN:* Heidenhain crescents

Heidenhain iron hematoxylin stain—an iron alum hematoxylin stain used for staining muscle striations and mitotic structures blue-black.

Heidenhain law—glandular secretion is always accompanied by an alteration in the structure of the gland.

Heidenhain pouch—a small sac or pouch of the stomach fashioned for the purpose of obtaining gastric juice and for studying gastric secretion in physiologic experiments.

Heilbronner, Karl, Dutch physician, 1869–1914.

Heilbronner thigh—in cases of organic paralysis, flattening and broadening of the thigh, when the patient lies supine on a hard mattress.

Heim, Ernst L., German physician, 1747–1834.

Heim-Kreysig sign—in adherent pericardium, an indrawing of the intercostal spaces, synchronous with cardiac systole. *SYN:* Kreysig sign

Heimlich, Harry J., U.S. thoracic surgeon, *1920.

Heimlich maneuver—a method used to expel an obstructing bolus of food from the throat.

Heimlich operation

Heimlich tube

Heimlich valve

Heine, Jacob von. See under von Heine.

Heine, Leopold, German ophthalmologist, 1870–1940.
 Heine operation—cyclodialysis.

Heineke, Walter, German surgeon, 1834–1901.
 Heineke colon resection
 Heineke gastroenterostomy
 Heineke hypospadias operation
 Heineke-Mikulicz herniorrhaphy
 Heineke-Mikulicz pyloroplasty—procedure in which a short longitudinal incision is made over the pylorus and closed transversely.

Heiner, Douglas C., U.S. pediatrician, *1925.
 Heiner syndrome—an infant's failure to thrive due to serum antibodies in cow's milk.

Heinz, Robert, German pathologist, 1865–1924.
 Heinz bodies—intracellular inclusions composed of denatured hemoglobin.
 Heinz body anemia
 Heinz body test—a test for glucose 6-phosphate dehydrogenase-deficient red blood cells.
 Heinz-Ehrlich body—*SYN:* Ehrlich inner body

Heister, Lorenz, German anatomist, 1683–1758.
 Heister diverticulum
 Heister valve—a series of crescentic folds of mucous membrane in the upper part of the cystic duct, arranged in a somewhat spiral manner. *SYN:* spiral fold of cystic duct

Hejna, Robert F., U.S. speech pathologist.
 Hejna test—measure of speech articulation.

Held, Hans, German anatomist, 1866–1942.
 Held bundle—a bundle of thick, heavily myelinated fibers that ends in the medial region of the anterior horn of the cervical spinal cord and appears to be involved in head movements during visual and auditory tracking. *SYN:* tectospinal tract
 Held decussation—the crossing of some of the fibers arising from the cochlear nuclei to form the lateral lemniscus.

Helie, Louis T., French gynecologist, 1804–1867.
 Helie bundle—a vertically arched bundle of fibers in the superficial layer of the myometrium.

Heller, Arnold L.G., German pathologist, 1840–1913.
 Heller plexus—plexus of small arteries in the wall of the intestine.

Heller, Ernst, German surgeon, 1877–1964.
 Heller operation—esophagomyotomy at the gastroesophageal region.

Hellin, Dyonizy, Polish pathologist, 1867–1935.
 Hellin law—law expressing the frequencies of twins and triplets.

NOTES

Helly, Konrad, Swiss pathologist, *1875.
   Helly fixative—a microanatomic fixative for cytoplasmic granules and nuclear staining.
   Helly fluid

Helmholtz, Hermann L.F. von, German physician, physicist, and physiologist, 1821–1894.
   Gibbs-Helmholtz equation—see under Gibbs
   Helmholtz axis ligament—a ligament forming the axis about which the malleus rotates. *SYN:* axis ligament of malleus
   Helmholtz coil
   Helmholtz energy—energy equivalent to the internal energy minus the entrophy contribution.
   Helmholtz keratometer
   Helmholtz ophthalmoscope
   Helmholtz theory of accommodation—the ciliary muscle relaxes for near vision and allows the anterior aspect of the lens to become more convex.
   Helmholtz theory of color vision—*SYN:* Young-Helmholtz theory of color vision
   Helmholtz theory of hearing—that the basilar membrane of the cochlea acts as a resonating structure, recording low tones from its apical turns and high tones from its basal turns. *SYN:* resonance theory of hearing
   Helmholtz-Gibbs theory—*SYN:* Gibbs-Helmholtz equation
   Young-Helmholtz theory of color vision—see under Young

Helmont, Jean B. van. See under van Helmont.

Helweg, Hans K.S., Danish physician, 1847–1901.
   Helweg bundle—a slender bundle of nerve fibers in the peripheral zone of the lateral funiculus of the spinal cord. *SYN:* olivospinal tract

Helweg-Larssen, Hans F., 20th century Danish dermatologist.
   Helweg-Larssen syndrome—familial anhidrosis present from birth, with neurolabyrinthitis developing in the fourth or fifth decade.

Hench, Philip S., U.S. physician, 1896–1965.
   Hench-Rosenberg syndrome—the sudden onset of arthritis, usually affecting a single joint with no appearance on x-ray examination. *SYN:* Rosenberg-Hench syndrome
   Rosenberg-Hench syndrome—*SYN:* Hench-Rosenberg syndrome

Henderson, Lawrence J., U.S. biochemist, 1879–1942.
   Henderson-Hasselbalch equation—a formula relating the pH value of a solution to the value of the acid in the solution and the ratio of the acid and the conjugate base concentrations.

Hendon, West Hendon Hospital, England
   Hendon arm—children's upper limb prosthesis. Created at England's West Hendon Hospital.

Henke, Wilhelm, German anatomist, 1834–1896.
   Henke space—retropharyngeal space.
   Henke triangle

Henle, Friedrich G.J., German anatomist, pathologist, and histologist, 1809–1885.
   crypts of Henle—infoldings of conjunctiva.
   Hassall-Henle bodies—see under Hassall

Henle ampulla—the dilation of the ductus deferens where it approaches its contralateral partner before it is joined by the duct of the seminal vesicle. *Syn:* ampulla of ductus deferens

Henle ansa—*Syn:* nephronic loop

Henle fenestrated elastic membrane—*Syn:* elastic laminae of arteries

Henle fiber layer—the layer of inner cone fibers in the central area of the retina.

Henle fissures—minute spaces filled with connective tissue between the muscular fasciculi of the heart.

Henle glands—accessory lacrimal glands. *Syn:* Baumgarten glands

Henle layer—the outer layer cells of the inner root sheath of the hair follicle.

Henle ligament

Henle loop—*Syn:* nephronic loop

Henle membrane—the transparent inner layer of the choroid in contact with the pigmented layer of the retina. *Syn:* lamina basalis choroideae

Henle nervous layer—the layer of the retina from the outer plexiform to the nerve fiber layer inclusive. *Syn:* entoretina

Henle reaction—dark brown staining of the medullary cells of the adrenal bodies when treated with the salts of chromium, the cortical cells remaining unstained.

Henle sheath—the delicate connective tissue enveloping individual nerve fibers within a peripheral nerve. *Syn:* endoneurium

Henle sphincter

Henle spine—small bony prominence anterior to the supramastoid pit at the posterosuperior margin of the bony external acoustic meatus. *Syn:* suprameatal spine

Henle tubules—the straight portions of the uriniferous tubules that form Henle loop, distinguished as the descending and ascending tubules of Henle.

Henle warts—*Syn:* Hassall-Henle bodies

Henneberg, Richard, German neurologist, 1868–1962.
    Henneberg reflex—reflex of the hard palate. *Syn:* Laehr-Henneberg reflex
    Laehr-Henneberg reflex—*Syn:* Henneberg reflex

Henning, Wilhelm, German physician, 1716–1794.
    Henning sign—stomach angle takes on a Gothic arch shape in the presence of chronic gastric ulcer.

Henoch, Eduard H., German pediatrician, 1820–1910.
    Henoch chorea—a disorder in which sudden spasmodic coordinated movements of certain muscles or groups of physiologically related muscles occur at irregular intervals. *Syn:* spasmodic tic
    Henoch purpura—*Syn:* Henoch-Schönlein purpura
    Henoch-Schönlein purpura—an eruption of nonthrombocytopenic purpuric lesions due to dermal leukocytoclastic vasculitis. *Syn:* Henoch-

(continued)

NOTES

Henoch (*continued*)
Schönlein syndrome; Schönlein disease; Schönlein purpura; Schönlein-Henoch purpura; acute vascular purpura; anaphylactoid purpura; Henoch purpura; purpura nervosa; purpura rheumatica
Henoch-Schönlein syndrome—*Syn:* Henoch-Schönlein purpura
Schönlein-Henoch syndrome—*Syn:* Henoch-Schönlein purpura

Henry, James Paget, U.S. physiologist, *1914.
Henry-Gauer response—inhibition of antidiuretic hormone secretion due to a rise in atrial pressure that stimulates atrial stretch receptors.

Henry, Joseph, U.S. physicist, 1797–1878.
Dalton-Henry law—see under Dalton

Henry, William, English chemist, 1775–1837.
Henry law—at equilibrium, at a given temperature, the amount of gas dissolved in a given volume of liquid is directly proportional to the partial pressure of that gas in the gas phase.

Henseleit, K., German internist, *1907.
Krebs-Henseleit cycle—see under Krebs

Hensen, Victor, German anatomist and physiologist, 1835–1924.
Hensen canal—a short membranous tube passing from the lower end of a saccule to the cochlear duct of the membranous labyrinth. *Syn:* uniting duct; Hensen duct
Hensen cell—one of the supporting cells in the organ of Corti.
Hensen disk—*Syn:* Hensen line
Hensen duct—*Syn:* Hensen canal
Hensen knot—a local thickening of the blastoderm at the cephalic end of the primitive streak of the embryo. *Syn:* Hensen node; primitive node
Hensen line—the paler area in the center of the A band of a striated muscle fiber, comprising the central portion of thick filaments that are not overlapped by thin filaments. *Syn:* Hensen disk; H band
Hensen node—*Syn:* Hensen knot
Hensen stripe—a band on the undersurface of the membrana tectoria of the cochlear duct.

Hensing, Friedrich W., German anatomist, 1719–1745.
Hensing ligament—the left superior colic ligament.

Herbert, Herbert, English ophthalmic surgeon, 1865–1942.
Herbert pits—corneal cavities.

Herbst, Ernst F.G., German anatomist, 1803–1893.
Herbst corpuscles—tactile corpuscles found in birds.

Herelle, var. of d'Herelle

Hering, Heinrich Ewald, German physiologist, 1866–1948.
Hering-Breuer reflex—inflation of the lungs arrests inspiration with expiration then ensuing; deflation of the lungs brings on inspiration.
sinus nerve of Hering—a branch of the glossopharyngeal nerve that innervates the baroreceptors in the wall of the carotid sinus and the chemoreceptors in the carotid body. *Syn:* carotid sinus nerve

Hering, Karl E.K., German physiologist, 1834–1918.
  canal of Hering—a ductule occurring between a bile canaliculus and an interlobular bile duct. *SYN:* cholangiole
  Hering test—a test of binocular vision.
  Hering theory of color vision—that there are three opponent visual processes: blue-yellow, red-green, and white-black.
  Semon-Hering theory—see under Semon, Richard
  Traube-Hering curves—see under Traube
  Traube-Hering waves—*SYN:* Traube-Hering curves

Herlitz, Gillis, Swedish pediatrician, *1902.
  Herlitz syndrome—epidermolysis bullosa in which the bullae are persistent, nonhealing, and often present in the oral mucosa and trachea. *SYN:* epidermolysis bullosa lethalis

Hermann, Friedrich, German anatomist, 1859–1920.
  Hermann fixative—a hardening fixative of glacial acetic acid, osmic acid, and platinum chloride.

Hermans, P.E., U.S. physician.
  Hermans syndrome—hyperplasia of the ileum caused by globulin deficiency and resulting in recurrent diarrhea and infections.

Herrenschwand, Friedrich von, German ophthalmologist, *1881.
  Herrenschwand syndrome—sympathetic lesions causing differences in color of the iris.

Herring, Percy T., English physiologist, 1872–1967.
  Herring bodies—accumulations of neurosecretory granules in dilated terminal endings of axons in the neurohypophysis.

Herrmann, Christian, Jr., U.S. physician, *1921.
  Herrmann syndrome—a nervous system disorder with photomyoclonus and hearing loss followed by diabetes mellitus, progressive dementia, pyelonephritis, and glomerulonephritis.

Hers, Henri-Géry, 20th century Belgian physiologist and biochemist.
  Hers disease—*SYN:* type 6 glycogenosis

Hershey, Alfred D., U.S. biologist, *1908, joint winner of the 1969 Nobel Prize for research on mechanisms and materials of virus inheritance.
  Hersman, C.F., U.S. physician.
  Hersman disease—progressive enlargement of the hands.

Herter, Christian A., U.S. physician, 1865–1910.
  Gee-Herter disease—*SYN:* Gee disease
  Herter disease—gluten sensitivity, manifested by diarrhea, malabsorption, steatorrhea, nutritional and vitamin deficiencies. *SYN:* celiac disease
  Herter-Heubner disease
  Heubner-Herter disease—*SYN:* Gee disease

H

NOTES

Hertwig, Richard, German zoologist, 1850–1937.
  Magendie-Hertwig sign—see under Magendie
  Magendie-Hertwig syndrome—*Syn:* Magendie-Hertwig sign

Hertwig, Wilhelm A.O., German embryologist, 1849–1922.
  Hertwig sheath—the merged outer and inner epithelial layers of the enamel organ which extends beyond the anatomical crown and initiates formation of dentin in the root of a developing tooth.

Hertz, Heinrich R., German physicist, 1857–1894.
  hertz—a unit of frequency equivalent to 1 cycle per second.
  hertzian experiments—experiments demonstrating that electromagnetic induction is propagated in waves analogous to waves of light but not affecting the retina.

Herxheimer, Karl, German dermatologist, 1861–1944.
  Herxheimer reaction—an inflammatory reaction in syphilitic tissues induced by specific treatment with Salvarsan, mercury, or antibiotics. *Syn:* Jarisch-Herxheimer reaction
  Herxheimer spiral
  Jarisch-Herxheimer reaction—*Syn:* Herxheimer reaction

Herying, Théodor, Polish otolaryngologist, 1847–1925.
  Herying sign—pus in a maxillary sinus causing a shadow under the eyes when tested with a flashlight in the mouth.

Heryng, Richard L., Austrian pathologist, 1824–1881.
  Heryng sign—infraorbital shadow related to diseases affecting the maxillary sinuses.

Herz, Max, Austrian physician, 1865–1936.
  Herz method—*Syn:* Herz system
  Herz system—a system of therapy consisting of baths, walks, and exercises. *Syn:* Herz method

Heschl, Richard L., Austrian pathologist, 1824–1881.
  Heschl gyri—two or three convolutions running transversely on the upper surface of the temporal lobe bordering on the sylvian fissure, separated from each other by the transverse temporal sulci. *Syn:* transverse temporal gyri

Hess, Alfred F., U.S. physician, 1875–1933.
  Hess test—*Syn:* Rumpel-Leede test

Hess, Carl von, German ophthalmologist, 1863–1923.
  Hess capsule iris forceps
  Hess expressor
  Hess eyelid operation
  Hess lens scoop
  Hess lens spoon
  Hess ptosis operation
  Hess screen—a screen used in the measurement of ocular deviation.
  Hess tonsil expressor

Hess, Walter R., Swiss physiologist and Nobel laureate, 1881–1973.
  trophotropic zone of Hess—an area in the hypothalamus concerned with positive rewarding bodily sensations.

Hesselbach, Franz K., German anatomist and surgeon, 1759–1816.
    Hesselbach fascia—the part of the superficial fascia of the thigh that covers the saphenous opening. *SYN:* cribriform fascia
    Hesselbach hernia—hernia with diverticula through the cribriform fascia, presenting a lobular outline.
    Hesselbach ligament—fibrous or muscular strands extending from the lower border of the transversus muscle to the lacunar ligament and pectineal fascia. *SYN:* interfoveolar ligament
    Hesselbach triangle—the triangular area in the lower abdominal wall bounded by the inguinal ligament, the border of the rectus abdominis, and the inferior epigastric vessels. *SYN:* inguinal triangle

Hessing, Friedrich von, German orthopedic surgeon, 1838–1918.
    Hessing brace—a brace of steel and molded leather designed to encase the body.

Heublein, Arthur C., U.S. radiologist, 1879–1932.
    Heublein method—use of low-dose ionizing irradiation over the whole body.

Heubner, Johann O.L., German pediatrician, 1843–1926.
    artery of Heubner—a cerebral artery. *SYN:* medial striate artery
    Heubner arteritis—inflammation of arteries within the circle of Willis secondary to chronic basal meningitis from tubercle bacillus or particular fungi.
    Heubner-Herter disease—*SYN:* Gee disease

Heuser, Chester, U.S. embryologist, 1885–1965.
    Heuser membrane—a layer of cells delaminated from the inner surface of the blastocystic cytotrophoblast and from the envelope of the primary yolk sac during the second week of embryonic life. *SYN:* exocelomic membrane

Hey, William, English surgeon, 1736–1819.
    Hey amputation—amputation of the foot in front of the tarsometatarsal joint.
    Hey hernia—*SYN:* Cooper hernia
    Hey internal derangement—dislocation of the semilunar cartilages of the knee joint.
    Hey ligament—the upper part of the falciform margin of the opening in the fascia lata through which the greater saphenous vein passes. *SYN:* superior horn of falciform margin of saphenous opening
    Hey skull saw

Heyer, W.T., U.S. scientist, *1902.
    Heyer-Pudenz valve—a valve used in the shunting procedure for hydrocephalus. *SYN:* Pudenz valve

Heymann, Walter, Belgian-U.S. physician, 1901–1985.
    Heymann nephritis—experimental membranous glomerulonephritis created in laboratory rats.

NOTES

H

Heymans, Corneille J.F., Belgian physiologist, 1892–1968.
    Heymans law—theory regarding stimuli.

Heyns, O.S., 20th century South African obstetrician.
    Heyns abdominal decompression apparatus—a vacuum chamber enclosing the abdomen of the pregnant woman, creating pressure during the first stage of labor.

Hibbs, Russell A., U.S. surgeon, 1869–1932.
    Hibbs approach
    Hibbs arthrodesis
    Hibbs biting forceps
    Hibbs blade
    Hibbs bone chisel
    Hibbs bone gouge
    Hibbs chisel elevator
    Hibbs costal elevator
    Hibbs foot procedure
    Hibbs fracture appliance
    Hibbs fracture frame
    Hibbs hammer
    Hibbs hip arthrodesis
    Hibbs laminectomy retractor
    Hibbs mallet
    Hibbs onlay graft fusion of the lumbar spine
    Hibbs operation—a type of spinal fusion.
    Hibbs osteotome
    Hibbs periosteal elevator
    Hibbs retractor
    Hibbs retractor blade
    Hibbs self-retracting retractor
    Hibbs spinal fusion
    Hibbs sponge
    Hibbs technique

Hicks, see under Braxton Hicks.

Higashi, Ototaka, Japanese physician.
    Chédiak-Higashi anomaly—*Syn:* Chédiak-Steinbrink-Higashi syndrome
    Chédiak-Higashi disease—*Syn:* Chédiak-Steinbrinck-Higashi syndrome
    Chédiak-Steinbrinck-Higashi anomaly—*Syn:* Chédiak-Steinbrinck-Higashi syndrome
    Chédiak-Steinbrinck-Higashi syndrome—see under Chédiak

Highmore, Nathaniel, English anatomist, 1613–1685.
    antrum of Highmore—the largest of the paranasal sinuses occupying the body of the maxilla, communicating with the middle meatus of the nose. *Syn:* maxillary sinus
    corpus highmori—*Syn:* Highmore body
    corpus highmorianum
    Highmore body—a mass of fibrous tissue continuous with the tunica albuginea, projecting into the testis from its posterior border. *Syn:* mediastinum testis; corpus highmori

Hildenbrand, Johann Valentin Edler, von, Austrian physician, 1763–1818.
  Hildenbrand disease—disease caused by Rickettsia, transmitted by body lice. *Syn:* camp fever; jail fever; ship fever

Hill, Archibald V., English biophysicist and Nobel laureate, 1886–1977.
  Hill equation—used to express the fractional saturation of a molecule with a ligand as a function of ligand concentration.
  Hill plot—a graphical representation of enzyme kinetic data or of binding phenomena to assess the degree of cooperativity of a system.

Hill, Harold A., U.S. radiologist, *1901.
  Hill-Sachs lesion—an irregularity seen in the head of the humerus following dislocation of the shoulder.

Hill, Lucius, U.S. thoracic surgeon, *1921.
  Hill operation—repair of hiatus hernia.

Hill, Robert, English plant physiologist, *1899.
  Hill reaction—that portion of the photosynthesis reaction that involves the photolysis of water and the liberation of oxygen and does not include carbon dioxide fixation.

Hill, Sir Leonard Erskine, English physiologist, 1866–1952.
  Hill phenomenon—*Syn:* Hill sign
  Hill sign—in aortic insufficiency, greater systolic blood pressure in the legs than in the arms. *Syn:* Hill phenomenon

Hillis, David S., U.S. obstetrician/gynecologist, 1873–1942.
  DeLee-Hillis stethoscope
  Hillis-Müller maneuver—manual pressure on the term fundus while a finger in the vagina determines the descent of the fetal head into the pelvis.

Hilton, John, English surgeon, 1804–1878.
  Hilton law—the nerve supplying a joint also supplies the muscles that move the joint and the skin covering the articular insertion of those muscles.
  Hilton method—division of the nerves supplying a part, for the relief of pain in ulcers.
  Hilton sac—a small diverticulum provided with mucous glands. *Syn:* saccule of larynx
  Hilton white line—a zone in the mucosa of the anal canal said to be palpable. *Syn:* white line of anal canal

Hines, Edgar A., U.S. physician, 1906–1978.
  Hines and Brown test—test for a lesion of central or sympathetic nervous system.

Hinman, Frank, Jr., U.S. urologist, *1915.
  Hinman syndrome—detrusor-sphincter incoordination. *Syn:* nonneurogenic neurogenic bladder

NOTES

H

Hinton, William A., U.S. physician, 1883–1959.
    Hinton test—a formerly widely used precipitin test for syphilis.
    Muller-Hinton agar—see under Muller

Hippel, Eugen von. See under von Hippel.

Hippocrates, Greek physician, 460–370 BC.
    Hippocrates bandage
    hippocratic—relating to, described by, or attributed to Hippocrates.
    hippocratic facies—sunken appearance of facial features seen in dehydration.
    hippocratic fingers—clubbing of the fingers.
    Hippocratic Oath—an oath demanded of physicians about to enter the practice of their profession.
    hippocratic splash—*SYN:* hippocratic succussion
    hippocratic succussion—a diagnostic procedure to test for obstruction of the pylorus of stomach. *SYN:* hippocratic splash
    hippocratism—a system of medicine attributed to Hippocrates and his disciples that is based on the imitation of nature's processes in the therapeutic management of disease.

Hirschberg, Julius, German ophthalmologist, 1843–1925.
    Hirschberg method—a method of measuring the amount of deviation of a strabismic eye.

Hirschfeld, Isador, U.S. dentist, 1881–1965.
    Hirschfeld canals—canals that extend vertically through alveolar bone between the roots of mandibular and maxillary incisor and maxillary bicuspid teeth. *SYN:* interdental canals
    Hirschfeld file
    Hirschfeld method
    Hirschfeld silver point

Hirschsprung, Harald, Danish physician, 1830–1916.
    Hirschsprung disease—congenital dilation and hypertrophy of the colon. *SYN:* congenital megacolon

His, Wilhelm, Jr., German physician, 1863–1934.
    His band—*SYN:* His bundle
    His bundle—modified cardiac muscle fibers. *SYN:* atrioventricular bundle; His band; Kent-His bundle; Kent bundle
    His bundle electrogram—an electrogram recorded from the His bundle.
    His bundle heart block
    His bundle recording
    His spindle—a fusiform dilation of the aorta immediately beyond the isthmus. *SYN:* aortic spindle
    His-Tawara system—the complex system of interlacing Purkinje fibers within the ventricular myocardium.
    Kent-His bundle—*SYN:* His bundle

His, Wilhelm, Sr., Swiss anatomist and embryologist in Germany, 1831–1904.
    His copula—a median elevation in the floor of the embryonic pharynx that is incorporated in the root of the tongue. *SYN:* hypobranchial eminence
    His line—a line dividing the face into an upper and a lower, or dental part.

His perivascular space—*SYN:* Virchow-Robin space

His rule—an obsolete calculation for the duration of pregnancy.

isthmus of His—the anterior portion of the rhombencephalon connecting with the mesencephalon. *SYN:* rhombencephalic isthmus

Hiskey, Marshall S., U.S. psychologist.
Hiskey-Nebraska Test of Learning Aptitude

Hiss, Philip, U.S. bacteriologist, 1868–1913.
Hiss stain—a stain for demonstrating the capsules of microorganisms, using gentian violet or basic fuchsin followed by a copper sulphate wash.

Hitchings, George H., joint winner of 1988 Nobel Prize for work related to drug treatment.

Hitzig, Eduard, German neurologist, 1838–1907.
Hitzig girdle—breast-level analgesia caused by tabes dorsalis.
Hitzig test—test of vestibular apparatus in the ear.

Hjärre, A., German pathologist, 1897–1958.
Hjärre disease—a granulomatous disease of the intestines and liver of chickens. *SYN:* coli granuloma

Hoboken, Nicholas van, Dutch anatomist and physician, 1632–1678.
Hoboken gemmules—*SYN:* Hoboken nodules
Hoboken nodules—gross dilations on the outer surface of the umbilical arteries. *SYN:* Hoboken gemmules
Hoboken valves—the flangelike protrusions into the lumen of the umbilical arteries where they are twisted or kinked in their course through the umbilical cord.

Hoche, Alfred E., German psychiatrist, 1865–1943.
Hoche bundle
Hoche tract

Hochenegg, Julius von, Austrian surgeon, 1859–1940.
Hochenegg operation—excision of the rectum, preserving the anal sphincter.
Hochenegg ulcer—hard tumor of the rectum resulting in defecation difficulty, fecal blood, colic, and mucus.

Hockey, Athel, Australian physician.
Hockey syndrome—genetic trait linked to mental retardation, precocious puberty, and obesity.

Hodara, Manehem, Turkish physician, d. 1926.
Hodara disease—condition of the scalp causing hair breakage.

Hodge, Hugh L., U.S. gynecologist, 1796–1873.
Hodge maneuver
Hodge obstetrical forceps
Hodge pessary—a double-curve oblong pessary employed for the correction of retrodeviations of the uterus.

NOTES

H

Hodgen, John T., U.S. surgeon, 1826–1882.
   Hodgen apparatus
   Hodgen splint—a suspension leg splint for fractures of the middle or lower end of the femur.

Hodgkin, Alan L., English physiologist and Nobel laureate, *1914.
   Goldman-Hodgkin-Katz equation—*Syn:* Goldman equation

Hodgkin, Thomas, English physician, 1798–1866.
   Hodgkin disease—malignant neoplasm of lymphoid cells of uncertain origin, associated with inflammatory infiltration of lymphocytes and eosinophilic leukocytes and fibrosis. *Syn:* lymphadenoma
   Hodgkin sarcoma
   Hodgkin-Key murmur—a musical diastolic murmur.
   non-Hodgkin lymphoma—a lymphoma other than Hodgkin disease.

Hodgkin, W.E.
   Rapp-Hodgkin syndrome—see under Rapp

Hodgson, Joseph, English physician, 1788–1869.
   Hodgson disease—dilation of the arch of the aorta associated with insufficiency of the aortic valve.

Hoeppli, Reinhard J.C., German parasitologist, *1893.
   Splendore-Hoeppli phenomenon—see under Splendore

Hofbauer, J. Isfred I., U.S. gynecologist, 1878–1961.
   Hofbauer cell—a large cell in the connective tissue of the chorionic villi.

Hoff, Jacobus H. van't. See under van't Hoff.

Hoffa, Albert, German surgeon, 1859–1908.
   Hoffa fat
   Hoffa operation—to relieve congenital dislocation of the hip.
   Hoffa tendon shortening

Hoffmann, August, German chemist, 1818–1892.
   Frei-Hoffmann reaction—*Syn:* Frei test

Hoffmann, Johann, German neurologist, 1857–1919.
   Hoffmann muscular atrophy—progressive dysfunction of the anterior horn cells in the spinal cord and brainstem cranial nerves. *Syn:* infantile spinal muscular atrophy
   Hoffmann phenomenon—excessive irritability of the sensory nerves to electrical or mechanical stimuli in tetany.
   Hoffmann reflex—*Syn:* Hoffmann sign
   Hoffmann sign—in latent tetany, mild mechanical stimulation of the trigeminal nerve causes severe pain. *Syn:* Hoffmann reflex
   Werdnig-Hoffmann disease—*Syn:* Werdnig-Hoffmann muscular atrophy
   Werdnig-Hoffmann muscular atrophy—see under Werdnig

Hoffmann, Moritz, German anatomist, 1622–1698.
   Hoffmann duct—the excretory duct of the pancreas. *Syn:* pancreatic duct

Hofmann, Georg von, Austrian bacteriologist, 1843–1890.
   Hofmann bacillus—a nonpathogenic species found in normal throats. *Syn: Corynebacterium pseudodiphtheriticum*

228

Hofmeister, Franz von, German surgeon, 1867–1926.
Hofmeister anastomosis
Hofmeister antecolic gastrojejunostomy
Hofmeister drainage bag
Hofmeister endometrial biopsy curet
Hofmeister gastrectomy—operation in which a portion of the stomach is removed and a retrocolic gastrojejunostomy is constructed.
Hofmeister gastroenterostomy
Hofmeister operation—partial gastrectomy with closure of a portion of the lesser curvature and retrocolic anastomosis of the remainder to jejunum.
Hofmeister technique
Hofmeister-Pólya anastomosis

Hofmeister, Franz, German biochemist, 1850–1922.
Hofmeister series—a series of cations and of anions. *SYN:* lyotropic series

Hogness, D.S., U.S. molecular biologist, *1925.
Grunstein-Hogness assay—a procedure for identifying plasmid clones by colony hybridization.
Hogness box

Hohmann, Georg, German surgeon, *1880.
Hohmann bunionectomy
Hohmann clamp
Hohmann osteotome
Hohmann osteotomy
Hohmann retractor
Hohmann tennis elbow procedure

Hoigne, Rolf V., Swiss physician, *1923.
Hoigne syndrome—neurologic disorders caused by injecting penicillin into the bloodstream.

Holden, Luther, English anatomist, 1815–1905.
Holden line—the crease or furrow of the skin of the groin caused by flexion of the thigh.

Holl, Mortiz, Austrian surgeon, 1852–1920.
Holl ligament—ligament joining the corpora cavernosa clitoridis in front of the urinary meatus.

Hollander, Franklin, U.S. physiologist, 1899–1966.
Hollander test—a test to determine the completeness of vagotomy for peptic ulcer. *SYN:* insulin hypoglycemia test

Hollenhorst, Robert W., U.S. ophthalmologist, *1913.
Hollenhorst plaques—glittering, orange-yellow, atheromatous emboli in the retinal arterioles that contain cholesterin crystals and originate in the carotid artery or great vessels.

Holley, Robert W., U.S. biochemist, *1928, joint winner of 1968 Nobel Prize for work related to genetic code.

NOTES

H

Holliday, R.
> **Holliday junction**—the cross-strand structure formed when two DNA duplexes cross in a recombination event. *Syn:* Holliday structure
> **Holliday structure**—*Syn:* Holliday junction

Holly, F., U.S. obstetrician.
> **Holly anemia**—anemia due to greatly depressed and inadequately functioning bone marrow, sometimes occurring during pregnancy.

Holmes, Sir Gordon M., English neurologist, 1876–1965.
> **Holmes-Adie pupil**—*Syn:* Adie syndrome
> **Holmes-Adie syndrome**—*Syn:* Adie syndrome
> **Stewart-Holmes sign**—see under Stewart, James Purves

Holmes, Thomas, U.S. psychiatrist, *1918.
> **Holmes-Rahe questionnaire**—*Syn:* Rahe-Holmes questionnaire
> **Rahe-Holmes questionnaire**—see under Rahe

Holmes, W.
> **Holmes stain**—a silver nitrate staining method for nerve fibers.

Holmgren, Alarik F., Swedish physiologist, 1831–1897.
> **Holmgren wool test**—a test for color blindness in which the subject matches variously colored skeins of wool.

Holmgrén, Emil A., Swedish histologist, 1866–1922.
> **Holmgrén-Golgi canals**—*Syn:* Golgi apparatus

Holt, Mary, 20th century English cardiologist.
> **Holt-Oram syndrome**—atrial septal defect in association with finger-like or absent thumb and other deformities of the forearm.

Holt, Sarah B., English physician.
> **Holt syndrome**—genetic trait resulting in supernumerary digits on hands and feet as well as abnormal shortness of metacarpal/metatarsal bones.

Holter, Norman, U.S. biophysicist, 1914–1983.
> **Holter monitor**—ambulatory monitoring technique used to obtain uninterrupted electrocardiographic signal readings.
> **Holter pump**
> **Holter shunt**
> **Holter tube**
> **Holter valve**

Holth, Sören, Norwegian ophthalmologist, 1863–1937.
> **Holth corneoscleral punch**
> **Holth forceps**
> **Holth iridencleisis**
> **Holth operation**—punch procedure done to remove sclera.
> **Holth punch forceps**
> **Holth sclerectomy**
> **Holth sclerectomy punch**

Holthouse, Carsten, English surgeon, 1810–1901.
> **Holthouse hernia**—inguinal hernia with extension of the loop of intestine along Poupart ligament.

Holzknecht, Guido, Austrian radiologist, 1872–1931.
    Holzknecht unit—an obsolete unit of x-ray dosage equal to one-fifth of the erythema dose.

Homans, John, U.S. surgeon, 1877–1954.
    Homans sign—slight pain at the back of the knee indicative of incipient or established thrombosis in the veins of the leg.

Home, Sir Everard, English surgeon, 1756–1832.
    Home lobe—the enlarged middle lobe of the prostate gland.

Hooke, Robert, English experimental physicist, 1635–1703.
    Hooke law—the stress applied to stretch or compress a body is proportional to the strain, or change in length thus produced.
    hookean behavior—the behavior of a perfectly elastic body.

Hooker, Charles W.
    Hooker-Forbes test—a test for compounds with progestational activity.

Hoover, Charles F., U.S. physician, 1865–1927.
    Hoover signs—in organic hemiplegia the patient attempts to lift a paralyzed leg, counterpressure will be made with the other heel, whether any movement occurs in the paralyzed limb or not.

Hope, James, English physician, 1801–1841.
    Hope murmur
    Hope resuscitator
    Hope sign—double heartbeat heard in presence of aortic aneurysm.

Hopf, Gustav, German dermatologist, 1900–1979.
    Hopf disease—*SYN:* Hopf keratosis
    Hopf keratosis—genetic trait resulting in wartlike nevi on the dorsum of hands and feet. *SYN:* Hopf disease

Hopkins, Sir Frederick G., English biochemist and Nobel laureate, 1861–1947.
    Benedict-Hopkins-Cole reagent—see under Benedict, Stanley

Hopmann, Carl M., German rhinologist, 1849–1925.
    Hopmann papilloma—a papillomatous overgrowth of the nasal mucous membrane. *SYN:* Hopmann polyp
    Hopmann polyp—*SYN:* Hopmann papilloma

Hoppe, Herman H., U.S. neurologist, 1867–1919.
    Hoppe-Goldflam disease—*SYN:* Goldflam disease

Horan, M.B.
    Nance-Horan syndrome—see under Nance

Horecker, Bernard L., U.S. biochemist, *1914.
    Warburg-Lipman-Dickens-Horecker shunt—*SYN:* Dickens shunt

Horne, Jan (Johannes) van. See under van Horne.

NOTES

H

Horner, Johann F., Swiss ophthalmologist, 1831–1886.

  Bernard-Horner syndrome—*SYN:* Horner syndrome

  Horner pupil—constricted pupil due to impairment of sympathetic nerve innervation of the dilator muscle of the pupil.

  Horner syndrome—ptosis, miosis, and anhidrosis on the side of the sympathetic palsy. *SYN:* ptosis sympathetica; Bernard-Horner syndrome; Bernard syndrome

  Horner-Trantas dots—evanescent white cellular infiltrates occurring in the bulbar form of vernal keratoconjunctivitis.

Horner, William E., U.S. anatomist, 1793–1853.

  Horner muscle—*SYN:* lacrimal part of orbicularis oculi muscle

  Horner teeth—incisor teeth having a horizontal hypoplastic groove.

Horsfall, Frank L., Jr., U.S. physician, 1906–1971.

  Tamm-Horsfall mucoprotein—see under Tamm

  Tamm-Horsfall protein

Horsley, Sir Victor A.H., English surgeon, 1857–1916.

  Horsley anastomosis

  Horsley bone cutter

  Horsley bone rongeur

  Horsley bone wax—a mixture of antiseptic agents, oil, and wax used to stop bleeding by plugging bone cavities or haversian canals. *SYN:* bone wax

  Horsley bone-cutting forceps

  Horsley cranial rongeur

  Horsley dural separator

  Horsley elevator

  Horsley forceps

  Horsley suture

  Horsley trephine

Hortega, Pio del Rio, Spanish neurohistologist in South America, 1882–1945.

  Hortega cells—small neuroglial cells that may become phagocytic in areas of neural damage or inflammation. *SYN:* microglia

  Hortega neuroglia stain—one of several silver carbonate methods to demonstrate astrocytes, oligodendroglia, and microglia.

Horton, Bayard T., U.S. physician, 1895–1980.

  Horton arteritis—a subacute, granulomatous arteritis involving the external carotid arteries, especially the temporal artery. *SYN:* temporal arteritis

  Horton cephalalgia—unilateral orbitotemporal headaches associated with ipsilateral photophobia, lacrimation, and nasal congestion. *SYN:* Horton headache; cluster headache

  Horton headache—*SYN:* Horton cephalalgia

Hounsfield, Godfrey N., English electronics engineer and Nobel laureate, *1919.

  Hounsfield number—a normalized value of the calculated x-ray absorption coefficient of a pixel in a computed tomogram. *SYN:* CT number

  Hounsfield unit—a normalized index of x-ray attenuation used in CT imaging.

Houssay, Bernardo A., Argentinian physiologist and Nobel laureate, 1887–1971.
  Houssay animal—an animal that has had its pancreas and hypophysis excised.
  Houssay phenomenon
  Houssay syndrome—the amelioration of diabetes mellitus by a destructive lesion in, or surgical removal of, the pituitary gland.

Houston, John, Irish physician, 1802–1845.
  Houston folds—*SYN:* transverse rectal folds
  Houston muscle—a variation of the bulbospongiosus muscle in the penis. *SYN:* compressor venae dorsalis penis
  Houston valves—*SYN:* transverse rectal folds

Hovius, Jacob, Dutch ophthalmologist, 1710–1786.
  canal of Hovius—an anastomotic circle between the anterior twigs of the venae vorticosae in the eyes of some animals, but not in normal human eyes.

Howard, John Eager, U.S. internist and endocrinologist, 1902–1985.
  Ellsworth-Howard test—see under Ellsworth
  Howard test—a differential ureteral catheterization test.

Howell, William, U.S. physiologist, 1860–1945.
  Howell unit—equivalent approximately to 0.002 mg of pure heparin. *SYN:* heparin unit
  Howell-Jolly bodies—spherical or ovoid eccentrically located granules occasionally observed in the stroma of circulating erythrocytes that occur most frequently after splenectomy or in megaloblastic or severe hemolytic anemia. *SYN:* Jolly bodies

Howship, John, English surgeon, 1781–1841.
  Howship lacunae—tiny depressions, pits, or irregular grooves in bone that are being resorbed by osteoclasts. *SYN:* resorption lacunae
  Romberg-Howship symptom—see under Romberg, Moritz

Hoyer, Heinrich F., Polish anatomist and histologist, 1834–1907.
  Hoyer anastomoses—*SYN:* Sucquet-Hoyer canals
  Hoyer canals—*SYN:* Sucquet-Hoyer canals
  Sucquet-Hoyer anastomoses—*SYN:* Sucquet-Hoyer canals
  Sucquet-Hoyer canals—see under Sucquet

Hubbard, Carl P., 20th century U.S. engineer.
  Hubbard tank—a tank designed for full-body immersion. *SYN:* full-body tank

Hubel, David H., Canadian-U.S. neurobiologist, *1926, joint winner of 1981 Nobel Prize for work related to vision.

Hubrecht, Ambrosius A.W., Dutch zoologist and comparative anatomist, 1853–1915.
  Hubrecht protochordal knot—a local thickening of the blastoderm at the cephalic end of the primitive streak of the embryo. *SYN:* primitive node

NOTES

H

Huchard, Henri, French physician, 1844–1910.
Huchard disease—hypertension that occurs without pre-existing renal disease or known cause. *SYN:* essential hypertension
Huchard sign—when patients with hypertension change from standing to supine position, the heart rate drop is less than that for normotensive patients.

Hudson, Arthur Cyril, English ophthalmologist, 1875–1962.
Hudson-Stähli line—a brown, horizontal line across the lower third of the cornea.

Huebner, O.
Nierhoff-Huebner syndrome—see under Nierhoff

Hueck, Alexander F., German anatomist, 1802–1842.
Hueck ligament—the network of fibers at the iridocorneal angle between the anterior chamber of the eye and the venous sinus of the sclera. *SYN:* trabecular reticulum

Huet, var. of Huët

Huët, G.J., Dutch physician, *1879.
Huët-Pelger anomaly—*SYN:* Pelger-Huët nuclear anomaly
Pelger-Huët nuclear anomaly—see under Pelger

Hueter, Karl, German surgeon, 1838–1882.
Hueter maneuver—pressing the patient's tongue downward and forward with the left forefinger in passing a stomach tube.
Hueter sign—in case of fracture, the vibration expected on tapping the bone is not transmitted when tissue intervenes between the fractured parts of bone.

Hüfner, Carl Gustav von, German physician, 1840–1908.
Hüfner equation—an equation expressing the relationship between myoglobin dissociation and oxygen partial pressure.

Huggins, Charles B., Canadian-U.S. surgeon and Nobel laureate, 1901–1994.
Huggins operation—orchidectomy performed for palliation or cure of cancer of the prostate. *SYN:* castration

Huguier, Pierre C., French surgeon, 1804–1873.
Huguier canal—a canal in the petrotympanic or glaserian fissure, near its posterior edge, through which the chorda tympani nerve issues from the skull. *SYN:* anterior canaliculus of chorda tympani
Huguier circle—anastomosis around the isthmus of the uterus between the right and left uterine arteries.
Huguier sinus—a depression on the medial wall of the middle ear which has the oval window in its lower portion. *SYN:* fossula fenestrae vestibuli

Huhner, Max, U.S. urologist, 1873–1947.
Huhner test—determination of sperm quantity and motility in specimens obtained from the cervical canal following coitus, performed around the time of ovulation.

Humm, Doncaster George, U.S. psychologist, 1887–1959.
Humm-Wadsworth Temperament Scale—personality inventory.

Hummelsheim, Eduard K.M.J., German ophthalmologist, 1868–1952.
 Hummelsheim operation—transplantation of a normal ocular rectus muscle, to substitute for a paralyzed muscle.

Humphry, Sir George M., English surgeon, 1820–1896.
 Humphry ligament—the ligamentous band that passes anterior to the posterior cruciate ligament, extending between the posterior portion of the lateral meniscus and the upper end of the anterior cruciate ligament. *SYN:* anterior meniscofemoral ligament

Hunermann, Carl, German physician.
 Conradi-Hunermann disease—*SYN:* Conradi disease

Hunner, Guy L., U.S. surgeon, 1868–1957.
 Fenwick-Hunner ulcer—*SYN:* Hunner ulcer
 Hunner stricture—bladder stricture produced by interstitial cystitis (Hunner ulcer).
 Hunner ulcer—a focal and often multiple lesion involving all layers of the bladder wall in chronic interstitial cystitis. *SYN:* elusive ulcer; Fenwick-Hunner ulcer

Hunt, James Ramsay, U.S. neurologist, 1872–1937.
 Hunt atrophy—obsolete term for atrophy of the small muscles of the hand, without sensory disturbances.
 Hunt neuralgia—a severe paroxysmal lancinating pain deep in the ear. *SYN:* geniculate neuralgia
 Hunt paradoxical phenomenon—in torsion dystonia, extension of the foot in response to passive flexion and flexion in response to attempted passive extension.
 Hunt syndrome—(1) an intention tremor beginning in one extremity and subsequently involving other parts of the body. *SYN:* progressive cerebellar tremor. (2) facial paralysis, otalgia, and herpes zoster resulting from viral infection of the seventh cranial nerve and geniculate ganglion. (3) a form of juvenile paralysis agitans associated with primary atrophy of the pallidal system. *SYN:* Ramsay Hunt syndrome (1); paleostriatal syndrome, pallidal syndrome.
 Ramsay Hunt syndrome—(1) *SYN:* Hunt syndrome (3); (2) herpes zoster oticus.

Hunt, William E., U.S. neurosurgeon, *1921.
 Hunt angled serrated ring forceps
 Hunt angled-tip forceps
 Hunt grasping forceps
 Tolosa-Hunt syndrome—see under Tolosa

Hunter, Charles, Canadian physician, 1872–1955.
 Hunter syndrome—an error of mucopolysaccharide metabolism. *SYN:* type II mucopolysaccharidosis

NOTES

H

235

Hunter, John, Scottish surgeon, anatomist, physiologist and pathologist, 1728–1793.

> **Hunter canal**—the space in the middle third of the thigh that gives passage to the femoral vessels and saphenous nerve. *Syn:* adductor canal
>
> **Hunter gubernaculum**—an obsolete term for gubernaculum testis.
>
> **Hunter operation**—ligation of the artery proximal and distal to an aneurysm.
>
> **Hunter-Schreger bands**—alternating light and dark lines seen in dental enamel. *Syn:* Hunter-Schreger lines; Schreger lines
>
> **Hunter-Schreger lines**—*Syn:* Hunter-Schreger bands
>
> **hunterian chancre**—chancre resulting from syphilis.
>
> **hunterian perforator**

Hunter, William, English pathologist, 1861–1937.

> **Hunter glossitis**—*Syn:* Moeller-Hunter syndrome

Hunter, William, Scottish anatomist and obstetrician, 1718–1783.

> **Hunter ligament**—*Syn:* round ligament of the uterus
>
> **Hunter line**—a fibrous band running vertically the entire length of the center of the anterior abdominal wall, receiving the attachments of the oblique and transverse abdominal muscles. *Syn:* linea alba
>
> **Hunter membrane**—the mucous membrane of the pregnant uterus. *Syn:* deciduous membrane

Huntington, George, U.S. physician, 1850–1916.

> **Huntington chorea**—an inherited degenerative disorder of the cerebral cortex and corpus striatum. *Syn:* Huntington disease; chronic progressive chorea; degenerative chorea; hereditary chorea
>
> **Huntington disease**—*Syn:* Huntington chorea

Hurler, Gertrud, Austrian pediatrician, 1889–1965.

> **Hurler disease**—*Syn:* Hurler syndrome
>
> **Hurler syndrome**—mucopolysaccharidosis with severe abnormality in development of skeletal cartilage and bone, corneal clouding, hepatosplenomegaly, mental retardation, and gargoyle-like facies. *Syn:* dysostosis multiplex; Hurler disease; lipochondrodystrophy; Pfaundler-Hurler syndrome; type IH mucopolysaccharidosis
>
> **Pfaundler-Hurler syndrome**—*Syn:* Hurler syndrome

Hürthle, Karl W., German histologist, 1860–1945.

> **Hürthle cell**—a large, granular eosinophilic cell derived from thyroid follicular epithelium by accumulation of mitochondria, e.g., in Hashimoto disease. *Syn:* Askanazy cell
>
> **Hürthle cell adenoma**—a follicular adenoma of the thyroid in which the epithelium has undergone metaplasia into Hürthle cells.
>
> **Hürthle cell carcinoma**—*Syn:* Hürthle cell tumor
>
> **Hürthle cell tumor**—neoplasm of the thyroid gland. *Syn:* Hürthle cell carcinoma

Huschke, Emil, German anatomist, 1797–1858.

> **Huschke auditory teeth**—tooth-shaped formations or ridges occurring on the vestibular lip of the limbus lamina spiralis of the cochlear duct. *Syn:* auditory teeth
>
> **Huschke canal**

Huschke cartilages—two horizontal cartilaginous rods at the edge of the cartilaginous septum of the nose.

Huschke foramen—an opening in the floor of the bony part of the external acoustic meatus near the tympanic membrane.

Huschke ligament

Huschke valve—a fold of mucous membrane guarding the lower opening of the nasolacrimal duct. *Syn:* lacrimal fold

Hutchinson, Sir Jonathan, English surgeon, 1828–1913.

Hutchinson crescentic notch—the semilunar notch on the incisal edge of Hutchinson teeth, encountered in congenital syphilis.

Hutchinson facies—the peculiar facial expression produced by drooping eyelids and motionless eyes in external ophthalmoplegia.

Hutchinson freckle—a brown or black mottled, irregularly outlined, slowly enlarging lesion. *Syn:* lentigo maligna

Hutchinson mask—the sensation experienced in tabetic neurosyphilis as if the face were covered with a mask or with cobwebs.

Hutchinson patch—interstitial or parenchymatous keratitis giving rise to neovascularization of the cornea. *Syn:* salmon patch

Hutchinson pupil—dilation of the pupil on the side of the lesion as part of a third nerve palsy.

Hutchinson teeth—the teeth of congenital syphilis in which the incisal edge is notched and narrower than the cervical area. *Syn:* notched teeth; screwdriver teeth; syphilitic teeth

Hutchinson triad—parenchymatous keratitis, labyrinthine disease, and Hutchinson teeth, significant of congenital syphilis.

Hutchinson-Gilford disease—a condition in which normal development in the first year is followed by gross retardation of growth, with dry wrinkled skin, total alopecia, and bird-like facies. *Syn:* progeria; Hutchinson-Gilford syndrome

Hutchinson-Gilford syndrome—*Syn:* Hutchinson-Gilford disease

Hutchinson, Sir Robert Grieve, English physician, 1871–1943.

Hutchinson disease—malignant adrenal gland tumor.

Hutchison, Sir Robert, English pediatrician, 1871–1960.

Hutchison syndrome—adrenal neuroblastoma of infants with metastasis to the orbit.

Hutinel, Victor H., French pediatrician, 1849–1933.

Hutinel disease—juvenile tuberculous pericarditis.

Huxley, Sir Andrew Fielding, English physiologist, *1917, joint winner of 1963 Nobel Prize for work related to nerve cell membrane.

Huxley, Thomas, English biologist, physiologist, and comparative anatomist, 1825–1895.

Huxley layer—the layer of cells interposed between Henle layer and the

(continued)

NOTES

H

Huxley *(continued)*
cuticle of the inner root sheath of the hair follicle. *Syn:* Huxley membrane; Huxley sheath
Huxley membrane—*Syn:* Huxley layer
Huxley sheath—*Syn:* Huxley layer

Huygens, Christian, Dutch physicist, 1629–1695.
Huygens ocular—the compound ocular of a microscope, composed of two planoconvex lenses so arranged that the plane side of each is directed toward the observer.
Huygens principle—used in ultrasound technology.

Hyde, James N., U.S. dermatologist, 1840–1910.
Hyde disease—an eruption of hard nodules in the skin caused by rubbing and accompanied by intense itching. *Syn:* prurigo nodularis; picker's nodules

Hynes, Wilfred, English plastic surgeon, *1903.
Anderson-Hynes pyeloplasty—see under Anderson, James
Hynes pharyngoplasty—an operation to narrow the pharynx in order to improve speech.

Hyrtl, Joseph, Austrian anatomist, 1810–1894.
Hyrtl anastomosis—*Syn:* Hyrtl loop
Hyrtl canal
Hyrtl epitympanic recess—the upper portion of the tympanic cavity above the tympanic membrane. *Syn:* epitympanic recess; Hyrtl recess
Hyrtl foramen—an occasional foramen in the sphenoid bone through which passes the motor portion of the trigeminal nerve. *Syn:* porus crotaphytico-buccinatorius
Hyrtl loop—a communicating loop between the right and left hypoglossal nerves. *Syn:* Hyrtl anastomosis
Hyrtl nerve
Hyrtl recess—*Syn:* Hyrtl epitympanic recess
Hyrtl sphincter—a band, generally incomplete, of circular muscular fibers in the rectum about 10 cm above the anus (upper rectal ampulla).

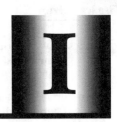

Iceland, an island in the North Atlantic where disease is prevalent.
  Iceland disease—chronic fatigue syndrome. *SYN:* epidemic neuromyasthenia

Ieshima, Atsushi, Japanese physician.
  Ieshima syndrome—genetic trait resulting in psychomotor retardation and multiple abnormalities.

Ilosvay, Lajos de, Hungarian chemist, *1851.
  Ilosvay reagent—test for nitrites.

Imerslund, Olga, Norwegian physician.
  Grasbeck-Imerslund syndrome—*SYN:* Imerslund-Grasbeck syndrome
  Imerslund-Grasbeck syndrome—familial enterocyte cobalamin malabsorption. *SYN:* malabsorption syndrome; Grasbeck-Imerslund syndrome

Imhoff, Karl, German engineer, 1876–1965.
  Imhoff tank—tank for digestion.

Imlach, Francis, Scottish anatomist and surgeon, 1819–1891.
  Imlach fat-pad—fat surrounding the round ligament of the uterus in the inguinal canal.
  Imlach ring—that part of the inguinal canal which lodges the round ligament of the uterus.

Imrie, C.W., Scottish surgeon.
  Imrie sign—flushing of the face during initial phase of acute pancreatitis. May be accompanied by gastrointestinal symptoms.

Ingrassia, Giovanni F., Italian anatomist, 1510–1580.
  Ingrassia apophysis—*SYN:* Ingrassia wing
  Ingrassia wing—one of a bilateral pair of triangular, pointed plates extending laterally from the anterolateral body of the sphenoid bone. *SYN:* lesser wing of sphenoid bone; Ingrassia apophysis

Iru Kandji, Australian aboriginal tribe.
  Iru Kandji syndrome—syndrome resulting from a jellyfish sting; produces shock and muscle pain as well as gastrointestinal symptoms.

Irvine, A. Ray, Jr., U.S. ophthalmologist, *1917.
  Irvine corneal scissors
  Irvine operation
  Irvine probe-pointed scissors
  Irvine-Gass syndrome—macular edema, aphakia, and vitreous humor adherent to incision for cataract extraction.

Isaacs, Hyam, South African neurophysiologist, *1927.
    Isaacs syndrome—peripheral nerve disease resulting in rigidity of the muscles. *Syn:* stiff man syndrome

Isambert, Emile, French physician, 1828–1876.
    Isambert disease—miliary tuberculosis.

Ishihara, Shinobu, Japanese ophthalmologist, 1879–1963.
    Ishihara I-Temp cautery
    Ishihara IV slit lamp
    Ishihara plate
    Ishihara test—a test for color vision deficiency.
    Ishihara test chart book

Israel, James Adolf, German urologist, 1848–1926.
    Actinomyces israelii

Itard, Jean M. G., French otologist, 1774–1838.
    Cholewa-Itard sign—*Syn:* Itard-Cholewa sign
    Itard-Cholewa sign—tympanic membrane anesthesia due to otosclerosis. *Syn:* Cholewa-Itard sign

Ito, Hayozo, Japanese physician, *1865.
    Ito-Reenstierna test—*Syn:* Ducrey test

Ito, Minor, 20th century Japanese dermatologist.
    hypomelanosis of Ito—inherited hypopigmented macules variably associated with epidermal nevi, alopecia, and ocular, skeletal, and neural abnormalities. *Syn:* incontinentia pigmenti achromians
    Ito nevus—pigmentation of skin innervated by lateral branches of the supraclavicular nerve and the lateral cutaneous nerve of the arm.

Ito, T., 20th century Japanese physician.
    Ito cells—fat-containing cells lining hepatic sinusoids.

Itsenko, N.M., Russian physician.
    Itsenko-Cushing syndrome—*Syn:* Cushing syndrome

Ivemark, Björn, Swedish pathologist, *1925.
    Ivemark syndrome—a possibly heritable disorder in which organs of the left side of the body are a mirror image of their counterpart on the right side, with associated splenic agenesis and cardiac malformations.

Ivy, Andrew Conway, U.S. physiologist, 1893–1978.
    Ivy bleeding time test

Ivy, Robert H., U.S. oral and plastic surgeon, 1881–1974.
    Ivy loop wiring—placement of a wire around two adjacent teeth to provide an attachment for intermaxillary elastics.

Izar, Guido, 20th century Italian pathologist.
    Izar reagent

J

Jabon, Marcel M.J., French physician, *1898.

    Jabon syndrome—gastrointestinal syndrome produced when antibiotic therapy destroys normal flora and allows specific strains of staphylococci to flourish.

Jaboulay, Mathieu, French surgeon, 1860–1913.

    Jaboulay amputation—amputation of an entire leg together with the os coxae. *Syn:* hemipelvectomy

    Jaboulay button

    Jaboulay method—anastomosis of arteries by splitting the cut ends a short distance, suturing the flaps together, and applying intima to intima. *Syn:* broad marginal confrontation method

    Jaboulay pyloroplasty—a side-to-side gastroduodenostomy.

Jaccoud, François Sigismond, French physician, 1830–1913.

    Jaccoud arthritis—a rare form of chronic arthritis, reported to occur after attacks of acute rheumatic fever. *Syn:* Jaccoud arthropathy

    Jaccoud arthropathy—*Syn:* Jaccoud arthritis

    Jaccoud syndrome

Jackson, Jabez N., U.S. surgeon, 1868–1935.

    Jackson anterior commissure laryngoscope

    Jackson approximation forceps

    Jackson broad staple forceps

    Jackson button forceps

    Jackson conventional foreign body forceps

    Jackson cross-action forceps

    Jackson double-prong forceps

    Jackson dull rotation forceps

    Jackson esophagoscope

    Jackson flexible upper lobe bronchus forceps

    Jackson globular object forceps

    Jackson membrane—a thin vascular membrane or veil-like adhesion covering the anterior surface of the ascending colon from the cecum to the right flexure. *Syn:* Jackson veil

    Jackson papilloma forceps

    Jackson pin-bending costophrenic forceps

    Jackson sharp-pointed rotation forceps

    Jackson spinal surgery and imaging table

    Jackson steel-stem woven filiform bougie

    Jackson triangular brass dilator

    Jackson veil—*Syn:* Jackson membrane

Jackson, John Hughlings, English neurologist, 1835–1911.

    Jackson law—loss of mental functions due to disease retraces in reverse order its evolutionary development.

    Jackson rule—after an epileptic attack, simple and quasiautomatic functions are less affected and more rapidly recovered than the more complex ones.

    Jackson sign—during quiet respiration the movement of the paralyzed side of the chest may be greater than that of the opposite side, while in forced respiration the paralyzed side moves less than the other.

    jacksonian epilepsy—*SYN:* jacksonian seizure

    jacksonian seizure—a seizure originating in or near the rolandic neocortex which clinically involves one part of the body. *SYN:* jacksonian epilepsy

Jacob, Arthur, Irish physician, 1790–1874.

    Jacob membrane

    Jacob ulcer

Jacob, François, French biologist, *1920, joint winner of 1965 Nobel Prize for work related to synthesis of viruses and enzymes.

Jacob, Octave, French physician.

    Jacob disease—inability to open the mouth secondary to mandibular constriction.

Jacobaeus, Hans C., Swedish surgeon, 1879–1937.

    Jacobaeus operation—obsolete term for pleurolysis.

    Jacobaeus thoracoscope

Jacobson, Julius, German ophthalmologist, 1828–1889.

    Jacobson neuralgia—*SYN:* Reichert syndrome

    Jacobson retinitis—*SYN:* syphilitic retinitis

Jacobson, Ludwig L., Danish anatomist, 1783–1843.

    Jacobson anastomosis—a portion of the tympanic plexus.

    Jacobson canal—a minute canal in the wedge of bone separating the jugular canal and carotid canal. *SYN:* tympanic canaliculus

    Jacobson cartilage—a narrow strip of cartilage located between the lower edge of the cartilage of the nasal septum and the vomer. *SYN:* cartilago vomeronasalis

    Jacobson nerve—*SYN:* tympanic nerve

    Jacobson organ—a fine vestigial horizontal canal ending in a blind pouch in the mucous membrane of the nasal septum. *SYN:* vomeronasal organ

    Jacobson plexus—a plexus on the promontory of the labyrinthine wall of the tympanic cavity, formed by the tympanic nerve, an anastomotic branch of the facial nerve, and sympathetic branches from the internal carotid plexus. *SYN:* tympanic plexus

    Jacobson reflex—flexion of the fingers elicited by tapping the flexor tendons over the wrist joint or the lower end of the radius.

Jacod, Maurice, French neurologist, *1880.

    Jacod syndrome—total ophthalmoplegia, blindness, and trigeminal neuralgia. *SYN:* Jacod triad

    Jacod triad—*SYN:* Jacod syndrome

Jacquart, Henri, 19th century French physician.
Jacquart facial angle—a facial angle with the intersection always at the nasal spine point.

Jacquemet, Marcel, French anatomist, 1872–1908.
Jacquemet recess—a pouch of peritoneum between the gallbladder and the liver.

Jacquemin, Emile, 19th century French chemist.
Jacquemin test—a test for phenol.

Jacques, James Archibald, manager of an English rubber company, 1815–1878.
Jacques catheter—urethral catheter.

Jacques, Paul, 19th century French physician.
Jacques plexus—a nerve plexus within the muscular coat of the fallopian tube.

Jacquet, Leonard L., French dermatologist, 1860–1914.
Jacquet erythema—diaper rash. *Syn:* diaper dermatitis

Jadassohn, Josef, German dermatologist in Switzerland, 1863–1936.
Borst-Jadassohn type intraepidermal epithelioma—see under Borst
Franceschetti-Jadassohn syndrome—*Syn:* Naegeli syndrome
Jadassohn nevus—congenital papillary acanthosis of the epidermis, with hyperplasia of sebaceous glands developing at puberty and presence of apocrine glands in nonapocrine areas of the skin. *Syn:* nevus sebaceus
Jadassohn-Lewandowski syndrome—ectodermal dysplasia of abnormal thickness and elevation of nail plates with palmar and plantar hyperkeratosis. *Syn:* pachyonychia congenta
Jadassohn-Pellizzari anetoderma—cutaneous atrophy preceded by erythematous or urticarial lesions of the trunk and upper portions of the extremities.
Jadassohn-Tièche nevus—a dark blue or blue-black nevus covered by smooth skin and formed by heavily pigmented spindle-shaped or dendritic melanocytes in the reticular dermis. *Syn:* blue nevus

Jadelot, Jean F. N., French physician, 1791–1830.
Jadelot furrows—*Syn:* Jadelot lines
Jadelot lines—facial lines in children. *Syn:* Jadelot furrows

Jaeger, Eduard, Ritter von Jaxthal, Austrian ophthalmologist, 1818–1884.
Jaeger hook
Jaeger keratome knife
Jaeger lid plate
Jaeger lid retractor
Jaeger reading chart
Jaeger strabismus hook
Jaeger test types—type of different sizes used for testing the acuity of near vision.

NOTES

Jaffe, Henry L., U.S. pathologist, 1896–1979
　　Jaffe-Lichtenstein disease—obsolete term for fibrous dysplasia of bone.

Jaffe, Max, German biochemist, 1841–1911.
　　Jaffe reaction—the basis of most routine creatinine tests.
　　Jaffe test—a qualitative test for the presence of indicanuria.

Jakob, Alfons M., German neuropsychiatrist, 1884–1931.
　　Creutzfeldt-Jakob disease—see under Creutzfeldt
　　Jakob-Creutzfeldt disease—*SYN:* Creutzfeldt-Jakob disease

James, George C.W., 20th century U.S. radiologist.
　　Swyer-James syndrome—see under Swyer
　　Swyer-James-Macleod syndrome—*SYN:* Swyer-James syndrome (2)

James, Thomas N., U.S. cardiologist and physiologist, *1925.
　　James fibers—atrio-His bundle connections thought to be the basis for the short P-R interval syndrome. *SYN:* James tracts
　　James tracts—*SYN:* James fibers

James, William, U.S. psychologist, 1842–1910.
　　James-Lange theory—that bodily changes, such as tachycardia or sweating, precede rather than follow the conscious perception of an emotion and by themselves evoke the emotional feeling.

Janet, Pierre M.F., French neurologist, 1859–1947.
　　Janet disease—psychasthenia.
　　Janet test—a test for functional or organic anesthesia.

Janeway, Edward G., U.S. physician, 1841–1911.
　　Janeway lesion—a small erythematous or hemorrhagic lesion seen in some cases of bacterial endocarditis.

Janeway, Theodore Caldwell, U.S. physician, 1872–1917.
　　Janeway sphygmomanometer

Jannetta, Peter J., U.S. neurosurgeon, *1932.
　　Jannetta aneurysm neck dissector
　　Jannetta bayonet forceps
　　Jannetta bayonet needle holder
　　Jannetta bayonet scissors
　　Jannetta dissector
　　Jannetta elevator
　　Jannetta microbayonet forceps
　　Jannetta needle holder
　　Jannetta posterior fossa retractor
　　Jannetta procedure—decompression of microvascular structures.
　　Jannetta sterilizing rack

Jansen, Albert, German otologist, 1859–1933.
　　Jansen bayonet nasal forceps
　　Jansen ear forceps
　　Jansen ear rongeur
　　Jansen mastoid raspatory
　　Jansen mouth gag
　　Jansen operation—an operation for frontal sinus disease, the lower wall

and lower portion of the anterior wall being removed and the mucous membrane curetted away.
Jansen scalp retractor
Jansen-Middleton punch forceps

Jansen, Murk, Dutch orthopedic surgeon, 1867–1935.
Jansen syndrome—rare congenital disease that causes anatomical abnormalities.

Jansky, Jan, Czech physician, 1873–1921.
Bielschowsky-Jansky disease—*Syn:* Jansky-Bielschowsky disease
Jansky classification—the classification of human blood groups now designated O, A, B, and AB.
Jansky-Bielschowsky disease—cerebral sphingolipidosis, early juvenile type. *Syn:* Bielschowsky-Jansky disease

Jaquet, Alfred, Swiss pharmacologist, 1865–1937.
Jaquet apparatus—apparatus for recording cardiac and venous impulses.

Jarcho, Julius, Russian-U.S. obstetrician, 1882–1963.
Jarcho pressometer—instrument used in hysterosalpingography.
Jarcho self-retaining uterine cannula
Jarcho uterine tenaculum

Jarcho, Saul, U.S. physician, *1906.
Jarcho syndrome—bone marrow metastatic carcinoma.

Jarisch, Adolf, Austrian dermatologist, 1850–1902.
Bezold-Jarisch reflex—see under Bezold
Jarisch-Herxheimer reaction—*Syn:* Herxheimer reaction

Jarjavay, Jean F., French anatomist and surgeon, 1815–1868.
Jarjavay ligament—a fold of peritoneum containing the rectouterine muscle. *Syn:* sacrouterine fold

Jaworski, Walery, Polish physician, 1849–1924.
Jaworski bodies—mucous shreds in the gastric contents in hyperchlorhydria.

Jeanselme, A. Edouard, French dermatologist, 1858–1935.
Jeanselme nodules—a form of tertiary yaws that is characterized by the occurrence of nodules on the arms and legs, situated usually near the joints. *Syn:* juxta-articular nodules

Jefferson, Sir Geoffrey, English neurologist, 1886–1961.
Jefferson syndrome—*Syn:* internal carotid artery aneurysm

Jeghers, Harold, U.S. physician, *1904.
Jeghers-Peutz syndrome—*Syn:* Peutz-Jeghers syndrome
Peutz-Jeghers syndrome—see under Peutz

Jellinek, Edward J., English physician, 1890–1963.
Jellinek formula—a method of estimating the prevalence of alcoholism in a nation's population.

NOTES

Jellinek, Stefan, Austrian physician, *1871.
> **Jellinek sign**—in Graves disease, a brownish pigmentation of the eyelids, especially the upper ones.

Jendrassik, Ernö, Hungarian physician, 1858–1921.
> **Jendrassik maneuver**—a method of emphasizing the patellar reflex: the subject hooks his hands together by the flexed fingers and pulls against them with all her strength.

Jenner, Harley D., Canadian physician, *1907.
> **Jenner-Kay unit**—that amount of phosphatase that liberates 1 mg of phosphorus.

Jenner, Louis, English physician, 1866–1904.
> **Jenner stain**—used for staining of blood smears.

Jensen, Carl O., Danish veterinary surgeon and pathologist, 1864–1934.
> **Jensen sarcoma**—a mouse tumor transmissible by inoculation.

Jensen, Edmund Z., Danish ophthalmologist, 1861–1950.
> **Jensen disease**—retinochoroiditis close to the optic disk. *SYN:* retinochoroiditis juxtapapillaris
> **Jensen intraocular lens forceps**
> **Jensen lens forceps**
> **Jensen polisher**
> **Jensen scratcher**
> **Jensen ties**

Jerne, Niels K., Danish immunologist, *1911, joint winner of the 1984 Nobel Prize for medicine and physiology.

Jervell, Anton, Norwegian cardiologist, *1901.
> **Jervell and Lange-Nielsen syndrome**—a prolonged Q-T interval recorded in the electrocardiogram of certain congenitally deaf children subject to Adams-Stokes seizures and ventricular fibrillation. *SYN:* surdocardiac syndrome

Jeune, Mathis, French pediatrician, *1910.
> **Jeune syndrome**—hereditary hypoplasia of the thorax, associated with pelvic skeletal abnormality. *SYN:* asphyxiating thoracic dysplasia

Jewett, Eugene Lyon, U.S. orthopedic surgeon, *1900.
> **Jewett bending iron**
> **Jewett bone extractor**
> **Jewett driver**
> **Jewett fracture appliance**
> **Jewett frame**
> **Jewett hip nail**
> **Jewett hyperextension brace**
> **Jewett nail plate**—orthopedic fixation device.
> **Jewett orthosis**
> **Jewett pickup screw**
> **Jewett prosthesis**
> **Jewett reamer**
> **Jewett thoracolumbosacral orthosis**

Jewett, Hugh, U.S. urologist, 1903–1990.
    Jewett and Strong staging—staging of bladder carcinoma (O, A through D).
    Jewett sound—a short straight sound for dilating the anterior urethra.

Jobert de Lamballe, Antoine, French surgeon, 1799–1867.
    Jobert de Lamballe fossa—the hollow just above the knee formed by the adductor magnus and the sartorius and gracilis.
    Jobert de Lamballe suture—an interrupted intestinal suture used for invaginating the margins of the intestines in circular enterorrhaphy.

Jobst, Conrad, U.S. engineer.
    Jobst boot—a device used to reduce limb edema. *SYN:* Jobst sleeve
    Jobst sleeve—*SYN:* Jobst boot
    Jobst stocking—an elastic stocking used to treat postphlebitic leg edema.

Joest, Ernst, German veterinary pathologist, 1873–1926.
    Joest bodies—intranuclear inclusion bodies (Cowdry type B) produced in certain nerve cells by Borna disease virus.

Joffroy, Alexis, French physician, 1844–1908.
    Joffroy reflex—twitching of the gluteal muscles when firm pressure is made on the buttocks, in cases of spastic paralysis. *SYN:* hip phenomenon
    Joffroy sign—immobility of the facial muscles when the eyeballs are rolled upward, in exophthalmic goiter; disorder of the arithmetical faculty in the early stages of organic brain disease.

Johne, H. Albert, German physician, 1839–1910.
    Johne bacillus—a species causing Johne disease, a chronic enteritis in cattle. *SYN: Mycobacterium paratuberculosis*
    Johne disease—a disease occurring in cattle and sheep, caused by infection with *Mycobacterium paratuberculosis. SYN:* paratuberculosis; chronic dysentery of cattle
    johnin—a diagnostic agent, analogous to tuberculin.

Johnson, Frank B., U.S. pathologist, *1919.
    Dubin-Johnson syndrome—see under Dubin

Johnson, Frank C., U.S. pediatrician, 1894–1934.
    Stevens-Johnson syndrome—see under Stevens, Albert

Johnson, Harry B., U.S. dentist.
    Johnson method—a method of filling the root canals of teeth by dissolving gutta-percha cones in a chloroform-rosin medium within the root canal. *SYN:* chloropercha method

Johnson, Treat Baldwin, U.S. chemist, 1875–1947.
    Wheeler-Johnson test—see under Wheeler, Henry

Johnston, Christopher, U.S. physician, *1891.
    Johnston organ—organ on fly antennae for sensing air flow during flight.

NOTES

Jolles, Adolf, Austrian chemist, 1863–1944.
    Jolles test—a test for bile.

Jolly, Friedrich, German neurologist, 1844–1904.
    Jolly reaction—rapid loss of response to faradic stimulation of a muscle with the galvanic response and the power of voluntary contraction retained. *SYN:* myasthenic reaction; Jolly test
    Jolly test—*SYN:* Jolly reaction

Jolly, Justin, French histologist, 1870–1953.
    Howell-Jolly bodies—see under Howell
    Jolly bodies—*SYN:* Howell-Jolly bodies

Jones, Ernest, English psychiatrist, 1879–1958.
    Ross-Jones test—see under Ross, Sir George

Jones, Henry Bence. See under Bence Jones.

Jones, Sir Robert, English orthopedic surgeon, 1858–1933.
    Jones abduction frame
    Jones arm splint
    Jones brace
    Jones first-toe repair
    Jones fracture
    Jones metacarpal splint
    Jones pin
    Jones position—position for treating humeral fracture.
    Jones resection arthroplasty
    Jones suspension traction
    Jones thoracic clamp
    Jones towel clamp
    Jones transfer
    Jones view

Jones, William A., U.S. dentist.
    Jones disease—genetic trait resulting in fullness of the face, suggestive of a cherub. *SYN:* Jones syndrome; cherubism
    Jones syndrome—*SYN:* Jones disease

Jonnesco, Thomas, Romanian surgeon, 1860–1926.
    Jonnesco fossa—a peritoneal recess extending upward behind the superior duodenal fold. *SYN:* superior duodenal recess

Jonston, Johns, Scottish physician in Poland, 1603–1675.
    Jonston alopecia—obsolete term for alopecia areata. *SYN:* Jonston area
    Jonston area—*SYN:* Jonston alopecia

Joseph, Jacques, German surgeon, 1865–1934.
    Joseph chisel
    Joseph clamp—used after rhinoplasty to maintain or improve the alignment of the bony support of the nose.
    Joseph double-edged knife
    Joseph knife—used in rhinoplasty to separate the overlying skin from the nasal dorsum.
    Joseph nasal knife
    Joseph nasal rasp

Joseph nasal raspatory
Joseph nasal saw
Joseph nasal scissors
Joseph perforator
Joseph periosteal elevator
Joseph punch
Joseph rhinoplasty—reduction and reshaping of the nose.
Joseph ruler
Joseph saw guide
Joseph septal bar
Joseph septal clamp
Joseph septal fracture appliance
Joseph septal frame
Joseph serrated scissors
Joseph single-prong hook

Joseph, R., French pediatrician.
Joseph syndrome—hereditary defect in renal tubules resulting in proteinuria with onset of epilepsy.

Joubert, Marie, 20th century Canadian neurologist.
Joubert syndrome—agenesis of the cerebellar vermis, characterized by tachypnea or prolonged apnea, abnormal eye movements, ataxia, and mental retardation.

Joule, James P., English physicist, 1818–1889.
joule—*SYN:* unit of heat
Joule equivalent—the dynamic equivalent of heat.

Jung, Carl Gustav, Swiss psychiatrist and psychologist, 1875–1961.
jungian psychoanalysis—the theory of psychopathology and the practice of psychotherapy. *SYN:* analytical psychology

Jung, Karl G., Swiss anatomist, 1793–1864.
Jung muscle—an occasional prolongation of the fibers of the tragicus to the spina helicis. *SYN:* pyramidal auricular muscle

Jungbluth, Hermann, 20th century German physician.
Jungbluth vessels—vessels under amnion of embryo.

Jüngling, Adolph O., German surgeon, 1884–1944.
Jüngling disease—an osteitis of tuberculous origin, marked by numerous small cavities in the osseous substance. *SYN:* osteitis tuberculosa multiplex cystica

Junius, Paul, German ophthalmologist, *1871.
Kuhnt-Junius degeneration—see under Kuhnt
Kuhnt-Junius disease—*SYN:* Kuhnt-Junius degeneration

Junod, Victor T., French physician, 1809–1881.
Junod boot—an airtight case used to divert a portion of the blood temporarily from the general circulation.

NOTES

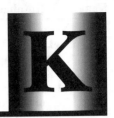

Kabat, Herman, U.S. physiatrist.
    Kabat method of exercise—system of therapeutic exercises designed for those with neuromuscular disabilities. *Syn:* Kabat-Knott method of exercise; Knott-Voss method of exercise
    Kabat-Knott method of exercise—*Syn:* Kabat method of exercise

Kader, Bronislaw, Polish surgeon, 1863–1937.
    Kader operation—a form of gastrostomy.

Kaes, Theodor, German neurologist, 1852–1913.
    band of Kaes-Bekhterev—band of horizontal myelinated fibers in the most superficial part of the third layer of the isocortex. *Syn:* Bekhterev band; layer of Bekhterev; line of Bekhterev; line of Kaes
    line of Kaes—*Syn:* band of Kaes-Bechterew

Kahlbaum, Karl L., German physician, 1828–1899.
    Kahlbaum-Wernicke syndrome

Kahler, Otto, Austrian physician, 1849–1893.
    Kahler bronchial forceps
    Kahler bronchus-grasping forceps
    Kahler disease—disease associated with anemia, hemorrhages, recurrent infections, and weakness; considered a malignant neoplasm. *Syn:* multiple myeloma
    Kahler forceps
    Kahler laryngeal forceps
    Kahler polyp forceps

Kahn, Eugen, German psychologist, *1887.
    Kahn Test of Symbol Arrangement—diagnostic psychological test.

Kahn, Reuben, U.S. bacteriologist, *1887.
    Kahn test—variation of Wasserman test for syphilis.

Kaiserling, Karl, German pathologist, 1869–1942.
    Kaiserling fixative—a method of preserving histologic and pathologic specimens without altering the color.

Kalischer, Siegfried, German physician, *1862.
    Sturge-Kalischer-Weber syndrome—*Syn:* Sturge-Weber syndrome

Kallmann, Franz Josef, U.S. medical geneticist and psychiatrist, 1897–1965.
    Kallmann syndrome—*Syn:* hypogonadism with anosmia

Kanavel, Allen B., U.S. surgeon, 1874–1938.
 Kanavel apparatus—used for finger, wrist, and forearm exercises. *Syn:* Kanavel table
 Kanavel brain-exploring cannula
 Kanavel cock-up splint
 Kanavel sign—tenderness of the lateral side of the palm, which may be secondary to bursitis of the ulna.
 Kanavel splint
 Kanavel table—*Syn:* Kanavel apparatus

Kandinsky, V.C., Russian psychiatrist, 1827–1899.
 Clérambault-Kandinsky complex—see under Clérambault
 Clérambault-Kandinsky syndrome—*Syn:* Clérambault-Kandinsky complex

Kandori, Fumio, Japanese ophthalmologist, *1904.
 fleck retina of Kandori—an autosomal-recessive disorder of the retinal pigment epithelium occurring among Japanese.

Kanner, Leo, Austrian psychiatrist in U.S., 1894–1991.
 Kanner syndrome—a severe emotional disturbance of childhood. *Syn:* infantile autism

Kantor, John L., U.S. radiologist, 1890–1949.
 Kantor string sign—luminal narrowing revealed on x-ray as a thin line of barium terminating at the ileocecal junction.

Kaplan, David M., U.S. physician, 1876–1952.
 Kaplan test—test for globulin-albumin in cerebrospinal fluid.

Kaposi, Moritz, (born Moritz Kohn), Hungarian dermatologist in Austria, 1837–1902.
 Kaposi sarcoma—a multifocal malignant neoplasm. *Syn:* multiple idiopathic hemorrhagic sarcoma
 Kaposi varicelliform eruption—a rare complication of vaccinia superimposed on atopic dermatitis, with generalized vesicles and vesicopapules and high fever. *Syn:* eczema vaccinatum

Karmen, Albert, U.S. internist and clinical pathologist, *1930.
 Karmen unit—a formerly used enzyme unit.

Karnofsky, D.A., 20th century U.S. physician.
 Karnofsky index
 Karnofsky scale—a performance scale used to evaluate a patient's progress after a therapeutic procedure.
 Karnofsky score

Karplus, Johann P., Austrian physician and physiologist, 1866–1936.
 Karplus sign—pleural effusion causes modification in vocal resonance.

Kartagener, Manes, Swiss physician, 1897–1975.
 Kartagener syndrome—complete situs inversus associated with bronchiectasis and chronic sinusitis. *Syn:* Kartagener triad; Zivert syndrome
 Kartagener triad—*Syn:* Kartagener syndrome

Kasabach, Haig H., U.S. physician, 1898–1943.
 Kasabach-Merritt syndrome—capillary hemangioma associated with

thrombocytopenic purpura. *Syn:* hemangioma-thrombocytopenia syndrome

Kasai, Morio, 20th century Japanese surgeon.
 Kasai operation—an operation for biliary atresia. *Syn:* portoenterostomy

Kasanin, Jacob S., U.S. psychologist, 1897–1946.
 Hanfmann-Kasanin Concept Formation Test—see under Hanfmann

Kashida, K., 20th century Japanese physician.
 Kashida sign

Kashin, Nikolai I., Russian orthopedist, 1825–1872.
 Kashin-Bek disease—a form of generalized osteoarthrosis believed to result from ingestion of wheat infected with the fungus *Fusarium sporotrichiella*.

Kast, Alfred, German physician, 1856–1903.
 Kast syndrome—benign neoplasm associated with vascular malformations containing cavernous hemangiomas.

Kasten, Frederick H., U.S. histochemist and cell biologist, *1927.
 Kasten fluorescent Feulgen stain—a fluorescent modification of the Feulgen stain.
 Kasten fluorescent PAS stain—a fluorescent modification of the periodic acid Schiff stain for polysaccharides that uses one of the Kasten fluorescent Schiff reagents.
 Kasten fluorescent Schiff reagents—used in cytochemical detection of DNA.

Katayama, Kunika, Japanese physician, 1856–1931.
 Katayama test—a qualitative colorimetric test for the presence of carboxyhemoglobin in the blood.

Katz, Sir Bernard, German-English neurophysiologist and Nobel laureate, *1911.
 Goldman-Hodgkin-Katz equation—*Syn:* Goldman equation

Kauffman, E., German physician, 1860–1931.
 Aberhalden-Kauffman-Lignac syndrome—see under Aberhalden

Kaveggia, E.F.
 Opitz-Kaveggia syndrome—see under Opitz

Kawasaki, Tomisaku, 20th century Japanese pediatrician.
 Kawasaki disease—a polymorphous erythematous febrile, sometimes epidemic, disease of unknown etiology occurring in children. *Syn:* Kawasaki syndrome; mucocutaneous lymph node syndrome
 Kawasaki syndrome—*Syn:* Kawasaki disease

Kay, Herbert D., English biochemist, *1893.
 Jenner-Kay unit—see under Jenner, Harley

Kay, Sir Andrew Watt, Scottish professor of surgery.
 Kay test—test related to peptic ulcers.

NOTES

Kayser, Bernhard, German physician, 1869–1954.
Kayser-Fleischer ring—a greenish-yellow pigmented ring encircling the cornea just within the corneoscleral margin, seen in hepatolenticular degeneration. *SYN:* Fleischer-Strümpell ring

Kazanjian, Varaztad H., Armenian otorhinolaryngologist in the U.S., 1879–1974.
Kazanjian scissors
Kazanjian nasal forceps
Kazanjian nasal hump forceps
Kazanjian operation—surgical extension of the vestibular sulcus of edentulous ridges to increase their height and to improve denture retention.
Kazanjian osteotome
Kazanjian splint

Kearns, Thomas P., U.S. ophthalmologist, *1922.
Kearns-Sayre syndrome—chronic progressive external ophthalmoplegia with associated cardiac conduction defects, short stature, and hearing loss.

Keating-Hart, Walter V., French physician, 1870–1922.
Keating-Hart method—fulguration in the treatment of external cancer or of the field of operation after removal of a malignant growth.

Keen, William W., U.S. surgeon, 1837–1932.
Keen operation—removal of sections of nerves as a cure for torticollis.
Keen sign—increased width at the malleoli in Pott fracture.

Keetley, Charles Robert Bell, English surgeon, 1848–1909.
Keetley-Torek operation—*SYN:* Torek operation

Kegel, A.H., 20th century U.S. gynecologist.
Kegel exercises—alternate contraction and relaxation of perineal muscles for treatment of urinary stress incontinence.

Kehr, Hans, German surgeon, 1862–1916.
Kehr incision
Kehr sign—violent pain in the left shoulder in a case of rupture of the spleen.
Kehr T-tube

Kehrer, Ferdinand A., German neurologist, 1883–1966.
Kehrer reflex—*SYN:* Kisch reflex

Keith, Sir Arthur, Scottish anatomist, 1866–1955.
Keith and Flack node—the mass of specialized cardiac muscle fibers that normally acts as the pacemaker of the cardiac conduction system. *SYN:* sinuatrial node; Flack node; Keith node
Keith bundle—modified cardiac muscle fibers. *SYN:* atrioventricular bundle
Keith node—*SYN:* Keith and Flack node

Keller, William Lordan, U.S. surgeon, 1874–1959.
Keller arthroplasty
Keller bunion osteotomy
Keller bunionectomy—excision of the proximal portion of the proximal phalanx of the first toe.
Keller hallux rigidus operation

Keller hallux valgus operation
Keller operation

Kellie, George, 18th century Scottish anatomist.
Monro-Kellie doctrine—*SYN:* Monro doctrine

Kelly, Adam B., English otolaryngologist, 1865–1941.
Paterson-Brown-Kelly syndrome—see under Paterson, Donald R.
Paterson-Kelly syndrome—*SYN:* Plummer-Vinson syndrome

K

Kelly, Howard A., U.S. gynecologist, 1858–1943.
Kelly clamp—a curved hemostat without teeth.
Kelly operation—correction of retroversion of the uterus; correction of
urinary stress incontinence.
Kelly placenta forceps
Kelly plication
Kelly rectal speculum
Kelly uterine dilator
Kelly uterine scissors
Kelly uterine tenaculum

Kelvin, Lord William Thomson, Scottish physicist, 1824–1907.
kelvin—a unit of thermodynamic temperature equal to 1/273.16 of the
thermodynamic temperature of the triple point of water.
Kelvin scale—temperature scale in which the triple point of water is
assigned the value of 273.16 K.
Kelvin thermometer

Kempner, Walter, U.S. physician, *1903.
Kempner rice diet—low-salt diet used to treat high blood pressure.

Kendall, Edward C., U.S. biochemist, 1886–1972, joint winner of the 1950 Nobel
Prize for research on the hormones of the adrenal cortex.
Kendall method—test to measure iodine in thyroid tissue.

Kennedy, Edward, U.S. dentist, *1883.
Kennedy classification—a listing of several forms of partially edentulous
jaws in accordance with the distribution of the missing teeth.

Kennedy, Robert Foster, U.S. neurologist, 1884–1952.
Foster Kennedy syndrome—*SYN:* Kennedy syndrome
Kennedy syndrome—ipsilateral optic atrophy with central scotoma and
contralateral choked disk or papilledema, caused by a meningioma of the
ipsilateral optic nerve. *SYN:* Foster Kennedy syndrome

Kennedy, William, U.S. neurologist.
Kennedy disease—an X-linked recessive disorder characterized by
progressive spinal and bulbar muscular atrophy.

Kenny, Frederic M., U.S. physician, *1929.
Kenny syndrome—genetic trait resulting in dwarfism and cortical
thickening of tubular bones.

NOTES

Kenny, Sister Elizabeth, Australian nurse, 1886–1952.
    Kenny crutch—a wooden forearm crutch.
    Kenny treatment—a method for the treatment of anterior poliomyelitis.

Kenny Rehabilitation Institute, Minneapolis, MN.
    Kenny rating—*Syn:* Kenny self-care evaluation
    Kenny score—*Syn:* Kenny self-care evaluation
    Kenny self-care evaluation—a system of numeric ratings for evaluating a patient's ability to perform 17 activities. *Syn:* Kenny rating; Kenny score

Kent, Albert F.S., English physiologist, 1863–1958.
    Kent bundle—*Syn:* His bundle
    Kent-His bundle—*Syn:* His bundle

Kerandel, Jean F., French physician, 1873–1934.
    Kerandel sign—a blow to a bony projection causing hyperesthesia and pain.
    Kerandel symptom—deep-seated hyperesthesia observed in cases of sleeping sickness.

Kergaradec, Jean Alexandre le Jameau, Vicomte de, French obstetrician-gynecologist, 1788–1877.
    Kergaradec sign—soft blowing sound synchronous with cardiac systole of mother, heard on auscultation of gravid uterus. *Syn:* uterine souffle; placental souffle

Kerley, Peter J., English radiologist, *1900.
    Kerley B lines—fine peripheral septal lines. *Syn:* costophrenic septal lines

Kernig, Vladimir, Russian physician, 1840–1917.
    Kernig sign—a failure of leg extension present in various forms of meningitis.

Kernohan, James W., Irish pathologist, 1897–1981.
    Kernohan notch—a notch in the cerebral peduncle due to displacement of the brainstem against the incisura of the tentorium by a transtentorial herniation.
    Kernohan-Woltman syndrome—cerebral lesion resulting in same-side hemiparesis. *Syn:* Woltman-Kernohan syndrome; Cruz phenomenon
    Woltman-Kernohan syndrome—*Syn:* Kernohan-Woltman syndrome

Kerr, Harry Hyland, U.S. surgeon, 1881–1963.
    Parker-Kerr basting suture
    Parker-Kerr operation
    Parker-Kerr suture—see under Parker, Edward

Kesling, Harold, D., U.S. orthodontist, *1901.
    Kesling appliance
    Kesling spring

Kestenbaum, U.S. ophthalmologist, 1890–1961.
    Kestenbaum number—the difference between the two pupil diameters when each eye is measured in bright light with the other eye tightly covered.
    Kestenbaum sign—a decrease in the number of arterioles crossing optic disk margins as a sign of optic neuritis.

Key, Ernst A.H., Swedish anatomist and physician, 1832–1901.
   foramen of Key-Retzius—one of the two lateral openings of the fourth ventricle into the subarachnoid space at the cerebellopontine angle. *SYN:* lateral aperture of the fourth ventricle
   Key-Retzius corpuscles—tactile corpuscles, resembling pacinian corpuscles, found in the beak of certain aquatic birds.
   sheath of Key and Retzius—the delicate connective tissue enveloping individual nerve fibers within a peripheral nerve. *SYN:* endoneurium

Khorana, Har G., Indian-U.S. chemist, *1922, joint winner of the 1968 Nobel Prize for discovering the process by which enzymes determine cell function in a genetic environment.

Kielland, var. of Kjelland

Kien, Alphonse M.J., 19th century German physician.
   Kussmaul-Kien respiration—*SYN:* Kussmaul respiration

Kienböck, Robert, Austrian radiologist, 1871–1953.
   Kienböck atrophy—acute atrophy of bone in an extremity following inflammation.
   Kienböck disease—osteolysis of the lunate bone following trauma to the wrist. *SYN:* lunatomalacia
   Kienböck dislocation—dislocation of semilunar bone.
   Kienböck unit—an obsolete unit of x-ray dosage equivalent to 1/10 the erythema dose.

Kiernan, Francis, English physician, 1800–1874.
   Kiernan space—interlobular space in the liver.

Kiesselbach, Wilhelm, German laryngologist, 1839–1902.
   Kiesselbach area—an area on the anterior portion of the nasal septum rich in capillaries (Kiesselbach plexus) and often the seat of epistaxis. *SYN:* Little area
   Kiesselbach plexus
   Kiesselbach triangle

Kikuchi, M.
   Kikuchi necrotizing lymphadenitis—nonmalignant disease primarily affecting cervical lymph nodes in females.

Kilian, Hermann F., German gynecologist, 1800–1863.
   Kilian line—a transverse line marking the promontory of the pelvis.

Kiliani, H., chemist, 1855–1945.
   Kiliani-Fischer reaction
   Kiliani-Fischer synthesis—a synthetic procedure for the extension of the carbon atom chain of aldoses by treatment with cyanide. *SYN:* feedback inhibition

NOTES

Killian, Gustav, German laryngologist, 1860–1921.
> **Killian antrum cannula**
> **Killian bundle**—*SYN:* inferior constrictor muscle of pharynx
> **Killian cannula**
> **Killian elevator**
> **Killian frontal sinus chisel**
> **Killian frontoethmoidectomy procedure**
> **Killian gouge**
> **Killian incision**
> **Killian nasal speculum**
> **Killian operation**—an operation for frontal sinus disease.
> **Killian septal compression forceps**
> **Killian septal elevator**
> **Killian septal speculum**
> **Killian tonsil knife**
> **Killian triangle**—the triangular-shaped area of the cervical esophagus. *SYN:* laimer triangle
> **Killian-Lynch suspension laryngoscope**

Kimmelstiel, Paul, German pathologist in the U.S., 1900–1970.
> **Kimmelstiel-Wilson disease**—*SYN:* Kimmelstiel-Wilson syndrome
> **Kimmelstiel-Wilson syndrome**—nephrotic syndrome and hypertension in diabetics, associated with diabetic glomerulosclerosis. *SYN:* Kimmelstiel-Wilson disease

Kimura, Tetsuji, 20th century Japanese pathologist.
> **Kimura disease**—solitary or multiple small benign cutaneous erythematous nodules. *SYN:* angiolymphoid hyperplasia with eosinophilia

Kindler, Werner, German otorhinolaryngologist, *1895.
> **Kindler-Zange syndrome**—*SYN:* Zange-Kindler syndrome
> **Zange-Kindler syndrome**—see under Zange

King, Earl J., Canadian biochemist, 1901–1962.
> **King unit**—the quantity of phosphatase that, acting upon disodium phenylphosphate in excess, at pH 9 for 30 minutes, liberates 1 mg of phenol. *SYN:* King-Armstrong unit
> **King-Armstrong unit**—*SYN:* King unit

Kingsbourne, M., English physician.
> **Kingsbourne syndrome**—neurologic disorder seen in children under the age of 3; results in ataxia, nystagmus and myoclonus.

Kingsley, Norman W., U.S. dentist, 1829–1913.
> **Kingsley splint**—a winged maxillary splint attached to a head appliance by elastics. *SYN:* reverse Kingsley splint
> **reverse Kingsley splint**—*SYN:* Kingsley splint

Kinyoun, Joseph J., U.S. physician, 1860–1919.
> **Kinyoun stain**—a method for demonstrating acid-fast microorganisms.

Kirchner, Wilhelm, Austrian otologist, 1849–1936.
> **Kirchner diverticulum**—eustachean tube diverticulum.

Kirk, Norman Thomas, U.S. Army surgeon, 1888–1960.
> **Kirk amputation**—amputation at the lower end of the femur, using the tendon of the quadriceps extensor to cover the end of the bone.

Kirk mallet
Kirk orthopedic hammer
Kirk technique

Kirkland, Olin, U.S. periodontist, 1876–1969.
Kirkland cement
Kirkland instrument
Kirkland knife—a heart-shaped knife used in gingival surgery.
Kirkland periodontal pack

K

Kirschner, Martin, German surgeon, 1879–1942.
Kirschner apparatus—*Syn:* Kirschner wire
Kirschner bone drill
Kirschner bow
Kirschner hip replacement system
Kirschner II-C shoulder system
Kirschner interlocking intramedullary nail
Kirschner Medical Dimension hip replacement
Kirschner pin fixation
Kirschner skeletal traction
Kirschner suture
Kirschner system
Kirschner total shoulder prosthesis
Kirschner traction
Kirschner wire—an apparatus for skeletal traction in long bone fracture.
Syn: Kirschner apparatus
Kirschner wire drill
Kirschner wire fixation
Kirschner wire inserter
Kirschner wire pin
Kirschner wire splint
Kirschner wire spreader
Kirschner wire tightener
Kirschner wire traction

Kirstein, Alfred, German physician, 1863–1922.
Kirstein method—examination of the larynx.

Kisch, Bruno, German physiologist, 1890–1966.
Kisch reflex—closure of the eye in response to stimulation of the skin at
the depth of the external auditory meatus. *Syn:* auriculopalpebral reflex;
Kehrer reflex

Kitasato, Shibasaburo, Baron, Japanese bacteriologist, 1856–1931.
Kitasato bacillus—a species causing plague. *Syn: Yersinia pestis*

Kjeldahl, Johan G.C., Danish chemist, 1849–1900.
Kjeldahl apparatus—an apparatus used in nitrogen analysis.

(continued)

NOTES

Kjeldahl (*continued*)
   Kjeldahl method
   macro-Kjeldahl method—a procedure for analyzing the content of nitrogenous compounds in urine, serum, or other specimens.
   micro-Kjeldahl method—a modification of the macro-Kjeldahl method designed for the analysis of nitrogenous compounds in relatively small quantities.

Kjelland, Christian, Norwegian obstetrician, 1871–1941.
   Kjelland blade
   Kjelland forceps—an obstetrical forceps having a sliding lock and little pelvic curve.
   Kjelland obstetrical forceps
   Kjelland rotation

Klapp, Rudolph, German surgeon, 1873–1949.
   Klapp creeping treatment—*SYN:* Klapp method
   Klapp exercises—*SYN:* Klapp method
   Klapp method—treatment of scoliosis by a series of systematic crawling movements whereby the spine is bent laterally and made more flexible. *SYN:* Klapp exercises; Klapp creeping treatment

Klatskin, Gerald, U.S. gastroenterologist, *1910.
   Klatskin biliary adenocarcinoma
   Klatskin cholangiocarcinoma
   Klatskin needle
   Klatskin tumor—carcinoma of the bile duct.

Klauder, Joseph V., U.S. dermatologist, 1888–1962.
   Klauder syndrome—acute inflammation of skin and mucous membranes.

Klebs, Theodor Albrecht Edwin, German physician, 1834–1913.
   Klebsiella—a genus of bacteria (family Enterobacteriaceae) that occurs in the respiratory, intestinal, and urogenital tracts of humans as well as in soil, water, and grain.
   Klebs disease
   Klebs-Loeffler bacillus—a species that causes diphtheria and produces a powerful exotoxin causing degeneration of various tissues, notably myocardium. *SYN: Corynebacterium diphtheriae*
   Klebsiella oxytoca

Klein, Edward E., Hungarian histologist, 1844–1925.
   Klein muscle—*SYN:* cutaneomucous muscle
   Klein-Gumprecht shadow nuclei—shadow nuclei in degenerating lymphoidocytes and macrolymphocytes in leukemia.

Kleine, Willi, 20th century German neuropsychiatrist.
   Kleine-Levin syndrome—a rare form of periodic hypersomnia associated with bulimia, behavioral disturbances, impaired thought processes, and hallucinations.

Klenzak, first name unknown, engineer and machinist, *1956.
   Klenzak ankle joint—a type of spring-loaded metal brace joint.
   Klenzak brace—brace used for footdrop.
   Klenzak double-channeled ankle joint

Klenzak joint—a metal joint used in a brace.
Klenzak knee joint

Kline, Benjamin S., U.S. pathologist, 1886–1968.
   Kline test—a test for syphilis.

Klinefelter, Harry F., Jr., U.S. physician, *1912.
   Klinefelter syndrome—a chromosomal anomaly in which patients are male in development but have seminiferous tubule dysgenesis, elevated urinary gonadotropins, variable gynecomastia, and eunuchoid habitus. *Syn:* XXY syndrome

Klippel, Maurice, French neurologist, 1858–1942.
   Feil-Klippel syndrome—*Syn:* Klippel-Feil syndrome
   Klippel-Feil syndrome—a congenital defect manifested as a short neck, extensive fusion of the cervical vertebrae, and abnormalities of the brainstem and cerebellum. *Syn:* cervical fusion syndrome; Feil-Klippel syndrome
   Klippel-Trenaunay-Weber syndrome—an anomaly of the extremity in which there is a combination of angiomatosis and anomalous development of the underlying bone and muscle, sometimes associated with localized gigantism. *Syn:* congenital dysplastic angiectasia; hemangiectatic hypertrophy; angio-osteohypertrophy syndrome

Kloepfer, H.W.
   Kloepfer syndrome—blindness beginning at the age of 2 months, arrested growth at 5 or 6, and progressive mental retardation.

Klotz, Henri P., French physician, *1910.
   Klotz syndrome—primary amenorrhea with concomitant poorly developed genitalia and reproductive organs.

Klumpke, Augusta Dejerine-. See under Dejerine-Klumpke.

Klüver, Heinrich, German-born U.S. neurologist, 1897–1979.
   Klüver-Barrera Luxol fast blue stain—in combination with cresyl violet, a stain useful for demonstrating myelin and Nissl substance.
   Klüver-Bucy syndrome—a syndrome mostly reported in monkeys, characterized by psychic blindness or hyperreactivity to visual stimuli, increased oral and sexual activity, and depressed drive and emotional reactions.

Knapp, Herman J., U.S. ophthalmologist, 1832–1911.
   Knapp cataract knife
   Knapp eye speculum
   Knapp iris hook
   Knapp iris knife needle
   Knapp iris repositor
   Knapp iris scissors
   Knapp iris spatula

(continued)

NOTES

Knapp *(continued)*
>**Knapp lacrimal sac retractor**
>**Knapp lens scoop**
>**Knapp lid operation**
>**Knapp pterygium operation**
>**Knapp streaks**—striae in Bruch membrane occurring in a variety of systemic disorders affecting elastic tissue. *SYN:* angioid streaks; Knapp striae
>**Knapp striae**—*SYN:* Knapp streaks

Knapp, Karl, German chemist, 1832–1911.
>**Knapp test**—a test for urine glucose.

Knaus, Hermann, Austrian gynecologist, *1892.
>**Ogino-Knaus rule**—see under Ogino

Kneipp, Sebastian, German pastor, 1821–1897.
>**Kneipp cure**—*SYN:* Kneipp treatment
>**Kneipp treatment**—a therapeutic system of treatment consisting of diet, walking barefoot in dewy grass or snow in the early morning, and cold-water applications. *SYN:* Kneipp cure; kneippism
>**kneippism**—*SYN:* Kneipp treatment

Knies, Max, German ophthalmologist, 1851–1917.
>**Knies sign**—pupil dilatation related to Graves disease.

Kniest, Wilhelm, 20th century German pediatrician.
>**Kniest syndrome**—a type of metatropic dwarfism.

Knight, James C., U.S. physician, 1810–1887.
>**Knight brace**—a thoracic, lumbar, sacral orthosis with abdominal flexible support. *SYN:* chairback brace

Knoll, Philipp, Bohemian physiologist, 1841–1900.
>**Knoll glands**—glands in the ventricular folds of the larynx (false vocal cords).

Knoop, Hedwig, German physician, *1908.
>**Knoop theory**—related to the catabolism of fatty acids.

Knott, Margaret, U.S. physical therapist, 1913–1978.
>**Kabat-Knott method of exercise**—*SYN:* Kabat method of exercise
>**Knott-Voss method of exercise**—*SYN:* Kabat method of exercise

Knowles, Frederick, U.S. orthopedic surgeon, 1888–1973.
>**Knowles pin nail**
>**Knowles pins**—femoral neck fracture fixation devices.
>**Knowles scissors**

Knox, Howard A., U.S. psychiatrist, *1885.
>**Knox Cube Test**—a performance test.

Kobelt, Georg L., German physician, 1804–1857.
>**Kobelt cyst**
>**Kobelt tubules**—remnants of the mesonephric tubules in the female. *SYN:* wolffian tubules

Kober, Philip A., U.S. chemist, *1884.
    Kober test—a test for naturally occurring estrogens.

Köbner, H., German dermatologist, 1838–1904.
    Köbner phenomenon—an isomorphic reaction seen in response to trauma in previously uninvolved sites of patients with skin diseases. *SYN:* isomorphic response

Koch, Robert, German bacteriologist and Nobel laureate, 1843–1910.
    Koch bacillus—(1) a species that causes tuberculosis. *SYN: Mycobacterium tuberculosis*; (2) a species that causes cholera. *SYN: Vibrio cholerae*
    Koch blue bodies—schizonts of *Theileria parva*, the causative agent of East Coast fever.
    Koch law—*SYN:* Koch postulates
    Koch old tuberculin
    Koch original tuberculin
    Koch phenomenon—infection immunity.
    Koch postulates—to establish the specificity of a pathogenic microorganism, it must be present in all cases of the disease; inoculations of its pure cultures must produce disease in animals, and from these it must be again obtained and be propagated in pure cultures. *SYN:* Koch law
    Koch-Weeks bacillus—a species found in the respiratory tract, causes acute respiratory infections. *SYN: Haemophilus influenzae*; Weeks bacillus

Koch, Walter, German surgeon, *1880.
    Koch node—the mass of specialized cardiac muscle fibers that normally acts as the "pacemaker" of the cardiac conduction system. *SYN:* sinuatrial node
    Koch triangle—a triangular area of the wall of the right atrium of the heart that marks the situation of the atrioventricular node.

Kocher, E. Theodor, Swiss surgeon and Nobel laureate, 1841–1917.
    Kocher elevator
    Kocher approach
    Kocher artery forceps
    Kocher biliary tract incision
    Kocher bladder retractor
    Kocher clamp—a heavy, straight hemostat.
    Kocher dissector
    Kocher forceps
    Kocher goiter dissector
    Kocher hemostat
    Kocher incision—an incision parallel with right costal margin.
    Kocher intestinal forceps
    Kocher kidney-elevating forceps
    Kocher maneuver
    Kocher periosteal dissector

(continued)

NOTES

(...ntinued)

...r retractor

...r sign—in Graves disease, on upward gaze the globe lags behind the movement of the upper eyelid.

Kocher spoon

Kocher ureterosigmoidostomy procedure

Kocher-Debré-Semelaigne syndrome—autosomal recessive inherited athyrotic cretinism associated with muscular pseudohypertrophy. *SYN:* Debré-Semelaigne syndrome

Kock, Nils G., Swedish surgeon, *1924.

Kock ileal reservoir

Kock ileostomy—*SYN:* Kock pouch

Kock nipple

Kock nipple valve

Kock pouch—a continent ileostomy with a reservoir and valved opening fashioned from doubled loops of ileum. *SYN:* Kock ileostomy

Koebner, Heinrich, German dermatologist, 1838–1904.

Koebner response—psoriasis due to trauma.

Koenig, Franz, German surgeon, 1832–1910.

Koenig syndrome—alternating attacks of constipation and diarrhea, with colic, meteorism, and gurgling in the right iliac fossa.

Koerber, Herman, German ophthalmologist, *1878.

Koerber-Salus-Elschnig syndrome—*SYN:* Parinaud I syndrome

Koerte, Werner, German surgeon, 1853–1937.

Koerte-Ballance operation—anastomosis of the facial and hypoglossal nerves for the treatment of facial paralysis.

Koettstorfer, J., 19th century German chemist.

Koettstorfer number—the number of milligrams of KOH required to saponify 1 g of fat. *SYN:* saponification number

Kofferath, Walter, German physician.

Kofferath syndrome—unilateral paralysis in newborns often caused by forceps during delivery.

Kogoj, Franz, Yugoslavian physician, *1894.

Kogoj abscess

spongiform pustule of Kogoj—an epidermal pustule formed by infiltration of neutrophils into necrotic epidermis in pustular psoriasis.

Köhler, Alban, German radiologist, 1874–1947.

Köhler disease—epiphysial aseptic necrosis of the tarsal navicular bone or of the patella.

Köhler, August, German microscopist, 1866–1948.

Köhler illumination—a method of illumination of microscopic objects.

Köhler, Georges J.F., German immunologist, *1946, joint winner of 1984 Nobel Prize for work related to the immune system.

Kohlrausch, Otto L.B., German physician, 1811–1854.

Kohlrausch muscle—the longitudinal muscles of the rectal wall.

Kohlrausch valves—*SYN:* transverse rectal folds

Kohn, Hans N., German pathologist, *1866.
Kohn one-step staining technique
Kohn pores—openings in the interalveolar septa of the lung. *Syn:* interalveolar pores

Kohnstamm, Oskar, German physician, 1871–1917.
Kohnstamm phenomenon—a slow, involuntary elevation of the arm after strong pressure against a firm object. *Syn:* after-movement

Kohs, Samuel C., U.S. psychologist, 1890–1977.
Kohs Block Design Test—intelligence test.

K

Kojewnikoff, Aleksei Y., Russian neurologist, 1836–1902.
Kojewnikoff epilepsy—simple partial motor status epilepticus of the rolandic cortex. *Syn:* epilepsia partialis continua

Kok, O., Dutch physician.
Kok disease—genetic trait associated with hypertonia in newborns.

Kölliker, Rudolph A. von, Swiss histologist, 1817–1905.
Kölliker layer—the layer of connective tissue in the iris.
Kölliker reticulum—non-neuronal cellular elements of the central and peripheral nervous system. *Syn:* neuroglia

Kollmann, Arthur, 19th century German urologist.
Kollmann dilator—a metallic expandable instrument used to dilate urethral strictures.

Kolmer, John A., U.S. pathologist, 1886–1962.
Kolmer test—a former standard quantitative method for the Wassermann test, with numerous modifications.

Kolodny, H.
Rebeitz-Kolodny-Richardson syndrome—see under Rebeitz

Kolopp, P., 20th century French dermatologist.
Woringer-Kolopp disease—see under Woringer

Kondoleon, Emmanuel, Greek surgeon, 1879–1939.
Kondoleon operation—excision of strips of subcutaneous connective tissue for the relief of elephantiasis.

König, Franz, German surgeon, 1832–1910.
König disease—complete or incomplete separation of joint cartilage and underlying bone, usually involving the knee. *Syn:* osteochondritis dissecans

Koplik, Henry, U.S. physician, 1858–1927.
Koplik spots—small red spots on buccal mucosa, occurring early in measles before skin eruption. *Syn:* Filatov spots; Flindt spots

Korff, Karl von, 20th century German anatomist and histologist.
Korff fibers—argyrophilic fibers that pass between odontoblasts at the periphery of the dental pulp and fan out into the dentin.

NOTES

Kornberg, A., U.S. biochemist and Nobel laureate, *1918.
    Kornberg enzyme—DNA polymerase I from *Escherichia coli.*

Kornsweig, var. of Kornzweig

Kornzweig, Abraham L., U.S. physician, *1900.
    Bassen-Kornzweig disease—*SYN:* Bassen-Kornzweig syndrome
    Bassen-Kornzweig syndrome—see under Bassen

Korotkoff, Nikolai S., Russian physician, 1874–1920.
    Korotkoff sounds—sounds heard over an artery when pressure over it is
    reduced below systolic arterial pressure, as when blood pressure is
    determined by the auscultatory method.
    Korotkoff test—a test of collateral circulation.

Korsakoff, Sergei S., Russian neurologist and psychiatrist, 1853–1900.
    Korsakoff psychosis—*SYN:* Korsakoff syndrome
    Korsakoff syndrome—an alcohol amnestic syndrome. *SYN:* amnestic
    psychosis; dysmnesic psychosis; Korsakoff psychosis; polyneuritic
    psychosis; amnestic syndrome
    Wernicke-Korsakoff encephalopathy
    Wernicke-Korsakoff syndrome—see under Wernicke

Korsakov, var. of Korsakoff

Koshland, Daniel E., U.S. biochemist, *1920.
    Adair-Koshland-Némethy-Filmer model—*SYN:* Koshland-Némethy-Filmer
    model
    Koshland-Némethy-Filmer model—a model to explain the allosteric form
    of cooperativity. *SYN:* induced fit model; Adair-Koshland-Némethy-Filmer
    model

Kossa, Julius von. See under von Kossa.

Kossel, Albrecht, German physiologist, 1853–1927.
    Kossel test—test for hypoxanthine.

Kostmann, Rolf, Swedish pediatrician, *1909.
    Kostmann disease—genetic predisposition for developing acute leukemia.
    SYN: Kostmann syndrome
    Kostmann syndrome—*SYN:* Kostmann disease

Kovalevsky, Alexander O., Russian embryologist, 1840–1901.
    Kovalevsky canal—canal connecting neural tube and archenteron in
    embryo.

Kowarsky, Albert, 20th century German physician.
    Kowarsky test—test for glucose in urine and diabetes in blood.

Koyanagi, Yosizo, Japanese ophthalmologist, 1880–1954.
    Vogt-Koyanagi syndrome—see under Vogt, Alfred

Krabbe, Knud H., Danish neurologist, 1885–1961.
    Christensen-Krabbe disease—see under Christensen
    Krabbe disease—a metabolic disorder of infancy. *SYN:* globoid cell
    leukodystrophy

Kraepelin, Emil, German psychiatrist, 1856–1926.
   Kraepelin-Morel disease—psychosis of schizophrenia.

Krantz, Kermit E., U.S. obstetrician-gynecologist, *1923.
   Marshall-Marchetti-Krantz operation—see under Marshall, Victor

Kraske, Paul, German surgeon, 1851–1930.
   Kraske operation—removal of the coccyx and excision of the left wing of the sacrum in order to afford approach for resection of the rectum for cancer or stenosis.
   Kraske parasacral approach
   Kraske position

Krause, Arlington C., U.S. ophthalmologist, *1896.
   Krause syndrome—retinopathy of prematurity combined with cerebral dysplasia. *SYN:* encephalo-ophthalmic dysplasia

Krause, Fedor, German surgeon, 1857–1937.
   Krause graft—a full-thickness skin graft. *SYN:* Krause-Wolfe graft
   Krause method
   Krause-Wolfe graft—*SYN:* Krause graft
   Wolfe-Krause graft—*SYN:* Wolfe graft

Krause, Karl F.T., German anatomist, 1797–1868.
   Krause glands—glands in the mucous membrane of the tympanic cavity.
   Krause ligament—the thickened anterior border of the urogenital diaphragm, formed by the fusion of its two fascial layers. *SYN:* transverse perineal ligament
   Krause muscle—*SYN:* cutaneomucous muscle

Krause, Wilhelm J.F., German anatomist, 1833–1910.
   Krause bone—small bone (secondary ossification center) in the triradiate cartilage between the ilium, the ischium, and the pubic bone in the growing acetabulum.
   Krause end bulbs—nerve terminals in skin, mouth, conjunctivae, and other parts generally believed to be sensitive to cold. *SYN:* bulboid corpuscles; corpuscula bulboidea
   Krause respiratory bundle—a slender, compact fiber bundle composed of primary sensory fibers that enter with the vagus, glossopharyngeal, and facial nerves. *SYN:* solitary tract
   Krause valve—*SYN:* Béraud valve

Krebs, Edwin G., U.S. biochemist, *1918, joint winner of 1992 Nobel Prize for work related to protein phosphorylation.

Krebs, Sir Hans Adolph, German biochemist in England and Nobel laureate, 1900–1981.
   Krebs cycle—together with oxidative phosphorylation, the main source of energy in the mammalian body and the end toward which carbohydrate, fat, and protein metabolism are directed. *SYN:* tricarboxylic acid cycle

(continued)

NOTES

267

Krebs *(continued)*

    Krebs-Henseleit cycle—the sequence of chemical reactions, occurring primarily in the liver, that results in the production of urea. *SYN:* urea cycle

    Krebs-Ringer solution—a modification of Ringer solution.

Kreibig, Wilhelm, German ophthalmologist.

    Kreibig opticomalacia—condition that causes unilateral sclerosis of retinal vessels and atrophy of optic nerve, resulting in blindness.

Kretschmann, Friederich, German otologist, 1858–1934.

    Kretschmann space—a slight depression in the epitympanic recess below the superior recess of the tympanic membrane.

Kretschmer, Ernst, German psychiatrist, 1888–1964.

    Kretschmer types—personality traits related to physical type.

Kreysig, Friedrich L., German physician, 1770–1839.

    Heim-Kreysig sign—see under Heim

    Kreysig sign—*SYN:* Heim-Kreysig sign

Krishaber, Maurice, French physician, 1836–1883.

    Krishaber disease—tachycardia with concomitant vertigo and insomnia.

Krisovski, Max, 19th century German physician.

    Krisovski sign—cicatricial mouth lines seen in cases of congenital syphilis.

Krogh, August, Danish physiologist and Nobel laureate, 1874–1949.

    Krogh spirometer—a water-sealed spirometer.

Kromayer, Ernst L.F., German dermatologist, 1862–1933.

    Aero-Kromayer lamp—air-cooled Kromayer lamp.

    Kromayer lamp—a quartz lamp of mercury vapor used in the treatment of skin diseases.

Kronecker, Karl H., Swiss physiologist, 1839–1914.

    Kronecker stain—a 5% sodium chloride stain rendered faintly alkaline with sodium carbonate, used in the examination of fresh tissues under the microscope.

Krönig, Georg, German physician, 1856–1911.

    Krönig isthmus—the narrow straplike portion of the resonant field that extends over the shoulder, connecting the larger areas of resonance over the pulmonary apex in front and behind.

    Krönig steps—extension of the lower part of the right border of absolute cardiac dullness in hypertrophy of the right heart.

Krönlein, Rudolf U., Swiss surgeon, 1847–1910.

    Krönlein hernia—a complicated hernia having a double sac, one part in the inguinal canal, the other projecting from the internal inguinal ring in the subperitoneal tissues. *SYN:* properitoneal inguinal hernia

    Krönlein operation—orbital decompression through the anterior lateral wall of the orbit.

Krukenberg, Adolph, German anatomist, 1816–1877.

    Krukenberg veins—the terminal branches of the hepatic veins that lie centrally in the hepatic lobules and receive blood from the liver sinusoids. *SYN:* central veins of liver

Krukenberg, Friedrich, German pathologist, 1871–1946.

    Krukenberg amputation—a cineplastic amputation at the carpus with the distal end of the forearm.

    Krukenberg pigment spindle forceps

    Krukenberg spindle—a vertical fusiform area of melanin pigmentation on the posterior surface of the central cornea.

    Krukenberg sponge

    Krukenberg tumor—metastatic carcinoma of the ovary.

Kruse, Walther, German bacteriologist, 1864–1943.

    Kruse brush—a bunch of fine platinum wires used to spread material over the surface of a culture medium.

    Shiga-Kruse bacillus—*SYN: Shigella dysenteriae*

Kuder, G. Frederic, U.S. psychologist.

    Kuder Preference Record—interest inventory test.

Kuersteiner, var. of Kürsteiner

Kufs, H., German psychiatrist, 1871–1955.

    Kufs disease—cerebral sphingolipidosis, adult type.

Kugelberg, Eric, Swedish neurologist, 1913–1983.

    Kugelberg-Welander disease—slowly progressive proximal muscular weakness with fasciculation and wasting. *SYN:* juvenile spinal muscular atrophy; Wohlfart-Kugelberg-Welander disease

    Müeller-Kugelberg syndrome—see under Müeller

    Wohlfart-Kugelberg-Welander disease—*SYN:* Kugelberg-Welander disease

Kuhlmann, Frederick, U.S. psychologist, 1876–1941.

    Kuhlmann-Anderson tests—general intelligence tests.

Kühne, Wilhelm (Willy) F., German physiologist and histologist, 1837–1900.

    Kühne fiber—artificial muscle fiber used to demonstrate the contractility of protoplasm.

    Kühne methylene blue—methylene blue in absolute alcohol and phenol solution.

    Kühne phenomenon—when a constant current is passed through a muscle, an undulation is seen to pass from the positive to the negative pole.

    Kühne plate—the endplate of a motor nerve fiber in a muscle spindle.

    Kühne spindle—a fusiform end organ in skeletal muscle in which afferent and a few efferent nerve fibers terminate. *SYN:* neuromuscular spindle

Kuhnt, Hermann, German ophthalmologist, 1850–1925.

    Kuhnt capsule forceps

    Kuhnt dacryostomy

    Kuhnt eyelid operation

    Kuhnt spaces—shallow diverticula or recesses between the ciliary body and ciliary zonule that open into the posterior chamber of the eye.

    Kuhnt-Junius degeneration—an obsolete eponym for disciform degeneration. *SYN:* Kuhnt-Junius disease

    Kuhnt-Junius disease—*SYN:* Kuhnt-Junius degeneration

NOTES

K

Kulchitsky, Nicholas, Russian histologist, 1856–1925.
　　Kulchitsky carcinoma—a small cell carcinoma of the esophagus composed of Kulchitsky cells with neurosecretory granules.
　　Kulchitsky cells—cells scattered throughout the digestive tract believed to produce at least 20 different gastrointestinal hormones and neurotransmitters. *SYN:* enteroendocrine cells

Külz, Rudolph E., German physician, 1845–1895.
　　Külz cylinder—a renal cast of strongly refracting granules said to be indicative of imminent diabetic coma. *SYN:* coma cast

Kümmell, Hermann, German surgeon, 1852–1937.
　　Kümmell spondylitis—late posttraumatic collapse of a vertebral body.

Kundrat, Hans, Austrian physician, 1845–1893.
　　Kundrat disease—lymphoid malignant tumor.

Kunkel, Henry George, U.S. physician, 1916–1983.
　　Bearn-Kunkel syndrome—see under Bearn
　　Bearn-Kunkel-Slater syndrome—*SYN:* Bearn-Kunkel syndrome
　　Kunkel syndrome—*SYN:* Bearn-Kunkel syndrome
　　Kunkel test

Küntscher, Gerhard, German surgeon, 1902–1972.
　　Küntscher cloverleaf nail
　　Küntscher driver
　　Küntscher femur guide pin
　　Küntscher intramedullary nail
　　Küntscher nail—an intramedullary nail used for internal fixation of a fracture.
　　Küntscher nail driver
　　Küntscher nail extender
　　Küntscher nail instrument
　　Küntscher nail set
　　Küntscher reamer
　　Küntscher rod
　　Küntscher shaft reamer
　　Küntscher traction apparatus

Kuntz, Albert, U.S. professor of histology, 1879–1957.
　　nerve of Kuntz

Kupffer, Karl W. von, German anatomist, 1829–1902.
　　Kupffer cell sarcoma
　　Kupffer cells—phagocytic cells of the mononuclear phagocyte series found on the luminal surface of the hepatic sinusoids. *SYN:* stellate cells of liver

Kurloff, Mikhail G., Russian physician, 1859–1932.
　　Kurloff bodies—palely basophilic, granular inclusions sometimes observed in the cytoplasm of the large mononuclear leukocytes of guinea pigs and certain other animals.

Kürsteiner, W., 19th century German anatomist.
　　Kürsteiner canals—a fetal complex of vesicular, canalicular, and glandlike structures derived from parathyroid, thymus, or thymic cord.

Kurz, Jaromir, Czech ophthalmologist, *1895.
Kurz syndrome—congenital blindness often followed later by mental retardation.

Kurzweil, Raymond C., 20th century U.S. inventor.
Kurzweil reading machine—computerized reading machine.

Küss, Georges, French physician, 1877–1967.
Küss disease—sigmoid and rectal stenosis caused by inflammation.

Kussmaul, Adolph, German physician, 1822–1902.
Kussmaul aphasia—mutism in psychosis.
Kussmaul breathing
Kussmaul coma—*Syn:* diabetic coma
Kussmaul disease—segmental inflammation, with infiltration by eosinophils, and necrosis of medium-sized or small arteries. *Syn:* polyarteritis nodosa
Kussmaul paradoxical pulse
Kussmaul pulse—reduction or disappearance of the pulse during inspiration.
Kussmaul respiration—deep, rapid respiration characteristic of diabetic or other causes of acidosis. *Syn:* Kussmaul-Kien respiration
Kussmaul sign—in constrictive pericarditis, a paradoxical increase in venous distention and pressure during inspiration. *Syn:* Kussmaul symptom
Kussmaul symptom—*Syn:* Kussmaul sign
Kussmaul-Kien respiration—*Syn:* Kussmaul respiration

Küster, Herman, early 20th century German gynecologist.
Mayer-Rokitansky-Küster-Hauser syndrome—see under Mayer
Rokitansky-Küster-Hauser syndrome—*Syn:* Mayer-Rokitansky-Küster-Hauser syndrome

Küstner, Heinz, German gynecologist, *1897.
Küstner suture
Küstner uterine tenaculum forceps
Prausnitz-Küstner antibody—see under Prausnitz
Prausnitz-Küstner reaction—see under Prausnitz
reversed Prausnitz-Küstner reaction—see under Prausnitz

Kveim, Morton A., Norwegian physician, *1892.
Kveim antigen—a saline suspension of human sarcoid tissue. *Syn:* Kveim-Stilzbach antigen
Kveim test—an intradermal test for the detection of sarcoidosis. *Syn:* Nickerson-Kveim test; Kveim-Stilzbach test
Kveim-Stilzbach antigen—*Syn:* Kveim antigen
Kveim-Stilzbach test—*Syn:* Kveim test
Nickerson-Kveim test—*Syn:* Kveim test

NOTES

Kwok, R.H.M., U.S. physician.

   Kwok quease—*SYN:* Chinese restaurant syndrome

Kyrle, J., German dermatologist, 1880–1926.

   Kyrle disease—discrete and confluent horny follicular plugs on crateriform base, often occurring on the arms and legs in diabetics with renal failure. *SYN:* hyperkeratosis follicularis et parafollicularis

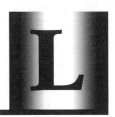

Laban von Varalja, Rudolf, German dancer, 1879–1958.
  labanotation—dance notation used in physical therapy.

Laband, Peter F., U.S. dentist, *1900.
  Laband syndrome—fibromatosis of the gingivae associated with hypoplasia of the distal phalanges, nail dysplasia, joint hypermotility, and sometimes hepatosplenomegaly.

Labbé, Ernest M., French physician, 1870–1939.
  Labbé neurocirculatory syndrome—an anxiety neurosis.

Labbé, Leon, French surgeon, 1832–1916.
  Labbé triangle—an area where the stomach is normally in contact with the abdominal wall.
  Labbé vein—an inconstant vein that passes from the superficial middle cerebral vein posteriorly over the lateral aspect of the temporal lobe to enter the transverse sinus. *Syn:* inferior anastomotic vein

Laborde, Jean B.V., French physician, 1830–1903.
  Laborde forceps
  Laborde method
  Laborde tracheal dilator

Ladd, William E., U.S. pediatric surgeon, 1880–1967.
  Ladd band—a peritoneal attachment of an incompletely rotated cecum, causing obstruction of the duodenum, found in malrotation of the intestine.
  Ladd calipers
  Ladd clamp
  Ladd elevator
  Ladd fiberoptic system
  Ladd intracranial pressure sensor
  Ladd knife
  Ladd operation—division of Ladd band to relieve duodenal obstruction in malrotation of the intestine.
  Ladd pressure monitor

Ladd-Franklin, Christine, U.S. psychologist, 1847–1930.
  Ladd-Franklin theory—a theory pertaining to color vision. *Syn:* molecular dissociation theory

Laënnec, René T.H., French physician, 1781–1826.
  Laënnec catarrh—asthmatic bronchitis with pearl-like expectoration.

(continued)

Laënnec *(continued)*
　　Laënnec cirrhosis—cirrhosis in which normal liver lobules are replaced by small regeneration nodules. *SYN:* portal cirrhosis; Laënnec disease
　　Laënnec disease—*SYN:* Laënnec cirrhosis
　　Laënnec pearls—obsolete term for small, round, translucent, tenacious bodies in the sputum of some persons with asthma.

Laffer, W.B., U.S. physician.
　　Laffer-Ascher syndrome

Lafora, Gonzalo Rodriguez, Spanish neurologist, 1887–1971.
　　Lafora body—an intraneural intracytoplasmic inclusion body seen in familial myoclonus epilepsy.
　　Lafora body disease—myoclonus epilepsy beginning at 11 to 18 years of age with progressive mental impairment. *SYN:* Lafora disease
　　Lafora disease—*SYN:* Lafora body disease

Lagrange, Pierre F., French ophthalmologist, 1857–1928.
　　Lagrange eye scissors
　　Lagrange sclerectomy

Lahey, Frank H., U.S. surgeon, 1880–1935.
　　Lahey bag
　　Lahey carrier
　　Lahey catheter
　　Lahey clamp
　　Lahey dissecting scissors
　　Lahey drain
　　Lahey forceps—thyroid forceps used to deliver the uterus in vaginal hysterectomy.
　　Lahey gall duct forceps
　　Lahey goiter retractor
　　Lahey goiter tenaculum
　　Lahey gouge
　　Lahey hemostatic forceps
　　Lahey hook
　　Lahey incision
　　Lahey ligature carrier
　　Lahey needle
　　Lahey osteotome
　　Lahey scissors
　　Lahey score
　　Lahey tenaculum
　　Lahey thoracic clamp
　　Lahey thoracic forceps
　　Lahey thyroid retractor
　　Lahey thyroid scissors
　　Lahey thyroid traction vulsellum forceps
　　Lahey trephine
　　Lahey tube
　　Lahey Y-tube

Lallemand, Claude F., French surgeon, 1790–1853.
    Lallemand bodies—(1) obsolete term for small gelatinoid concretions sometimes observed in seminal fluid; (2) old term for Bence Jones cylinders. *SYN:* Trousseau-Lallemand bodies.
    Trousseau-Lallemand bodies—*SYN:* Lallemand bodies (2)

Lallouette, Pierre, French physician, 1711–1792.
    Lallouette pyramid—an inconstant narrow lobe of the thyroid gland that marks the point of continuity with the thyroglossal duct. *SYN:* pyramidal lobe of thyroid gland

Lamarck, Jean-Baptiste P.A., French botanist, zoologist, and biological philosopher, 1744–1829.
    lamarckian theory—that acquired characteristics may be transmitted to descendants and that experience, not biology alone, can change and thereby influence genetic transmission.

Lamaze, Fernand, French obstetrician, 1890–1957.
    Lamaze method—a technique of psychoprophylactic preparation for childbirth. *SYN:* Lamaze technique
    Lamaze technique—*SYN:* Lamaze method

Lambert, Edward H., U.S. physician, *1915.
    Eaton-Lambert syndrome—*SYN:* Lambert-Eaton syndrome
    Lambert-Eaton syndrome—progressive proximal muscle weakness in patients with carcinoma, caused by antibodies directed against motor-nerve axon terminals. *SYN:* Eaton-Lambert syndrome

Lambert, Johann Heinrich, German mathematician and physicist, 1728–1777.
    Beer-Lambert law—see under Beer, August
    Lambert cosine law—mathematical measure of the intensity of radiation.

Lambrinudi, Constantine, English orthopedic surgeon, 1890–1943.
    Lambrinudi operation—a form of triple arthrodesis done in such a manner as to prevent footdrop. *SYN:* Lambrinudi triple arthrodesis
    Lambrinudi osteotomy
    Lambrinudi splint
    Lambrinudi technique
    Lambrinudi triple arthrodesis—*SYN:* Lambrinudi operation

Lamy, Maurice, French physician, 1895–1975.
    Maroteaux-Lamy I syndrome—see under Maroteaux
    Maroteaux-Lamy II syndrome—see under Maroteaux
    Maroteaux-Lamy syndrome—see under Maroteaux

Lancefield, Rebecca Craighill, U.S. bacteriologist, *1895.
    Lancefield classification—a serologic classification dividing hemolytic streptococci into groups which bear a definite relationship to their sources.

NOTES

Lancereaux, Étienne, French physician, 1829–1910.
   Lancereaux diabetes
   Lancereaux law

Lancisi, Giovanni M., Italian physician, 1654–1720.
   Lancisi sign—a large systolic jugular venous wave.
   striae lancisi—the lateral longitudinal stria and the medial longitudinal stria.

Landau, A., German pediatrician.
   Landau reflex—test for hypertonia or hypotonia in infants. *SYN:* Landau response
   Landau response—*SYN:* Landau reflex

Landing, B.H.
   Norman-Landing syndrome—see under Norman

Landis, Eugene M., U.S. physiologist, *1901.
   Landis-Gibbon test—a test for vascular disease.

Landolt, Edmund, French ophthalmologist, 1846–1926.
   Landolt bodies—bipolar nerve cells lying between the retinal rods and cones in amphibia, reptiles, and birds.
   Landolt circles
   Landolt enucleation scissors
   Landolt eye knife
   Landolt eyelid reconstruction
   Landolt keratome
   Landolt operation
   Landolt ring—instrument used for testing of visual acuity.

Landouzy, Louis T.J., French neurologist, 1845–1917.
   Dejerine-Landouzy dystrophy—*SYN:* Landouzy-Dejerine dystrophy
   Dejerine-Landouzy myopathy—*SYN:* Landouzy-Dejerine dystrophy
   Landouzy-Dejerine dystrophy—a relatively benign type of muscular dystrophy commencing in childhood and slowly progressive. *SYN:* facioscapulohumeral muscular dystrophy; Dejerine-Landouzy dystrophy; Dejerine-Landouzy myopathy
   Landouzy-Grasset law—in lesions of one hemisphere, the patient's head is turned to the side of the affected muscles if there is spasticity and to that of the cerebral lesion if there is paralysis. *SYN:* Grasset law

Landry, Jean B.O., French physician, 1826–1865.
   Landry paralysis—*SYN:* Landry syndrome
   Landry syndrome—marked by paresthesia of the limbs and muscular weakness or a flaccid paralysis. *SYN:* acute idiopathic polyneuritis; Landry-Guillain-Barré syndrome; Landry paralysis
   Landry-Guillain-Barré syndrome—*SYN:* Landry syndrome

Landsteiner, Karl, Austrian-U.S. pathologist and Nobel laureate, 1868–1943.
   Donath-Landsteiner cold autoantibody—see under Donath
   Donath-Landsteiner phenomenon—see under Donath
   Landsteiner-Donath test

Landström, John, Swedish surgeon, 1869–1910.
   Landström muscle—microscopic muscle fibers in the fascia behind and about the eyeball.

Landzert, T., 19th century German anatomist.
 Gruber-Landzert fossa—see under Gruber, Wenzel
 Landzert fossa—a fossa formed by two peritoneal folds enclosing the left colic artery and the inferior mesenteric vein at the side of the duodenum

Lane, Sir W. Arbuthnot, English surgeon, 1856–1943.
 Lane band—a congenital band on the distal ileum causing stasis. *SYN:* Lane kink
 Lane bone-holding clamp
 Lane bone-holding forceps
 Lane catheter
 Lane clamp
 Lane disease—asymptomatic symmetrical palmar erythema. *SYN:* erythema palmare hereditarium
 Lane dissector
 Lane elevator
 Lane forceps
 Lane kink—*SYN:* Lane band
 Lane mouth gag
 Lane needle
 Lane plates—flattened, narrow, metal plates used to hold the fragments of a fractured bone in apposition.
 Lane retractor
 Lane rongeur
 Lane screwdriver
 Murphy-Lane bone skid

Lang, Basil T., English ophthalmologist, 1880–1928.
 Lang dissector
 Lang eye speculum
 Lang knife
 Lang scoop
 Lang suture

Lange, Carl F.A., German biochemist, 1883–1953.
 Lange solution—a colloidal gold solution used to demonstrate protein abnormalities in spinal fluid.
 Lange test—an obsolete, nonspecific test for altered proteins in spinal fluid. *SYN:* gold sol test; Zsigmondy test

Lange, Carl G., Danish psychologist, 1834–1900.
 James-Lange theory—see under James, William

Lange, Cornelia de. See under de Lange.

Lange-Nielsen, F., 20th century Norwegian cardiologist.
 Jervell and Lange-Nielsen syndrome—see under Jervell

Langenbeck, Bernhard R.K. von, German surgeon, 1810–1887.
 Langenbeck amputation

(continued)

NOTES

Langenbeck (*continued*)
   Langenbeck elevator
   Langenbeck flap
   Langenbeck forceps
   Langenbeck incision
   Langenbeck knife
   Langenbeck needle holder
   Langenbeck periosteal elevator
   Langenbeck raspatory
   Langenbeck retractor
   Langenbeck saw
   Langenbeck triangle—formed by lines drawn from the anterior superior iliac spine to the surface of the great trochanter and to the surgical neck of the femur.

Langendorff, Oscar, German physiologist, 1853–1908.
   Langendorff method—perfusion of the isolated mammalian heart by carrying fluid under pressure into the sectioned aorta and thus into the coronary system.

Langer, Carl (Ritter von Edenberg), Austrian anatomist, 1819–1887.
   Langer arch—*SYN:* axillary arch muscle
   Langer lines—lines which can be extrapolated by connecting linear openings made when a round pin is driven into the skin of a cadaver. *SYN:* cleavage lines
   Langer muscle—*SYN:* axillary arch muscle

Langerhans, Paul, German anatomist, 1847–1888.
   islets of Langerhans—cellular masses composed of different cell types that comprise the endocrine portion of the pancreas and are the source of insulin and glucagon. *SYN:* Langerhans islands; pancreatic islands; pancreatic islets; islet tissue
   Langerhans cell granulomatosis
   Langerhans cells—dendritic clear cells in the epidermis that are active participants in cutaneous delayed hypersensitivity.
   Langerhans granule—a small membrane-bound granule first reported in Langerhans cells of the epidermis. *SYN:* Birbeck granule
   Langerhans islands—*SYN:* islets of Langerhans

Langhans, Theodor, German pathologist, 1839–1915.
   Langhans cells—multinucleated giant cells seen in tuberculosis and other granulomas. *SYN:* cytotrophoblastic cells; Langhans-type giant cells
   Langhans layer—the inner layer of the trophoblast. *SYN:* cytotrophoblast
   Langhans stria—fibrinoid that accumulates on the chorionic plate between the bases of placental villi during the first half of pregnancy.
   Langhans-type giant cells—*SYN:* Langhans cells

Langley, John N., English physiologist, 1852–1925.
   Langley granules—granules in serous secreting cells.

Langmuir, Irving, U.S. chemist and Nobel laureate, 1881–1957.
   Langmuir trough—a trough with a movable surface barrier for studying the compression of surface films.

Lannelongue, Odilon M., French surgeon and pathologist, 1840–1911.
  Lannelongue foramina—a number of fossae in the wall of the right atrium, containing the openings of minute intramural veins. *Syn:* foramina of the venae minimae
  Lannelongue ligaments—fibrous bands that pass from the pericardium to the sternum. *Syn:* sternopericardial ligament

Lanquepin, Anne, 20th century French pediatrician.
  Fèvre-Lanquepin syndrome—see under Fèvre

Lanterman, A.J., 19th century U.S. anatomist in Germany.
  Lanterman incisures—*Syn:* Schmidt-Lanterman incisures
  Lanterman segments—the divisions of the nerve fiber between the Schmidt-Lanterman incisures.
  Schmidt-Lanterman clefts—*Syn:* Schmidt-Lanterman incisures
  Schmidt-Lanterman incisures—see under Schmidt, Henry

L

Lanz, Otto, Swiss surgeon in Holland, 1865–1935.
  Lanz incision
  Lanz line—a horizontal plane marking the boundary between the lateral and umbilical regions superiorly and the inguinal and pubic regions inferiorly. *Syn:* interspinal plane
  Lanz low-pressure cuff endotracheal tube
  Lanz operation
  Lanz point
  Lanz tracheostomy tube

Lapicque, Louis, French physiologist, 1866–1952.
  Lapicque law—the chronaxie is inversely proportional to the diameter of an axon.

Laplace, Ernest, U.S. surgeon, 1861–1924.
  Laplace forceps—a forceps for approximating intestines during surgical anastomosis.
  Laplace liver retractor

Laplace, Pierre S. de, French mathematician, 1749–1827.
  Laplace law—the equilibrium relationship between transmural pressure difference, wall tension, and radius of curvature in a concave surface.

Laquer, Ernst, German physiologist, *1910.
  Laquer stain for alcoholic hyalin

Laron, Zvi, Israeli pediatric endocrinologist, *1927.
  Laron-type dwarfism—dwarfism associated with absent or very low levels of somatomedin C (insulin-like growth factor I) or abnormalities in receptor activity.

Laroyenne, Lucien, French surgeon, 1831–1902.
  Laroyenne operation—puncture of Douglas pouch to evacuate pus and to secure drainage in cases of pelvic suppuration.

NOTES

Larrey, Baron Dominique Jean de, French surgeon, 1766–1842.
Larrey amputation—amputation at the shoulder joint.
Larrey cleft—a muscular defect in the diaphragm between the costal and the sternal portions. *SYN:* trigonum sternocostale
Larrey ligation—a ligation of the femoral artery immediately below the inguinal ligament.
Larrey-Weil disease—*SYN:* Weil disease

Larsen, Loren J., U.S. orthopedic surgeon, *1914.
Larsen syndrome—characterized by multiple congenital dislocations with osseous anomalies, including characteristic flattened facies and cleft soft palate.

Larsson, Tage Konrad Leopold, Swedish scientist, *1905.
Sjögren-Larsson syndrome—see under Sjögren, Torsten

Lasègue, Ernest C., French physician, 1816–1883.
Lasègue disease—obsolete eponym for delusions of persecution.
Lasègue maneuver
Lasègue sign—when patient is supine with hip flexed, dorsiflexion of the ankle causes pain or muscle spasm in the posterior thigh indicates lumbar root or sciatic nerve irritation.
Lasègue syndrome—in conversion hysteria, inability to move an anesthetic limb except under control of the sight.

Lash, Abraham Fae, U.S. obstetrician-gynecologist, *1898.
Lash hysterectomy
Lash operation—removal of a wedge of the internal cervical os with suturing of the internal os into a tighter canal structure.
Lash technique

Lassar, Oskar, German dermatologist, 1849–1907.
Lassar paste—preparation used for eczema.

Latarget, André, French anatomist, 1877–1947.
Latarget nerve—terminal branch of anterior vagal trunk which runs along lesser curvature of the stomach. *SYN:* superior hypogastric plexus
Latarget vein—a tributary of the right gastric vein that passes anterior to the pylorus at its junction with the duodenum. *SYN:* prepyloric vein

Latham, Peter M., English physician, 1789–1875.
Latham circle—area of cardiac dullness between left nipple and sternum.

Latzko, Wilhelm, Austrian obstetrician, 1863–1945.
Latzko cesarean section
Latzko closure
Latzko colpocleisis
Latzko fistula repair
Latzko radical hysterectomy
Latzko repair of vesicovaginal fistula

Lauber, Hans, Swiss ophthalmologist, *1876.
Lauber disease—defective vision in the presence of bright light associated with white spots in deep layers of retinal tissue.

Laugier, Stanislas, French surgeon, 1799–1872.
    Laugier hernia—a hernia passing through an opening in the lacunar ligament.
    Laugier sign—in fracture of the lower portion of the radius, the styloid processes of the radius and of the ulna are on the same level.

Laumonier, Jean B.P.N.R., French surgeon, 1749–1818.
    Laumonier ganglion—a small ganglionic swelling on filaments from the internal carotid plexus, lying on the undersurface of the carotid artery in the cavernous sinus. *SYN:* carotid ganglion

Launois, Pierre E., French physician, 1856–1914.
    Launois-Bensaude syndrome—accumulation and progressive enlargement of collections of adipose tissue in the subcutaneous tissue of the head, neck, upper trunk, and upper portions of the upper extremities. *SYN:* multiple symmetric lipomatosis
    Launois-Cléret syndrome—*SYN:* Fröhlich syndrome

Laurence, John Zachariah, English ophthalmologist, 1830–1874.
    Laurence-Moon-Biedl syndrome—mental retardation, pigmentary retinopathy, hypogenitalism, and spastic paraplegia.

Laurer, Johann F., German pharmacologist, 1798–1873.
    Laurer canal—a tube originating on the surface of the ootype of trematodes.

Lauth, Ernst A., German physician, 1803–1837.
    Lauth canal—the vascular structure encircling the anterior chamber of the eye and through which the aqueous is returned to the blood circulation. *SYN:* sinus venosus sclerae

Lauth, Thomas, German anatomist and surgeon, 1758–1826.
    Lauth ligament—*SYN:* transverse ligament of the atlas

Lavdovsky, Michail D., Russian histologist, 1846–1902.
    Lavdovsky nucleoid—a set of radiating microtubules extending outward from the cytocentrum and centrosphere of a dividing cell. *SYN:* astrosphere

Laveran, Charles Louis Alphonse, French protozoologist and Nobel laureate, 1845–1922.

Lawrence, Robert D., English physician, 1912–1964.
    Lawrence-Seip syndrome—loss of subcutaneous fat associated with hepatomegaly, excessive bone growth, and insulin-resistant diabetes. *SYN:* lipoatrophy

Laxová, Renata
    Neu-Laxová syndrome—see under Neu

Le Bel, Joseph Achille, French chemist, 1847–1930.
    Le Bel-van't Hoff rule—the number of stereoisomers of an organic compound is $2n$ where n represents the number of asymmetric carbon atoms unless there is an internal plane of symmetry.

NOTES

Le Chatelier, Henri, French physical chemist, 1850–1936.

    Le Chatelier law—if external factors such as temperature and pressure disturb a system in equilibrium, adjustment occurs in such a way that the effect of the disturbing factors is reduced to a minimum. *SYN:* Le Chatelier principle

    Le Chatelier principle—*SYN:* Le Chatelier law

Le Fort, Léon C., French surgeon and gynecologist, 1829–1893.

    Le Fort amputation—a modification of Pirogoff amputation.

    Le Fort bougie

    Le Fort catheter

    Le Fort classification—classification of bone fractures (I, II, III).

    Le Fort dilator

    Le Fort follower

    Le Fort I fracture—*SYN:* Guérin fracture

    Le Fort II fracture—*SYN:* pyramidal fracture

    Le Fort III fracture—*SYN:* craniofacial dysjunction fracture

    Le Fort osteotomy—osteomy often done to correct a maxillary skeletal deformity.

    Le Fort reconstruction

    Le Fort repair

    Le Fort sound—a curved sound used for dilation of urethral strictures in the male.

    Le Fort speculum

    Le Fort suture

Leber, Theodor, German ophthalmologist, 1840–1917.

    amaurosis congenita of Leber—an autosomal recessive cone-rod abiotrophy causing blindness or severely reduced vision at birth.

    Leber hereditary optic atrophy—hereditary degeneration of the optic nerve and papillomacular bundle, resulting in rapid loss of central vision.

    Leber idiopathic stellate neuroretinitis—a unilateral neuroretinitis with perifoveal exudates in Henle nerve fiber layer producing a macular star and spontaneous regression in a few months. *SYN:* stellate neuroretinitis

    Leber plexus—a small venous plexus in the eye between the venous sinuses of the sclera (of Schlemm) and the spaces of the iridocorneal angle (of Fontana).

Lecat, Claude N., French surgeon, 1700–1768.

    Lecat gulf—the hollow portion of the bulbous urethra.

Ledderhose, Georg, German physician, 1855–1925.

    Ledderhose syndrome—clawfoot.

Lederberg, Joshua, U.S. biochemist, *1925, joint winner of 1958 Nobel Prize for work related to genetics.

Lederer, Max, U.S. pathologist, 1885–1952.

    Lederer anemia—obsolete term for a form of acute acquired hemolytic anemia associated with abnormal hemolysins and sometimes with hemoglobinuria.

Ledermann, Sully, French psychiatrist.

    Ledermann formula—the formula used to estimate the prevalence of various degrees of alcohol dependency.

Lee, Robert, English physician, 1793–1877.
Lee ganglion—a gangliated autonomic plexus on each side of the cervix of the uterus, derived from the inferior hypogastric plexus. *SYN:* uterovaginal plexus

Lee, Roger I., U.S. physician, *1881.
Lee-White method—a method for determining coagulation time of venous blood in tubes of standard bore at body temperature.

Leede, Carl S., U.S. physician, *1882.
Leede-Rumpel phenomenon—*SYN:* Rumpel-Leede phenomenon
Rumpel-Leede phenomenon—see under Rumpel
Rumpel-Leede sign—*SYN:* Rumpel-Leede test
Rumpel-Leede test—see under Rumpel

Leeuwenhoek, Anton van, Dutch microscopist, 1632–1723.
Leeuwenhoek canals—*SYN:* haversian canals

Lefèvre, Paul, 20th century French dermatologist.
Papillon-Lefèvre syndrome—see under Papillon

Legal, Emmo, German physician, 1859–1922.
Legal test—a test for acetone.

Legendre, Gaston J., French physician, *1887.
Legendre function
Legendre sign—in facial hemiplegia of central origin, when the examiner raises the lids of the actively closed eyes, the resistance is less on the affected side.

Legg, Arthur T., U.S. surgeon, 1874–1939.
Legg osteotome
Legg-Calvé-Perthes disease—epiphysial aseptic necrosis of the upper end of the femur. *SYN:* pseudocoxalgia; coxa plana; Calvé-Perthes disease; Perthes disease; quiet hip disease

Lehmann, J.O. Orla, Swedish physician, *1927.
Börjeson-Forssman-Lehmann syndrome—see under Börjeson

Leichtenstern, Otto, German physician, 1845–1900.
Leichtenstern phenomenon—*SYN:* Leichtenstern sign
Leichtenstern sign—gently tapping one of the bones of the extremities causes the patient to draw back violently in cases of cerebrospinal meningitis. *SYN:* Leichtenstern phenomenon

Leigh, Denis, English psychiatrist, *1915.
Leigh disease—subacute encephalomyelopathy affecting infants. *SYN:* subacute necrotizing encephalomyelopathy; necrotizing encephalomyelopathy
Leigh syndrome

NOTES

Leiner, Karl, Austrian pediatrician, 1871–1930.
> **Leiner disease**—severe, extensive seborrheic dermatitis with exfoliative dermatitis, generalized lymphoadenopathy, and diarrhea in the newborn. *Syn:* erythroderma desquamativum

Leishman, Sir William B., Scottish surgeon, 1865–1926.
> *Leishmania*—a genus of digenetic, asexual, protozoan flagellates.
> **Leishman chrome cells**—basophilic granular leukocytes (basophils) observed in the circulating blood of some persons with blackwater fever.
> **Leishman stain**—a polychromed eosin-methylene blue stain used in the examination of blood films.
> **Leishman-Donovan body**—the intracytoplasmic, nonflagellated leishmanial form of certain intracellular parasites. *Syn:* amastigote; L-D body
> **leishmaniasis**—tropical disease that is spread by sandflies.

Leiter, Russell G., U.S. psychologist, *1901.
> **Leiter International Performance Scale**—a nonverbal test for measuring intelligence.

Lejeune, Jerôme J.L.M., French cytogeneticist, *1926.
> **Lejeune syndrome**—a disorder characterized by microcephaly, antimongoloid palpebral fissures, epicanthal folds, micrognathia, strabismus, mental and physical retardation, and a characteristic high-pitched catlike whine. *Syn:* cri-du-chat syndrome

Leksell, Lars, Swedish physician, 1907–1986.
> **Leksell bone rongeur**
> **Leksell cardiovascular rongeur**
> **Leksell director**
> **Leksell forceps**
> **Leksell frame**
> **Leksell punch**
> **Leksell sternal approximator**
> **Leksell sternal spreader**
> **Leksell trephine**

Leloir, Henri Camille, French physician, 1855–1896.
> **Leloir disease**—*Syn:* lupus erythematosus

Lembert, Antoine, French surgeon, 1802–1851.
> **Czerny-Lembert suture**—see under Czerny
> **Lembert suture**—an inverting suture for intestinal surgery.

Lemli, Luc, 20th century U.S. pediatrician.
> **Smith-Lemli-Opitz syndrome**—see under Smith, David W.

Lendrum, A.C., 20th century Scottish pathologist.
> **Fraser-Lendrum stain for fibrin**—see under Fraser
> **Lendrum phloxine-tartrazine stain**—a stain for demonstrating acidophilic inclusion bodies.

Lenègre, Jean, 20th century French cardiologist.
> **Lenègre disease**—*Syn:* Lenègre syndrome
> **Lenègre syndrome**—isolated damage of the cardiac conduction system as a result of a sclerodegenerative lesion. *Syn:* Lenègre disease

Lenhossék, Michael (Mihály) von, Hungarian anatomist, 1863–1937.
    Lenhossék processes—short processes possessed by some ganglion cells.

Lenier, Karl, Austrian physician, 1871–1930.
    Lenier dermatitis—skin disorder of newborns.

Lennert, K.
    Lennert classification—classification of non-Hodgkin lymphoma. *SYN:* Kiel classification
    Lennert lesion—*SYN:* Lennert lymphoma
    Lennert lymphoma—malignant lymphoma with a high proportion of diffusely scattered epithelioid cells, tonsillar involvement, and an unpredictable course. *SYN:* Lennert lesion

Lennhoff, Rudolf, German physician, 1866–1933.
    Lennhoff sign—when liver is infected with a tapeworm, a furrow forms between liver cyst and lowest rib on deep inspiration.

Lennox, William G., U.S. neurologist, 1884–1960.
    Lennox syndrome—*SYN:* Lennox-Gastaut syndrome
    Lennox-Gastaut syndrome—a generalized myoclonic astatic epilepsy in children, with mental retardation. *SYN:* Lennox syndrome

Lenoir, Camille A.H., French anatomist, *1867.
    Lenoir facet—the medial articular surface of the patella.

Lenz, Widukind, German physician, *1919.
    Lenz syndrome—inherited X-linked trait consisting of multiple abnormalities.

Leonardi, Giuseppe, Italian physician.
    Magrassi-Leonardi syndrome—see under Magrassi

Leopold, Christian G., German physician, 1846–1911.
    Leopold maneuvers—four maneuvers employed to determine fetal position.

Lepehne, Georg, German physician, *1887.
    Lepehne-Pickworth stain—a staining technique for hemoglobin.

Lerch, Otto, U.S. physician, *1894.
    Lerch percussion

Leri, André, French orthopedic surgeon, 1875–1930.
    Leri pleonosteosis—*SYN:* dyschondrosteosis
    Leri sign—voluntary flexion of the elbow is impossible in a case of hemiplegia when the wrist on that side is passively flexed.
    Leri-Weill disease—*SYN:* dyschondrosteosis
    Leri-Weill syndrome—*SYN:* dyschondrosteosis
    Marie-Leri syndrome—see under Marie, Pierre

L

NOTES

Leriche, René, French surgeon, 1879–1955.
    Leriche forceps
    Leriche operation—sympathetic denervation by arterial decortication. *SYN:* periarterial sympathectomy
    Leriche sympathectomy
    Leriche syndrome—aortoiliac occlusive disease producing distal ischemic symptoms and signs.

Lermoyez, Marcel, French otolaryngologist, 1858–1929.
    Lermoyez nasal punch
    Lermoyez syndrome—increasing deafness interrupted by a sudden attack of dizziness after which the hearing improves. *SYN:* labyrinthine angiospasm

Lerner, I.M., U.S. population geneticist, 1910–1967.
    Lerner homeostasis—the restorative mechanisms that tend to correct perturbations in the genetic composition of a population. *SYN:* genetic homeostasis

Leroy, Edgar August, French physician, *1883.
    Fiessinger-Leroy-Reiter syndrome—*SYN:* Reiter syndrome

Lesch, Michael, U.S. pediatrician, *1939.
    Lesch-Nyhan syndrome—a genetic disorder marked by choreoathetosis, mental retardation, and self-mutilation.

Leser, Edmund, German surgeon, 1828–1916.
    Leser-Trélat sign—the sudden appearance and rapid increase in the number and size of seborrheic keratoses with pruritus, associated with internal malignancy.

Lesser, Ladislaus Leo, German surgeon born in Poland, 1846–1925.
    Lesser triangle—the space between the bellies of the digastric muscle and the hypoglossal nerve.

Lesshaft, Pjotr F., Russian physician, 1836–1909.
    Lesshaft triangle—*SYN:* Grynfeltt triangle

Letterer, Erich, German pathologist, *1895.
    Letterer-Siwe disease—the acute disseminated form of Langerhans cell histiocytosis. *SYN:* nonlipid histiocytosis

Leudet, Théodor E., French physician, 1825–1887.
    Leudet tinnitus—a dry spasmodic click heard in catarrhal inflammation of the eustachian tube.

Lev, Maurice, U.S. pathologist, *1908.
    Lev disease—*SYN:* Lev syndrome
    Lev syndrome—bundle branch block in a patient with normal myocardium and normal coronary arteries resulting from fibrosis or calcification including the conducting system. *SYN:* Lev disease

Levaditi, Constantin, Romanian bacteriologist in Paris, 1874–1928.
    Levaditi method
    Levaditi stain—a silver nitrate stain for blackening spirochetes in tissue sections.

LeVeen, Harry H., U.S. surgeon, *1914.
    LeVeen ascites shunt
    LeVeen catheter
    LeVeen dialysis shunt
    LeVeen endarterectomy
    LeVeen inflation syringe
    LeVeen inflator with pressure gauge
    LeVeen peritoneal shunt
    LeVeen peritoneovenous shunt
    LeVeen shunt—a plastic tube used to transport ascitic fluid from the abdomen via a jugular vein to the superior vena cava.
    LeVeen valve

Leventhal, Michael L., U.S. obstetrician-gynecologist, 1901–1971.
    Stein-Leventhal syndrome—see under Stein, Irving

Lévi, E. Leopold, French endocrinologist, 1868–1933.
    dominantly inherited Lévi disease—dominantly inherited dwarfism characterized by low birth weight, snub nose, and stocky build. *SYN:* snub-nose dwarfism
    Lorain-Lévi dwarfism—see under Lorain
    Lorain-Lévi infantilism—*SYN:* Lorain-Lévi dwarfism
    Lorain-Lévi syndrome—*SYN:* Lorain-Lévi dwarfism

Levi-Montalcini, Rita, Italian neurobiologist, *1909, joint winner of 1986 Nobel Prize for work related to growth factors.

Levin, Abraham, U.S. physician, 1880–1940.
    Levin tube—a tube introduced through the nose into the upper alimentary canal to facilitate intestinal decompression.
    Levin tube catheter

Levin, Max, U.S. neurologist, *1901.
    Kleine-Levin syndrome—see under Kleine

Levine, Samuel A., U.S. cardiologist, 1891–1966.
    Lown-Ganong-Levine syndrome—see under Lown

Levret, André, French obstetrician, 1703–1780.
    Levret forceps—a modification of the Chamberlen forceps, curved to correspond to the curve of the parturient passage.
    Mauriceau-Levret maneuver—*SYN:* Mauriceau maneuver

Lévy, Gabrielle, French neurologist, 1886–1935.
    Roussy-Lévy disease—see under Roussy
    Roussy-Lévy syndrome—*SYN:* Roussy-Lévy disease

Lewandowski, Felix, German dermatologist, 1879–1921.
    Jadassohn-Lewandowski syndrome—see under Jadassohn
    nevus elasticus of Lewandowski—obsolete term for plaques now known to be a collagenous nevus.

NOTES

Lewey, var. of Lewy

Lewis, Edward B., joint winner of 1995 Nobel Prize for work related to genetics and early development of embryo.

Lewis, Gilbert N., U.S. chemist, 1875–1946.
Lewis acid—an acid that is an electron pair acceptor.

Lewy, Frederic H., German neurologist in the U.S., 1885–1950.
Lewy bodies—intracytoplasmic inclusion bodies especially noted in pigmented brainstem neurons and seen in Parkinson disease.

Leyden, Ernst V. von, German physician, 1832–1910.
Charcot-Leyden crystals—see under Charcot
Leyden ataxia—*SYN:* Westphal-Leyden syndrome
Leyden crystals—*SYN:* Charcot-Leyden crystals
Leyden disease
Leyden neuritis—fatty degeneration of the fibers of the affected nerve.
Leyden-Möbius muscular dystrophy—*SYN:* limb-girdle muscular dystrophy

Leydig, Franz von, German anatomist, 1821–1908.
Leydig cell adenoma—small benign tumors of the testis that often produce testosterone, causing endocrine symptoms. *SYN:* interstitial cell tumor of testis
Leydig cells—cells between the seminiferous tubules of the testis that secrete testosterone. *SYN:* interstitial cells
Leydig drain

Lhermitte, Jean, French neurologist, 1877–1959.
Lhermitte sign—sudden electric-like shocks extending down the spine on flexing the head.

Li, Frederick P., 20th century epidemiologist.
Li-Fraumeni cancer syndrome—familial breast cancer in young women, with soft tissue sarcomas in children and other cancers in close relatives.

Libman, Emanuel, U.S. physician, 1872–1946.
Libman-Sacks endocarditis—verrucous endocarditis sometimes associated with disseminated lupus erythematosus. *SYN:* atypical verrucous endocarditis; nonbacterial verrucous endocarditis; Libman-Sacks syndrome
Libman-Sacks syndrome—*SYN:* Libman-Sacks endocarditis

Liborius, Paul, 19th century Russian bacteriologist.
Liborius method—a method for culturing anaerobic bacteria.

Lichtenstein, Louis, U.S. physician, 1906–1977.
Jaffe-Lichtenstein disease—see under Jaffe, Henry

Lichtheim, Ludwig, German physician, 1845–1928.
Dejerine-Lichtheim phenomenon—*SYN:* Lichtheim sign
Lichtheim sign—in subcortical aphasia, the patient can indicate by use of the fingers the number of syllables of a word but cannot speak. *SYN:* Dejerine-Lichtheim phenomenon
Lichtheim syndrome

Liddell, Edward G.T., English neurophysiologist, 1895–1981.
Liddell-Sherrington reflex—tonic contraction of the muscles in response to

a stretching force due to stimulation of muscle proprioceptors. *Syn:* myotatic reflex

Lieberkuhn, var. of Lieberkühn

Lieberkühn, Johann N., German anatomist and physician, 1711–1756.
    Lieberkühn crypts—*Syn:* Lieberkühn glands
    Lieberkühn follicles—*Syn:* Lieberkühn glands
    Lieberkühn glands—the tubular glands in the mucous membrane of the small and large intestines. *Syn:* intestinal glands; Lieberkühn crypts; Lieberkühn follicles

Liebermann, Leo von S., Hungarian physician, 1852–1926.
    Burchard-Liebermann reaction—see under Burchard
    Liebermann-Burchard test—a calorimetric test for unsaturated sterols, notably cholesterol.

Liebermeister, Carl von, German physician, 1833–1901.
    Liebermeister rule—in adult febrile tachycardia, about eight pulse beats correspond to an increase of 1°C.

Liebig, Baron Justus von, German chemist, 1803–1873.
    Liebig theory—that the hydrocarbons that oxidize readily and burn are nutritive material that produce the greatest quantity of animal heat.

Liebow, Averill A., Austrian-U.S. pulmonary pathologist, 1911–1978.
    usual interstitial pneumonia of Liebow—a progressive inflammatory condition of the lung. *Syn:* Hamman-Rich syndrome; idiopathic interstitial fibrosis; fibrosing alveolitis

Liéou, Young C., French physician.
    Barré-Liéou syndrome—see under Barré
    Liéou-Barré syndrome—*Syn:* Barré-Liéou syndrome

Liepmann, Hugo K., German neurologist, 1863–1925.
    Liepmann disease—*Syn:* apraxia

Liesegang, Ralph E., German chemist, 1869–1947.
    Liesegang rings—colored rings of precipitated silver chromate formed when a drop of concentrated silver nitrate is added to the surface of a gel containing potassium dichromate.

Lieutaud, Joseph, French anatomist and pathologist, 1703–1780.
    Lieutaud body—*Syn:* Lieutaud trigone
    Lieutaud triangle—*Syn:* Lieutaud trigone
    Lieutaud trigone—a triangular smooth area at the base of the bladder between the openings of the two ureters and that of the urethra. *Syn:* trigone of bladder; Lieutaud body; Lieutaud triangle
    Lieutaud uvula—a slight projection into the cavity of the bladder marking the location of the middle lobe of the prostate. *Syn:* uvula of bladder

NOTES

Lightwood, Reginald, 20th century English pediatrician.
    Lightwood disease—hypercalciuria in infants.
    Lightwood syndrome—tubular acidosis of the kidney.

Lignac, George O.E., Dutch pediatrician, 1891–1954.
    Aberhalden-Kauffman-Lignac syndrome—see under Aberhalden
    Lignac disease
    Lignac-Fanconi syndrome—the most common of a group of diseases with characteristic renal tubular dysfunction disorders. *SYN:* cystinosis

Likert, Rensis, U.S. social psychologist, *1903.
    Likert scale—a method of measuring attitudes.

Lillie, Ralph D., U.S. pathologist, 1896–1979.
    Glenner-Lillie stain for pituitary—see under Glenner
    Lillie allochrome connective tissue stain
    Lillie azure-cosin stain
    Lillie ferrous iron stain
    Lillie sulfuric acid Nile blue stain
    Lillie-Crow test

Lilly, John C., U.S. physiologist, *1915.
    Silverman-Lilly pneumotachograph—see under Silverman, Leslie

Lindau, Arvid, Swedish pathologist, 1892–1958.
    Lindau disease—*SYN:* von Hippel-Lindau syndrome
    Lindau tumor—a benign cerebellar neoplasm. *SYN:* hemangioblastoma
    von Hippel-Lindau syndrome—see under von Hippel

Lindbergh, Charles A., U.S. aviator, 1902–1974.
    Carrel-Lindbergh pump—see under Carrel

Lindemann, Edward E., U.S. surgeon, 1879–1919.
    Lindemann cannula—a cannula used in blood transfusion.

Lindner, Karl, Austrian ophthalmologist, 1883–1961.
    Lindner bodies—initial bodies resembling inclusion bodies found in scrapings of epithelial cells infected with trachoma.
    Lindner corneoscleral suture
    Lindner cyclodialysis spatula
    Lindner cyclodialysis spoon
    Lindner sclerotomy
    Lindner spatula

Lindqvist, Johan Torsten, Swedish physician, *1906.
    Fahraeus-Lindqvist effect—see under Fahraeus

Lindsay, P.G., U.S. physician.
    Lindsay nails—the distal portion of the fingernails develop brown pigmentation due to chronic renal failure. *SYN:* half-and-half nails

Lineweaver, Hans, U.S. physical chemist, *1907.
    Lineweaver-Burk equation—rearrangement of the Michaelis-Menten equation.
    Lineweaver-Burk plot—graphical representation of enzyme kinetic data. *SYN:* double-reciprocal plot

Ling, Per Henrik, Swedish hygienist, 1776–1839.
   Ling method—gymnastic exercises without the use of apparatus. *Syn:* lingism

Linné, Carl von, Swedish botanist and physician, 1707–1778.
   linnaean system of nomenclature—the system of nomenclature in which the names of species are composed of genus and species. *Syn:* binary nomenclature

Lipmann, Fritz A., German-U.S. biochemist in the U.S. and Nobel laureate, 1899–1986.
   Warburg-Lipmann-Dickens-Horecker shunt—*Syn:* Dickens shunt

Lipschütz, Benjamin, Austrian physician, 1878–1931.
   Lipschütz cell—a cell whose protoplasm contains single and double granules of varying size, stainable with hematoxylin. *Syn:* centrocyte
   Lipschütz erythema—*Syn:* Afzelius erythema
   Lipschütz ulcer—a simple acute ulceration of the vulvae or lower vagina of nonvenereal origin. *Syn:* ulcus vulvae acutum

Lisch, Karl, Austrian ophthalmologist, *1907.
   Lisch nodule—iris hamartomas typically seen in type 1 neurofibromatosis. *Syn:* Sakurai-Lisch nodule
   Sakurai-Lisch nodule—*Syn:* Lisch nodule

Lisfranc, Jacques, French surgeon, 1790–1847.
   Lisfranc amputation—amputation of the foot at the tarsometatarsal joint, the sole being preserved to make the flap. *Syn:* Lisfranc operation
   Lisfranc dislocation
   Lisfranc fracture
   Lisfranc joints—the three synovial joints between the tarsal and metatarsal bones. *Syn:* tarsometatarsal joints
   Lisfranc ligaments—ligaments that pass from the cuneiform bones to the metatarsals, the one from the first cuneiform to the second metatarsal being the strongest. *Syn:* interosseous cuneometatarsal ligaments
   Lisfranc operation—*Syn:* Lisfranc amputation
   scalene tubercle of Lisfranc—a small spine on the inner edge of the first rib, giving attachment to the scalenus anterior muscle. *Syn:* scalene tubercle

Lison, Lucien, Belgian scientist, *1907.
   Lison-Dunn stain—a technique using leuco patent blue V and hydrogen peroxidase to demonstrate hemoglobin peroxidase on time sections and smears.

Lison, Michael, Israeli physician.
   Lison syndrome—genetic trait resulting in premature graying of hair, sharp facial features, vitiligo, and other abnormalities.

NOTES

Lissauer, Heinrich, German neurologist, 1861–1891.
    column of Spitzka-Lissauer—*Syn:* Spitzka marginal tract
    Lissauer bundle—*Syn:* Lissauer fasciculus
    Lissauer column—*Syn:* Lissauer fasciculus
    Lissauer fasciculus—a longitudinal bundle of thin, unmyelinated and
    poorly myelinated fibers capping the apex of the posterior horn of the
    spinal gray matter. *Syn:* dorsolateral fasciculus; Lissauer bundle; Lissauer
    column; Lissauer marginal zone; Lissauer tract
    Lissauer marginal zone—*Syn:* Lissauer fasciculus
    Lissauer paralysis
    Lissauer tract—*Syn:* Lissauer fasciculus
    Lissauer zone

Lisser, Hans, U.S. physician, *1888.
    Escamilla-Lisser syndrome—see under Escamilla
    Escamilla-Lisser-Shepardson syndrome

Lister, Joseph (Lord Lister), English surgeon, 1827–1912.
    Listeria—a genus of aerobic to microaerophilic, motile, peritrichous
    bacteria.
    Lister dressing—the first type of antiseptic dressing, one of gauze
    impregnated with carbolic acid.
    Lister forceps
    Lister knife
    Lister method—antiseptic surgery as first advocated by Lister in 1867.
    Syn: listerism
    Lister scissors
    Lister tubercle—a small prominence on the dorsal aspect of the distal end
    of the radius that serves as a trochlea or pulley for the tendon. *Syn:*
    dorsal tubercle of radius
    Listerella—in bacteriology, a rejected generic name sometimes cited as a
    synonym of *Listeria*. The type species is *Listerella hepatolytica*.
    Listerine—antiseptic mouthwash.
    listerism—*Syn:* Lister method

Listing, Johann B., German physiologist, 1808–1882.
    Listing law—when the eye leaves one object and fixes upon another it
    revolves about an axis perpendicular to a plane cutting both the former
    and the present lines of vision.
    Listing reduced eye—a representation that simplifies calculations of retinal
    imagery.

Liston, Robert, English surgeon, 1794–1847.
    Liston bone-cutting forceps
    Liston knives—long-bladed knives of various sizes used in amputations.
    Liston shears—strong shears for cutting plaster of Paris bandages.
    Liston splint—a long splint extending from the axilla to the sole of the
    foot.

Little, James, U.S. surgeon, 1836–1885.
    Little area—*Syn:* Kiesselbach area

Little, William J., English surgeon, 1810–1894.
    Little disease—a type of cerebral palsy in which there is bilateral

spasticity, with the lower extremities more severely affected. *Syn:* spastic diplegia

Littré, Alexis, French anatomist, 1658–1726.
   Littré glands—numerous mucous glands in the wall of the penile urethra. *Syn:* glands of the male urethra
   Littré hernia—a hernia in which only a portion of the wall of the intestine is engaged. *Syn:* parietal hernia

Litzmann, Karl K.T., German gynecologist, 1815–1890.
   Litzmann obliquity—inclination of the fetal head so that the posterior parietal bone presents to the parturient canal. *Syn:* posterior asynclitism

Livierato, P., Italian physician, 1860–1936.
   Livierato sign—cardiac sign.

Lobo, Jorge, 20th century Brazilian physician.
   Lobo disease—a chronic localized mycosis of the skin. *Syn:* lobomycosis
   lobomycosis—*Syn:* Lobo disease

Lobry de Bruyn, Cornelius A., Dutch chemist, 1857–1904.
   Lobry de Bruyn-van Ekenstein transformation—the base-catalyzed interconversion of an aldose and a ketose.

Lobstein, Johann F.G., German pathologist, 1777–1835.
   Lobstein ganglion—a small sympathetic ganglion often present in the course of the greater splanchnic nerve. *Syn:* splanchnic ganglion

Locke, Frank S., English physiologist, 1871–1949.
   Cabot-Locke murmur—see under Cabot
   Locke solutions—solutions used for irrigating and culturing mammalian heart and other tissues in laboratory experiments.
   Locke-Ringer solution—a solution used in the laboratory for physiological and pharmacological experiments.

Lockwood, Charles B., English anatomist and surgeon, 1858–1914.
   ligament of Lockwood—*Syn:* suspensory ligament of eyeball
   Lockwood clamp
   Lockwood forceps
   Lockwood ligament—*Syn:* suspensory ligament of eyeball
   Lockwood tendon

Loeb, Leo, U.S. pathologist, 1869–1959.
   Loeb deciduoma—mass of decidual tissue produced in the uterus, in the absence of a fertilized ovum, by means of mechanical or hormonal stimulation.

Loeffler, Friedrich A.J., German bacteriologist and surgeon, 1852–1915.
   Klebs-Loeffler bacillus—see under Klebs

(continued)

NOTES

Loeffler *(continued)*
>   **Loeffler bacillus**—a species that causes diphtheria. *Syn: Corynebacterium diphtheriae*
>   **Loeffler blood culture medium**—a culture medium for the isolation of *Corynebacterium diphtheriae.*
>   **Loeffler caustic stain**—a stain for flagella, utilizing an aqueous solution of tannin and ferrous sulfate with the addition of an alcoholic fuchsin stain.
>   **Loeffler methylene blue**—a stain for diphtheria organisms.
>   **Loeffler stain**—a stain for flagella.

Loevit, Moritz, Austrian pathologist, 1851–1918.
>   **Loevit cell**—originally a term denoting all forms of human red blood cells containing a nucleus, both pathologic and normal. *Syn:* erythroblast

Loewenthal, Wilhelm, German physician, 1850–1894.
>   **Loewenthal bundle**—a bundle of thick, heavily myelinated fibers that ends in the medial region of the anterior horn of the cervical spinal cord and appears to be involved in head movements during visual and auditory tracking. *Syn:* tectospinal tract; Loewenthal tract
>   **Loewenthal reaction**—the agglutinative reaction in relapsing fever.
>   **Loewenthal tract**—*Syn:* Loewenthal bundle

Loewi, Otto, German-U.S. physiologist and pharmacologist, 1873–1961, joint winner of 1936 Nobel prize for work related to nerve impulse chemical transmission.

Löffler, var. of Loeffler

Löffler, Wilhelm, Swiss physician, 1887–1972.
>   **Löffler disease**—*Syn:* Löffler endocarditis
>   **Löffler endocarditis**—fibroplastic parietal endocarditis with eosinophilia, an endocarditis of obscure cause characterized by progressive congestive heart failure, multiple systemic emboli, and eosinophilia. *Syn:* Löffler disease; Löffler syndrome (2)
>   **Löffler parietal fibroplastic endocarditis**—sclerosis of the endocardium in the presence of a high eosinophil count.
>   **Löffler pneumonia**—eosinophilic pneumonia.
>   **Löffler syndrome**—(1) *Syn:* simple pulmonary eosinophilia; (2) *Syn:* Löffler endocarditis.

Löfgren, Sven, Swedish physician, 1910–1978.
>   **Löfgren syndrome**—related to sarcoidosis.

Logan, William H.G., early 20th century U.S. plastic surgeon.
>   **Logan bow**—heavy stainless steel wire bent in an arc and taped to both cheeks to protect the incision and to relieve tension on a freshly repaired cleft lip.

Lombard, Etienne, French physician, 1868–1920.
>   **Lombard voice-reflex test**—a test useful in assessing functional hearing loss.

Lombroso, Cesare, Italian criminologist and professor, 1835–1909.
>   **characterology**—Lombroso was a proponent of the theory that attempted to establish a correlation between physical characteristics and criminal behavior.

Londe, P.F.L., 1865–1944.
   Fazio-Londe atrophy—see under Fazio
   Fazio-Londe disease—*Syn:* Fazio-Londe atrophy

London, Fritz, German-U.S. physicist, 1900–1954.
   London forces—*Syn:* van der Waals forces

Long, John H., U.S. physician, 1856–1927.
   Long coefficient—*Syn:* Long formula
   Long formula—a formula for estimating from the specific gravity of a specimen of urine the approximate amount of solids in grams per liter. *Syn:* Long coefficient

Longmire, William P., Jr., U.S. surgeon, *1913.
   Longmire anastomosis
   Longmire operation—intrahepatic cholangiojejunostomy with partial hepatectomy for biliary obstruction.

Looney, Joseph M., U.S. biochemist, *1896.
   Folin-Looney test—see under Folin

Looser, Emil, Swiss physician, 1877–1936.
   Looser lines—radiolucent bands in the cortex of a bone. *Syn:* Looser zones
   Looser zones—*Syn:* Looser lines

Lorain, Paul, French physician, 1827–1875.
   Lorain disease—dwarfism generally associated with hypogonadism. *Syn:* idiopathic infantilism
   Lorain-Lévi dwarfism—a rare form of dwarfism caused by the absence of a functional anterior pituitary gland. *Syn:* pituitary dwarfism; Lorain-Lévi infantilism; Lorain-Lévi syndrome
   Lorain-Lévi infantilism—*Syn:* Lorain-Lévi dwarfism
   Lorain-Lévi syndrome—*Syn:* Lorain-Lévi dwarfism

Lorenz, Adolf, Austrian surgeon, 1854–1946.
   Lorenz sign—an obsolete term for stiffness of the thoracic spine in early pulmonary tuberculosis.

Lorenz, Konrad, Austrian zoologist, *1903, joint winner of 1973 Nobel Prize for work related to social behavior.

Loschmidt, Joseph (Johann), Czech chemist and physicist, 1821–1895.
   Loschmidt number—the number of molecules in 1 cm^3q of ideal gas at 0°C and 1 atmosphere of pressure.

Lotheissen, Georg, Austrian surgeon, 1868–1941.
   Lotheissen herniorrhaphy
   Lotheissen operation

L

NOTES

Louis, Pierre C.A., French physician, 1787–1872.
    Louis angle—the angle between the manubrium and the body of the sternum at the manubriosternal junction. *SYN:* sternal angle
    Louis law—tuberculosis in any organ is associated with tuberculosis in the lung.

Louis-Bar, Denise, mid-20th century French physician.
    Louis-Bar syndrome—an autosomal recessive disorder characterized by cerebellar ataxia and telangiectasia. *SYN:* ataxia telangiectasia

Lovén, Otto C., Swedish physician, 1835–1904.
    Lovén reflex—a reaction in which a local dilation of vessels accompanies a general vasoconstriction.

Low, George C., English physician, 1872–1952.
    Castellani-Low sign—see under Castellani

Lowe, Charles U., U.S. pediatrician, *1921.
    Lowe syndrome—a congenital syndrome with hydrophthalmia, cataracts, mental retardation, aminoaciduria, reduced ammonia production by the kidney, and vitamin D-resistant rickets. *SYN:* oculocerebrorenal syndrome; Lowe-Terrey-MacLachlan syndrome
    Lowe-Terrey-MacLachlan syndrome—*SYN:* Lowe syndrome

Löwenberg, Benjamin B., French laryngologist, 1836–1905.
    Löwenberg canal—*SYN:* cochlear duct
    Löwenberg forceps—forceps for the removal of adenoid growths in the nasopharynx.
    Löwenberg scala—*SYN:* cochlear duct

Löwenstein, L.W.
    Buschke-Löwenstein tumor—see under Buschke

Lower, Richard, English anatomist and physiologist, 1631–1691.
    Lower ring—one of four fibrous rings that form part of the fibrous skeleton of the heart. *SYN:* fibrous ring of heart
    Lower tubercle—the slight projection on the wall of the right atrium between the orifices of the venae cavae. *SYN:* intervenous tubercle

Lowman, Charles LeRoy, U.S. orthopedist, 1879–1977.
    Lowman bone-holding clamp
    Lowman bone-holding forceps
    Lowman clamp
    Lowman flatfoot procedure
    Lowman forceps
    Lowman retractor
    Lowman rongeur
    Lowman sling procedure

Lown, Bernard, U.S. cardiologist, *1921.
    Lown cardioverter
    Lown technique
    Lown-Ganong-Levine syndrome—electrocardiographic syndrome of a short P-R interval with normal duration of the QRS complex.

Lowry, Oliver H., U.S. biochemist, *1910.
Lowry protein assay—a method for determining protein concentrations using the Folin-Ciocalteu reagent. *Syn:* Lowry-Folin assay
Lowry-Folin assay—*Syn:* Lowry protein assay

Lowry, R. Brian, 20th century Irish medical geneticist in Canada.
Coffin-Lowry syndrome—*Syn:* Coffin-Siris syndrome

Lowsley, Oswald S., U.S. urologist, 1884–1955.
Lowsley forceps
Lowsley hemostat
Lowsley lithotrite
Lowsley needle
Lowsley nephropexy
Lowsley prostate retractor
Lowsley retractor
Lowsley ribbon-gut needle
Lowsley stone crusher
Lowsley tractor—instrument used in perineal prostatectomy.
Lowsley urethroscope

Lubarsch, Otto, German pathologist, 1860–1933.
Lubarsch crystals—intracellular crystals in the testis resembling sperm crystals.

Luc, Henri, French laryngologist, 1855–1925.
Caldwell-Luc operation—see under Caldwell, George
Luc forceps
Luc operation—*Syn:* Caldwell-Luc operation
Ogston-Luc operation—see under Ogston

Lucas, Richard C., English anatomist and surgeon, 1846–1915.
Lucas groove—a faint groove occasionally caused by the chorda tympani nerve on the spine of the sphenoid. *Syn:* stria spinosa

Lucas-Champonnière, Justin M.M., French surgeon, 1843–1913.
Lucas-Champonnière disease—a form of bronchitis.

Luciani, Luigi, Italian physiologist, 1842–1919.
Luciani syndrome—syndrome of the cerebellum associated with lack of muscle tone, lack of strength, and incoordination. *Syn:* Luciani triad
Luciani triad—*Syn:* Luciani syndrome

Lucio, R., Mexican physician, 1819–1866.
Lucio leprosy—an acute form occurring in pure diffuse lepromatous leprosy. *Syn:* Lucio leprosy phenomenon; lazarine leprosy
Lucio leprosy phenomenon—*Syn:* Lucio leprosy

Lucké, Balduin, U.S. pathologist, 1889–1954.
Lucké adenocarcinoma—*Syn:* Lucké carcinoma

(continued)

NOTES

Lucké *(continued)*
> **Lucké carcinoma**—a herpesvirus-associated adenocarcinoma of the kidney in adult frogs. *SYN:* Lucké adenocarcinoma
> **Lucké virus**—a herpesvirus associated with Lucké carcinoma.

Lücke, George A., German surgeon, 1829–1894.
> **Lücke test**—a test for hippuric acid.

Ludloff, Karl, German surgeon, 1864–1945.
> **Ludloff sign**—(1) swelling and ecchymosis appearing at the base of Scarpa triangle; (2) inability to raise the thigh in the sitting posture.

Ludwig, Daniel, German anatomist, 1625–1680.
> **Ludwig angle**—the angle between the manubrium and the body of the sternum at the manubriosternal junction. *SYN:* sternal angle

Ludwig, Karl F.W., German anatomist and physiologist, 1816–1895.
> **depressor nerve of Ludwig**—*SYN:* Ludwig nerve
> **Ludwig ganglion**—a small collection of parasympathetic nerve cells in the interatrial septum.
> **Ludwig labyrinth**—proximal and distal convoluted tubules and the associated renal corpuscles supplied by branches of the interlobular arteries. *SYN:* convoluted part of kidney lobule
> **Ludwig nerve**—a branch of the vagus which ends in the aortic arch and base of the heart. *SYN:* aortic nerve; depressor nerve of Ludwig
> **Ludwig stromuhr**—one of the first devices for measuring flow in blood vessels.

Ludwig, Kurt, German anatomist, *1922.
> **Klinger-Ludwig acid-thionin stain for sex chromatin**—a method using a preliminary acid treatment on buccal smears prior to staining with buffered thionin, to differentiate Barr body.

Ludwig, Wilhelm Friedrich von, German surgeon, 1790–1865.
> **Ludwig angina**—cellulitis, usually of odontogenic origin, bilaterally involving the submaxillary, sublingual, and submental spaces.
> **Ludwig applicator**
> **Ludwig sinus applicator**

Luebering, J.
> **Rapoport-Luebering shunt**—see under Rapoport

Luer, German instrument maker, d. 1883.
> **Luer curet**
> **Luer forceps**
> **Luer needle**
> **Luer reconstruction plate**
> **Luer retractor**
> **Luer rongeur**
> **Luer scoop**
> **Luer speculum**
> **Luer suction cannula adapter**
> **Luer syringe**—a glass syringe used for hypodermic and intravenous purposes. *SYN:* Luer-Lok syringe
> **Luer tracheal cannula**

Luer tube
Luer-Lok syringe—*Syn:* Luer syringe

Luetscher, John A., U.S. physician, *1913.
Luetscher syndrome—excessive aldosterone causing renal, liver, and heart disease.

Luft, John H., U.S. histologist, *1927.
Luft potassium permanganate fixative—a fixative useful in electron microscopy for cytologic preservation of lipoprotein complexes in membranes and myelin, because of its oxidative properties.

Luft, Rolf, 20th century Swedish endocrinologist.
Luft disease—a metabolic disease.

Lugol, Jean G.A., French physician, 1786–1851.
Lugol iodine solution—an iodine-potassium iodide solution used as an oxidizing agent, for removal of mercurial fixation artifacts, and also in histochemistry and to stain amebas.

Lumsden, Thomas W., English physician, 1874–1953.
Lumsden pneumotoxic center

Luna, Lee G., 20th century U.S. medical technologist.
Luna-Ishak stain—a staining method using celestine blue and acid fuchsin in which bile canaliculi stain pink to red.

Luria, Salvador E., Italian-U.S. biologist, 1912–1991, joint winner of 1969 Nobel Prize for work related to viruses.

Luschka, Hubert, German anatomist, 1820–1875.
foramen of Luschka—one of the two lateral openings of the fourth ventricle into the subarachnoid space at the cerebellopontine angle. *Syn:* lateral aperture of the fourth ventricle
Luschka bursa—a cystic notochordal remnant found inconstantly in the posterior wall of the nasopharynx at the lower end of the pharyngeal tonsil. *Syn:* pharyngeal bursa
Luschka cartilage—a small cartilaginous nodule sometimes found in the anterior portion of the vocal cord.
Luschka crypt
Luschka cystic glands—small mucous tubuloalveolar glands in the mucosa of the larger bile ducts, especially in the neck of the gallbladder. *Syn:* glands of biliary mucosa
Luschka ducts—glandlike tubular structures in the wall of the gallbladder, especially in the part covered with peritoneum.
Luschka ganglion
Luschka gland—*Syn:* Luschka tonsil
Luschka joints—small synovial joints between adjacent lateral lips of the bodies of the lower cervical vertebrae. *Syn:* uncovertebral joints

(continued)

NOTES

Luschka *(continued)*

Luschka ligaments—fibrous bands that pass from the pericardium to the sternum. *Syn:* sternopericardial ligament

Luschka muscles

Luschka nerve

Luschka sinus—venous sinus in the petrosquamous suture.

Luschka tonsil—a collection of more or less closely aggregated lymphoid nodules on the posterior wall and roof of the nasopharynx. *Syn:* pharyngeal tonsil; Luschka gland

Luse, Sarah A., 20th century U.S. physician.

Luse bodies—collagen fibers with abnormally long spacing between electron-dense bands.

Lust, Franz A., 20th century German pediatrician.

Lust phenomenon—abduction with dorsal foot flexion related to latent tetany. *Syn:* Lust sign; peroneal sign; peroneal nerve phenomenon

Lutembacher, René, French cardiologist, 1884–1916.

Lutembacher syndrome—a congenital cardiac abnormality consisting of a defect of the interatrial septum, mitral stenosis, and enlarged right atrium.

Lutz, Alfredo, Brazilian physician, 1855–1940.

Lutz-Splendore-Almeida disease—a chronic mycosis caused by *Paracoccidioides brasiliensis. Syn:* paracoccidioidomycosis

Luys, Jules B., French physician, 1828–1897.

centre médian de Luys—*Syn:* centromedian nucleus

corpus luysi—*Syn:* subthalamic nucleus

Luys body—*Syn:* subthalamic nucleus

Luys body syndrome

nucleus of Luys—*Syn:* subthalamic nucleus

Lwoff, André, French virologist and microbiologist, *1902, joint winner of 1965 Nobel Prize for work related to synthesis of viruses and enzymes.

Lyell, Alan, 20th century dermatologist.

Lyell disease—a disease affecting infants in which large areas of skin peel off as a result of upper respiratory staphylococcal infection. *Syn:* staphylococcal scalded skin syndrome; Ritter disease; Ritter syndrome

Lyell syndrome—a syndrome in which a large portion of the skin becomes intensely erythematous with epidermal necrosis, and peels off. *Syn:* toxic epidermal necrolysis

Lyme, city in Connecticut where disease was first recognized.

Lyme arthritis—the arthritic manifestations of Lyme disease.

Lyme disease—infectious disease spread by tick.

Lynch, Henry T., U.S. oncologist, *1928.

Lynch syndrome I—familial predisposition to colon cancer.

Lynch syndrome II—familial predisposition for other primary cancers in addition to the predisposition for colon cancer; site is often female reproductive organs.

Lynen, Feodor, German biochemist, 1911–1979, joint winner of 1964 Nobel Prize for work related to cholesterol and metabolism of fatty acids.

Lyon, B.B. Vincent, U.S. physician, 1880–1953.
 Meltzer-Lyon test—see under Meltzer

Lyon, Mary F., English cytogeneticist, *1925.
 Lyon hypothesis—*Syn:* lyonization
 lyonization—the normal phenomenon that wherever there are two or more haploid sets of X-linked genes in each cell all but one of the genes are inactivated apparently at random and have no phenotypic expression. *Syn:* X-inactivation; Lyon hypothesis

L

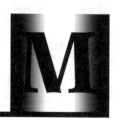

M'Dowel, Benjamin G., Irish anatomist, 1829–1885.
  frenulum of M'Dowel—tendinous fasciculi passing from the tendon of the pectoralis major muscle across the bicipital groove.

M'Naghten, Daniel, English criminal, tried in March, 1843.
  M'Naghten rule—the classic English test of criminal responsibility.

MacConkey, Alfred T., English bacteriologist, 1861–1931.
  MacConkey agar—a medium used to identify Gram-negative bacilli and characterize them according to their status as lactose fermenters. *SYN:* MacConkey medium
  MacConkey medium—*SYN:* MacConkey agar

Macewen, Sir William, Scottish surgeon, 1848–1924.
  Macewen classification
  Macewen drill
  Macewen herniorrhaphy
  Macewen operation
  Macewen osteotomy
  Macewen saw
  Macewen sign—percussion of the skull gives a cracked-pot sound in cases of hydrocephalus. *SYN:* Macewen symptom
  Macewen symptom—*SYN:* Macewen sign
  Macewen triangle—*SYN:* suprameatal triangle

Mach, Ernst, Austrian scientist, 1838–1916.
  Mach band—a relatively bright or dark band.
  Mach number—the ratio between the speed of an object moving through a fluid medium and the speed of sound in the same medium.

Mach, Rene Sigmund, Swiss physician, 1904.
  Mach syndrome—adrenal hyperplasia.

Machiavelli, Niccolo, Italian author and statesman, 1469–1527.
  Mach scale—used to determine an individual's use of manipulation.
  machiavellianism—a personality trait of one who manipulates others to achieve goals.

Machover, Karen Alper, U.S. psychologist, *1902.
  Machover draw-a-person test—a test used in psychology and psychiatry.

Macintosh, Charles, Scottish chemist, 1766–1843.
  Macintosh blockers—a system of tubes used during thoracic operations to block one lung or lobe from the other.

Mackay, R. Stuart, U.S. physicist, *1924.
Mackay-Marg tonometer—a recording electronic applanation tonometer.

Mackenrodt, Alwin K., German gynecologist, 1859–1925.
Mackenrodt incision
Mackenrodt ligament—*Syn:* cardinal ligament
Mackenrodt operation

Mackenzie, Richard J., Scottish surgeon, 1821–1854.
Mackenzie amputation—a modification of Syme amputation at the ankle joint, the flap being taken from the inner side.

Mackenzie, Sir James, Scottish physician in England, 1853–1925.
Mackenzie polygraph—an instrument formerly used in the clinical investigation of cardiac arrhythmias.

MacLachlan, Elsie A., 20th century researcher.
Lowe-Terrey-MacLachlan syndrome—*Syn:* Lowe syndrome

Maclennan, A.
Maclennan syndrome—sphincter pain. *Syn:* Thaysen syndrome.

MacLeod, John James Richard, joint winner of 1923 Nobel Prize for discovering insulin.

Macleod, Roderick, Scottish physician, 1795–1852.
Macleod rheumatism—rheumatoid arthritis with abundant serous effusion in the affected joints.

Macleod, William Mathieson, English physician, 1911–1977.
Macleod syndrome—*Syn:* Swyer-James syndrome (1)
Swyer-James-Macleod syndrome—*Syn:* Swyer-James syndrome (2)

MacNeal, Ward J., U.S. bacteriologist, 1881–1946.
MacNeal tetrachrome blood stain—a stain for blood smears.
Novy and MacNeal blood agar—a nutrient agar suitable for the cultivation of a number of trypanosomes.

MacQuarrie, Thomas William, U.S. psychologist.
MacQuarrie test for mechanical ability—test used in psychology and psychiatry.

MacWilliams, John Alexander, English physician, 1857–1937.
MacWilliams test—a urine test.

Maddox, Ernest E., English ophthalmologist, 1860–1933.
Maddox prism
Maddox rod
Maddox rod occluder
Maddox rod test—used to test eye muscle balance.

Madelung, Otto W., German surgeon, 1846–1926.
Madelung deformity—a distal radial ulnar subluxation due to relative deficiency of axial growth of the medial side of the distal radius. *Syn:* carpus curvus
Madelung disease—accumulation and progressive enlargement of adipose tissue in the subcutaneous tissue of the head, neck, upper trunk, and

upper portions of the upper extremities. *Syn:* multiple symmetric lipomatosis

Madelung lipoma—fatty tumor.

Madelung neck—multiple symmetric lipomatosis confined to the neck.

Madelung subluxation—incomplete dislocation or luxation.

Madlener, Max, German surgeon, 1868–1951.

Madlener operation—tubal sterilization by clamp and tie.

Madsen, Thorvald J.M., *1870.

Arrhenius-Madsen theory—see under Arrhenius

Maffucci, Angelo, Italian physician, 1847–1903.

Maffucci syndrome—enchondromatosis with multiple cavernous hemangiomas. *Syn:* dyschondroplasia with hemangiomas

Magendie, François, French physiologist, 1783–1855.

Bell-Magendie law—*Syn:* Bell law

Magendie foramen—*Syn:* medial aperture of the fourth ventricle

Magendie law—*Syn:* Bell law

Magendie spaces—space between the pia and arachnoid at the level of the fissures of the brain.

Magendie-Hertwig sign—skew deviation of the eyes in acute cerebellar lesions. *Syn:* Magendie-Hertwig syndrome

Magendie-Hertwig syndrome—*Syn:* Magendie-Hertwig sign

M

Magill, Sir Ivan Whiteside.

Magill band

Magill circuit

Magill endotracheal tube

Magill forceps

Magill laryngoscope

Magill Pain Questionnaire

Magnan, Valentin J.J., French psychiatrist, 1835–1916.

Magnan sign—paresthesia in the psychosis of cocaine addicts.

Magnan trombone movement—involuntary forward and back movement of the tongue when it is drawn out of the mouth in several basal ganglia disorders.

Magnus, I.A.

Magnus syndrome—protoporphyrin in bone marrow.

Magnus, Rudolph, German physiologist, 1873–1927.

Magnus sign—an obsolete sign: after death, constriction of a limb or one of its segments is not followed by venous congestion of the distal part.

Magoss, I.V., U.S. physician.

Magoss-Walshe syndrome—preaortic renal vein compression.

Magrassi, Flaviano, Italian physician, *1908.

Magrassi-Leonardi syndrome—eosinophilic pneumonia.

NOTES

Mahaim, I.
   Mahaim fibers—paraspecific fibers originating from the A-V node, the His bundle, or the bundle branches and inserting into the ventricular myocardium. *Syn:* nodoventricular fibers

Mahler, Richter A., German obstetrician, 1863–1941.
   Mahler sign—increased pulse rate with no elevation of temperature, indicating thrombosis.

Maier, Rudolf, German physician, 1824–1888.
   Maier sinus—an infundibuliform depression on the internal surface of the lacrimal sac which receives the lacrimal canaliculi.

Main, Thomas Forrest, English psychiatrist.
   Main syndrome—psychotic female health professional who exploits her background to obtain health care.

Maisonneuve, Jules Germain François, French surgeon, 1809–1897.
   Maisonneuve amputation
   Maisonneuve bandage
   Maisonneuve fracture
   Maisonneuve sign
   Maisonneuve urethrotome

Maissiat, Jacques H., French anatomist, 1805–1878.
   Maissiat band—a fibrous reinforcement of the fascia lata on the lateral surface of the thigh. *Syn:* iliotibial tract
   Maissiat ligament

Maixner, Emmerich, Austrian physician, 1847–1920.
   Maixner cirrhosis—hemorrhagic liver cirrhosis.

Majocchi, Domenico, Italian dermatologist, 1849–1929.
   Majocchi disease—asymptomatic annular lesions, principally of the lower extremities of adolescent males. *Syn:* purpura annularis telangiectodes; Majocchi syndrome
   Majocchi granulomas—erythematous papules due to a deep follicular fungal infection, most frequently seen on shaved legs of women. *Syn:* tinea profunda
   Majocchi purpura
   Majocchi syndrome—*Syn:* Majocchi disease

Makeham, William Matthew, English actuary, d. 1892.
   Makeham hypothesis—assumption that death is the consequence of two generally coexisting causes: (1) chance; (2) a deterioration or increased inability to withstand destruction.

Malacarne, Michele V.G., Italian surgeon, 1744–1816.
   Malacarne pyramid—a lobule on the undersurface of the cerebellum, the posterior portion of the vermis.
   Malacarne space—the bottom of the interpeduncular fossa at the base of the midbrain. *Syn:* posterior perforated substance

Malan, Edmond, U.S. physician.
   Malan syndrome—vascular disorder of the foot and leg.

Malassez, Louis C., French physiologist, 1842–1910.
    Malassezia—a genus of fungi (family Cryptococcaceae) of low
      pathogenicity.
    Malassez disease—testicular cyst.
    Malassez epithelial rests—epithelial remains of Hertwig root sheath in the
      periodontal ligament.

Malecot, Achille-Etienne, French surgeon, *1852.
    Malecot catheter—a two- or four-winged catheter.
    Malecot drain
    Malecot tube

Malgaigne, Joseph F., French surgeon, 1806–1865.
    Malgaigne amputation—amputation of the foot in which only the
      astragalus is retained. *Syn:* subastragalar amputation
    Malgaigne apparatus
    Malgaigne bulging
    Malgaigne clamp
    Malgaigne fossa—a space containing the bifurcation of the common
      carotid artery. *Syn:* carotid triangle; Malgaigne triangle
    Malgaigne fracture
    Malgaigne hernia—infantile inguinal hernia prior to the descent of the
      testis.
    Malgaigne hook
    Malgaigne luxation—longitudinal subluxation of the radial head from the
      annular ligament. *Syn:* nursemaid's elbow
    Malgaigne swelling
    Malgaigne triangle—*Syn:* Malgaigne fossa

M

Malherbe, Albert, French physician, 1845–1915.
    Malherbe calcifying epithelioma—a benign solitary hair follicle tumor.
      Syn: pilomatrixoma
    Malherbe syndrome—dermal tumor. *Syn:* Malherbe-Chenantais syndrome
    Malherbe-Chenantais syndrome—*Syn:* Malherbe syndrome

Mall, Franklin Paine, U.S. anatomist and embryologist, 1862–1917.
    Mall formula—the age in days of a human embryo calculated as the
      square root of its length.
    Mall ridges—rarely used term for pulmonary ridges.
    periportal space of Mall—a tissue space between the limiting lamina and
      the portal canal in the liver.

Mallory, Frank B., U.S. pathologist, 1862–1941.
    Mallory aniline blue stain—*Syn:* Mallory trichrome stain
    Mallory bodies—large, poorly defined accumulations of eosinophilic
      material in the cytoplasm of damaged hepatic cells in certain forms of
      cirrhosis. *Syn:* alcoholic hyaline bodies
    Mallory collagen stain
    Mallory iodine stain

(continued)

NOTES

Mallory *(continued)*
>**Mallory phloxine stain**
>**Mallory phosphotungstic acid hematoxylin stain**
>**Mallory stain for actinomyces**
>**Mallory stain for hemofuchsin**
>**Mallory trichrome stain**—a method especially suitable for studying connective tissue. *SYN:* Mallory triple stain; Mallory aniline blue stain
>**Mallory triple stain**—*SYN:* Mallory trichrome stain
>**picro-Mallory trichrome stain**—a modification of Mallory trichrome stain that involves the addition of picric acid.

Mallory, G. Kenneth, U.S. pathologist, *1900.
>**Mallory syndrome**—gastroesophageal junction mucosal laceration.
>**Mallory-Weiss lesion**—laceration of the gastric cardia, as seen in the Mallory-Weiss syndrome. *SYN:* Mallory-Weiss tear
>**Mallory-Weiss syndrome**—laceration of the lower end of the esophagus, associated with bleeding, caused usually by severe retching and vomiting.
>**Mallory-Weiss tear**—*SYN:* Mallory-Weiss lesion

Malpighi, Marcello, Italian anatomist, histologist, and embryologist, 1628–1694.
>**malpighian bodies**—small nodular masses of lymphoid tissue attached to the sides of the smaller arterial branches. *SYN:* splenic lymph follicles; malpighian glands; malpighian nodules
>**malpighian capsule**—*SYN:* glomerular capsule
>**malpighian cell**—a cell of the stratum spinosum of the epidermis.
>**malpighian corpuscles**—*SYN:* renal corpuscle
>**malpighian glands**—*SYN:* malpighian bodies
>**malpighian glomerulus**—a tuft formed of capillary loops at the beginning of each nephric tubule in the kidney. *SYN:* malpighian tuft
>**malpighian layer**—*SYN:* malpighian stratum
>**malpighian nodules**—*SYN:* malpighian bodies
>**malpighian pyramid**—*SYN:* renal pyramid
>**malpighian rete**—*SYN:* malpighian stratum
>**malpighian stigmas**—the points of entrance of the smaller veins into the larger veins of the spleen.
>**malpighian stratum**—the living layer of the epidermis comprising the stratum basale, stratum spinosum, and stratum granulosum. *SYN:* malpighian layer; malpighian rete
>**malpighian tubules**—in insects, slender tubular or hairlike excretory structures.
>**malpighian tuft**—*SYN:* malpighian glomerulus
>**malpighian vesicles**—the minute air-filled vesicles on the surface of an expanded lung.

Malthus, Thomas R., English statistician and clergyman, 1766–1834.
>**malthusianism**—the theory that the world's population will outgrow the food supply.

Manchester, England, where the operation was developed.
>**Manchester operation**—a vaginal operation for prolapse of the uterus, consisting of cervical amputation and parametrial fixation (cardinal ligaments) anterior to the uterus. *SYN:* Fothergill operation

Manhold, John H., U.S. dentist, *1919.
  Volpe-Manhold Index—see under Volpe

Mankowsky, Boris Nikitich, Russian physician, 1883–1962.
  Mankowsky syndrome—familial bone disorders. *SYN:* familial dysplastic
    osteopathy

Mann, Frank C., U.S. surgeon, 1887–1962.
  Mann-Bollman fistula—a fistula used in experimental investigations of the
    digestive tract.
  Mann-Whitney U test
  Mann-Williamson operation—an operation performed on experimental
    animals in research on peptic ulcer.
  Mann-Williamson ulcer

Mann, John Dixon, English physician, 1840–1912.
  Dixon Mann sign—*SYN:* Mann sign
  Mann sign—seen in Graves disease. *SYN:* Dixon Mann sign

Mann, Ludwig, German physician, 1866–1936.
  Mann syndrome—brain contusion accompanied by coordination disorders.
  Wernicke-Mann hemiplegia—*SYN:* Wernicke-Mann paralysis
  Wernicke-Mann paralysis—*SYN:* Wernicke-Mann hemiplegia

M

Mannkopf, Emil W., German physician, 1836–1918.
  Mannkopf sign—acceleration of the pulse when a painful point is pressed
    upon.

Manson, Sir Patrick, English authority on tropical medicine, 1844–1922.
  Schistosoma mansoni—a disease-causing parasite transmitted by snails.
  Mansonella—a genus of filaria, widely distributed in tropical Africa and
    South America.
  Mansonia—a genus of brown or black medium-sized mosquitoes.
  Manson disease—*SYN:* schistosomiasis mansoni
  Manson eye worm—a widely distributed spiruroid nematode parasite of
    fowl. *SYN: Oxyspirura mansoni*
  Manson pyosis—obsolete term for a superficial pyogenic infection. *SYN:*
    pemphigus contagiosus
  Manson schistosomiasis—*SYN:* schistosomiasis mansoni
  Manson syndrome—pulmonary obliterative arteriolitis.
  schistosomiasis mansoni—infection with *Schistosoma mansoni. SYN:*
    Manson disease; intestinal schistosomiasis; Manson schistosomiasis

Mantel, Nathan, U.S. biostatistician, *1927.
  Mantel-Haenszel test—a summary chi-square test for stratified data, used
    when controlling for confounding.

Mantoux, Charles, French physician, 1877–1947.
  Mantoux method

(continued)

NOTES

Mantoux *(continued)*
>   **Mantoux pit**—shallow depressions of the palms and soles in basal cell nevus syndrome.
>   **Mantoux test**

Maranon, Gregorio, Spanish physician, 1887–1960.
>   **Maranon I syndrome**—spinal disorder.
>   **Maranon II syndrome**—muscle lipomas.
>   **Maranon III syndrome**—thyrotoxic state.
>   **Maranon IV syndrome**—testicular hypertrophy and gynecomastia.

Marburg, city in Germany.
>   **Marburg disease**—acute febrile illness; high mortality. *Syn:* green monkey disease; African hemorrhagic disease; Marburg virus
>   **Marburg virus**—*Syn:* Marburg disease

Marcacci, Arturo, Italian physiologist, 1854–1915.
>   **Marcacci muscle**—a sheet of smooth muscle fibers underlying the areola and nipple of the mammary gland.

Marchand, Felix, German pathologist, 1846–1928.
>   **Marchand adrenals**—small collections of accessory adrenal tissue in the broad ligament of the uterus or in the testes. *Syn:* Marchand rest
>   **Marchand cell**
>   **Marchand rest**—*Syn:* Marchand adrenals
>   **Marchand syndrome**—liver cirrhosis.
>   **Marchand wandering cell**—a cell of the mononuclear phagocyte system.

Marchant, Gérard T.J., French surgeon, 1850–1903.
>   **Marchant zone**—the area on the sphenoid and occipital bones at the base of the skull.

Marchesani, Oswald, German ophthalmologist, 1900–1952.
>   **Marchesani syndrome**—recessive autosomal inheritance disorder. *Syn:* Weill-Marchesani syndrome
>   **Weill-Marchesani syndrome**—*Syn:* Marchesani syndrome

Marchetti, Andrew A., U.S. obstetrician and gynecologist, 1901–1970.
>   **Marchetti operation**
>   **Marshall-Marchetti-Krantz operation**—see under Marshall, Victor

Marchi, Vittorio, Italian physician, 1851–1908.
>   **Marchi fixative**—used to demonstrate degenerating myelin.
>   **Marchi reaction**—failure of the myelin sheath of a nerve to blacken when submitted to the action of osmic acid.
>   **Marchi stain**—a staining method for demonstrating fat and degenerating nerve fibers.
>   **Marchi tract**—a bundle of thick, heavily myelinated fibers originating in the deep layers of the superior colliculus. *Syn:* tectospinal tract

Marchiafava, Ettore, Italian pathologist, 1847–1935.
>   **Marchiafava syndrome**—*Syn:* Marchiafava-Bignami syndrome
>   **Marchiafava-Bignami disease**—a disorder consisting of demyelination of the corpus callosum and cortical laminar necrosis involving the frontal and temporal lobes. *Syn:* Marchiafava syndrome
>   **Marchiafava-Micheli anemia**—*Syn:* Marchiafava-Micheli syndrome

Marchiafava-Micheli syndrome—an infrequent disorder with insidious onset and chronic course, characterized by episodes of hemolytic anemia, hemoglobinuria, pallor, icterus or bronzing of the skin, a moderate degree of splenomegaly, and sometimes hepatomegaly. *SYN:* paroxysmal nocturnal hemoglobinuria; Marchiafava-Micheli anemia

Marcille, Maurice, 1871–1941.
Marcille triangle—an area bounded by the medial border of the psoas major, the lateral margin of the vertebral column, and the iliolumbar ligament below.

Marden, Philip M., U.S. physician.
Marden-Walker syndrome—autosomal recessive trait.

Marek, Josef, Hungarian veterinarian and pathologist, 1867–1952.
Marek disease—*SYN:* avian lymphomatosis
Marek disease virus—the herpesvirus that causes avian lymphomatosis. *SYN:* avian neurolymphomatosis virus

Marey, Étienne Jules, French physiologist, 1830–1904.
Marey law—the pulse rate varies inversely with the blood pressure.

Marfan, Antoine Bernard-Jean, French pediatrician, 1858–1942.
Dennie-Marfan syndrome—see under Dennie
Marfan disease—*SYN:* Marfan syndrome
Marfan law—the healing of localized tuberculosis protects against subsequent development of pulmonary tuberculosis.
Marfan syndrome—a syndrome of congenital changes in the mesodermal and ectodermal tissues, skeletal changes, ectopia lentis, and vascular defects. *SYN:* Marfan disease

M

Marg, Elwin, U.S. physicist, *1918.
Mackay-Marg tonometer—see under Mackay

Marghescu, S., German physician.
Marghescu and Braun-Falco syndrome—congenital poikiloderma, autosomal recessive trait.

Marie, Pierre, French neurologist, 1853–1940.
Bamberger-Marie disease—*SYN:* Bamberger-Marie syndrome
Bamberger-Marie syndrome—see under Bamberger, Eugen
Brissaud-Marie syndrome—see under Brissaud
Charcot-Marie-Tooth disease—see under Charcot
Debré-Marie syndrome—see under Debré
Foix-Cavany-Marie syndrome—see under Foix
Marie ataxia—obsolete term for a variety of non-Friedreich hereditary ataxias.
Marie I syndrome—*SYN:* Menzel syndrome
Marie II syndrome—endocrine and neurologic disorders.

(continued)

NOTES

Marie *(continued)*
   Marie-Leri syndrome—swelling of deformed joints.
   Marie-Sainton syndrome—excessive head development. *Syn:* cleidocranial
      dysplasia; cleidocranial dysostosis; Hulkcrantz anosteoplasia
   Marie-Strümpell disease—*Syn:* Strümpell-Marie disease
   Nonne-Marie syndrome—*Syn:* Menzel syndrome
   Strümpell-Marie disease—see under Strümpell

Marin Amat, Manuel, Spanish opthalmologist, *1879.
   Marin Amat syndrome—involuntary eye closure. *Syn:* Mueller-Kannberg
      syndrome

Marinesco, Georges, Romanian neurologist, 1863–1938.
   Marinesco succulent hand—edema of the hand with coldness and lividity
      of the skin, observed in syringomyelia. *Syn:* main succulente
   Marinesco-Radovici reflex—*Syn:* Radovici sign
   Marinesco-Sjögren syndrome—development and mental retardation. *Syn:*
      hereditary oligophrenic cerebellolental degeneration; oligophrenic
      cerebellolenticular degeneration; Garland-Moorhause syndrome; Sjögren
      II syndrome; Torsten syndrome
   Marinesco-Sjögren-Garland syndrome—a rare neurologic disorder
      characterized by cerebellolental degeneration with mental retardation.
      Syn: cataract-oligophrenia syndrome; Torsten Sjögren syndrome

Marion, Georges, French urologist, 1869–1932.
   Marion disease—a congenital obstruction of the posterior urethra.

Mariotte, Edmé, French physicist, 1620–1684.
   Mariotte blind spot—an oval area of the ocular fundus devoid of light
      receptors where the axons of the retinal ganglion cell converge to form
      the optic nerve head. *Syn:* optic disk
   Mariotte bottle—a stoppered bottle with bottom outlet, used as a
      reservoir for constant infusions.
   Mariotte experiment—an experiment that proves the absence of
      photoreceptors where the optic nerve enters the eye.
   Mariotte law—*Syn:* Boyle law

Marjolin, Jean N., French physician, 1780–1850.
   Marjolin syndrome—*Syn:* Marjolin ulcer
   Marjolin ulcer—well-differentiated but aggressive squamous cell
      carcinoma occurring in cicatricial tissue at the epidermal edge of a sinus
      draining underlying osteomyelitis. *Syn:* Marjolin syndrome; epidermoid
      ulcer

Markoe, Thomas Masters, U.S. physician, 1819–1901.
   Markoe abscess—chronic bone abscess.

Markoff, var. of Markov

Markov, Andrei, Russian mathematician, 1865–1922.
   Markov chain—number of steps or events in sequence.
   Markov chaining—a theory used in psychiatry.
   Markov process—a process such that the conditional probability
      distribution for the state at any future instant, given the present state, is
      unaffected by any additional knowledge of the past history of the system.

Markovits, A.S.
    Markovits syndrome—ocular pain.

Marlow, Frank William, U.S. ophthalmologist, 1858–1942.
    Marlow test—a test for heterophoria.

Maroteaux, Pierre, French medical geneticist, *1926.
    Maroteaux syndrome—metaphyseal dysostosis of the knees.
    Maroteaux-Lamy I syndrome—multiple genetic defects.
    Maroteaux-Lamy II syndrome—multiple genetic defects.
    Maroteaux-Lamy syndrome—an error of mucopolysaccharide metabolism characterized by excretion of dermatan sulfate in the urine, growth retardation, and skeletal deformities. *Syn:* type VI mucopolysaccharidosis; polydystrophic dwarfism
    Maroteaux-Spranger-Wiedemann syndrome—genetic defects.

Marshall, Don, U.S. ophthalmologist, *1905.
    Marshall syndrome—autosomal dominant trait.

Marshall, Eli K., U.S. pharmacologist, 1889–1966.
    Marshall method—a quantitative procedure for estimating free and conjugated sulfanilamide in body fluids.

Marshall, John, English anatomist, 1818–1891.
    Marshall oblique vein—a small vein on the posterior wall of the left atrium which merges with the great cardiac vein to form the coronary sinus. *Syn:* oblique vein of left atrium
    Marshall syndrome—inflamed edematous papules.
    Marshall vestigial fold—a pericardial fold containing the obliterated remains of the left superior vena cava. *Syn:* fold of left vena cava

Marshall, Richard E., U.S. physician.
    Marshall syndrome—clinical growth disorder. *Syn:* Marshall-Smith syndrome
    Marshall-Smith syndrome—*Syn:* Marshall syndrome

Marshall, Victor F., U.S. urologist, *1913.
    Marshall-Marchetti-Krantz operation—an operation for urinary stress incontinence, performed retropubically.

Marshall, Wallace, U.S. physician.
    Marshall-White syndrome—ischemic angiospastic spots on the palms of the hands. *Syn:* Bier syndrome; Bier spots

Martegiani, J., 19th century Italian anatomist.
    Martegiani area—*Syn:* Martegiani funnel
    Martegiani funnel—the funnel-shaped dilation on the optic disk that indicates the beginning of the hyaloid canal. *Syn:* Martegiani area

Martin, A.
    Bosviel-Martin syndrome—*Syn:* Martin syndrome
    Martin syndrome—hemorrhage of the uvula. *Syn:* apoplexia uvulae; Bosviel-Martin syndrome; staphylohematoma

NOTES

Martin, August E., German gynecologist, 1847–1933.
> **Martin tube**—a drainage tube with a cross piece near the extremity to keep it from slipping out of a cavity.
> **Martin-Gruber anastomosis**—a nerve anomaly in the forearm, consisting of a median to ulnar nerve communication.
> **Martin-Albright syndrome**—hereditary defects. *Syn:* Albright IV syndrome

Martin, Henry A., U.S. surgeon, 1824–1884.
> **Martin bandage**—a roller bandage of soft rubber used to make compression on a limb in the treatment of varicose veins or ulcers.
> **Martin cartilage clamp**
> **Martin disease**—a periosteoarthritis of the foot from excessive walking.
> **Martin incision**
> **Martin vigorimeter**

Martin, J.E.
> **Thayer-Martin agar**—see under Thayer
> **Thayer-Martin medium**—*Syn:* Thayer-Martin agar

Martin de Gimard, Jules Louis Alexandre, French physician, *1858.
> **Martin de Gimard syndrome**—necrotic purpura in children. *Syn:* de Gimard syndrome; Gimard syndrome

Martin du Pan, Charles, Swiss physician, 1878–1948.
> **Martin du Pan-Rutishauser syndrome**—joint ankylosis. *Syn:* laminar osteochondritis

Martinotti, Giovanni, Italian physician, 1857–1928.
> **Martinotti cell**—a small multipolar nerve cell of the cerebral cortex.

Martorell, Fernando Otzet, Spanish cardiologist, *1906.
> **Martorell syndrome**—atheromatous and/or thrombotic obliteration of the branches of the aortic arch. *Syn:* aortic arch syndrome

Martorell, R.
> **Martorell I syndrome**—above-the-ankle ulceration. *Syn:* hypertensive ischemic ulcer

Mashburn, Neely Cornelius, U.S. physician, *1886.
> **Mashburn complex coordinator**—instrument used in measuring eye-hand and foot coordination

Masini, Giulio, Italian physician, 1874–1937.
> **Masini sign**—a marked degree of dorsal extension of the fingers on the metacarpals and of the toes on the metatarsals, noted in children with mental instability.

Maslow, Abraham H., U.S. psychologist, 1908–1970.
> **Maslow hierarchy**—a ranking of needs that a human presumably fills successively in the order of lowest to highest: physiological needs, love and belonging, self-esteem, and self-actualization.
> **Maslow pyramid of needs**
> **Maslow theory of human motivation**

Mason, Edward E., U.S. surgeon, *1920.
> **Mason operation**—high division of the stomach used for treatment of morbid obesity. *Syn:* gastric bypass

Masselon, M. Julián, French physician, 1844–1917.
    Masselon glasses
    Masselon spectacles—spectacles that keep the upper eyelid raised above the pupil in cases of paralytic blepharoptosis. *SYN:* lid crutch spectacles

Masset, Alfred Auguste, French physician, *1870.
    Masset test—a test to show the presence of bile pigments.

Masshoff, Johann Wilhelm, German physician, *1908.
    Masshoff syndrome—mesenteric lymphadenitis.

Masson, C.L. Pierre, Canadian pathologist, 1880–1959.
    Fontana-Masson silver stain—*SYN:* Masson-Fontana ammoniacal silver stain
    Masson argentaffin stain
    Masson body—macrophages and fibrin found in pulmonary alveoli in organizing pneumonia.
    Masson pseudoangiosarcoma—a benign florid papillary endothelial proliferation within the veins of the skin or subcutis. *SYN:* intravascular papillary endothelial hyperplasia
    Masson trichrome stain
    Masson-Fontana ammoniacal silver stain—a stain used to demonstrate melanin and argentaffin granules. *SYN:* Fontana-Masson silver stain

M

Masson, W., scientist.
    Masson disk—measures threshold of brightness vision.

Master, Arthur M., U.S. physician, 1895–1973.
    Master test—a test requiring the subject to ascend and descend two nine-inch steps repeatedly, the number of trips determined from age- and sex-specific tables. *SYN:* Master two-step exercise test
    Master two-step exercise test—*SYN:* Master test

Masters, William H., U.S. gynecologist, *1915.
    Allen-Masters syndrome—see under Allen, Willard

Masugi, Matazo, Japanese pathologist, 1896–1947.
    Masugi nephritis—glomerulonephritis produced by injecting into rats a rabbit antiserum prepared against rat kidney tissue suspensions.

Matas, Rudolph, U.S. surgeon, 1860–1957.
    Matas operation—obsolete term for aneurysmoplasty.

Mathes, Paul, Austrian physician, 1871–1923.
    Mathes syndrome—breast pain with nursing. *SYN:* puerperal mastitis

Matsoukas, J.
    Matsoukas syndrome—genetic defects.

Matzenauer, Rudolf, Austrian dermatologist, *1861.
    Matzenauer-Pollard syndrome—spontaneous inflammatory skin lesions affecting women with dysmenorrhea. *SYN:* dermatitis symmetrica dysmenorrhagica

NOTES

Mauchart, Burkhard D., German anatomist, 1696–1751.
Mauchart ligaments

Maugeri, Salvatore, Italian physician, *1905.
Maugeri syndrome—cardiopulmonary symptoms associated with silicate exposure. *Syn:* silicotic mediastinopathy

Maumené, Edme Jules, French chemist, 1818–1891.
Maumené test—urine test for glucose.

Maumenee, A.E.
Maumenee syndrome—opacified and thickened corneas.

Maunoir, Jean Pierre, French physician, 1768–1861.
Maunoir hydrocele—serous dilatation of cervical cleft, duct, or cervical lymph space. *Syn:* cervical hydrocele
Maunoir iris scissors
Maunoir scissors

Maurer, Georg, German physician in Sumatra, *1909.
Maurer clefts—*Syn:* Maurer dots
Maurer dots—finely granular precipitates or irregular cytoplasmic particles that usually occur diffusely in red blood cells infected with the trophozoites of *Plasmodium falciparum. Syn:* Maurer clefts

Mauriac, Charles Marie Tamarelle, French physician, 1832–1905.
Mauriac syndrome—tertiary syphilis manifestation. *Syn:* erythema nodosum syphiliticum

Mauriac, Pierre, French physician, *1882.
Mauriac syndrome—complications of juvenile-onset diabetes mellitus. *Syn:* Pierre Mauriac syndrome
Pierre Mauriac syndrome—*Syn:* Mauriac syndrome

Mauriceau, François, French obstetrician, 1637–1709.
Mauriceau maneuver—a method of assisted breech delivery. *Syn:* Mauriceau-Levret maneuver
Mauriceau-Levret maneuver—*Syn:* Mauriceau maneuver

Mauthner, Ludwig, Austrian ophthalmologist, 1840–1894.
Mauthner cell—a large neuron of the spinal cord with its cell body located in the metencephalon of fish and amphibia.
Mauthner fiber—an axon.
Mauthner sheath—the plasma membrane of the axon. *Syn:* axolemma
Mauthner test—an obsolete test for color perception similar to Holmgren test, but made with vials filled with pigments instead of with skeins of wool.

Maxcy, Kenneth Fuller, U.S. bacteriologist, *1889.
Maxcy disease—a type of typhoid fever endemic in the southern United States.

Maxim, Charles Hiram, U.S. physician, 1839–1887.
Maxim-Gilbert sequencing—a method of sequencing DNA using dimethyl sulfate and hydrazinolysis.

Maximow, Alexander A., Russian physician in U.S., 1874–1928.
Maximow stain for bone marrow

Maxwell, Patrick William, Irish ophthalmologist, 1856–1917.
    Maxwell ring—a small faint ring in the visual field.

May, Duane L., 20th century U.S. physician.
    May-White syndrome—autosomal dominant trait causing progressive myoclonus epilepsy with lipomas, deafness, and ataxia.

May, Richard, German physician, 1863–1936.
    May-Hegglin anomaly—*SYN:* Hegglin anomaly
    May-Hegglin syndrome—*SYN:* Hegglin syndrome

Maydl, Karl, Austrian physician, 1853–1903.
    Maydl colostomy
    Maydl disease
    Maydl hernia
    Maydl operation
    Maydl pessary

Mayer, Karl, Austrian neurologist, 1862–1932.
    Mayer reflex—apposition and adduction of the thumb. *SYN:* basal joint reflex

Mayer, Karl, W., German gynecologist, 1795–1868.
    Mayer pessary—elastic ring pessary. *SYN:* Dumontpallier pessary
    Mayer position
    Mayer speculum

Mayer, Paul, German histologist, 1848–1923.
    Mayer hemalum stain—a progressive nuclear stain also used as a counterstain.
    Mayer mucicarmine stain
    Mayer mucihematein stain
    Mayer-Rokitansky-Küster-Hauser syndrome—congenital absence of the vagina. *SYN:* Rokitansky-Küster-Hauser syndrome

Mayo, Charles H., U.S. surgeon, 1865–1939.
    Mayo bunionectomy—excision of the head of the first metatarsal.
    Mayo cannula
    Mayo carpal instability classification
    Mayo carrier
    Mayo clamp
    Mayo elbow prosthesis
    Mayo forceps
    Mayo hemostat
    Mayo herniorrhaphy
    Mayo hook
    Mayo instrument table
    Mayo knife
    Mayo needle
    Mayo needle holder

M

(continued)

NOTES

Mayo (*continued*)
>**Mayo nerve block**
>**Mayo probe**
>**Mayo resection arthroplasty**
>**Mayo retractor**
>**Mayo scissors**
>**Mayo scoop**
>**Mayo semiconstrained elbow prosthesis**
>**Mayo stripper**
>**Mayo suture**
>**Mayo total ankle prosthesis**
>**Mayo total elbow arthroplasty**
>**Mayo-Gibbon heart-lung machine**
>**Mayo-Hegar needle holder**

Mayo, William J., U.S. surgeon, 1861–1939.
>**Mayo operation**—an operation for the radical cure of umbilical hernia.
>**Mayo vein**—*Syn:* prepyloric vein

Mayo-Robson, Sir Arthur W., English surgeon, 1853–1933.
>**Mayo-Robson point**—a point just above and to the right of the umbilicus, where tenderness on pressure exists in disease of the pancreas.
>**Mayo-Robson position**—a supine position used in gallbladder operations.

Mayou, Marmaduke Stephen, English ophthalmologist, 1876–1934.
>**Batten-Mayou disease**—*Syn:* Batten disease

Mazzoni, Vittorio, Italian physician, 1880–1940.
>**Golgi-Mazzoni corpuscle**—see under Golgi
>**Mazzoni corpuscle**—a tactile corpuscle apparently identical with Krause end bulb.

McArdle, Brian, 20th century English neurologist.
>**McArdle disease**—*Syn:* McArdle syndrome
>**McArdle syndrome**—glycogenosis due to muscle glycogen phosphorylase deficiency, resulting in accumulation of glycogen of normal chemical structure in muscle. *Syn:* type 5 glycogenosis; Cori syndrome; McArdle-Schmid-Pearson syndrome; McArdle disease
>**McArdle-Schmid-Pearson disease**—*Syn:* McArdle syndrome

McBride, Earl D., U.S. orthopedic surgeon, *1891.
>**McBride bunion repair**—*Syn:* McBride bunionectomy
>**McBride bunionectomy**—removal of a bunion. *Syn:* McBride bunion repair; McBride operation
>**McBride cup**
>**McBride femoral prosthesis**
>**McBride operation**—*Syn:* McBride bunionectomy
>**McBride pin**
>**McBride plate**
>**McBride procedure**
>**McBride prosthesis**
>**McBride tripod**
>**McBride tripod pin traction**

McBurney, Charles, U.S. surgeon, 1845–1913.

    McBurney incision—an incision parallel with the course of the external oblique muscle, one or two inches cephalad to the anterior superior spine of the ilium.

    McBurney inguinal herniorrhaphy—*Syn:* McBurney operation

    McBurney operation—surgery to repair inguinal hernia. *Syn:* McBurney inguinal herniorrhaphy

    McBurney point—a point where pressure elicits tenderness in acute appendicitis.

    McBurney retractor

    McBurney sign—tenderness at site two-thirds of the distance between the umbilicus and the anterior-superior iliac spine seen in appendicitis.

McCarthy, Daniel J., U.S. neurologist, 1874–1958.

    McCarthy reflexes—(1) contraction of the adductors of the thigh upon tapping the spinal column. *Syn:* spinoadductor reflex; (2) contraction of the orbicularis oculi muscle induced by tapping the supraorbital nerve. *Syn:* supraorbital reflex.

    McCarthy scales of children's abilities—used to test children's comprehension between 2–1/2 and 8–1/2 years of age.

McCarthy, Joseph Francis, U.S. urologist, 1874–1965.

    McCarthy catheter

    McCarthy coagulation electrode

    McCarthy cystoscope

    McCarthy electrotome

    McCarthy evacuator

    McCarthy forceps

    McCarthy panendoscope

    McCarthy resectoscope

    McCarthy telescope

M

McClintock, Barbara, winner of 1983 Nobel Prize for work related to genetics.

McCrea, Lowrain E., U.S. urologist, *1896.

    McCrea cystoscope

    McCrea sound

McCune, Donovan James, U.S. pediatrician, 1902–1976.

    McCune-Albright syndrome—polyostotic fibrous dysplasia with irregular brown patches of cutaneous pigmentation and endocrine dysfunction, especially precocious puberty in girls. *Syn:* Albright disease; Albright syndrome (1)

McDonald, Ellice, U.S. gynecologist, 1876–1955.

    McDonald cerclage

    McDonald clamp

    McDonald maneuver—measurement of uterus to approximate gestational age in weeks.

(continued)

NOTES

McDonald *(continued)*
> **McDonald measurement**
> **McDonald pelvimetry**
> **McDonald procedure**
> **McDonald rule**—a rule to determine the lunar months of pregnancy.

McEvedy, Peter George, English surgeon, 1890–1951.
> **McEvedy approach**—an approach used in femoral herniorrhaphy.

McFarlane, D.C.
> **Oliver-McFarlane syndrome**—see under Oliver

McGoon, Dwight C., U.S. surgeon, *1925.
> **McGoon technique**—plastic reconstruction of an incompetent mitral valve.

McIndoe, Sir Archibald Hector, English surgeon, 1900–1960.
> **McIndoe chisel**
> **McIndoe elevator**
> **McIndoe forceps**
> **McIndoe incision**
> **McIndoe operation**
> **McIndoe rasp**
> **McIndoe retractor**
> **McIndoe scissors**
> **McIndoe vaginal creation**
> **McIndoe vaginal reconstruction**

McIntosh, James, English pathologist and bacteriologist, *1916.
> **McIntosh-Fildes jar**

McKee, George Kenneth, English orthopedic surgeon, *1930.
> **McKee brace**
> **McKee femoral prosthesis**
> **McKee line**
> **McKee prosthesis**
> **McKee table**
> **McKee totally constrained elbow prosthesis**
> **McKee tri-fin nail**
> **McKee-Farrar acetabular cup**
> **McKee-Farrar hip prosthesis**

McKittrick, Leland Sterling, U.S. physician, *1892.
> **McKittrick syndrome**—colon and rectal villous adenoma, with electrolyte imbalance. *Syn:* McKittrick-Wheelock syndrome
> **McKittrick-Wheelock syndrome**—*Syn:* McKittrick syndrome

McKusick, Victor Almon, U.S. physician, *1921.
> **Cross-McKusick-Breen syndrome**
> **McKusick syndrome**—dwarfism; autosomal recessive trait. *Syn:* McKusick-Cross syndrome
> **McKusick-Cross syndrome**—*Syn:* McKusick syndrome
> **McKusick-Dungy-Kaufman syndrome**—*Syn:* McKusick-Kaufman syndrome
> **McKusick-Kaufman syndrome**—autosomal recessive trait. *Syn:* Kaufman syndrome; McKusick-Dungy-Kaufman syndrome

McLean, Malcolm, U.S. obstetrician, 1848–1924.
    Tucker-McLean forceps—see under Tucker

McMurray, Thomas P., English surgeon, *1889.
    McMurray knife
    McMurray maneuver
    McMurray osteotomy
    McMurray sign
    McMurray test—rotation of the tibia on the femur.

McNemar, Quinn, U.S. psychologist and statistician, *1900.
    Terman-McNemar test of mental ability—see under Terman

McPhail, M.K., Canadian physiologist, *1907.
    McPhail test—a test for progesterone.

McQuarrie, I.
    McQuarrie syndrome—signs of hypoglycemia.

McReynolds, John O., U.S. ophthalmologist, 1865–1942.
    McReynolds eye spatula
    McReynolds keratome
    McReynolds operation
    McReynolds pterygium knife
    McReynolds pterygium scissors
    McReynolds pterygium transplant
    McReynolds technique

McVay, Chester B., U.S. surgeon, *1911.
    McVay herniorrhaphy—*SYN:* McVay operation
    McVay incision
    McVay operation—repair of inguinal and femoral hernias. *SYN:* McVay
    herniorrhaphy

MD Anderson, cancer research hospital in Houston, Texas.
    MD Anderson grading system

Meadows, William Robert, U.S. cardiologist, *1919.
    Meadows syndrome—postpartum myocardiopathy.

Mean, James Howard, U.S. endocrinologist, 1885–1967.
    Mean sign—lag of the eyeball on upward gaze.

Mechnikov, Ilya Ilyich, 1908 joint winner of Nobel Prize for work related to
immunity.

Meckel, Johann F., the elder, German anatomist and obstetrician, 1714–1774.
    Meckel band—the portion of the anterior ligament of the malleus that
    extends from the base of the anterior process through the petrotympanic
    fissure, to attach to the spine of the sphenoid. *SYN:* Meckel ligament
    Meckel cave

(continued)

M

NOTES

Meckel *(continued)*

 Meckel cavity—*Syn:* Meckel space

 Meckel ganglion—a small parasympathetic ganglion in the upper part of the pterygopalatine fossa. *Syn:* pterygopalatine ganglion

 Meckel ligament—*Syn:* Meckel band

 Meckel space—the cleft in the meningeal layer of dura of the middle cranial fossa that encloses the roots of the trigeminal nerve and the trigeminal ganglion. *Syn:* trigeminal cave; Meckel cavity

 Meckel sphenopalatine ganglionectomy

Meckel, Johann F., the younger, German anatomist and embryologist, 1781–1833.

 Meckel cartilage—a temporary supporting structure in the embryonic mandible. *Syn:* mandibular cartilage

 Meckel diverticulum—the remains of the yolk stalk of the embryo.

 Meckel plane—a craniometric plane cutting the alveolar and the auricular points.

 Meckel scan—use of technetium-99m pertechnetate in a scan of the gastric mucosa to detect ectopic gastric mucosa in Meckel diverticulum.

 Meckel syndrome—*Syn:* Meckel-Gruber syndrome

 Meckel-Gruber syndrome—a malformation syndrome. *Syn:* dysencephalia splanchnocystica; Meckel syndrome

Medawar, Sir Peter Brian, joint winner of 1960 Nobel Prize for work related to immunology.

Medea, from Greek mythology: Medea killed the children fathered by Jason after he left her for a younger woman.

 Medea complex—a mother's compulsion to kill her children as revenge against their father.

Medin, Karl O., Swedish physician, 1847–1927.

 Medin poliomyelitis

Medusa, in Greek mythology, a Gorgon who turned men to stone.

 caput Medusae—(1) varicose veins radiating from the umbilicus; (2) dilated ciliary arteries girdling the corneoscleral limbus in rubeosis iridis. *Syn:* head of Medusa

 head of Medusa—*Syn:* caput Medusae

Meeh, K., 19th century German physiologist.

 Meeh formula—*Syn:* Meeh-Dubois formula

 Meeh-DuBois formula—a formula for predicting surface area. *Syn:* Meeh formula

Mees, R.A., 20th century Dutch physician.

 Mees lines—transverse white lines that appear in the nails that occur after poisoning or severe systemic disorders.

Meesmann, Alois, German ophthalmologist, 1888–1969.

 Meesmann dystrophy—corneal dystrophy; autosomal dominant trait. *Syn:* Meesmann-Wilke syndrome; Meesmann-Wilke disease; Meesmann syndrome

 Meesmann syndrome—*Syn:* Meesmann dystrophy

 Meesmann-Wilke disease—*Syn:* Meesmann dystrophy

 Meesmann-Wilke syndrome—*Syn:* Meesmann dystrophy

Méglin, J.A., French physician, 1756–1824.
Méglin point—where the greater palatine nerve emerges from the great palatine foramen.

Meibom, Hendrik (Heinrich), German anatomist, 1638–1700.
meibomian conjunctivitis—an obsolete term for a conjunctivitis associated with chronic inflammation of the meibomian glands, with swollen tarsal plates and frothy seborrheic secretion. *Syn:* seborrheic blepharoconjunctivitis
meibomian cyst—a chronic inflammatory granuloma of a meibomian gland. *Syn:* chalazion
meibomian glands—sebaceous glands embedded in the tarsal plate of each eyelid, discharging at the edge of the lid near the posterior border. *Syn:* tarsal glands
meibomian sty—an acute purulent infection of a meibomian (tarsal) gland. *Syn:* hordeolum internum

Meier, Georg, German serologist, *1875.
Porges-Meier test—see under Porges

Meier, Norman Charles, U.S. psychologist, 1893–1967.
Meier art judgment test—used to determine an individual's artistic abilities.

Meige, Henri, French physician, 1866–1940.
Meige disease—autosomal dominant lymphedema.
Nonne-Milroy-Meige syndrome—see under Nonne

Meigs, Joseph V., U.S. gynecologist, 1892–1963.
Demons-Meigs syndrome—*Syn:* Meigs syndrome
Meigs curet
Meigs hemostat
Meigs operation
Meigs retractor
Meigs suture
Meigs syndrome—adnexal mass; uterine prolapse. *Syn:* Demons-Meigs syndrome; Meigs-Cass syndrome
Meigs-Cass syndrome—*Syn:* Meigs syndrome

Meinicke, Ernst, German physician, 1878–1945.
Meinicke test—the first successful application of immune precipitation to diagnosis of syphilis, now obsolete.

Meissner, Georg, German histologist, 1829–1905.
Meissner corpuscle—one of numerous oval bodies found in the papillae of the skin, especially those of the fingers and toes. *Syn:* tactile corpuscle
Meissner ganglion
Meissner plexus—a gangliated plexus of unmyelinated nerve fibers. *Syn:* submucosal plexus

M

NOTES

Meleney, Frank L., U.S. surgeon, 1889–1963.
    Meleney gangrene—*Syn:* Meleney ulcer
    Meleney infection
    Meleney ulcer—undermining ulcer of the skin and subcutaneous tissues, usually following an operation. *Syn:* Meleney gangrene; progressive bacterial synergistic gangrene

Melkersson, Ernst G., Swedish physician, 1898–1932.
    Melkersson syndrome—*Syn:* Melkersson-Rosenthal syndrome
    Melkersson-Rosenthal syndrome—cheilitis granulomatosum, fissured tongue, and facial nerve paralysis. *Syn:* Melkersson syndrome; Miescher cheilitis

Melnick, John C., U.S. radiologist, *1928.
    Melnick-Needles syndrome—a generalized skeletal dysplasia with prominent forehead and small mandible. *Syn:* osteodysplasty

Melotte, George W., U.S. dentist, 1835–1915.
    Melotte metal—a soft, fusable alloy.

Meltzer, Martin, U.S. physician, *1930.
    Meltzer syndrome—vascular, renal, and arthritic disturbances.

Meltzer, Samuel J., U.S. physiologist, 1851–1920.
    Meltzer law—all living functions are continually controlled by two opposite forces: augmentation and inhibition. *Syn:* law of contrary innervation
    Meltzer sign—loss of second sound on auscultation of the heart after swallowing.
    Meltzer-Lyon test—a test used in diagnosis of gallbladder conditions.

Mendel, Gregor J., Austrian geneticist, 1822–1884.
    Mendel first law—factors that affect development retain their individuality from generation to generation, do not become contaminated when mixed in a hybrid, and become sorted out from one another when the next generation of gametes is formed. *Syn:* law of segregation
    Mendel second law—different hereditary factors assort independently when the gametes are formed. *Syn:* law of independent assortment
    mendelian character—an inherited character under the control of a single locus.
    mendelian inheritance—inheritance in which stable and undecomposable characters controlled by a single genetic locus are transmitted over many generations. *Syn:* alternative inheritance
    mendelian ratio—the ratio of progeny with a particular phenotype or genotype expected in accordance with Mendel law among the offspring of matings specified as to genotype or phenotype.

Mendel, Kurt, German neurologist, 1874–1946.
    Bekhterev-Mendel reflex—see under Bekhterev, Vladimir
    Mendel instep reflex—the foot being firmly supported on its inner side, a sharp tap on the dorsal tendons causes extension of the second to the fifth toes. *Syn:* back of foot reflex
    Mendel-Bekhterev reflex—*Syn:* Bekhterev-Mendel reflex

Mendeléeff, Dimitri (Dmitri) I., Russian chemist, 1834–1907.
Mendeléeff law—the properties of elements are periodical functions of their atomic weights. *SYN:* periodic law
mendelevium—an element, atomic No. 101, atomic weight 258.1, prepared in 1955 by bombardment of einsteinium with alpha particles.

Mendelson, Curtis L., U.S. obstetrician, *1913.
Mendelson syndrome—aspiration pneumonia in obstetrical patients.

Mendes Da Costa, S.
Mendes Da Costa syndrome—edema.

Ménétrier, Pierre E., French physician, 1859–1935.
Ménétrier disease—gastric mucosal hyperplasia. *SYN:* hypertrophic gastritis; giant hypertrophy of gastric mucosa; Ménétrier syndrome
Ménétrier syndrome—*SYN:* Ménétrier disease

Menge, Karl, German gynecologist, 1864–1945.
Menge operation
Menge pessary—a ring pessary.

Mengo, a region of Uganda where virus was discovered in animals in 1948.
Mengo encephalomyelitis—*SYN:* Mengo virus
Mengo virus—a strain of encephalomyocarditis. *SYN:* Mengo encephalomyelitis

Ménière, Prosper, French physician, 1799–1862.
Ménière disease—characterized by vertigo, nausea, vomiting, tinnitus, and progressive deafness due to swelling of the endolymphatic duct. *SYN:* endolymphatic hydrops; Ménière syndrome; auditory vertigo; labyrinthine vertigo
Ménière syndrome—*SYN:* Ménière disease

Menkes, John H., U.S. neurologist, *1928.
Menkes disease
Menkes syndrome—congenital defect of copper metabolism. *SYN:* kinky-hair disease; steely-hair syndrome

Mennell, James Beaver, English physician, 1880–1957.
Mennell sign—a test for sensitive ligaments.

Mensendieck, Bess M., U.S. physician, 1861–1957.
Mensendieck exercises—physical education system.

Menten, Maud L., Canadian pathologist in U.S., 1879–1960.
Michaelis-Menten constant—*SYN:* Michaelis constant
Michaelis-Menten equation—see under Michaelis
Michaelis-Menten hypothesis—see under Michaelis
Victor-Michaelis-Menten equation—*SYN:* Michaelis-Menten equation

Menzel, P.
Menzel syndrome—cerebellar ataxia. *SYN:* Marie I syndrome; Nonne-Marie syndrome; Sanger-Brown syndrome

M

NOTES

Mercier, Louis A., French urologist, 1811–1882.
>**median bar of Mercier**—a prominent band of fibromuscular tissue involving the interureteric ridge or neck of the urinary bladder.
>**Mercier bar**—a fold of mucous membrane extending from the orifice of the ureter of one side to that of the other side. *Syn:* interureteric fold
>**Mercier catheter**
>**Mercier sound**—a catheter the beak of which is short and bent almost at a right angle.
>**Mercier valve**—an occasional fold of mucosa of the bladder partially occluding the ureteral orifice.

Merendino, K. Alvin, U.S. surgeon, *1914.
>**Merendino technique**—plastic reconstruction of an incompetent mitral valve.

Meretoja, J., 20th century Finnish physician.
>**Meretoja syndrome**—interstitial amyloid accumulation. *Syn:* amyloidosis

Merkel, Friedrich S., German anatomist and physiologist, 1845–1919.
>**Merkel cell tumor**—a rare malignant cutaneous tumor. *Syn:* trabecular carcinoma; primary neuroendocrine carcinoma of the skin
>**Merkel corpuscle**—a specialized tactile sensory nerve ending in the epidermis. *Syn:* tactile meniscus; Merkel tactile cell; Merkel tactile disk
>**Merkel tactile cell**—*Syn:* Merkel corpuscle
>**Merkel tactile disk**—*Syn:* Merkel corpuscle

Merkel, Julius, German psychologist.
>**Merkel law**—principle used in psychology.

Merkel, Karl L., German anatomist and laryngologist, 1812–1876.
>**Merkel filtrum ventriculi**—a groove between the two prominences in each lateral wall of the vestibule of the larynx. *Syn:* filtrum ventriculi
>**Merkel fossa**—a groove in the posterolateral wall of the vestibule of the larynx between the corniculate and cuneiform cartilages.
>**Merkel muscle**—a fasciculus from the posterior cricoarytenoid muscle inserted into the inferior horn of the thyroid cartilage. *Syn:* ceratocricoid muscle

Merrifield, R. Bruce, U.S. biochemist and Nobel laureate, *1921.
>**Merrifield synthesis**—the synthesis of peptides and proteins via an automated system on carrier polymers.

Merritt, Katharine K., U.S. pediatrician, *1886.
>**Kasabach-Merritt syndrome**—see under Kasabach

Merten, David F., U.S. radiologist.
>**Singleton-Merten syndrome**—see under Singleton

Merwarth, H.R.
>**Merwarth syndrome**—progressive hemiplegia due to venous occlusion. *Syn:* cerebral venous thrombosis

Méry, Jean, French anatomist, 1645–1722.
>**Méry gland**—one of two small compound racemose glands that discharge through a small duct into the spongy portion of the urethra. *Syn:* bulbourethral gland

Merzbacher, Ludwig, German physician in Argentina, 1875–1942.
Merzbacher-Pelizaeus disease—*SYN:* Pelizaeus-Merzbacher disease
Pelizaeus-Merzbacher disease—see under Pelizaeus

Mesmer, Franz Anton, Austrian physician, 1733–1815.
mesmeric crisis—reaction technique *SYN:* magnetic crisis; grand crisis
mesmerism—the use of hypnotism as practiced by Mesmer.

Metchnikoff, Elie, Russian biologist in France and Nobel laureate, 1845–1916.
Metchnikoff cellular immunity theory
Metchnikoff theory—the theory that the body is protected against infection by leukocytes and other cells.

Mett, Emil Ludwig Paul, German physician, *1867.
Mett test—a test for digestion.
Mett tube—glass tube filled with coagulated egg white.

Meyenburg, H. von, Swiss pathologist, *1877.
Meyenburg complex—clusters of small bile ducts occurring in polycystic livers, separate from the portal areas.
Meyenburg disease—a degenerative disease of cartilage. *SYN:* relapsing polychondritis; Meyenburg-Altherr-Uehlinger syndrome; von Meyenburg disease
Meyenburg-Altherr-Uehlinger syndrome—*SYN:* Meyenburg disease
von Meyenburg disease—*SYN:* Meyenburg disease

M

Meyer, Adolf, U.S. psychiatrist, 1866–1950.
Meyer temporal loop
Meyer-Archambault loop—the fibers of the visual radiation that loop around the tip of the temporal horn.

Meyer, Edmund V., German laryngologist, 1864–1931.
Meyer cartilages—the anterior sesamoid cartilages at the anterior attachments of the vocal ligaments.

Meyer, Georg H., Swiss anatomist, 1815–1892.
Meyer line—a line through the axis of the big toe and passing the midpoint of the heel in a normal foot.
Meyer posture—normal posture of standing subject.
Meyer sinus—a small concavity in the floor of the external auditory canal near the tympanic membrane.

Meyer, Hans H., German pharmacologist, 1853–1939.
Meyer-Overton rule—because inhalation agents act via the lipid-rich central nervous system cells, anesthetic potency increases with lipid solubility.
Meyer-Overton theory of narcosis—that narcotic efficiency parallels the coefficient of partition between oil and water, and that lipoids in the cell and on the cell membrane absorb the drug because of this affinity. *SYN:* lipoid theory of narcosis

NOTES

Meyer, Willy, U.S. surgeon, 1854–1932.
Meyer reagent—a solution to detect minute traces of blood.

Meyer-Betz, Friedrich, 20th century German physician.
Meyer-Betz disease—*SYN:* Meyer-Betz syndrome
Meyer-Betz syndrome—excretion of myoglobin in the urine resulting from muscle degeneration. *SYN:* myoglobinuria; Meyer-Betz disease

Meyer-Schwickerath, Gerhard Rudolph Edmund, German ophthalmologist, *1920.
Meyer-Schwickerath coagulator

Meyerhof, Otto F., German-U.S. biochemist and Nobel laureate, 1884–1951.
Embden-Meyerhof pathway—see under Embden
Embden-Meyerhof-Parnas pathway—*SYN:* Embden-Meyerhof pathway
Meyerhof oxidation quotient—an index for the effect of oxygen on glycolysis and on fermentation.

Meynert, Theodor H., Austrian neurologist, 1833–1892.
Meynert cells—solitary pyramidal cells found in the cortex in the region of the calcarine fissure.
Meynert commissures—the commissural fibers that lie above and behind the optic chiasm. *SYN:* commissurae supraopticae
Meynert decussation
Meynert fasciculus—a compact bundle of fibers in the midbrain. *SYN:* retroflex fasciculus; Meynert retroflex bundle
Meynert layer—layer three of the cortex cerebri. *SYN:* pyramidal cell layer
Meynert retroflex bundle—*SYN:* Meynert fasciculus

Meynet, Paul Claude Hyacinthe, French physician, 1831–1892.
Meynet nodes—nodules in joint capsules and tendons in rheumatic disorders.

Mibelli, Vittorio, Italian dermatologist, 1860–1910.
Mibelli angiokeratomas—telangiectatic small papules of the extremities, common in adolescent girls.
Mibelli disease—*SYN:* Mibelli syndrome
Mibelli syndrome—eruption of miliary translucent papules. *SYN:* porokeratosis; Mibelli disease

Michaelis, Leonor, German-U.S. chemist, 1875–1949.
Michaelis buffer
Michaelis constant—the true dissociation constant for the enzyme-substrate binary complex in a single-substrate rapid equilibrium enzyme-catalyzed reaction. *SYN:* Michaelis-Menten constant
Michaelis-Gutmann body—a rounded homogenous body containing calcium and iron found within macrophages in the bladder wall in malakoplakia.
Michaelis-Menten constant—*SYN:* Michaelis constant
Michaelis-Menten equation—an initial-rate equation for a single-substrate noncooperative enzyme-catalyzed reaction relating the initial velocity to the initial substrate concentration. *SYN:* Victor-Michaelis-Menten equation
Michaelis-Menten hypothesis—that a complex is formed between an enzyme and its substrate (the O'Sullivan-Tompson hypothesis), which

complex then decomposes to yield free enzyme and the reaction products (Brown hypothesis), the latter rate determining the overall rate of substrate-product conversion.

Victor-Michaelis-Menten equation—*Syn:* Michaelis-Menten equation

Michel, Gaston, French surgeon, 1874–1937.
Michel clip
Michel deformity
Michel forceps
Michel malformation
Michel mirror
Michel pick
Michel spur
Michel trephine

Micheli, Ferdinando, Italian physician, 1872–1936.
Marchiafava-Micheli anemia—*Syn:* Marchiafava-Micheli syndrome
Marchiafava-Micheli syndrome—see under Marchiafava

Michotte, L.J., French physician.
Michotte syndrome—*Syn:* Baastrup syndrome

Middeldorpf, K., German physician.
Middeldorpf splint
Middeldorpf triangle
Middeldorpf tumor—congenital sacral tumor.

Miehlke, A.
Miehlke-Partsch syndrome—deformities of neonates which are caused by thalidomide. *Syn:* thalidomide-induced phocomelia

Mierzejewski, Jan Lucian, Polish neurologist and psychiatrist, 1839–1908.
Mierzejewski effect—development of excessive gray brain matter.

Miescher, Guido, Swiss dermatologist, 1877–1961.
Miescher cheilitis—*Syn:* Melkersson-Rosenthal syndrome
Miescher I syndrome—benign velvety warty growths. *Syn:* acanthosis nigricans
Miescher II syndrome—inflammatory granulomas of the lips. *Syn:* granulomatous cheilitis
Miescher trichofolliculoma—benign tumor of the hair follicle *Syn:* hair follicle tumor
Miescher-Leder syndrome—reddish granulomatous plaques. *Syn:* granuloma disciformis; necrobiosis maculosa

Miescher, Johann F., Swiss pathologist, 1811–1887.
Miescher elastoma—circinate groups of hyperkeratotic papules associated with pseudoxanthoma elasticum.

(continued)

NOTES

329

Miescher *(continued)*
    Miescher granuloma—an annular eruption on sun-exposed skin. *SYN:* actinic granuloma
    Miescher tubes—elongate fusiform or cylindrical bodies forming the encapsulated cystic intramuscular stage of the protozoan *Sarcocystis.*

Mietens, Carl, German physician.
    Mietens-Weber syndrome—autosomal recessive defects.

Migula, Walter, German naturalist, 1863–1938.
    Migula classification—a bacteria classification.

Mikaelian, (origin unknown).
    Mikaelian syndrome—probable autosomal recessive trait. *SYN:* ectodermal dysplasia with hearing loss

Mikity, Victor G., U.S. radiologist, *1919.
    Wilson-Mikity syndrome—see under Wilson, Miriam

Mikulicz, Johannes von-Radecki, Polish surgeon in Germany, 1850–1905.
    Heineke-Mikulicz herniorrhaphy—see under Heineke
    Heineke-Mikulicz pyloroplasty—see under Heineke
    Mikulicz angle
    Mikulicz aphthae—a severe form of aphthae. *SYN:* aphthae major
    Mikulicz cells
    Mikulicz clamp
    Mikulicz crusher
    Mikulicz disease—benign swelling of the lacrimal, and usually also of the salivary glands, in consequence of an infiltration of and replacement of the normal gland structure by lymphoid tissue.
    Mikulicz drain
    Mikulicz forceps
    Mikulicz incision
    Mikulicz operation
    Mikulicz pack
    Mikulicz pad
    Mikulicz retractor
    Mikulicz sponge
    Mikulicz syndrome—symptoms characteristic of Mikulicz disease occurring as a complication of some other disease, such as lymphoma or leukemia.
    Mikulicz-Vladimiroff amputation—an osteoplastic resection of the foot. *SYN:* Vladimiroff-Mikulicz amputation
    Vladimiroff-Mikulicz amputation—*SYN:* Mikulicz-Vladimiroff amputation

Miles, William E., English surgeon, 1869–1947.
    Miles clamp
    Miles clip
    Miles operation—combined abdominoperineal resection for rectal carcinoma. *SYN:* Miles resection
    Miles punch biopsy forceps
    Miles resection—*SYN:* Miles operation
    Miles retractor

Milian, Gaston Auguste, French physician, 1871–1945.
    Milian disease—*SYN:* Milian syndrome

Milian erythema—*SYN:* Milian syndrome
Milian syndrome—reaction to arsenophenamine compounds. *SYN:* ninth-day erythema; Milian erythema; Milian disease

Milkman, Louis A., U.S. radiologist, 1895–1951.
Milkman fracture
Milkman syndrome—osteomalacia with multiple pseudofractures.

Millar, John, Scottish physician, 1733–1805.
Millar asthma—stridorous laryngismus.

Millard, Auguste L.J., French physician, 1830–1915.
Millard-Gubler syndrome—*SYN:* Gubler syndrome

Millard, Henry B., U.S. physician, 1832–1893.
Millard test—a test for albumin.

Miller, James Q., U.S. physician.
Miller-Dieker syndrome—arrested brain development. *SYN:* lissencephaly; Norman-Roberts syndrome

Miller, Thomas Grier, U.S. physician, *1886.
Miller-Abbott catheter—*SYN:* Miller-Abbott tube
Miller-Abbott tube—a double-lumen tube used for intestinal decompression. *SYN:* Abbott tube; Miller-Abbott catheter

Miller, Willoughby D., U.S. dentist, 1853–1907.
Miller chemicoparasitic theory—that dental caries is caused by microorganisms of the mouth fermenting dietary carbohydrates and producing acids that demineralize the teeth.

Millikan, Clark Harold, U.S. neurologist, *1915.
Millikan-Siekert syndrome—stenosis of proximal subclavian artery. *SYN:* basilar artery insufficiency

Millin, Terence John, English and Irish surgeon, *1890.
Millin clamp
Millin forceps
Millin operation
Millin prostatectomy
Millin retractor
Millin tube

Millon, Auguste N.E., French chemist, 1812–1867.
Millon reaction—used to test for proteins.
Millon reagent—mercuric nitrate and nitric acid as used in the Millon reaction.
Millon-Nasse test—a test for protein.

Mills, Charles Karsner, U.S. physician, 1845–1931.
Mills disease—slowly progressive paralysis. *SYN:* ascending hemiplegia

M

NOTES

Milroy, William F., U.S. physician, 1855–1942.
Milroy disease—the congenital type of autosomal dominant lymphedema.
Nonne-Milroy-Meige syndrome—see under Nonne

Milstein, César, Argentinian-English immunologist, joint winner of 1984 Nobel Prize for work related to immune system.

Milton, John L., English dermatologist, 1820–1898.
Milton disease—recurrent large circumscribed areas of subcutaneous edema of sudden onset, usually disappearing within 24 hours. *Syn:* angioedema

Minamata, bay in Japan where condition first observed.
Minamata syndrome—paresthesias and degenerative changes caused by ingestion of fish contaminated by methyl mercury. *Syn:* alkyl mercury poisoning

Minerva, Roman goddess of warfare and memory.
Minerva cast
Minerva collar
Minerva jacket—plaster cast made for stabilization of the vertebra.

Minkowski, Oskar, German physician, 1858–1931.
Minkowski-Chauffard syndrome—familial blood disorder; autosomal dominant trait.

Minkowsky, var. of Minkowski

Minor, Lazar Salomonovich, Russian physician, 1855–1942.
Minor syndrome—paralysis caused by hemorrhage into the spinal cord. *Syn:* central hematomyelia; Minor-Oppenheim syndrome
Minor-Oppenheim syndrome—*Syn:* Minor syndrome

Minot, George Richards, U.S. physician and Nobel laureate, 1885–1950.
Minot-Murphy diet—the use of large amounts of raw liver in the treatment of pernicious anemia.

Mirizzi, P.L., 20th century Argentinian physician.
Mirizzi syndrome—stenosis of hepatic duct. *Syn:* hepatic duct obstruction

Mitchell, Charles L., U.S. orthopedic surgeon, *1901.
Mitchell bunionectomy
Mitchell distal osteotomy
Mitchell operation
Mitchell osteotomy

Mitchell, Silas Weir, U.S. neurologist, poet, and novelist, 1829–1914.
Gerhardt-Mitchell disease—see under Gerhardt, Carl
Mitchell disease—*Syn:* Gerhardt-Mitchell disease
Mitchell treatment—treatment of mental illness by rest, nourishing diet, and a change of environment. *Syn:* Weir Mitchell treatment
Weir Mitchell disease—*Syn:* Gerhardt-Mitchell disease
Weir Mitchell treatment—*Syn:* Mitchell treatment

Mitsuda, Kensuke, Japanese physician, *1876.
Mitsuda antigen—an autoclaved suspension of human tissue naturally infected with *Mycobacterium leprae*.
Mitsuda reaction—a delayed hypersensitivity lepromin reaction, in the

form of erythematous papular nodules, at the site of intradermal injection of Mitsuda antigen in a lepromin test.
Mitsuda test—lepromin test by intradermal injection.

Mitsuo, Gentaro, Japanese ophthalmologist, 1876–1913.
Mitsuo phenomenon—restoration of the normal color of the fundus with dark adaptation in Oguchi disease.

Miura, Noboru, Japanese dentist.
Cooperman-Miura syndrome—see under Cooperman
Miura-Cooperman syndrome—*SYN:* Cooperman-Miura syndrome

Mixter, Samuel Jason, U.S. surgeon, 1855–1926.
Mixter clamp
Mixter dilating probe
Mixter dilator
Mixter forceps
Mixter hemostat
Mixter irrigating probe
Mixter needle
Mixter probe
Mixter punch
Mixter scissors
Mixter-Paul hemostatic forceps
Paul-Mixter tube

M

Miyagawa, Yoneji, Japanese bacteriologist, 1885–1959.
Miyagawa bodies—a term previously used to refer to *Chlamydia trachomatis* (*Miyagawanella lymphogranulomatosis*), the elementary bodies that develop in the intracytoplasmic microcolonies of lymphogranuloma venereum.
Miyagawanella—formerly considered a genus of Chlamydiaceae, but now synonymous with *Chlamydia.*

Mobitz, Woldemar, German cardiologist, *1889.
Mobitz types of atrioventricular block—type I, the dropped beat of the Wenckebach phenomenon; type II, a dropped cardiac cycle that occurs without alteration in the conduction of the preceding intervals.

Möbius, Paul J., German physician, 1853–1907.
Leyden-Möbius muscular dystrophy—see under Leyden
Möbius I syndrome—moderate migraine accompanied by extraocular palsy. *SYN:* ophthalmoplegic migraine; occasional oculomotor paralysis
Möbius II syndrome—facial paralysis. *SYN:* congenital facial diplegia; developmental bilateral facial paralysis
Möbius sign—impairment of ocular convergence in Graves disease.
Möbius syndrome—a developmental bilateral facial paralysis usually associated with oculomotor or other neurological disorders. *SYN:* congenital facial diplegia

NOTES

Moe, John H., U.S. surgeon, *1905.
   Moe alar hook
   Moe hook
   Moe impactor
   Moe intertrochanteric plate—*Syn:* Moe plate
   Moe nail
   Moe plate—plate used for internal fixation of intertrochanteric femoral fracture. *Syn:* Moe intertrochanteric plate
   Moe procedure
   Moe rod
   Moe spinal fusion
   Moe system

Moeller, Alfred, German bacteriologist, *1868.
   Moeller grass bacillus—a species found in soil and dust and on plants. *Syn: Mycobacterium phlei*

Moeller, Julius O.L., German surgeon, 1819–1887.
   Moeller glossitis—*Syn:* Moeller-Hunter syndrome
   Moeller-Hunter syndrome—red, swollen, and painful tongue. *Syn:* atrophic glossitis; Hunter glossitis; Moeller glossitis

Moënckeberg, var. of Mönckeberg
   Moersch, F.P.
   Moersch-Woltmann syndrome—prodromal occasional aching and tightness of muscles. *Syn:* muscular rigidity

Mohr, O.L.
   Mohr finger splint
   Mohr syndrome—autosomal dominant inheritance. *Syn:* acrocephalosyndactyly IV

Mohrenheim, Joseph J. Freiherr von, Austrian-Russian surgeon, 1755–1799.
   Mohrenheim fossa—a triangular depression bounded by the clavicle and the adjacent borders of the deltoid and pectoralis major muscles. *Syn:* infraclavicular fossa; Mohrenheim space
   Mohrenheim space—*Syn:* Mohrenheim fossa

Mohs, Frederick E., U.S. surgeon, *1910.
   Mohs chemosurgery—a microscopically controlled technique for removal of skin tumors. *Syn:* Mohs surgery; Mohs micrographic surgery; microscopically controlled surgery
   Mohs fresh tissue chemosurgery technique—chemosurgery in which superficial cancers are excised after fixation in vivo.
   Mohs micrographic surgery—*Syn:* Mohs chemosurgery
   Mohs surgery—*Syn:* Mohs chemosurgery
   Mohs technique

Mohs, Friedrich, German mineralogist, 1773–1839.
   Mohs hardness number—a number on a mineralogic scale.
   Mohs scale—a qualitative scale in which minerals are classified in order of their increasing hardness. *Syn:* hardness scale

Molisch, Hans, Austrian chemist, 1856–1937.
   Molisch test—a color test for sugar.

Moll, Jacob A., Dutch oculist, 1832–1914.
   Moll glands—a number of modified apocrine sudoriferous glands in the eyelids, with ducts that usually open into the follicles of the eyelashes. *SYN:* ciliary glands

Mollaret, Pierre, French neurologist, *1898.
   Mollaret meningitis—*SYN:* Mollaret syndrome.
   Mollaret syndrome—recurrent benign viral infection. *SYN:* recurrent meningitis; Mollaret meningitis

Moloney, John B., 20th century U.S. oncologist.
   Moloney virus—a lymphoid leukemia retrovirus of mice, in the subfamily Oncovirinae.

Moloney, Paul J., Canadian physician, 1870–1939.
   Moloney test—a test to detect a high degree of sensitivity to diphtheria toxoid.

Moloy, Howard C., U.S. obstetrician, 1903–1953.
   Caldwell-Moloy classification—see under Caldwell, William E.

Monakow, Constantin von, Swiss histologist, 1853–1930.
   Monakow bundle—*SYN:* Monakow tract
   Monakow fasciculus—*SYN:* Monakow tract
   Monakow fibers—*SYN:* Monakow tract
   Monakow nucleus—a cell group lateral to the cuneate nucleus which receives posterior root fibers corresponding to the proprioceptive innervation of the arm and hand. *SYN:* accessory cuneate nucleus
   Monakow syndrome—contralateral hemiplegia, hemianesthesia, and homonymous hemianopsia due to occlusion of the anterior choroidal artery.
   Monakow tract—indirect increase in flexor muscle tone. *SYN:* rubrospinal tract; Monakow bundle; Monakow fasciculus; Monakow fibers

Mönckeberg, Johann G., German pathologist, 1877–1925.
   Mönckeberg arteriosclerosis—arteriosclerosis involving the peripheral arteries with deposition of calcium in the medial coat but with little or no encroachment on the lumen. *SYN:* medial arteriosclerosis; Mönckeberg calcification; Mönckeberg degeneration; Mönckeberg sclerosis; Mönckeberg medial calcification; Mönckeberg syndrome
   Mönckeberg calcification—*SYN:* Mönckeberg arteriosclerosis
   Mönckeberg degeneration—*SYN:* Mönckeberg arteriosclerosis
   Mönckeberg sclerosis—*SYN:* Mönckeberg arteriosclerosis
   Mönckeberg syndrome—*SYN:* Mönckeberg arteriosclerosis

Moncrieff, Alan Aird, English physician, *1901.
   Moncrieff cannula
   Moncrieff discission
   Moncrieff irrigator

(continued)

M

NOTES

Moncrieff *(continued)*
Moncrieff operation
Moncrieff syndrome—autosomal recessive trait. *Syn:* Moncrieff-Wilkinson syndrome
Moncrieff-Wilkinson syndrome—*Syn:* Moncrieff syndrome

Mondini, C., Italian physician, 1729–1803.
Mondini deafness—congenital deafness.
Mondini deformity

Mondonesi, Filippo, Italian physician.
Mondonesi reflex—in a case of coma from severe apoplexy, pressure on the eyeballs causes contraction of the facial muscles of expression on the side opposite to the lesion; in coma due to diabetes, uremia, or other toxic cause, the reflex is present on both sides. *Syn:* bulbomimic reflex

Mondor, Henri J.J., French surgeon, 1885–1962.
Mondor disease—*Syn:* Mondor syndrome
Mondor phlebitis—*Syn:* Mondor syndrome
Mondor syndrome—thoracoepigastric vein phlebitis. *Syn:* thrombophlebitis of the breast and chest wall; Mondor disease; Mondor phlebitis

Monge Medrano, Carlos, Peruvian professor of medicine and high altitude specialist, 1884–1970.
Monge disease—loss of high-altitude tolerance after prolonged exposure. *Syn:* chronic mountain sickness; Monge syndrome
Monge syndrome—*Syn:* Monge disease

Moniz, Antonio Caetano de Abgreu Freire Egas, Portuguese neurosurgeon and diplomat, 1874–1955, joint winner of 1949 Nobel Prize for work related to prefrontal lobotomy for treatment of certain psychoses.

Monneret, Jules Auguste Edward, French physician, 1810–1868.
Monneret pulse—slow, soft, and full pulse.

Monod, Jacques L., French biochemist and Nobel laureate, 1910–1976.
Monod-Wyman-Changeux model—a model used to explain the allosteric form of cooperativity. *Syn:* concerted model

Monro, Alexander, Jr., Scottish anatomist, 1733–1817.
foramen of Monro—*Syn:* Monro foramen
Monro doctrine—a doctrine that states that the cranial cavity is a closed box and that a change in the quantity of intracranial blood can occur only through the displacement of or replacement by cerebrospinal fluid. *Syn:* Monro-Kellie doctrine
Monro foramen—the short passage that connects the third ventricle of the diencephalon with the lateral ventricles of the cerebral hemispheres. *Syn:* interventricular foramen; foramen of Monro
Monro line—*Syn:* Monro-Richter line
Monro sulcus—*Syn:* hypothalamic sulcus
Monro-Kellie doctrine—*Syn:* Monro doctrine
Monro-Richter line—a line passing from the umbilicus to the anterior superior iliac spine. McBurney point occurs on this line. *Syn:* Monro line; Richter-Monro line
Richter-Monro line—*Syn:* Monro-Richter line

Monro, Alexander, Sr., Scottish anatomist and surgeon, 1697–1767.
    bursa of Monro—*Syn:* intratendinous bursa of elbow
    Monro bursa—*Syn:* intratendinous bursa of elbow

Monson, George S., U.S. dentist, 1869–1933.
    anti-Monson curve—in dentistry, a curve of occlusion which is convex upward. *Syn:* reverse curve
    Monson curve—the curve of occlusion in which each cusp and incisal edge touches or conforms to a segment of the surface of a sphere 8 inches in diameter, with its center in the region of the glabella.

Monteggia, Giovanni B., Italian surgeon, 1762–1815.
    Monteggia dislocation
    Monteggia fracture—fracture of the ulna with dislocation of the radial head.
    Monteggia lesion
    reverse Monteggia fracture

Montessori, Maria, Italian psychiatrist and educator, 1870–1952.
    Montessori school—school with program on self-education with emphasis on practical living.

Montgomery, William F., Irish obstetrician, 1797–1859.
    Montgomery follicles—*Syn:* Montgomery glands
    Montgomery glands—a number of small mammary glands forming small rounded projections from the surface of the areola of the breast. *Syn:* areolar glands; Montgomery follicles
    Montgomery strap
    Montgomery tubercles—elevated reddened areolar glands.
    Montgomery vaginal speculum

M

Moon, Henry, English surgeon, 1845–1892.
    Moon molars—small dome-shaped first molar teeth occurring in congenital syphilis.

Moon, Robert C., U.S. ophthalmologist, 1844–1914.
    Laurence-Moon-Biedl syndrome—see under Laurence

Moon, William, English inventor, 1818–1894.
    Moon system—a touch-type alphabet for the blind. *Syn:* Moon type
    Moon type—*Syn:* Moon system

Moore, Austin Talley, U.S. orthopedist and surgeon, 1899–1963.
    Austin Moore arthroplasty
    Austin Moore bone reamer
    Austin Moore calipers
    Austin Moore chisel
    Austin Moore corkscrew
    Austin Moore extractor
    Austin Moore pin

(continued)

NOTES

Moore *(continued)*
    Austin Moore prosthesis
    Austin Moore rasp

Moore, Charles H., English surgeon, 1821–1870.
    Moore method—treatment of aneurysm.

Moore, Edward Mott, U.S. physician, 1814–1902.
    modified Moore hip-locking prosthesis
    Moore approach
    Moore bone drill
    Moore bone reamer
    Moore bone retractor
    Moore button
    Moore direction finder
    Moore driver
    Moore elevator
    Moore extractor
    Moore femoral neck prosthesis
    Moore fixation pin
    Moore forceps
    Moore fracture
    Moore hip endoprosthesis system
    Moore hip prosthesis
    Moore hollow chisel
    Moore measuring rod
    Moore nail
    Moore osteotomy-osteoclasis
    Moore pin
    Moore prosthesis extractor
    Moore prosthesis-mortising chisel
    Moore rasp
    Moore raspatory
    Moore sliding nail plate
    Moore spinal fusion gouge
    Moore stem
    Moore technique
    Moore template
    Moore tibial plateau fracture classification
    Moore tube
    Moore-Blount driver
    Moore-Blount screwdriver

Moore, Matthew T., U.S. neuropsychiatrist, *1901.
    Moore syndrome—painful abdominal symptoms that may be followed by seizures. *SYN:* abdominal epilepsy; visceral epilepsy

Moore, Robert Foster, English ophthalmologist, 1878–1963.
    Moore lightning streaks—photopsia manifested by vertical flashes of light caused by the involutional shrinkage of vitreous humor.

Mooren, Albert, German ophthalmologist, 1828–1899.
    Mooren ulcer—chronic inflammation of the peripheral cornea that slowly progresses centrally with corneal thinning and sometimes perforation.

Mooser, Hermann, Swiss pathologist in Mexico, *1891.
  Mooser bodies—a term used to refer to the rickettsiae found in the exudate and in tissue from the tunica vaginalis in endemic typhus fever (caused by *Rickettsia typhi*).
  Mooser cell

Morand, Sauveur F., French surgeon, 1697–1773.
  Morand foot—a foot having eight toes.
  Morand spur—the lower of two elevations on the medial wall of the posterior horn of the lateral ventricle of the brain. *SYN:* calcar avis

Morax, Victor, French ophthalmologist, 1866–1935.
  Moraxella anatipestifer
  Moraxella bovis
  Moraxella lacunata—a species causing conjunctivitis. *SYN:* Morax-Axenfeld diplobacillus
  Moraxella liquefaciens
  Moraxella lwoffi
  Moraxella—a genus of obligately aerobic nonmotile bacteria (family Neisseriaceae) parasitic on the mucous membranes of humans and other mammals.
  Morax keratoplasty
  Morax operation
  Morax-Axenfeld conjunctivitis—conjunctivitis caused by diplobacillus.
  Morax-Axenfeld diplobacillus—*SYN: Moraxella lacunata*

M

Morel, Bénédict A., French psychiatrist, 1809–1873.
  Morel disease—alcohol withdrawal. *SYN:* delirium tremens
  Morel ear—a large, misshapen, outstanding auricle with obliterated grooves and thinned edges.
  Stewart-Morel syndrome—*SYN:* Morgagni syndrome

Morel, Ferdinand, Swiss physician, 1888–1957.
  Morel-Wildi syndrome—frontal cerebral cortex dysgenesis.

Morelli, F., 20th century Italian physician.
  Morelli test—*SYN:* Moritz test

Morgagni, Giovanni B., Italian anatomist and pathologist, 1682–1771.
  frenulum of Morgagni—a fold running from the junction of the two commissures of the ileocecal valve on either side along the inner wall of the cecocolic junction. *SYN:* frenulum of ileocecal valve; Morgagni frenulum; Morgagni retinaculum
  Morgagni appendix—an inconstant narrow lobe of the thyroid gland. *SYN:* pyramidal lobe of thyroid gland
  Morgagni cartilage—a small nonarticulating rod of elastic cartilage in the aryepiglottic fold anterolateral and somewhat superior to the corniculate cartilage. *SYN:* cuneiform cartilage; Morgagni tubercle

(continued)

NOTES

Morgagni *(continued)*

Morgagni caruncle—the portion of the prostate lying between the urethra and the ejaculatory ducts. *Syn:* middle lobe of prostate

Morgagni cataract—a hypermature cataract in which the nucleus gravitates within the capsule. *Syn:* sedimentary cataract

Morgagni columns—a number of vertical ridges in the mucous membrane of the upper half of the anal canal. *Syn:* anal columns

Morgagni concha—the upper thin, spongy, bony plate projecting from the lateral wall of the nasal cavity and separating the superior meatus from the sphenoethmoidal recess. *Syn:* superior nasal concha

Morgagni crypts—the grooves between the anal columns. *Syn:* anal sinuses

Morgagni disease—*Syn:* Adams-Stokes syndrome

Morgagni foramen—congenital defect in the fusion of sternal and costal elements of the diaphragmatic anlage that is the site of a parasternal hernia. *Syn:* foramen cecum of tongue

Morgagni fossa—the terminal dilated portion of the urethra in the glans penis. *Syn:* navicular fossa of urethra; Morgagni fovea

Morgagni fovea—*Syn:* Morgagni fossa

Morgagni frenulum—*Syn:* frenulum of Morgagni

Morgagni globules—vesicles beneath the capsule and between lens fibers in early cataract. *Syn:* Morgagni spheres

Morgagni hernia

Morgagni humor—*Syn:* Morgagni liquor

Morgagni hydatid—a vestigial remnant of the embryonic mesonephric duct. *Syn:* vesicular appendices of uterine tube

Morgagni lacuna—one of a number of little recesses in the mucous membrane of the spongy urethra into which empty the ducts of the urethral glands. *Syn:* urethral lacuna

Morgagni liquor—a fluid found postmortem between the epithelium and the fibers of the lens, resulting from the liquefaction of a semifluid material existing there during life. *Syn:* Morgagni humor

Morgagni nodule—a nodule at the center of the free border of each semilunar valve at the beginning of the pulmonary artery and aorta. *Syn:* nodule of semilunar valve

Morgagni prolapse—chronic inflammation of laryngeal ventricle.

Morgagni retinaculum—*Syn:* frenulum of Morgagni

Morgagni sinus—*Syn:* anal sinuses; prostatic utricle; laryngeal ventricle

Morgagni spheres—*Syn:* Morgagni globules

Morgagni syndrome—hyperostosis frontalis interna in elderly women, with obesity and neuropsychiatric disorders. *Syn:* metabolic craniopathy; Stewart-Morel syndrome

Morgagni tubercle—*Syn:* Morgagni cartilage

Morgagni valves—delicate crescent-shaped mucosal folds that pass between the lower ends of neighboring anal columns. *Syn:* anal valves

Morgagni ventricle—the recess in each lateral wall of the larynx between the vestibular and vocal folds and into which the layrngeal sacculus opens. *Syn:* laryngeal ventricle

Morgagni-Adams-Stokes syndrome—*Syn:* Adams-Stokes syndrome

morgagnian cyst—a vestigial remnant of the embryonic mesonephric duct. *Syn:* vesicular appendices of uterine tube

Morgan, Campbell De. See under De Morgan.

Morgan, Harry de R., English physician, 1863–1931.
    Morgan bacillus—type (and only) species of the genus *Morganella*. *SYN:*
    Morganella morganii

Morgan, Thomas Hunt, U.S. zoologist, 1866–1945, 1933 Nobel Prize winner for
work related to chromosomes and their relation to heredity.

Morison, James R., English surgeon, 1853–1939.
    Morison incision
    Morison method
    Morison pouch—the deep recess of the peritoneal cavity on the right side.
    SYN: hepatorenal recess

Morita, Shomei, 20th century Japanese physician.
    Morita therapy—psychotherapy based on elements of conduct in Zen
    Buddhism.

Moritz, Friedrich Heinrich Ludwig, German physician, 1861–1938.
    Moritz reaction—*SYN:* Moritz test
    Moritz test—test to determine the difference between a transudate and an
    exudate. *SYN:* Moritz reaction; Rivalata reaction; Morelli test

Mörner, Karl A.H., Swedish chemist, 1855–1917.
    Mörner test—for cysteine and tyrosine.

Moro, Ernst, German physician, 1874–1951.
    Moro reflex—the reflex response of an infant when allowed to drop a
    short distance through the air or startled by a sudden noise or jolt. *SYN:*
    startle reflex

Morquio, Louis, Uruguayan physician, 1867–1935.
    Brailsford-Morquio disease—*SYN:* Morquio syndrome
    Morquio disease—*SYN:* Morquio syndrome
    Morquio sign
    Morquio syndrome—an error of mucopolysaccharide metabolism
    characterized by severe skeletal defects. *SYN:* Brailsford-Morquio disease;
    Morquio disease; Morquio-Ullrich disease; type IVA, B
    mucopolysaccharidosis
    Morquio-Ullrich disease—*SYN:* Morquio syndrome

Morris, Sir Henry, English surgeon, 1844–1926.
    Morris biphase screw
    Morris cannula
    Morris catheter
    Morris clamp
    Morris drain
    Morris incision
    Morris retractor
    Morris splint

Morrison, Ashton B., Irish pathologist in the U.S., *1922.
    Verner-Morrison syndrome—see under Verner

M

NOTES

Morrow, P.A.
    Morrow-Brooke syndrome—*Syn:* Brooke disease (2)

Morsier, G. de. See under de Morsier.

Mortensen, Ole, Danish physician.
    Mortensen syndrome—*Syn:* Di Guglielmo syndrome

Mortimer, female patient for whom the malady is named.
    Mortimer disease—*Syn:* Mortimer malady
    Mortimer malady—skin disease. *Syn:* Mortimer disease

Morton, Dudley J., U.S. orthopedist, 1884–1960.
    Morton syndrome—congenital shortening of the first metatarsal, causing metatarsalgia.

Morton, Richard, English physician, 1637–1698.
    Morton cough—cough associated with tuberculosis.

Morton, Samuel G., U.S. physician, 1799–1851.
    Morton plane—a plane passing through the summits of the parietal and occipital protuberances.

Morton, Thomas G., U.S. physician, 1835–1903.
    Morton bandage
    Morton disease—*Syn:* Morton neuralgia
    Morton foot—*Syn:* Morton neuralgia
    Morton interdigital neuroma
    Morton nerve entrapment syndrome—*Syn:* Morton neuralgia
    Morton neuralgia—neuralgia of an interdigital nerve. *Syn:* Morton disease; Morton foot; Morton neuroma; Morton nerve entrapment syndrome; Morton toe
    Morton neuroma—*Syn:* Morton neuralgia
    Morton ophthalmoscope
    Morton sign
    Morton test
    Morton toe—*Syn:* Morton neuralgia
    Morton toe support

Morvan, Augustin, French physician, 1819–1897.
    Morvan chorea—continuous involuntary quivering of muscles at rest. *Syn:* myokymia
    Morvan disease—the presence of longitudinal cavities in the spinal cord. *Syn:* syringomyelia; Morvan syndrome
    Morvan syndrome—*Syn:* Morvan disease

Moschcowitz, Alexis Victor, U.S. surgeon, 1865–1933.
    Moschcowitz enterocele repair
    Moschcowitz operation—femoral hernia repair.

Moschowitz, Eli, U.S. physician, 1879–1964.
    Moschowitz disease—*Syn:* hemolytic thrombocytopenic purpura
    Moschowitz syndrome—acute febrile pleiochromic anemia with hyaline thrombosis of terminal arterioles and capillaries *Syn:* Baehr-Schiffrin disease; Moschowitz-Singer-Symmers syndrome
    Moschowitz test—a test for arteriosclerosis.
    Moschowitz-Singer-Symmers syndrome—*Syn:* Moschowitz syndrome

Mosher, Clelia D., U.S. physician, 1863–1940.
Mosher exercises—exercises for dysmenorrhea.

Mosler, Karl F., German physician, 1831–1911.
Mosler diabetes—inosituria with excretion of large quantities of water.
Mosler sign—tenderness over the sternum in a patient with acute myeloblastic anemia.

Moss, Gerald, U.S. physician, *1931.
Moss decompression feeding catheter
Moss G-tube PEG kit
Moss PEG kit
Moss T-anchor needle
Moss tube

Moss, Melvin L., U.S. oral pathologist, *1923.
Gorlin-Chaudhry-Moss syndrome—see under Gorlin, Robert

Moss, William Lorenzo, U.S. physician, 1876–1957.
Moss classification—a classification of ABO blood types.

Mosse, Max, German physician, *1873.
Mosse polycythemia—*Syn:* Mosse syndrome
Mosse syndrome—cirrhosis of the liver with polycythemia vera. *Syn:* Mosse polycythemia; liver cirrhosis

M

Mosso, Angelo, Italian physiologist, 1846–1910.
Mosso ergograph—an instrument used to obtain a graphic record of flexion of a finger, hand, or arm.
Mosso sphygmomanometer—an apparatus for measuring the blood pressure in the digital arteries.

Moszkowicz, Ludwig, Austrian surgeon, 1873–1945.
Moszkowicz test—a test for arteriosclerosis. *Syn:* hyperemia test

Motais, Ernst, French ophthalmologist, 1845–1913.
Motais operation—transplantation of the middle third of the tendon of the superior rectus muscle of the eyeball into the upper lid to supplement the action of the levator muscle in ptosis.

Mounier-Kuhn, P., 20th century French physician.
Mounier-Kuhn syndrome—congenital widening of trachea and bronchi. *Syn:* tracheobronchomegaly

Moynihan, Lord Berkeley George Andrew, English surgeon, 1865–1936.
Moynihan clamp
Moynihan clip
Moynihan forceps
Moynihan gutter—right paracolic gutter.
Moynihan incision
Moynihan position

(continued)

NOTES

Moynihan *(continued)*
> **Moynihan probe**
> **Moynihan respirator**
> **Moynihan scoop**
> **Moynihan speculum**

Mozart, Wolfgang Amadeus, Austrian composer, 1756–1791.
> **Mozart ear**—fusion of the large portion of the anthelix with the helix.

Much, Hans C.R., German physician, 1880–1932.
> **Much bacillus**—said to be the form present in the tuberculous skin lesions.

Mucha, Victor, Austrian dermatologist, 1877–1919.
> **Mucha-Habermann disease**—an acute dermatitis affecting children and young adults. *SYN:* pityriasis lichenoides et varioliformis acuta; Mucha-Habermann syndrome
> **Mucha-Habermann syndrome**—*SYN:* Mucha-Habermann disease

Muckle, T.J., 20th century Canadian pediatrician.
> **Muckle-Wells syndrome**—a syndrome characterized by familial amyloidosis.

Muehrcke, Robert C.
> **Muehrcke lines**—white lines parallel with the lanula and separated from each other by normal pink areas, associated with hypoalbuminemia.

Müeller, R.
> **Müeller-Kugelberg syndrome**—muscle degeneration caused by steroid use. *SYN:* steroid myopathy

Muir, E.G. English physician.
> **Muir-Torre syndrome**—*SYN:* Torre syndrome

Mulder, Gerardus Johann, Dutch chemist, 1802–1880.
> **Mulder test**—a test for glucose. *SYN:* xanthroproteic reaction.

Mulder, Johannes, Dutch anatomist, 1769–1810.
> **Mulder angle**—a facial angle.

Mules, Philip H., English ophthalmologist, 1843–1905.
> **Mules eye implant**
> **Mules graft**
> **Mules operation**—evisceration of the eyeball followed by the insertion within the sclera of a spherical prosthesis to support an artificial eye.
> **Mules prosthesis**
> **Mules scoop**

Muller, Hermann Joseph, U.S. biologist and geneticist, 1890–1967, winner of the 1947 Nobel Prize for work related to x-ray mutations.
> **Muller-Hinton agar**—medium containing beef infusion, peptone, and starch used primarily for the disk-agar diffusion method for antimicrobial susceptibility testing.

Müller, Friedrich von, German physician, 1858–1941.
> **Müller sign**—rhythmic movements of the uvula, accompanied by redness and swelling of the velum palati and tonsils in aortic insufficiency.

Müller, Heinrich, German anatomist, 1820–1864.
Müller fibers—(1) *Syn:* circular fibers; (2) sustentacular neuroglial cells of the retina. *Syn:* Müller radial cells
Müller muscle—*Syn:* orbitalis muscle; circular fibers; superior tarsal muscle
Müller radial cells—*Syn:* Müller fibers (2)
Müller trigone—the floor of the supraoptic recess of the third ventricle.

Müller, Hermann F., German histologist, 1866–1898.
formol-Müller fixative—contains 2% commercial formalin.

Müller, Johannes P., German anatomist, physiologist, and pathologist, 1801–1858.
Müller capsule—the expanded beginning of a nephron composed of an inner and outer layer. *Syn:* glomerular capsule
Müller duct—either of the two paired embryonic tubes extending along the mesonephros. *Syn:* paramesonephric duct
Müller law—each type of sensory nerve ending gives rise to its own specific sensation. *Syn:* law of specific nerve energies
Müller maneuver—the reverse of the Valsalva maneuver.
Müller tubercle—the first evidence of the embryonic uterus and vagina. *Syn:* sinus tubercle

Müller, Peter, German obstetrician, 1836–1922.
Hillis-Müller maneuver—see under Hillis

Müller, Walther, 20th century German physicist.
Geiger-Müller counter—see under Geiger
Geiger-Müller tube

M

Münchausen, Baron Karl Friedrich Hieronymus von, German soldier and adventurer, 1720–1797.
Munchausen by proxy syndrome—a parent, usually knowledgeable about or experienced in health care, harming a child in order to gain the attention of healthcare providers.
Munchausen syndrome—repeated fabrication of clinically convincing simulations of disease for the purpose of gaining medical attention.

Munk, Fritz, German physician, *1879.
Munk disease—kidney disease.

Munro, John C., U.S. surgeon, 1858–1910.
Munro point—a point at the right edge of the rectus abdominis muscle where pressure elicits tenderness in appendicitis.

Munro, William J., 19th century Australian dermatologist.
Munro abscess—*Syn:* Munro microabscess
Munro microabscess—a microscopic collection of polymorphonuclear leukocytes found in the stratum corneum in psoriasis. *Syn:* Munro abscess

NOTES

Munro Kerr, John Martin, Scottish obstetrician and gynecologist, 1868–1955.
    Munro Kerr cesarean section—*Syn:* Munro Kerr section
    Munro Kerr incision
    Munro Kerr maneuver
    Munro Kerr section—cesarean section that opens the lower uterine segment transversely without displacing the bladder. *Syn:* Munro Kerr cesarean section

Munsell, Albert Henry, U.S. painter, 1858–1918.
    Farnsworth-Munsell color test—see under Farnsworth
    Munsell color system—method of color notation.

Munsell, Hazel E., U.S. chemist, *1891.
    Sherman-Munsell unit—see under Sherman, Henry

Munson, Edward Sterling, U.S. ophthalmologist, *1933.
    Munson sign—abnormal bulging of the lower eyelid.

Münzer, Egmont, Austrian physician, 1865–1924.
    tract of Münzer and Wiener—a fiber bundle arising in the superior colliculus and ending in the lateral part of the gray matter of the ventral part of the pons. *Syn:* tectopontine tract

Murat, Louis, French physician, *1874.
    Murat sign—a test given to tuberculosis patients.

Murchison, Charles, English physician, 1830–1879.
    Murchison-Pel-Ebstein syndrome—multiple symptoms of fever, sweats, etc., generally related to malignancy. *Syn:* Murchison-Saunderson syndrome
    Murchison-Saunderson syndrome—*Syn:* Murchison-Pel-Ebstein syndrome

Muret, Paul-Louis, French physician, *1878.
    Quénu-Muret sign—see under Quénu

Murphy, John B., U.S. surgeon, 1857–1916.
    Murphy approach
    Murphy bone lever
    Murphy bone skid
    Murphy brace
    Murphy button
    Murphy chisel
    Murphy dilator
    Murphy drip—*Syn:* proctoclysis
    Murphy forceps
    Murphy gouge
    Murphy hook
    Murphy knife
    Murphy light
    Murphy method
    Murphy needle
    Murphy percussion—*Syn:* piano percussion
    Murphy punch
    Murphy reamer
    Murphy retractor
    Murphy scissors

Murphy sign—right upper quadrant pain on inspiration.
Murphy splint
Murphy tube
Murphy-Lane bone skid

Murphy, William Parry, U.S. physician, *1892, joint winner of 1934 Nobel Prize for work related to anemia.
Minot-Murphy diet

Murray, John, English physician.
Murray syndrome—rare autosomal recessive trait. *SYN:* Murray-Puretic-Drescher syndrome
Murray-Puretic-Drescher syndrome—*SYN:* Murray syndrome

Murray, Joseph E., U.S. plastic surgeon, *1919, joint winner of 1990 Nobel Prize for work related to cell and organ transplantation.

Murray Valley, location in Australia where epidemics occurred in 1950 and 1951.
Murray Valley disease—*SYN:* Murray Valley encephalitis
Murray Valley encephalitis—a severe encephalitis with high mortality. *SYN:* Murray Valley disease; Australian X disease; Australian X encephalitis
Murray Valley virus—a group B arbovirus that causes Murray Valley encephalitis. *SYN:* Australian X disease virus; MVE virus

Murri, A.
Murri disease
Murri syndrome—cerebellar degeneration. *SYN:* cerebellar ataxia

Musset, L.C. Alfred de, French poet, 1810–1857.
de Musset sign—*SYN:* Musset sign
Musset sign—in incompetence of the aortic valve, rhythmical nodding of the head, synchronous with the heart beat. *SYN:* de Musset sign

Mustard, William T., Canadian thoracic surgeon, *1914.
Mustard operation—correction, at the atrial level, of hemodynamic abnormality due to transposition of the great arteries. *SYN:* Mustard procedure
Mustard procedure—*SYN:* Mustard operation

Myerson, Abraham, U.S. neurologist, 1881–1948.
Myerson sign—a sign of Parkinson disease.

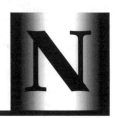

Naboth, Martin, German anatomist and physician, 1675–1721.
  Naboth cyst
  Naboth follicle
  Naboth gland
  Naboth vesicle
  nabothian cyst—a retention cyst that develops when a mucous gland of the cervix uteri is obstructed. *SYN:* nabothian follicle
  nabothian follicle—*SYN:* nabothian cyst
  nabothian gland

Naegeli, Oskar, Swiss physician, 1885–1959.
  Naegeli syndrome—reticular skin pigmentation, diminished sweating, hypodontia, and hyperkeratosis of the palms and soles. *SYN:* Franceschetti-Jadassohn syndrome

Naegeli, Otto, Swiss physician, 1871–1938.
  Naegeli monocytic leukemia—a variant of granulocytic leukemia with monocytosis in the peripheral blood. *SYN:* myelomonocytic leukemia

Naffziger, Howard C., U.S. surgeon, 1884–1961.
  Naffziger operation—orbital decompression for severe malignant exophthalmos.
  Naffziger syndrome—*SYN:* Adson syndrome (1) ; scalenus-anticus syndrome
  Naffziger test

Nagel, Willibald A., German ophthalmologist and physiologist, 1870–1911.
  Nagel test—a test for color vision.

Nägele, Franz K., German obstetrician, 1777–1851.
  Nägele maneuver
  Nägele obliquity—inclination of the fetal head in cases of flat pelvis, the anterior parietal bone presenting to the parturient canal. *SYN:* anterior asynclitism
  Nägele pelvis—an obliquely contracted or unilateral synostotic pelvis.
  Nägele rule—means of estimating date of delivery by counting back three months from the first day of the last menstrual period and adding seven days.

Nageotte, Jean, French histologist, 1866–1948.
  Babinski-Nageotte syndrome—see under Babinski
  Nageotte bracelets
  Nageotte cells—cells found in the cerebrospinal fluid.

Nager, Felix Robert, Swiss otorhinolaryngologist, 1877–1959.
Nager acrofacial dysostosis
Nager sign
Nager syndrome
Nager-Reynier syndrome—*Syn:* Treacher Collins syndrome

Nagler, F.P.O., 20th century Australian bacteriologist.
Nagler reaction

Nagler, Joseph, Austrian radiologist, *1910.
Nagler effect
Nagler test

Nagyrapolt, Albert Szent-György Von, winner of Nobel Prize in 1937 for work related to regulation of respiration.

Najjar, Victor A., U.S. physician and biochemist, *1914.
Crigler-Najjar disease—*Syn:* Crigler-Najjar syndrome
Crigler-Najjar syndrome—see under Crigler

Nakanishi, K., Japanese physician.
Nakanishi stain—a method for vital staining of bacteria.

Nance, Walter E., U.S. physician
Nance deafness—*Syn:* Nance syndrome
Nance dwarfism—*Syn:* Nancy-Sweeney syndrome
Nance syndrome—X-linked characteristic of multiple otologic abnormalities. *Syn:* Nance deafness
Nance-Horan syndrome—X-linked trait; multiple congenital abnormalities. *Syn:* X-linked cataract-dental syndrome
Nance-Sweeney syndrome—autosomal recessive inheritance. *Syn:* Nance dwarfism

Napalkov, A.V., Russian neurophysiologist.
Napalkov phenomenon—conditioned reflex response in which fear increases instead of decreases when stimulus is removed.

Nasmyth, Alexander, London dentist, d. 1847.
Nasmyth cuticle—two extremely thin layers covering the entire crown of newly erupted teeth and subsequently abraded by mastication. *Syn:* enamel cuticle; Nasmyth membrane
Nasmyth membrane—*Syn:* Nasmyth cuticle

Nasse, Christian Friedrich, German physician, 1788–1851.
Millon-Nasse test—see under Millon

Nathans, Daniel, joint winner of 1978 Nobel Prize for work related to restriction enzymes.
Nauheim, Bad Nauheim, German spa.
Nauheim bath—*Syn:* Nauheim treatment
Nauheim treatment—treatment of certain cardiac affections by baths in water through which carbonic acid gas is bubbling, followed by resistance exercises. *Syn:* Nauheim bath; Schott treatment

Nauta, Walle J.H., U.S. neuroscientist, *1916.
Nauta stain—a stain for degenerating axons.

Necker, Louis, Swiss physicist and mathematician, 1730–1804.
    Necker cube—line drawing in which 12 angles of the cube are visible.

Needles, Carl F., U.S. pediatrician, *1935.
    Melnick-Needles syndrome—see under Melnick

Needles, J.W., U.S. dentist.
    Needles split cast method—a procedure for placing indexed casts on an articulator to facilitate their removal and replacement on the instrument. *SYN:* split cast method

Neel, A.V., Scandinavian physician.
    Bing-Neel syndrome—see under Bing

Neelsen, Friedrich K.A., German pathologist, 1854–1894.
    Ziehl-Neelsen stain—see under Ziehl

Neftel, William B., U.S. neurologist, 1830–1906.
    Neftel disease—paresthesia of the head and trunk and extreme discomfort in any but the recumbent position.

Negri, Adelchi, Italian physician, 1876–1912.
    Negri bodies—pathognomonic inclusion bodies found in the cytoplasm of certain nerve cells containing the virus of rabies. *SYN:* Negri corpuscles
    Negri corpuscles—*SYN:* Negri bodies

Negro, Camillo, Italian neurologist, 1861–1927.
    Negro cogwheel rigidity—*SYN:* Negro phenomenon
    Negro phenomenon—a sudden brief halt in usually smooth respiration or other motor activity. *SYN:* cogwheel phenomenon; Negro rigidity; Negro cogwheel rigidity
    Negro rigidity—*SYN:* Negro phenomenon

Neher, Erwin, German biophysicist, *1944, joint winner of 1991 Nobel Prize for work related to ion channels in the cell.

Neisser, Albert L.S., German physician, 1855–1916.
    Neisseria catarrhalis
    Neisseria flavescens
    Neisseria gonorrhoeae—a species that causes gonorrhea in humans. *SYN:* Neisser coccus
    Neisseria lactamica
    Neisseria meningitidis
    Neisseria sicca
    Neisseria subflava
    Neisseria—a genus of aerobic to facultatively anaerobic bacteria (family Neisseriaceae) that are parasites of animals.
    Neisseria **mucosa**
    Neisser coccus—*SYN:* Neisseria gonorrhoeae
    Neisser diplococcus
    Neisser syringe—a urethral syringe used in treatment of gonococcal urethritis.

NOTES

Neisser, Max, German bacteriologist, 1869–1938.
  Neisser stain—a stain for the polar nuclei of the diphtheria bacillus.

Nélaton, Auguste, French surgeon, 1807–1873.
  Nélaton bullet probe
  Nélaton catheter
  Nélaton dislocation—wedging of the astragalus between the widely
    separated tibia and fibula, usually complicated with fracture.
  Nélaton drain
  Nélaton fibers—*SYN:* Nélaton sphincter
  Nélaton fold
  Nélaton line—a line drawn from the anterior superior iliac spine to the
    tuberosity of the ischium. *SYN:* Roser-Nélaton line
  Nélaton operation
  Nélaton sphincter—the middle rectal fold. *SYN:* Nélaton fibers
  Nélaton syndrome—hereditary neuropathy. *SYN:* Denny-Brown syndrome
  Roser-Nélaton line—*SYN:* Nélaton line

Nelson, Don H., U.S. internist, *1925.
  Nelson syndrome—a syndrome of hyperpigmentation, third nerve damage,
    and enlarging sella turcica caused by pituitary adenomas that become
    symptomatic following adrenalectomy. *SYN:* postadrenalectomy syndrome
  Nelson tumor—a pituitary tumor causing the symptoms of Nelson
    syndrome.

Némethy, George, Hungarian-U.S. biochemist, *1934.
  Adair-Koshland-Némethy-Filmer model—*SYN:* Koshland-Némethy-Filmer
    model
  Koshland-Némethy-Filmer model—see under Koshland

Nencki, Marcellus von, Polish physician, 1847–1901.
  Nencki test—a test for indole.

Neri, Vincenzo, Italian neurologist, *1882.
  Neri sign—a sign of organic hemiplegia.

Nernst, Walther, German physicist and Nobel laureate, 1864–1941.
  Nernst equation—the equation relating the electrical potential and
    concentration gradient of an ion across a permeable membrane at
    equilibrium.
  Nernst potential
  Nernst theory—that the passage of an electric current through the tissues
    causes a dissociation of the ions.

Nessler, A., German chemist, 1827–1905.
  Nessler reagent—a solution of potassium hydroxide, mercuric iodide, and
    potassium iodide.

Netherton, Earl W., U.S. dermatologist, *1893.
  Netherton syndrome—brittle hair; atopic manifestations. *SYN:* congenital
    icthyosiform erythroderma

Nettleship, Edward, English ophthalmologist and dermatologist, 1845–1913.
  Nettleship dilator
  Nettleship iris repositor

Nettleship syndrome—pigmented nodules or macules. *Syn:* urticaria pigmentosa

Neu, Richard L., U.S. scientist.
Neu syndrome—*Syn:* Neu-Laxová syndrome
Neu-Laxová syndrome—multiple birth defects *Syn:* Neu syndrome

Neubauer, Johann E., German anatomist, 1742–1777.
Neubauer artery—*Syn:* thyroid ima artery
Neubauer ruled hemacytometer

Neufeld, Alonzo John, U.S. orthopedic surgeon, *1906.
Neufeld apparatus
Neufeld cast
Neufeld driver
Neufeld dynamic method
Neufeld femoral nail plate
Neufeld nail
Neufeld pin
Neufeld plate
Neufeld screw
Neufeld traction
Neufeld tractor

Neufeld, Fred, German bacteriologist, 1869–1945.
Neufeld capsular swelling—increase in opacity and visibility of the capsule of capsulated organisms exposed to specific agglutinating anticapsular antibodies. *Syn:* quellung phenomenon; Neufeld reaction; quellung reaction; quellung test
Neufeld reaction—*Syn:* Neufeld capsular swelling

N

Neuhauser, Edward Blaine, U.S. physician, *1908.
Neuhauser-Berenberg syndrome—excessive vomiting in children. *Syn:* cardioesophageal relaxation syndrome

Neumann, Ernst F.C., German histologist, anatomist, and pathologist, 1834–1918.
Neumann cells—nucleated cells in the bone marrow developing into red blood cells.
Neumann sheath—a layer of tissue relatively resistant to the action of acids, which forms the walls of the dentinal tubules. *Syn:* dentinal sheath
Neumann syndrome—muscle cell tumor in infants *Syn:* neonatal myoblastoma
Rouget-Neumann sheath—see under Rouget, Charles

Neumann, Franz E., German physicist, 1798–1895.
Neumann law—in compounds of analogous chemical constitution, the molecular heat, or the product of the specific heat by the atomic weight, is always the same.

NOTES

Neumann, Isidor Edler von Heilwart, Austrian dermatologist, 1832–1906.
> **Neumann disease**—a form of pemphigus vulgaris in which vegetations develop on the eroded surfaces left by ruptured bullae. *SYN:* pemphigus vegetans

Neumann, M.A.
> **Neumann syndrome**—inherited dementia. *SYN:* familial dementia

Neumann-Neurode, Detleff, German physical educator, 1879–1945.
> **Neumann-Neurode exercises**—exercises for children from the age of 4 months.

Neusser, Edmund von, Austrian physician, 1852–1912.
> **Neusser granules**—tiny basophilic granules sometimes observed in an indistinct zone about the nucleus of a leukocyte.

Neve, Ernest Frederic, English physician, 1861–1941.
> **Neve cancer**—epithelioma caused by heat and substances of kangri when worn against the skin. *SYN:* kangri burn cancer

Newcastle, a community in England, near the location where Newcastle disease was first observed.
> **Newcastle disease**—an influenza-like disease of birds that is transmissible to man if in contact with diseased birds. *SYN:* avian influenza

Newton, Sir Isaac, English physicist, 1642–1727.
> **newton**—derived unit of force in the SI system.
> **Newton disk**—a disk on which there are seven colored sectors, which, when rapidly rotated, appear white.
> **Newton law**—the attractive force between any two bodies is proportional to the product of their masses and inversely proportional to the square of the distance between their centers. *SYN:* law of gravitation
> **Newton rings**—colored rings on thin surfaces.
> **newtonian aberration**—the difference in focus or magnification of an image arising because of a difference in the refraction of different wavelengths composing white light. *SYN:* chromatic aberration
> **newtonian constant of gravitation**—a universal constant relating the gravitational force, attracting two masses toward each other when they are separated by a distance.
> **newtonian flow**—the type of flow characteristic of a newtonian fluid.
> **newtonian fluid**—a fluid in which flow and rate of shear are always proportional to the applied stress.
> **newtonian viscosity**—the viscosity characteristics of a newtonian fluid.

Nezelof, C., French pathologist, *1922.
> **Nezelof syndrome**—type of thymic alymphoplasia. *SYN:* cellular immunodeficiency with abnormal immunoglobulin synthesis
> **Nezelof type of thymic alymphoplasia**—*SYN:* cellular immunodeficiency with abnormal immunoglobulin synthesis

Nicol, William, Scottish physicist, 1768–1851.
> **Nicol prism**—a prism that transmits only polarized light.

Nicolas, Joseph, French physician, 1868–1960.
    Nicolas-Favre disease—a venereal infection usually caused by *Chlamydia trachomatis*. *SYN:* venereal lymphogranuloma
    Nicolas-Moutot-Charlet syndrome—congenital mucocutaneous disease.

Nicolau, Stefan George, Romanian physician
    Nicolau syndrome—accidental intra-arterial injection resulting in embolization.

Nicolle, J.H., French microbiologist and Nobel laureate, 1866–1936.
    Nicolle stain for capsules—stain in a mixture of a saturated solution of gentian violet in alcohol-phenol.
    Nicolle white mycetoma—mycetoma caused by a species of *Aspergillus*.

Nielsen, Holger, Danish army officer, 1866–1955.
    Nielsen method—a method of artificial respiration.

Nielsen, Johannes Mygaard, U.S. physician, 1890–1969.
    Nielsen I syndrome—excessive weakness caused by physical exhaustion. *SYN:* neuromuscular exhaustion
    Nielsen II syndrome—apathy, akinesia, mutism, and incontinence.

Niemann, Albert, German physician, 1880–1921.
    Niemann disease—*SYN:* Niemann-Pick disease
    Niemann splenomegaly—enlargement of spleen occurring in Niemann-Pick disease.
    Niemann-Pick cell—*SYN:* Pick cell
    Niemann-Pick disease—lipid histiocytosis that occurs most commonly in Jewish infants and leads to early death. *SYN:* sphingomyelin lipidosis; Niemann disease

Nierhoff, H.
    Nierhoff-Huebner syndrome—convulsion, somnolence, and muscular flaccidity. *SYN:* endochondral dysostosis

Nievergelt, Kurt, Swiss physician, *1913.
    Nievergelt syndrome—rare bone disease characterized by multiple deformities. *SYN:* Nievergelt-Erb syndrome; Nievergelt-Pearlman syndrome
    Nievergelt-Erb syndrome—*SYN:* Nievergelt syndrome
    Nievergelt-Pearlman syndrome—*SYN:* Nievergelt syndrome

Niewenglowski, Gaston H., 19th century French scientist.
    Niewenglowski rays—radiation emitted from a phosphorescent body after exposure to sunlight.

Nikiforoff, Mikhail, Russian dermatologist, 1858–1915.
    Nikiforoff method—for the fixing of blood films.

Nikolsky, Pyotr V., Russian dermatologist, 1858–1940.
    Nikolsky sign—a peculiar vulnerability of the skin in pemphigus vulgaris.

N

NOTES

Nirenberg, Marshall W., U.S. biochemist, *1927, joint winner of 1968 Nobel Prize for work related to genetic code.

Nisbet, William, English physician, 1759–1822.
Nisbet chancre—chancre with lymphangitis; abscesses of the penis.

Nishimoto, A., Japanese physician.
Nishimoto disease—vascular syndrome. *SYN:* Nishimoto-Takeuchi syndrome
Nishimoto-Takeuchi syndrome—*SYN:* Nishimoto disease

Nissen, Rudolf, Swiss surgeon, *1896.
Nissen forceps
Nissen fundoplication
Nissen gastrectomy
Nissen hiatal hernia repair
Nissen operation
Nissen procedure
Nissen rib spreader
Nissen suture

Nissl, Franz, German neurologist, 1860–1919.
Nissl bodies—*SYN:* Nissl substance
Nissl degeneration—degeneration of the cell body occurring after transection of the axon.
Nissl granules—*SYN:* Nissl substance
Nissl methods—staining techniques.
Nissl stain—a method for staining nerve cells.
Nissl substance—the material consisting of granular endoplasmic reticulum and ribosomes that occurs in nerve cell bodies and dendrites. *SYN:* Nissl bodies; Nissl granules; tigroid bodies; substantia basophilia; basophil substance

Nitabuch, Raissa, 19th century German physician.
Nitabuch layer—*SYN:* Nitabuch membrane
Nitabuch membrane—a layer of fibrin between the boundary zone of compact endometrium and the cytotrophoblastic shell in the placenta. *SYN:* Nitabuch layer; Nitabuch stria
Nitabuch stria—*SYN:* Nitabuch membrane

Noack, Margot, German physician, *1909.
Noack syndrome—multiple congenital malformations. *SYN:* acrocephalopolysyndactyly

Noble, Charles P., U.S. gynecologist, 1863–1935.
Noble position—patient standing and bent slightly forward.

Noble, Robert L., Canadian physiologist, *1910.
Noble-Collip procedure—obsolete procedure in which shock in rats is induced by rotating them in a drum.

Nocard, Edmund I.E., French veterinarian, 1850–1903.
Nocardia—a genus of aerobic nonmotile actinomycetes (family Nocardiaceae, order Actinomycetales), transitional between bacteria and fungi, which are mainly saprophytic but may produce disease in human beings and other animals.

Nocardia **dacryoliths**—white pseudoconcretions, composed of masses of *Nocardia* species found in the lacrimal canaliculi. *Syn:* Desmarres dacryoliths

Nocardiaceae—a family of acid-fast, Gram-positive, aerobic bacteria (order Actinomycetales) that includes the genus *Nocardia*.

Preisz-Nocard bacillus—see under Preisz

Noguchi, Hideyo, Japanese pathologist, 1876–1928.
Noguchi test—a test for globulin.

Nomarski, Georges, 20th century French optical inventor.
Nomarski optics—an optical system for differential interference contrast microscopy.

Nonne, Max, German physician, 1861–1959.
Nonne-Marie syndrome—*Syn:* Menzel syndrome
Nonne-Milroy-Meige syndrome—ankle edema. *Syn:* congenital elephantiasis; tropholymphedema

Nonnenbruch, Wilhelm, German physician, 1887–1955.
Nonnenbruch syndrome—oliguria. *Syn:* extrarenal kidney syndrome

Noonan, Jacqueline A., U.S. pediatric cardiologist, *1921.
Noonan syndrome—the male phenotype of Turner syndrome, characterized by congenital heart disease.

Nordau, Max Simon, German scientist, 1849–1923.
Nordau disease—degeneration of the mind and body.

Norman, Margaret G., Canadian physician.
Norman-Roberts syndrome—*Syn:* Miller-Dieker syndrome

Norman, R.M., English physician.
Norman-Landing syndrome—genetic defects. *Syn:* beta-galactosidase deficiency

Norrie, Gordon, Danish ophthalmologist, 1855–1941.
Norrie disease—congenital bilateral masses of tissue arising from the retina or vitreous and resembling glioma (pseudoglioma), usually with atrophy of iris and development of cataract, associated mental retardation and deafness. *Syn:* Norrie syndrome; Norrie-Warburg syndrome
Norrie syndrome—*Syn:* Norrie disease
Norrie-Warburg syndrome—*Syn:* Norrie disease

Norris, Richard, English physiologist, 1831–1916.
Norris corpuscles—decolorized red blood cells that are invisible or almost invisible in the blood plasma unless they are appropriately stained.

Norton, U.F., U.S. obstetrician.
Norton operation—extraperitoneal cesarean section by a paravesical approach.

N

NOTES

Norum, K.R.
    Norum syndrome—corneal defects.

Nothnagel, C.W. Hermann, Austrian physician, 1841–1905.
    Nothnagel acroparesthesia—vasomotor disorders which cause acroparesthesias. *Syn:* vasomotor acroparesthesia
    Nothnagel acroparesthesia—abnormal sensation in the extremities accompanied by circulatory disorders.
    Nothnagel syndrome—dizziness, staggering, and rolling gait, with irregular forms of oculomotor paralysis and often nystagmus, seen in cases of tumor of the midbrain.
    Nothnagel II syndrome—midbrain lesion. *Syn:* Brun syndrome

Novy, Frederick G., U.S. bacteriologist, 1864–1957.
    Novy and MacNeal blood agar—a nutrient agar suitable for the cultivation of a number of trypanosomes.
    Novy rat disease—a viral disease among experimental rats.

Nowakowski, H.
    Nowakowski-Lenz syndrome—male pseudohermaphroditism.

Nuck, Anton, Dutch anatomist, 1650–1692.
    canal of Nuck—a persistent processus vaginalis in the female.
    Nuck diverticulum—a peritoneal diverticulum in the embryonic lower anterior abdominal wall. *Syn:* processus vaginalis of peritoneum
    Nuck hydrocele—accumulation of serous fluid in the labium majus or in Nuck canal. *Syn:* hydrocele feminae

Nuel, Jean P., Belgian ophthalmologist and otologist, 1847–1920.
    Nuel space—an interval in the spiral organ (of Corti) between the outer pillar cells on one side and the phalangeal cells and hair cells on the other.

Nuhn, Anton, German anatomist, 1814–1889.
    Nuhn gland—one of the small mixed glands deeply placed near the apex of the tongue on each side of the frenulum. *Syn:* anterior lingual gland

Nussbaum, Johann von, German surgeon, 1829–1890.
    Nussbaum bracelet—an appliance designed for use with writer's cramp.

Nussbaum, Moritz, German histologist, 1850–1915.
    Nussbaum experiment—exclusion of the glomeruli of the kidney from the circulation by ligation of the renal artery.

Nüsslein-Volhard, Christiane, joint winner of 1995 Nobel Prize for work related to genetics and early development of embryo.

Nygaard, Kaare Kristiaan, U.S. physician.
    Nygaard-Brown syndrome—*Syn:* Trousseau syndrome

Nyhan, William L. U.S. pediatrician, *1926.
    Lesch-Nyhan syndrome—see under Lesch

Nyssen, Rene, Belgian physician.
    Nyssen-van Bogaert-Meyer syndrome—autosomal recessive trait, with multiple defects.

Nysten, Pierre H., French physician, 1771–1818.
    Nysten law—rigor mortis affects first the muscles of the head and spreads toward the feet.

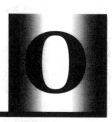

O'Beirne, James, Irish surgeon, 1786–1862.
   O'Beirne sphincter—a circular band of muscular fibers at the rectosigmoid junction. *Syn:* rectosigmoid sphincter
   O'Beirne tube

O'Brien, Cecil Starling, U.S. ophthalmologist, 1889–1977.
   O'Brien akinesia
   O'Brien block
   O'Brien cataract
   O'Brien scissors

O'Donnell, F.E., Jr.
   O'Donnell-Pappas syndrome—*Syn:* Karsch-Neugenbauer syndrome

O'Dwyer, Joseph P., U.S. physician, 1841–1898.
   O'Dwyer tube—a metal tube formerly used for intubation of the larynx in diphtheria.

O'Hara, Michael, Jr., U.S. surgeon, 1869–1926.
   O'Hara forceps—two slender clamp forceps used in intestinal anastomosis.
   O'Hara operation

Obal, Adalbert, U.S. physician.
   Obal syndrome—ocular disorders associated with malnutrition.

Ober, Frank Roberts, U.S. orthopedic surgeon, 1881–1960.
   Ober anterior transfer
   Ober exercise—an exercise developed to stretch a tight fascia lata.
   Ober incision
   Ober operation
   Ober posterior drainage
   Ober release
   Ober technique
   Ober tendon passer
   Ober test—test used to determine the degree of tightness of the fascia lata.

Obermayer, Friedrich, Austrian physician, 1861–1925.
   Obermayer test—a test for indican.

Obermeier, Otto H.F., German physician, 1843–1873.
   Obermeier spirillum—a species causing relapsing fever, transmitted by bedbugs and lice. *Syn:* Borrelia recurrentis

Obersteiner, H., Austrian neurologist, 1847–1922.
    Obersteiner-Redlich line—*Syn:* Obersteiner-Redlich zone
    Obersteiner-Redlich zone—marks the true boundary between the central
    and the peripheral nervous system. *Syn:* Obersteiner-Redlich line

Occam, Willliam of, English philosopher.
    Occam razor—in principle of scientific parsimony, the simplest explanation
    is always preferable.

Ochoa, Severo, Spanish-U.S. biochemist and Nobel laureate, *1905.
    Ochoa law—the content of the X-chromosome tends to be
    phylogenetically conserved.

Ochsner, Albert J., U.S. surgeon, 1858–1925.
    Ochsner cartilage forceps
    Ochsner clamp—a straight hemostat with teeth.
    Ochsner forceps
    Ochsner hemostat
    Ochsner hook
    Ochsner method—an obsolete treatment for appendicitis.
    Ochsner muscle
    Ochsner retractor
    Ochsner ring
    Ochsner scissors
    Ochsner tissue forceps
    Ochsner trocar
    Ochsner tube
    Oshsner ring

Ockuly, O.E.
    Ockuly-Montgomery syndrome—small brownish lesions.

Oddi, Ruggero, Italian physician; 1864–1913.
    Oddi sphincter—*Syn:* sphincter of Oddi
    sphincter of Oddi—the smooth muscle sphincter of the hepatopancreatic
    ampulla within the duodenal papilla. *Syn:* Oddi sphincter; sphincter of
    hepatopancreatic ampulla

Oeckerman, P.A.
    Oeckerman syndrome—multiple genetic defects.

Oedipus, character from Greek mythology.
    oedipism—(1) self-infliction of injury to the eyes; (2) manifestation of the
    Oedipus complex.
    Oedipus complex—a phase of psychosexual development in which the
    child is erotically attached to parent of the opposite sex and has feelings
    of aggression toward the same-sex parent.
    Oedipus period—the time of a child's development characterized by erotic
    attachment to the parent of the opposite sex.

Oehl, Eusebio, Italian anatomist, 1827–1903.
    Oehl muscles—strands of muscle fibers in the chordae tendineae of the
    left atrioventricular valve.

Oehler, Johannes, German physician, *1879.
    Oehler symptom—a sudden pallor and coldness in the arm, with slight
    disability, occurring on lifting a heavy weight.

Ogilvie, Sir William H., English surgeon, 1887–1971.
Ogilvie herniorrhaphy
Ogilvie syndrome—motility disturbance of the intestines.

Ogino, Kyusaka, 20th century Japanese physician.
Ogino-Knaus rule—the basis for the rhythm method of contraception.

Ogston, Sir Alexander, Scottish surgeon, 1844–1929.
Ogston line—a guide to resection of the medial condyle for knock-knees.
Ogston-Luc operation—an operation for frontal sinus disease.

Oguchi, Chita, Japanese ophthalmologist, 1875–1945.
Oguchi disease—a rare congenital, nonprogressive night blindness.

Ogura, Joseph H., U.S. otolaryngologist, *1915.
Ogura cartilage forceps
Ogura fossa
Ogura operation—orbital decompression by removal of the floor of the orbit through an opening made in the supradental fossa.
Ogura saw
Ogura technique
Ogura tissue forceps

Ohara, Shoichiro, 20th century Japanese physician.
Ohara disease—tularemia.

Ohm, Georg S., German physicist, 1787–1854.
ohm—The practical unit of electrical resistance.
Ohm law—in an electric current passing through a wire, the intensity of the current in amperes equals the electromotive force in volts divided by the resistance in ohms.

Okazaki, Reiji and Tuneko, 20th century Japanese biochemists.
Okazaki fragment—short pieces of DNA formed during DNA synthesis.

Oldfield, Michael C., 20th century English physician.
Oldfield syndrome—familial colon polyposis.

Oliver, G.L.
Oliver-McFarlane syndrome—genetic defects. *Syn:* Gray syndrome

Oliver, William Silver, English physician, 1836–1908.
Oliver sign—tracheal tugging.
Oliver test—a test for albumin.

Ollendorf, Helene, German dermatologist.
Buschke-Ollendorf syndrome—see under Buschke

Ollier, Louis X.E.L., French surgeon, 1830–1900.
Ollier approach
Ollier disease—proliferation of cartilage in the metaphyses of several
(continued)

NOTES

Ollier *(continued)*
>bones, causing distorted growth in length or pathological fractures. *SYN:* enchondromatosis
>**Ollier graft**—a thin split-thickness graft, usually in small pieces. *SYN:* Thiersch graft; Ollier-Thiersch graft
>**Ollier incision**
>**Ollier layer**
>**Ollier method**
>**Ollier operation**
>**Ollier rake retractor**
>**Ollier raspatory**
>**Ollier retractor**
>**Ollier technique**
>**Ollier theory**—a theory of compensatory growth.
>**Ollier-Thiersch graft**—*SYN:* Ollier graft

Olshausen, Robert von, German obstetrician, 1835–1915.
>**Olshausen operation**—surgery done for retroversion of the uterus.
>**Olshausen sign**
>**Olshausen suspension**

Olshevsky, Dimitry E., U.S. physician, *1900.
>**Olshevsky tube**

Olszewski, Jerzy, Polish-Canadian neuropathologist, d. 1966.
>**Steele-Richardson-Olszewski disease**—*SYN:* Steele-Richardson-Olszewski syndrome
>**Steele-Richardson-Olszewski syndrome**—see under Steele

Ombrédanne, Louis, French surgeon, 1871–1956.
>**Ombrédanne forceps**
>**Ombrédanne mallet**
>**Ombrédanne operation**—*SYN:* transseptal orchiopexy

Omenn, Gilbert S., U.S. internist, *1941.
>**Omenn syndrome**—a rapidly fatal autosomal recessive immunodeficiency disease.

Ommaya, Ayub K., U.S. neurosurgeon, *1930.
>**Ommaya cerebrospinal fluid reservoir**
>**Ommaya intraventricular reservoir system**
>**Ommaya reservoir**
>**Ommaya reservoir implant material**
>**Ommaya reservoir prosthesis**
>**Ommaya reservoir transensor**
>**Ommaya retromastoid reservoir**
>**Ommaya shunt**
>**Ommaya side-port flat-bottomed reservoir**
>**Ommaya suboccipital reservoir**
>**Ommaya tube**
>**Ommaya ventricular reservoir**

Ondine, German mythological character.
>**Ondine curse**—alveolar hyperventilation.

Onufrowicz, Wladislaus, Swiss anatomist, 1836–1900.
   Onuf nucleus—small somatic motor neurons in the ventral horn of the spinal cord at level S2.

Opalski, Adam, Polish physician, 1897–1963.
   Opalski cell—a characteristically altered glial cell in the basal ganglia and thalamus, found in hepatocerebral degeneration and Wilson disease.

Opitz, John M., U.S. pediatrician, *1935.
   Opitz-Frias syndrome—males affected from birth; swallowing problems with recurrent aspiration, stridorous breathing, and hoarse cry.
   Opitz-Kaveggia syndrome—in males; X-linked recessive syndrome of multiple congenital anomalies and mental retardation. *SYN:* Keller syndrome
   Smith-Lemli-Opitz syndrome—see under Smith, David W.

Opitz, Z.
   Opitz syndrome—thrombophlebitis of the splenic vein.

Oppenheim, Hermann, German neurologist, 1858–1919.
   Minor-Oppenheim syndrome—*SYN:* Minor syndrome
   Oppenheim brace
   Oppenheim congenital hypotonia
   Oppenheim disease—*SYN:* Oppenheim syndrome
   Oppenheim gait
   Oppenheim reflex—extension of the toes induced by scratching of the inner side of the leg, a sign of cerebral irritation.
   Oppenheim sign—suggests pyramidal tract disease.
   Oppenheim splint
   Oppenheim spring wire splint
   Oppenheim stroke test
   Oppenheim syndrome—congenital atonic pseudoparalysis, observed especially in infants. *SYN:* amyotonia congenita; Oppenheim disease
   Ziehen-Oppenheim disease—see under Ziehen

Oppenheimer, A.
   Oppenheimer syndrome—limitation of spinal motion. *SYN:* physiologic vertebral ligamentous calcification

Oram, S., 20th century English cardiologist.
   Holt-Oram syndrome—see under Holt, Mary

Orbeli, Leon A., Russian physiologist, 1882–1958.
   Orbeli effect—the fatigue of a muscle stimulated by its nerve is reduced by concurrent stimulation of sympathetic fibers to the muscle.
   Orbeli phenomenon

Ormond, John K., U.S. urologist, *1886.
   Ormond disease—*SYN:* retroperitoneal fibrosis
   Ormond syndrome—*SYN:* Gerota fascitis

O

NOTES

Ornish, Dean, U.S. physician, *1953.
    Ornish reversal diet—a diet designed to reverse coronary artery disease.

Orr, Hiram Winnett, U.S. orthopedic surgeon, 1877–1956.
    Orr forceps
    Orr incision
    Orr method
    Orr technique
    Orr treatment

Orsi, Francesco, Italian physician, 1828–1890.
    Orsi-Grocco method—palpatory percussion of the heart.

Orth, Johannes J., German pathologist, 1847–1923.
    Orth fixative—formalin added to Müller fixative, used for bringing out chromaffin, studying early degenerative processes and necrosis and for demonstrating rickettsiae and bacteria.
    Orth stain—a lithium carmine stain for nerve cells and their processes.

Ortner, Norbert, Austrian physician, 1865–1935.
    Ortner syndrome—laryngeal paralysis that is associated with heart disease.
    Ortolani

Ortolani, Marius, 20th century Italian orthopedic surgeon.
    Ortolani click
    Ortolani maneuver
    Ortolani sign
    Ortolani test—test for congenital hip dislocation.

Orton, S.T., U.S. neurologist, 1879–1975.
    Wolf-Orton bodies—see under Wolf

Orzechowski, K.
    Orzechowski syndrome—involuntary oscillations of the eyes in horizontal and vertical directions; tremulousness; sign of encephalitis.

Osebold, W.R.
    Osebold-Remondini syndrome—middle phalanges of all digits are hypoplastic or absent; autosomal dominant inheritance. *Syn:* brachydactyly

Osgood, Robert B., U.S. orthopedic surgeon, 1873–1956.
    Osgood femoral supracondylar osteotomy
    Osgood modified technique
    Osgood operation
    Osgood rotational osteotomy
    Osgood-Schlatter disease—epiphysial aseptic necrosis of the tibial tubercle. *Syn:* apophysitis tibialis adolescentium; Schlatter disease; Schlatter-Osgood disease
    Schlatter-Osgood disease—*Syn:* Osgood-Schlatter disease

Osler, Sir William, Canadian physician in U.S. and England, 1849–1919.
    Osler II syndrome—recurrent episodes of colic pain. *Syn:* ball-valve gallstone
    Osler disease—a chronic form of polycythemia. *Syn:* polycythemia vera
    Osler node—a tender cutaneous lesion characteristic of subacute bacterial endocarditis.

Osler sign—in acute bacterial endocarditis, circumscribed painful erythematous swelling in the skin and subcutaneous tissues of the hands and feet.
Osler triad
Rendu-Osler-Weber syndrome—see under Rendu

Ostertag, B.
Ostertag syndrome—*Syn:* hereditary amyloid nephropathy

Ostwald, Friedrich Wilhelm, German physical chemist and Nobel laureate, 1853–1932.
Ostwald solubility coefficient—the milliliters of gas dissolved per milliliter of liquid and per atmosphere partial pressure of the gas at any given temperature.

Osuntokun, B.O.
Osuntokun syndrome—congenital analgesia and deafness. *Syn:* pain indifference-deafness

Ota, Masao T., Japanese dermatopathologist, 1885–1945.
Ota nevus—pigmentation of the conjunctiva and skin around the eye, usually unilateral. *Syn:* oculodermal melanosis
Ota syndrome—onset in childhood; asymptomatic. *Syn:* oculodermal melanocytosis

Othello, one of Shakespeare's characters.
Othello syndrome—delusions of infidelity of one's sexual partner; onset usually in 4th decade of life; may be a feature of depressive psychosis, epilepsy, or alcoholism. *Syn:* erotic jealousy

Otis, Arthur Brooks, U.S. respiratory physiologist, *1913.
Rahn-Otis sample—see under Rahn

Otto, Adolph W., German surgeon, 1786–1845.
Otto disease—a disease characterized by an inward bulging of the acetabulum into the pelvic cavity, resulting from arthritis of the hip joints, usually due to rheumatoid arthritis. *Syn:* Otto pelvis; protrusio acetabuli; arthrokatadysis
Otto forceps
Otto pelvis—*Syn:* Otto disease

Ottoson, David, 20th century Swedish physiologist.
Ottoson potential—an electronegative wave of potential occurring on the surface of the olfactory epithelium in response to stimulation by an odor. *Syn:* electro-olfactogram

Ouchterlony, Orjan, Swedish bacteriologist, *1914.
Ouchterlony immunodiffusion
Ouchterlony method—*Syn:* Ouchterlony test
Ouchterlony technique—*Syn:* Ouchterlony test
Ouchterlony test—double (gel) diffusion test in two dimensions. *Syn:* Ouchterlony technique; Ouchterlony method

NOTES

Oudin, Paul, French electrotherapist, 1851–1923.
    Oudin current—a high-frequency current.
    Oudin resonator—a special wire coil.

Overton, Charles E., German biologist in Sweden, 1865–1933.
    Meyer-Overton rule—see under Meyer, Hans
    Meyer-Overton theory of narcosis—see under Meyer, Hans

Owen, Sir Richard, English anatomist, 1804–1892.
    contour lines of Owen—*Syn:* Owen lines
    interglobular space of Owen—one of a number of irregularly branched spaces near the periphery of the dentin of the crown of a tooth. *Syn:* interglobular space
    Owen lines—accentuated incremental lines in the dentin thought to be due to disturbances in the mineralization process. *Syn:* contour lines of Owen

Owren, Paul A., Norwegian hematologist, *1905.
    Owren disease—a congenital deficiency of factor V, resulting in prolongation of prothrombin time and coagulation time.

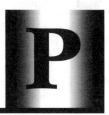

Paas, Herman R., German physician, *1900.
    Paas disease—familial skeletal deformities.

Pacchioni, Antonio, Italian anatomist, 1665–1726.
    pacchionian bodies—tufted prolongations of pia-arachnoid. *SYN:* arachnoid granulations; pacchionian corpuscles; pacchionian glands; pacchionian granulations
    pacchionian corpuscles—*SYN:* pacchionian bodies
    pacchionian depressions—pits on the inner surface of the skull in which are lodged the arachnoidal granulations. *SYN:* granular pits
    pacchionian glands—*SYN:* pacchionian bodies
    pacchionian granulations—*SYN:* pacchionian bodies

Pachon, Michel V., French physiologist, 1867–1938.
    Pachon method—cardiography carried out with the patient lying on the left side.
    Pachon test—in a case of aneurysm, determination of the collateral circulation by estimation of the blood pressure.

Pacini, Filippo, Italian anatomist, 1812–1883.
    Pacini bodies
    pacinian corpuscles—*SYN:* Vater corpuscles
    Vater-Pacini corpuscles—*SYN:* Vater corpuscles

Padgett, Earl Calvin, U.S. surgeon, 1893–1946.
    Padgett blade
    Padgett cannula
    Padgett dermatome
    Padgett graft
    Padgett implant
    Padgett prosthesis

Page, I.H.
    Page syndrome—periodic appearance of blotchy flushes covered by beads of perspiration on the face, upper chest, and abdomen.

Pagenstecher, Alexander, German ophthalmologist, 1828–1879.
    Pagenstecher circle—around the point of attachment of a freely movable abdominal tumor.

Paget, Sir James, English surgeon, 1814–1899.
    extramammary Paget disease—*SYN:* Paget disease

(continued)

Paget (*continued*)

   Paget abscess syndrome—an abscess recurrence at the same site after apparent cure.

   Paget associated osteogenic sarcoma

   Paget cells—relatively large neoplastic epithelial cells.

   Paget disease—an intraepidermal form of mucinous adenocarcinoma, most commonly in the anogenital region. *SYN:* extramammary Paget disease

   Paget disease of bone—osteitis deformans *SYN:* Paget II syndrome

   Paget disease of the nipple—duct carcinoma.

   Paget disease of the penis—carcinoma that develops after balanitis.

   Paget I syndrome—relationship to or possible extension of mammary duct carcinoma.

   Paget II syndrome—*SYN:* Paget disease of bone

   Paget juvenile syndrome—*SYN:* familial osteoectasia

   Paget necrosis—necrosis in the superficial layers of the shaft of a long bone.

   Paget quiet necrosis

   Paget test—a test to determine whether a mass is a solid tumor or a cyst.

   Paget-von Schrötter syndrome—stress thrombosis or spontaneous thrombosis of the subclavian or axillary vein. *SYN:* effort-induced thrombosis

Paget, Sir Richard, English physical scientist, 1869–1955.

   Paget sign language—a sign language for the hearing impaired. *SYN:* Paget-Gorman sign language

   Paget-Gorman sign language—*SYN:* Paget sign language

Pagon, R.A.

   Pagon syndrome—anemia from birth (in males); ataxia evident by age 1 year; clonus and positive Babinski sign. *SYN:* sideroblastic anemia; spinocerebellar ataxia

Paine, R.S.

   Paine retinaculatome

   Paine syndrome—males only; onset at birth; physical and mental retardation; seizures. *SYN:* microcephaly

   Paine-Efron syndrome—pain in the back and thigh followed by slowly progressive ataxia. *SYN:* ataxia-telangiectasia variant

Pajot, Charles, French obstetrician, 1816–1896.

   Pajot hook

   Pajot law—a law governing a fetus' rotating movements during labor.

   Pajot maneuver—obsolete term for method to bring the fetal head down in the axis of the birth canal.

Pal, Jacob, Austrian physician, 1863–1936.

   Pal stain—stain used to study myelinated nerves.

Palade, George E., Romanian-U.S. cell biologist and Nobel laureate, *1912.

   Palade granule—a granule of ribonucleoprotein, the site of protein synthesis from aminoacyl-tRNAs as directed by mRNAs. *SYN:* ribosome

   Weibel-Palade bodies—see under Weibel

Palant, D.I.

   Palant-Feingold-Berkman syndrome—in females from birth, short stature, midline cleft palate, bilateral camptodactyly of 4th and 5th fingers, broad distal phalanges of toes, syndactyly of 2nd and 3rd toes, feet have valgus deformity, eyes are deep set and almond shaped (mongoloid slant), bulbous nose, epicanthal folds. *Syn:* unusual face, mental retardation, limb abnormality, cleft palate

Palfyn, Jean, Belgian surgeon and anatomist, 1650–1730.
Palfyn sinus—a space within the crista galli of the ethmoid described as communicating with the ethmoidal and frontal sinuses.
Palfyn suture

Pallister, P.D.
Pallister syndrome—autosomal dominant inheritance affecting both sexes.

Palmer, Walter L., U.S. physician, *1896.
Palmer acid test for peptic ulcer—in duodenal ulcer, the administration of acid by duodenal tube causes severe pain.

Pancoast, Henry K., U.S. radiologist, 1875–1939.
Pancoast syndrome—lower trunk brachial plexopathy and Horner syndrome due to malignant tumor in the region of the superior pulmonary sulcus.
Pancoast tumor—an adenocarcinoma of a lung apex causing Pancoast syndrome. *Syn:* superior pulmonary sulcus tumor

Pancoast, Joseph, U.S. surgeon, 1805–1882.
Pancoast operation
Pancoast suture—in plastic surgery, union of two edges by a tongue-and-groove arrangement.

Pandy, Kalman, Hungarian neurologist, *1868.
Pandy reaction—a test to determine the presence of proteins in the spinal fluid. *Syn:* Pandy test
Pandy test—*Syn:* Pandy reaction

Paneth, Josef, Austrian physician, 1857–1890.
Paneth granular cells—cells located at the base of intestinal glands of the small intestine that contain large acidophilic refractile granules and may produce lysozyme. *Syn:* Davidoff cells

Panizza, Bartolomeo, Italian anatomist, 1785–1867.
Panizza plexus—lymph vessel plexuses located in the prepuce's lateral fossae.

Panner, H.J., Danish radiologist, 1871–1930.
Panner disease—epiphyseal aseptic necrosis of the capitellum of the humerus.

Pansch, Adolf, German anatomist, 1841–1887.
Pansch fissure—a sulcus cerebral fissure running from the lower extremity of the central fissure nearly to the end of the occipital lobe.

NOTES

Panum, Peter L., Danish physiologist, 1820–1885.
    Panum area—the area in and about the macula retinae in which stimulation of noncorresponding retinal points results in stereoscopic vision. *Syn:* fusion area

Papanicolaou, George N., Greek-U.S. physician, anatomist, and cytologist, 1883–1962.
    Pap smear—a smear of vaginal or cervical cells obtained for cytological study. *Syn:* Papanicolaou smear
    Pap test—examination of cells stained with Papanicolaou stain. *Syn:* Papanicolaou smear test; Papanicolaou test
    Papanicolaou examination
    Papanicolaou smear—*Syn:* Pap smear
    Papanicolaou smear test—*Syn:* Pap test
    Papanicolaou stain—a multichromatic stain used in cancer screening, especially of gynecologic smears.
    Papanicolaou test—*Syn:* Pap test

Papas, C.V., Greek physician.
    Bartsocas-Papas syndrome—see under Bartsocas

Papez, James W., U.S. anatomist, 1883–1958.
    Papez circle—network of nerve fibers and centers.
    Papez circuit—a long circuitous conduction chain in the mammalian forebrain.
    Papez theory of emotions—theory that emotions are controlled by Papez circle.

Papillon, M.M., 20th century French dermatologist.
    Papillon-Lefèvre syndrome—a congenital hyperkeratosis of the palms and soles, with progessive destruction of alveolar bone about the deciduous and permanent teeth.

Papillon-Léage, E., 20th century French dentist.
    Papillon-Léage and Psaume syndrome—an inherited syndrome, lethal in males, with varying combinations of defects of the oral cavity, face, and hands, and, frequently, mental retardation. *Syn:* orodigitofacial dysostosis

Pappas, H.R.
    O'Donnell-Pappas syndrome—*Syn:* Karsch-Neugenbauer syndrome

Pappenheim, Artur, German physician, 1870–1916.
    Pappenheim stain—a method for differentiating tubercle and smegma bacilli.
    Unna-Pappenheim stain—see under Unna

Paracelsus, Aureolus Theophrastus Bombastus von Hohenheim, Swiss physician, 1493–1541.
    paracelsian method—the use of chemical agents only in the treatment of disease.

Pardee, Harold Ensign Bennett, U.S. physician, *1886.
    Pardee sign—ST segment elevation on electrocardiogram.

Paré, Ambroise, French surgeon, 1510–1590.
    Paré suture—the approximation of the edges of a wound by pasting strips of cloth to the surface and stitching them instead of the skin.

Parham, Frederick William, U.S. surgeon, 1856–1927.
   Parham band—a metallic ribbon used to repair fractured long bones.
   Parham support

Parinaud, Henri, French ophthalmologist, 1844–1905.
   Parinaud conjunctivitis—a chronic necrotic inflammation of the
      conjunctiva characterized by large, irregular, reddish follicles and
      regional lymphadenopathy.
   Parinaud I syndrome—retraction nystagmus; systemic hypertension;
      Babinski sign; extraocular palsy; pupils usually normal in size but have
      poor reaction to light and near vision. *SYN:* divergence paralysis;
      Koerber-Salus-Elschnig syndrome
   Parinaud oculoglandular syndrome—unilateral conjunctival granuloma
      with preauricular adenopathy in tularemia, chancre, and tuberculosis.
   Parinaud ophthalmoplegia—*SYN:* Parinaud syndrome
   Parinaud syndrome—paralysis of conjugate upward gaze with a lesion at
      the level of the superior colliculi. *SYN:* Parinaud ophthalmoplegia

Paris, city in France.
   plaster of Paris—a gypsum material used for making casts.

Park, Henry, English surgeon, 1744–1831.
   Park aneurysm—an arteriovenous aneurysm in which the brachial artery
      communicates with the brachial and median basilic veins.

Park, William H., U.S. bacteriologist, 1863–1939.
   Park-Williams bacillus—a special strain of *Corynebacterium diphtheriae*
      used for toxin production.
   Park-Williams fixative—a fixative for spirochetes, comprised of a 2%
      solution of osmic acid; the bacteria are exposed to the fumes of the
      solution for a few seconds.

Parker, Edward Mason, U.S. surgeon, 1860–1941.
   Parker clamp
   Parker discission knife
   Parker fixation forceps
   Parker incision
   Parker needle
   Parker retractor
   Parker serrated discission knife
   Parker-Heath anterior chamber syringe
   Parker-Heath cautery
   Parker-Heath electrocautery
   Parker-Heath piggyback probe
   Parker-Kerr basting suture
   Parker-Kerr operation
   Parker-Kerr suture—a continuous inverting suture used to close an open
      end of intestine.

NOTES

Parker, George Howard, U.S. zoologist, 1864–1955.
   Parker fluid—formaldehyde and alcohol.

Parker, R.W.
   Parker syndrome—onset under the age of 10 years, either sex; possible association with various congenital deformities. *SYN:* adrenal medullary neuroblastoma

Parkinson, James, English physician, 1755–1824.
   Parkinson disease—a neurological syndrome usually resulting from deficiency of the neurotransmitter dopamine as the consequence of degenerative, vascular, or inflammatory changes in the basal ganglia. *SYN:* parkinsonism (1)
   Parkinson facies—the expressionless or masklike facies characteristic of parkinsonism. *SYN:* masklike face; Parkinson sign
   Parkinson sign—*SYN:* Parkinson facies
   Parkinson triangle
   parkinsonism—(1) *SYN:* Parkinson disease; (2) syndrome similar to Parkinson disease appearing as a side effect of certain drugs.

Parkinson, Sir John, English cardiologist, *1885.
   Wolff-Parkinson-White syndrome—see under Wolff

Parnas, Jakob Karol, Polish physiologic chemist, 1884–1955.
   Embden-Meyerhof-Parnas pathway—*SYN:* Embden-Meyerhof pathway

Parona, Francesco, Italian surgeon, 1861–1910.
   Parona space—a space between the pronator quadratus deep and the overlying flexor tendons of the forearm. *SYN:* space of Parona
   space of Parona—*SYN:* Parona space

Parrot, Jules, French physician, 1829–1883.
   Bednar-Parrot syndrome—*SYN:* Parrot I syndrome
   Parrot atrophy of the newborn
   Parrot disease—pseudoparalysis in infants due to syphilitic osteochondritis; cachexia, primarily due to prolonged dietary deficiency of protein and calories. *SYN:* marasmus
   Parrot I syndrome—pseudoparalysis; periarticular swelling, onset seldom after 3 months of age. *SYN:* Bednar-Parrot syndrome; Parrot syphilitic osteochondritis
   Parrot II syndrome—failure to thrive, emaciation, edema, dry skin, with subcutaneous fat loss, abdomen flat or distended, hypothermia, slow pulse, decreased metabolic rate. *SYN:* marasmus; infantile atrophy; inanition; athrepsia
   Parrot nodes—*SYN:* Parrot sign
   Parrot pseudoparalysis—syphilitic osteochondritis in newborns causing pseudoparalysis in one or more extremities. *SYN:* syphilitic pseudoparalysis
   Parrot sign—indicates congenital syphilis in newborns. *SYN:* Parrot nodes
   Parrot syphilitic osteochondritis—*SYN:* Parrot I syndrome

Parry, Caleb H., English physician, 1755–1822.
   Parry disease—*SYN:* Graves disease

Pascal, Blaise, French scientist, 1623–1662.
    pascal—a derived unit of pressure or stress in the SI system.
    Pascal law—fluids at rest transmit pressure equally in every direction.

Pascheff, Constantin (Konstantin), Bulgarian ophthalmologist, 1873–1961.
    Pascheff conjunctivitis—a unilateral, suppurative, necrotic inflammation of the conjunctiva. *SYN:* necrotic infectious conjunctivitis

Paschen, Enrique, German pathologist, 1860–1936.
    Paschen bodies—particles of virus observed in relatively large numbers in squamous cells of the skin, or the cornea of experimental animals, in variola (smallpox) or vaccinia. *SYN:* Paschen corpuscles; Paschen granules
    Paschen corpuscles—*SYN:* Paschen bodies
    Paschen granules—*SYN:* Paschen bodies

Pasini, Augustine, 20th century Argentinian dermatologist.
    atrophoderma of Pasini and Pierini—a form of slate-colored atrophy of the skin occurring in discrete 2-cm or larger lesions.
    Pasini syndrome—small, firm, white perifollicular papules that appear primarily on the lumbosacral region. *SYN:* albopapuloid epidermolysis bullosa
    Pasini variant
    Pasini-Pierini syndrome—slight depression below the level of normal skin of different shapes, colors, and dimensions. *SYN:* atrophic morphea variant

Pasqualini, R.Q.
    Pasqualini syndrome—having no libido or potency. *SYN:* pseudoeunuchoidism

Passavant, Philippas G., German physician, 1815–1893.
    Passavant bar—*SYN:* Passavant cushion
    Passavant cushion—a prominence on the posterior wall of the nasopharynx formed by contraction of the superior constrictor of the pharynx during swallowing. *SYN:* Passavant pad; Passavant bar; Passavant ridge
    Passavant pad—*SYN:* Passavant cushion
    Passavant ridge—*SYN:* Passavant cushion

Passey, R.D., 20th century English pathologist.
    Harding-Passey melanoma—see under Harding

Passow, A.
    Passow syndrome—multiple congenital anomalies. *SYN:* Bremer status dysraphicus

Passwell, J.H.
    Passwell syndrome—ichthyosis, mental retardation, and dwarfism from birth.

P

NOTES

Pasteur, Louis, French chemist and bacteriologist, 1822–1895.
> *Pasteurella*
> **Pasteur effect**—the inhibition of fermentation by oxygen, first observed by Pasteur.
> **Pasteur pipette**—a cotton-plugged, glass tube drawn out to a fine tip, used for the sterile transfer of small volumes of fluid.
> **Pasteur vaccine**
> **pasteurellosis**—infection with bacteria of *Pasteurella.*
> **pasteurization**—bacteria destruction process.
> **pasteurizer**—pasteurization apparatus.

Pastia, Chessec, Romanian physician, *1878.
> **Pastia lines**
> **Pastia sign**—the presence of pink or red transverse lines at the bend of the elbow in the pre-eruptive stage of scarlatina. *Syn:* Thomson sign

Patau, Klaus, 20th century U.S. cytogeneticist.
> **Patau syndrome**—a syndrome usually fatal within two years, characterized by mental retardation, malformed ears, and multiple organ anomalies. *Syn:* trisomy 13 syndrome

Patein, G., French physician, 1857–1928.
> **Patein albumin**—a substance resembling serum albumin but soluble in acetic acid. *Syn:* acetosoluble albumin

Patella, Vincenzo, Italian physician, 1856–1928.
> **Patella disease**—pyloric stenosis in tuberculosis patients.

Paterson, Donald R., English otolaryngologist, 1863–1939.
> **Paterson cannula**
> **Paterson forceps**
> **Paterson-Brown-Kelly syndrome**—limited elevation of the eye in adduction, due to fascia contracting the superior oblique muscle on the same side. *Syn:* tendon sheath syndrome
> **Paterson-Kelly syndrome**—*Syn:* Plummer-Vinson syndrome

Patey, David H., English surgeon, 1899–1977.
> **Patey axillary node dissection**
> **Patey mastectomy**
> **Patey modified radical mastectomy**
> **Patey operation**—modified radical mastectomy.

Patrick, Hugh T., U.S. neurologist, 1860–1938.
> **Patrick drill**
> **Patrick maneuver**
> **Patrick sign**
> **Patrick test**—a test to determine the presence or absence of sacroiliac disease.
> **Patrick trigger area**

Paul, Frank Thomas, English surgeon, 1851–1941.
> **Mixter-Paul hemostatic forceps**
> **Paul-Mixter tube**

Paul, Gustav, Austrian physician, 1859–1935.
> **Paul reaction**—formerly a test for smallpox. *Syn:* Paul test

Paul test—*SYN:* Paul reaction

Paul-Bunnell test—test for detection of heterophil antibodies in infectious mononucleosis.

Pauli, Wolfgang, Austrian-U.S. physicist and Nobel laureate, 1900–1958.

Pauli exclusion principle—the theory limiting the number of electrons in the orbit or shell of an atom.

Pauling, Linus C., U.S. chemist and Nobel laureate, 1901–1994.

Pauling theory—a theory of narcosis pertaining to nonhydrogen-bonding agents. *SYN:* hydrate microcrystal theory of anesthesia

Pauling-Corey helix—the helical (commonly right-handed) form present in many proteins. *SYN:* α helix

Pautrier, Lucien M.A., French dermatologist, 1876–1959.

Pautrier abscess—*SYN:* Pautrier microabscess

Pautrier microsbscess—a microscopic lesion in the epidermis, seen in mycosis fungoides. *SYN:* Pautrier abscess

Pauzat, Jean E., 19th century French physician.

Pauzat disease—osteoplastic periostitis or fatigue fractures of the metatarsal bones, caused by excessive marching.

Pavlov, Ivan, Russian physiologist and Nobel laureate, 1849–1936.

Pavlov behavorial theory

Pavlov method—the method of studying conditioned reflex activity by the observation of a motor indicator, such as the salivary or electroencephalographic response.

Pavlov pouch—a section of the stomach of a dog used in studies of gastric secretions. *SYN:* miniature stomach; Pavlov stomach

Pavlov reflex—peripheral vasoconstriction and a rise in blood pressure in response to a fall in pressure in the great veins. *SYN:* auriculopressor reflex

Pavlov stomach—*SYN:* Pavlov pouch

Pavlov theory of schizophrenia—Pavlov's belief that symptoms of schizophrenia result from an inhibited state of the cerebral cortex.

pavlovian conditioning—a type of conditioning in which a previously neutral stimulus elicits a response as a result of pairing it a number of times with an unconditioned stimulus for that response. *SYN:* respondent conditioning

Pavy, Frederick W., English physician, 1829–1911.

Pavy disease—cyclic or recurrent physiologic albuminuria.

Paxton, Francis V., English physician, 1840–1924.

Paxton disease—*Corynebacterium* infection of axillary and pubic hairs. *SYN:* trichomycosis axillaris

Payne, J. Howard, U.S. surgeon, *1916.

Payne operation—a jejunoileal bypass for morbid obesity.

Payne retractor

P

NOTES

Payr, Erwin, German surgeon, 1871–1946.
Payr clamp—a clamp used in gastrectomy or enterectomy.
Payr disease—constipation, with left upper quadrant pain. *SYN:* splenic flexure syndrome
Payr forceps
Payr gastrectomy
Payr membrane—a fold of peritoneum that crosses over the left flexure of the colon.
Payr rectractor
Payr sign—pain on pressure over the sole of the foot, a sign of thrombophlebitis.
Payr syndrome—occurs in approximately 20% of patients with irritable bowel, usually postprandially.

Péan, Jules Émile, French surgeon, 1830–1898.
Péan amputation
Péan clamp
Péan forceps
Péan incision
Péan operation
Péan position
Péan scissors

Pearson, H.A.
Pearson syndrome—refractory sideroblastic anemia; malabsorption or other pancreatic exocrine insufficiency.

Pearson, Karl, English mathematician, 1857–1936.
McArdle-Schmid-Pearson disease—*SYN:* McArdle syndrome
Poisson-Pearson formula—see under Poisson

Pecquet, Jean, French anatomist, 1622–1674.
Pecquet cistern—*SYN:* Pecquet reservoir
Pecquet duct—the largest lymph vessel in the body. *SYN:* thoracic duct
Pecquet reservoir—a dilated sac at the lower end of the thoracic duct into which the intestinal trunk and two lumbar lymphatic trunks open. *SYN:* cisterna chyli; Pecquet cistern; receptaculum pecqueti
receptaculum pecqueti—*SYN:* Pecquet reservoir

Pedersen, E.
Pedersen syndrome—abrupt onset of vertigo, nausea, vomiting. *SYN:* Dix-Hallpike; neurolabyrinthitis

Peiffer, J., German physician, *1922.
Hirsch-Peiffer stain—a stain used for cytologic demonstration of metachromatic leukodystrophy.

Pel, Pieter K., Dutch physician, 1852–1919.
Murchison-Pel-Ebstein syndrome—see under Murchison
Pel crises—ocular crises.
Pel-Ebstein disease—*SYN:* Pel-Ebstein fever
Pel-Ebstein fever—the remittent fever common in Hodgkin disease. *SYN:* Pel-Ebstein disease

Pelger, Karel, Dutch physician, 1885–1931.
Huët-Pelger anomaly—*SYN:* Pelger-Huët nuclear anomaly

Pelger-Huët nuclear anomaly—congenital inhibition of lobulation in the nuclei of neutrophilic leukocytes. *Syn:* Huët-Pelger anomaly

Pelizaeus, Friedrich, German neurologist, 1850–1917.
Merzbacher-Pelizaeus disease—*Syn:* Pelizaeus-Merzbacher disease
Pelizaeus-Merzbacher disease—a sudanophilic leukodystrophy with a tigroid appearance of the myelin resulting from patchy demyelination. *Syn:* Merzbacher-Pelizaeus disease

Pellegrini, Augusto, Italian surgeon, *1877.
Pellegrini disease—a calcific density in the medial collateral ligament and/or bony growth at the internal condyle of the femur. *Syn:* Pellegrini-Stieda disease
Pellegrini-Stieda disease—*Syn:* Pellegrini disease

Pellizzari, Pietro, Italian dermatologist, 1823–1892.
Jadassohn-Pellizzari anetoderma—see under Jadassohn

Pellizzi, G.B., 19th-20th century Italian physician.
Pellizzi syndrome—a disorder in which gonadal maturation and the adolescent growth spurt in bodily height occur in the first decade of life. *Syn:* macrogenitosomia praecox

Pena, S.D.J.
Pena-Shokeir II syndrome—onset from birth of vomiting, failure to thrive.

Pendred, Vaughan, English surgeon, 1869–1946.
Pendred syndrome—a type of familial goiter.

Penfield, W.
Penfield syndrome—onset 6 to 7 years of age, primarily in males, of seizures accompanied by vegetative manifestations.

Penrose, Charles B., U.S. gynecologist, 1862–1925.
Penrose drain—a soft tube-shaped rubber drain.
Penrose tourniquet
Penrose tube

Penzoldt, Franz, German physician, 1849–1927.
Penzoldt test—a test for acetone.

Pepper, William, Jr., U.S. physician, 1874–1947.
Pepper syndrome—obsolete term for neuroblastoma of the adrenal gland with metastases in the liver.

Pereyra, Armand Joseph, U.S. gynecologist and obstetrician, *1904.
Pereyra bladder suspension
Pereyra cannula
Pereyra needle
Pereyra operation—*Syn:* Pereyra procedure
Pereyra paraurethral suspension

P

(continued)

NOTES

Pereyra *(continued)*
> **Pereyra procedure**—surgical procedure for the correction of incontinence. *Syn:* Pereyra operation; Pereyra technique
> **Pereyra technique**—*Syn:* Pereyra procedure
> **Pereyra vesicourethral suspension**

Perez, Bernard, French physician, 1836–1903.
> **Perez reflex**—running a finger down the spine of an infant held supported in a prone position will normally cause the whole body to become extended.
> **Perez-Castro forceps**

Perez, George V., Spanish physician, d. 1920.
> **Perez sign**—rales common in cases of fibrous mediastinitis and also of aneurysm of the aortic arch.

Perheentupa, J.
> **Perheentupa syndrome**—failure to grow, amblyopia. *Syn:* Mulibrey dwarfism

Perkins, Elisha, U.S. physician, 1741–1799.
> **perkinism**—a form of quackery purporting to treat disease by applying metals with magnetic and magic properties.

Perkins, George, English orthopedic surgeon, 1892–1979.
> **Perkins elevator**
> **Perkins formula**
> **Perkins line**
> **Perkins retractor**
> **Perkins test**
> **Perkins tonometer**
> **Perkins traction**
> **Perkins tractor**

Perkoff, G.T.
> **Perkoff syndrome**—poststeroid myopathy. *Syn:* Slocumb syndrome

Perlia, Richard, 19th century German ophthalmologist.
> **convergence nucleus of Perlia**—*Syn:* Perlia nucleus
> **Perlia nucleus**—a small cell group located between the somatic cell columns of the oculomotor nuclei. *Syn:* convergence nucleus of Perlia; Spitzka nucleus

Perls, Max, German pathologist, 1843–1881.
> **Perls Prussian blue stain**—a stain for ferric iron.
> **Perls test**—a test for hemosiderin, utilizing Perls prussian blue stain.

Perlstein, Meyer Aaron, U.S. pediatrician, 1902–1969.
> **Perlstein brace**—*Syn:* Perlstein orthosis
> **Perlstein joint**—*Syn:* Perlstein orthosis
> **Perlstein orthosis**—children's ankle-foot orthosis. *Syn:* Perlstein brace; Perlstein joint

Perrin, Maurice, French surgeon, 1826–1889.
> **Perrin-Ferraton disease**—hip snap.

Perroncito, Aldo, Italian histologist, 1882–1929.
    apparatus of Perroncito—*Syn:* Perroncito apparatus
    Perroncito apparatus—fibrils in the form of spirals which occur during nerve regeneration. *Syn:* Perroncito spirals; apparatus of Perroncito
    Perroncito spirals—*Syn:* Perroncito apparatus

Perry, Murle, 20th century U.S. colostomy patient.
    Perry bag—a type of colostomy bag.

Perthes, Georg C., German surgeon, 1869–1927.
    Calvé-Perthes disease—*Syn:* Legg-Calvé-Perthes disease
    Legg-Calvé-Perthes disease—see under Legg
    Perthes disease—*Syn:* Legg-Calvé-Perthes disease
    Perthes incision
    Perthes lesion
    Perthes sling—used primarily for patients with Legg-Calvé-Perthes disease to support the leg in partial flexion. *Syn:* Sam Brown sling
    Perthes test—a test for patency of the deep femoral vein.

Pertik, Otto, Hungarian pathologist, 1852–1913.
    Pertik diverticulum—an abnormally deep pharyngeal recess.

Peters, Albert, German physician, 1862–1938.
    Peters anomaly—a congenital disorder originating from faulty separation of embryonic structures. *Syn:* anterior chamber cleavage syndrome

Peters, Hubert, Austrian obstetrician, 1859–1934.
    Peters ovum—one of very few young human embryos recovered in good condition; its study furnished many facts regarding early embryonic changes.
    Peters tissue forceps

Petersen, Christian F., German surgeon, 1845–1908.
    Petersen bag—an obsolete device consisting of a rubber bag introduced into the rectum and inflated to push up the bladder to facilitate suprapubic cystotomy.
    Petersen lithotomy
    Petersen operation

Petit, Alexis T., French physicist, 1791–1820.
    Dulong-Petit law—see under Dulong

Petit, Antoine, French surgeon and anatomist, 1718–1794.
    Petit ligament—a fold of peritoneum containing the rectouterine muscle. *Syn:* sacrouterine fold

Petit, François du, French surgeon and anatomist, 1664–1741.
    Petit canals—the spaces between the fibers of the ciliary zonule at the equator of the lens of the eye. *Syn:* zonular spaces
    Petit sinus—the space between the superior aspect of each cusp of the aortic valve and the dilated portion of the wall of the ascending aorta. *Syn:* aortic sinus

P

NOTES

Petit, Jean L., French surgeon, 1674–1750.
   Petit hernia—lumbar hernia occurring in Petit triangle.
   Petit herniotomy—herniotomy without incision into the sac.
   Petit ligament
   Petit lumbar triangle—an area in the posterior abdominal wall. *SYN:* lumbar triangle

Petit, Paul, French anatomist, *1889.
   Petit aponeurosis—the posterior layer of the broad ligament of the uterus.

Pétrequin, Joseph Pierre Eléonor, French surgeon, 1809–1896.
   Pétrequin ligament

Petri, Julius, German bacteriologist, 1852–1921.
   Petri dish—a small shallow plate used especially in microbiology for the cultivation of microorganisms on solid media. *SYN:* Petri plate
   Petri plate—*SYN:* Petri dish
   Petri test—a test for proteins.

Pette, H.H. German neuropathologist, 1887–1964.
   Pette-Döring disease—probably a form of subacute sclerosing panencephalitis. *SYN:* nodular panencephalitis

Pettenkofer, Max Josef von, German chemist, 1818–1901.
   Pettenkofer test—a test for bile acids in urine.

Pettit, Auguste, French physician, 1869–1939.
   Bachman-Pettit test—see under Bachman, George

Petzetakis, M.
   Petzetakis syndrome—possible virus of *Chlamydia*. *SYN:* cat-scratch fever
   Petzetakis-Takos syndrome—break in corneal epithelium

Peutz, John L.A., Dutch physician, 1886–1957.
   Jeghers-Peutz syndrome—*SYN:* Peutz-Jeghers syndrome
   Peutz syndrome—*SYN:* Peutz-Jeghers syndrome
   Peutz-Jeghers syndrome—generalized hamartomatous multiple polyposis of the intestinal tract, consistently involving the jejunum, associated with melanin spots of the lips, buccal mucosa, and fingers. *SYN:* Peutz syndrome; Jeghers-Peutz syndrome

Peyer, Johann K., Swiss anatomist, 1653–1712.
   Peyer glands—*SYN:* Peyer patches
   Peyer nodules—solitary lymph nodes
   Peyer patches—collections of many lymphoid follicles closely packed together, forming oblong elevations on the mucous membrane of the small intestine. *SYN:* Peyer glands; aggregated lymphatic nodules; agmen peyerianum; aggregated lymphatic follicles; folliculi lymphatici aggregati; aggregate glands

Peyronie, Francois de la, French surgeon, 1678–1747.
   Peyronie disease—plaques or strands of dense fibrous tissue surrounding the corpus cavernosum of the penis, causing deformity and painful erection. *SYN:* van Buren disease; penile fibromatosis
   Peyronie-like plaque

Peyrot, Jean J., French surgeon, 1843–1918.
> **Peyrot thorax**—an obliquely oval deformity of the chest in cases of a very large pleural effusion.

Pezzer, Oscar M.B. de. See under de Pezzer.

Pfannenstiel, Hermann Johann, German gynecologist, 1862–1909.
> **Pfannenstiel incision**—an incision made transversely and through the external sheath of the recti muscles, about an inch above the pubes.
> **Pfannenstiel transverse approach**

Pfaundler, Meinhard von, German physician, 1872–1947.
> **Pfaundler-Hurler syndrome**—*SYN:* Hurler syndrome

Pfeiffer, Emil, German physician, 1846–1921.
> **Pfeiffer disease**—infectious mononucleosis. *SYN:* glandular fever

Pfeiffer, Richard F.J., German physician, 1858–1945.
> *Pfeifferella*—an obsolete genus of bacteria.
> **Pfeiffer bacillus**—a species found in the respiratory tract that causes acute respiratory infections, acute conjunctivitis, bacterial meningitis, and purulent meningitis. *SYN: Haemophilus influenzae*
> **Pfeiffer blood agar**—solid agar, with a few drops of human blood smeared on the surface.
> **Pfeiffer phenomenon**—bacteriolysis.
> **Pfeiffer syndrome**—*SYN:* type V acrocephalosyndactyly

Pflüger, Eduard F.W., German anatomist and physiologist, 1829–1910.
> **Pflüger cords**—ovarian tubes. *SYN:* Pflüger tubes
> **Pflüger law**—a given segment of a nerve is irritated by the development of catelectrotonus and the disappearance of anelectrotonus, but the reverse does not hold. *SYN:* law of polar excitation
> **Pflüger tubes**—*SYN:* Pflüger cords

Pfuhl, Eduard, German physician, 1852–1905.
> **Pfuhl sign**—the pressure of pus within a subphrenic abscess rises during inspiration and falls during expiration, the reverse of what happens in the case of a purulent collection above the diaphragm.

Phalen, George S., U.S. orthopaedist, *1911.
> **Phalen maneuver**—a maneuver done to check for carpal tunnel abnormality. *SYN:* Phalen test; Phalen sign
> **Phalen position**
> **Phalen sign**—*SYN:* Phalen maneuver
> **Phalen test**—*SYN:* Phalen maneuver

Phelps, Abel Mix, U.S. surgeon, 1851–1902.
> **Phelps brace**
> **Phelps gracilis test**
> **Phelps operation**—surgery for talipes.
> **Phelps orthosis**
> **Phelps splint**

P

NOTES

Phelps, Winthrop Morgan, U.S. orthopedic surgeon, 1894–1971.
Phelps method of exercise—a method of exercise used to treat individuals with central nervous system lesions.
Phelps neurectomy
Phelps partial resection
Phelps scalpulectomy

Phemister, Dallas B., U.S. surgeon, 1882–1951.
Phemister acromioclavicular pin fixation
Phemister approach
Phemister biopsy trephine
Phemister brace
Phemister elevator
Phemister graft—an autogenous onlay bone graft used in treating delayed union of fractures.
Phemister incision
Phemister medial approach
Phemister onlay bone graft
Phemister punch
Phemister rasp
Phemister raspatory
Phemister reamer
Phemister splint

Philadelphia, city in Pennsylvania.
Philadelphia chromosome—an abnormal minute chromosome formed by a rearrangement of chromosomes 9 and 22, found in cultured leukocytes of many patients with chronic granulocytic leukemia.
Philadelphia cocktail—*SYN:* Rivers cocktail

Philip, Sir Robert W., Scottish physician, 1857–1939.
Philip glands—enlarged deep glands just above the clavicle, found in children with pulmonary tuberculosis.

Philippe, Claudien, French pathologist, 1866–1903.
Philippe triangle

Phillips, Charles, French urologist, 1809–1871.
Phillips bougie
Phillips catheter—a urethral catheter with a filiform guide for the urethra.
Phillips clamp
Phillips dilator
Phillips forceps

Phocas, B. Gerasime, French surgeon, 1861–1937.
Phocas disease—chronic glandular mastitis.

Physick, Philip Syng, U.S. surgeon, 1768–1837.
Physick operation
Physick pouches—proctitis with mucous discharge and burning pain, involving especially the sacculations between the rectal valves.

Pick, Arnold, Czech psychiatrist, 1851–1924.
Arnold Pick syndrome—inability to focus reflexively on objects due to aperceptive blindness.
Pick bundle—a bundle of nerve fibers recurring rostralward from the

pyramidal tract in the medulla oblongata and believed to consist of corticonuclear fibers.

Pick, Friedel, German physician, 1867–1926.
  Pick atrophy—*Syn:* Pick disease
  Pick bodies—intracytoplasmic argentophilic inclusion bodies seen in neurons in Pick disease.
  Pick disease—a rare type of cerebral degenerative disorder manifested primarily as dementia. *Syn:* progressive circumscribed cerebral atrophy; Pick syndrome; Pick atrophy
  Pick syndrome—*Syn:* Pick disease

Pick, Ludwig, German physician, 1868–1935.
  Niemann-Pick cell—*Syn:* Pick cell
  Niemann-Pick disease—see under Niemann
  Pick cell—a relatively large mononuclear cell widely distributed in the spleen and other tissues in patients with Niemann-Pick disease. *Syn:* Niemann-Pick cell
  Pick tubular adenoma—a testicular tumor. *Syn:* androblastoma

Pickworth, F.A.
  Lepehne-Pickworth stain—see under Lepehne

Pierini, Luigi, 20th century Argentinian dermatologist.
  atrophoderma of Pasini and Pierini—see under Pasini
  Pasini-Pierini syndrome—see under Pasini

Pignet, Maurice-C.J., French surgeon, *1871.
  Pignet formula

Piltz, Jan, Polish neurologist, 1870–1931.
  Piltz reflex—a pupil's attention reflex.
  Piltz sign—constriction of both pupils when an effort is made to close eyelids forcibly held apart. *Syn:* eye-closure pupil reaction; Westphal-Piltz phenomenon; Westphal pupillary reflex
  Westphal-Piltz phenomenon—*Syn:* Piltz sign

Pinard, Adolphe, French obstetrician, 1844–1934.
  Pinard fetoscope
  Pinard maneuver—for management of a frank breech presentation.
  Pinard sign

Pindborg, Jens J., Danish oral pathologist, *1921.
  Pindborg tumor—a benign epithelial odontogenic neoplasm. *Syn:* calcifying epithelial odontogenic tumor

Pinel, Philippe, French psychiatrist, 1745–1826.
  Haslam-Pinel syndrome—see under Haslam
  Pinel system—the abolition of forcible restraint in the treatment of the mental hospital patient.
  Pinel-Haslam syndrome—*Syn:* Haslam-Pinel syndrome

NOTES

P

Pins, Emil, Austrian physician, 1845–1913.
    Pins sign—*Syn:* Ewart sign
    Pins syndrome—dullness, diminution of vocal fremitus and of the vesicular murmur, and a slight distant blowing sound heard in the posteroinferior region of the chest on the left side in cases of pericardial effusion.

Pintner, Rudolf, U.S. psychologist, 1884–1942.
    Pintner-Paterson scale of performance tests—series of 15 performance tests.

Piper, E.B., U.S. obstetrician-gynecologist, 1881–1935.
    Piper forceps—obstetrical forceps used to facilitate delivery of the head in breech presentation.
    Piper lateral wall retractor

Pirie, George A., Scottish radiologist, 1864–1929.
    Pirie bone—an anomalous bone of the foot located near the head of the talus. *Syn:* dorsal talonavicular bone

Pirogoff, Nikolai I., Russian surgeon, 1810–1881.
    Pirogoff amputation—amputation of the foot.
    Pirogoff angle—the junction of the internal jugular and subclavian veins; in neuroradiology, the angle of union of the superior thalamostriate vein with the internal cerebral vein. *Syn:* venous angle
    Pirogoff operation
    Pirogoff triangle—a triangle formed by the intermediate tendon of the digastric muscle, the posterior border of the mylohyoid muscle, and the hypoglossal nerve.

Pirquet von Cesenatico, Clemens P., Austrian physician, 1874–1929.
    Pirquet reaction—*Syn:* Pirquet test
    Pirquet test—a cutaneous tuberculin test. *Syn:* dermotuberculin reaction; Pirquet reaction

Piskacek, Ludwig, Austrian obstetrician, 1854–1933.
    Piskacek sign—asymmetrical enlargement of the corpus uteri.

Pitkin, George, U.S. surgeon, 1885–1934.
    Pitkin dermatome
    Pitkin needle—*Syn:* Pitkin syringe
    Pitkin syringe—a self-filling syringe used to administer anesthesia. *Syn:* Pitkin needle

Pitot, Henri, French engineer, 1695–1771.
    Pitot tube—a stationary L-shaped tube inserted in a fluid stream and used for measuring the velocity of fluid movement.

Pitres, Jean A., French physician, 1848–1927.
    Pitres area—prefrontal cortex of the cerebral hemisphere.
    Pitres rule—a multilingual person who recovers from aphasia will recover the language that was most fluent at the time of the event.
    Pitres section—six coronal sections through the brain.
    Pitres sign—diminished sensation in the testes and scrotum in tabes dorsalis; pain is caused by slight touch. *Syn:* haphalgesia

Placido da Costa, Antonio, Portuguese ophthalmologist, 1848–1916.
   Placido da Costa disk—an instrument marked with lines or circles, used to observe the corneal reflex. *SYN:* Placido keratoscope; Placido disk
   Placido disk—*SYN:* Placido da Costa disk
   Placido keratoscope—*SYN:* Placido da Costa disk

Planck, Max, German physicist and Nobel laureate, 1858–1947.
   Planck constant—a natural constant occurring in many physical formulas.
   Planck theory—that energy can be emitted, transmitted, and absorbed only in discrete quantities. *SYN:* quantum theory

Plateau, Joseph Antoine Ferdinand, Belgian physicist, 1801–1883.
   Plateau-Talbot law—when successive light stimuli follow each other sufficiently rapidly to become fused, their apparent brightness is diminished.

Plato, Greek philosopher, 427–347 B.C.
   platonic love—a love in which there is no sexual desire.

Platt, Sir Harry, English surgeon, *1886.
   Putti-Platt arthroplasty
   Putti-Platt director
   Putti-Platt instrumentation
   Putti-Platt operation—see under Putti
   Putti-Platt procedure—*SYN:* Putti-Platt operation
   Putti-Platt shoulder procedure
   reverse Putti-Platt procedure

Plaut, Hugo K., German physician, 1858–1928.
   Plaut bacillus—*Fusobacterium nucleatum.*

Pleasure, Max A., U.S. dentist.
   Pleasure curve—a curve of occlusion which when viewed in sagittal section conforms to a line that is convex upward, except for the last molars.

Plimmer, Henry G., English protozoologist, 1857–1918.
   Plimmer bodies—obsolete term for cancer bodies.

Plotz, Harry, U.S. physician, 1890–1947.
   Plotz bacillus—a small, Gram-positive bacterium suggested as the pathogenic agent of typhus fever.

Plugge, Pieter Cornelis, Dutch biochemist, 1847–1897.
   Plugge test—a test for phenol.

Plummer, Henry S., U.S. physician, 1874–1937.
   Plummer bag—*SYN:* Plummer dilator
   Plummer bougie

(continued)

P

NOTES

Plummer *(continued)*

Plummer dilator—an instrument for dilating the lower end of the esophagus in cardiospasm. *Syn:* Plummer bag

Plummer disease—hyperthyroidism resulting from a nodular toxic goiter, usually not accompanied by exophthalmos.

Plummer sign—a sign of Graves disease.

Plummer-Vinson syndrome—iron deficiency anemia, dysphagia, esophageal web, and atrophic glossitis. *Syn:* sideropenic dysphagia; Paterson-Kelly syndrome

Pohl, John F., U.S. orthopedic surgeon, 1903–1981.

method of Pohl—locomotor rehabilitation system for individuals with central nervous system lesions.

Pohl, Julius Heinrich, late 19th century German pharmacologist.

Pohl test—a test for globulins.

Poirier, Paul J., French surgeon, 1853–1907.

Poirier gland—a lymph node on the uterine artery where it crosses the ureter.

Poirier line—a line extending from the nasion to the lambda.

space of Poirier

Poiseuille, Jean Léonard Marie, French physiologist and physicist, 1797–1869.

poise—the unit of viscosity equal to 1 dyne-second per square centimeter and to 0.1 pascal-second.

Poiseuille equation

Poiseuille law—describes the volume flow rate of a liquid through a tube.

Poiseuille space—the layer of the bloodstream next to the wall of the capillary vessel that flows slowly and transports the white blood cells. *Syn:* still layer

Poiseuille viscosity coefficient—an expression of the viscosity as determined by the capillary tube method.

Poisson, Siméon Denis, French mathematician, 1781–1840.

Poisson distribution—a discontinuous distribution important in statistical work.

Poisson ratio

Poisson-Pearson formula—a formula to determine the statistical error in calculating the endemic index of malaria.

Poland, Alfred, English physician, 1820–1872.

Poland anomaly—*Syn:* Poland syndrome

Poland syndrome—absence of a portion of the pectoralis major muscle and syndactyly. *Syn:* Poland anomaly

Politzer, Adam, Austrian otologist, 1835–1920.

Politzer bag—a pear-shaped rubber bag used for forcing air through the eustachian tube by the Politzer method.

Politzer ear perforator

Politzer knife

Politzer luminous cone—a triangular area at the anterior inferior part of the tympanic membrane. *Syn:* pyramid of light

Politzer method—inflation of the eustachian tube and tympanum by forcing air into the nasal cavity at the instant the patient swallows. *SYN:* politzerization

Politzer operation
Politzer otoscope
Politzer speculum
Politzer test—a test for deafness in one ear.
politzerization—*SYN:* Politzer method

Polland, var. of Poland

Polya, var. of Pólya

Pólya, Jenö (Eugene), Hungarian surgeon, 1876–1944.
Hofmeister-Pólya anastomosis
Pólya anastomosis
Pólya femoral herniorrhaphy
Pólya gastrectomy—partial gastrectomy with retrocolic anastomosis of the full width of stomach to jejunum. *SYN:* Pólya operation
Pólya gastroenterostomy
Pólya gastrojejunostomy
Pólya operation—*SYN:* Pólya gastrectomy
Pólya technique
Reichel-Pólya stomach resection—see under Reichel, Friedrich

Pomeroy, Ralph H., U.S. obstetrician-gynecologist, 1867–1925.
Pomeroy operation—excision of a ligated portion of the fallopian tubes.
Pomeroy salpingectomy
Pomeroy sterilization
Pomeroy syringe
Pomeroy tubal ligation

Pompe, Johann C., 20th century Dutch physician.
Pompe disease—glycogenosis due to lysosomal alpha-1,4-glucosidase deficiency. *SYN:* type 2 glycogenosis; Pompe syndrome
Pompe syndrome—*SYN:* Pompe disease

Poncet, Antonin, French surgeon, 1849–1913.
Poncet disease—*SYN:* Poncet rheumatism
Poncet rheumatism—tuberculous arthritis. *SYN:* Poncet disease

Ponfick, Emil, German pathologist, 1844–1913.
Ponfick shadow—a hypochromic, crescent-shaped erythrocyte. *SYN:* achromocyte

Pontiac, city in Michigan, where an outbreak of Legionella occurred in 1968.
Pontiac fever—a strain of *Legionella pneumophila.*

Pool, Eugene H., U.S. surgeon, 1874–1949.
Pool phenomenon—in tetany, spasm of the extensor muscles of the knee and of the calf muscles when the extended leg is flexed at the hip; in

(continued)

P

NOTES

Pool *(continued)*
tetany, contraction of the arm muscles following the stretching of the brachial plexus resembles the contraction resulting from stimulation of the ulnar nerve. *SYN:* Pool-Schlesinger sign; Schlesinger sign
Pool-Schlesinger sign—*SYN:* Pool phenomenon

Porges, Otto, Austrian bacteriologist, *1879.
Porges method—a method of destroying the capsule of bacteria by heating with N/4 hydrochloric acid and neutralizing with NaOH.
Porges-Meier test—an early flocculation test for syphilis.

Porro, Edoardo, Italian obstetrician, 1842–1902.
Porro cesarean hysterectomy—*SYN:* Porro hysterectomy
Porro hysterectomy—cesarean section followed by hysterectomy. *SYN:* Porro cesarean hysterectomy; Porro operation
Porro operation—*SYN:* Porro hysterectomy

Porter, Curt C., U.S. biochemist, *1914.
Porter-Silber chromogens—used chiefly to determine plasma cortisol concentrations and the urinary output of 17-hydroxycorticoids.
Porter-Silber chromogens test—a urine test used as a measure of adrenocortical function. *SYN:* 17-hydroxycorticosteroid test
Porter-Silber reaction—the basis of the 17-hydroxycorticosteroid test.

Porter, Rodney R., English biochemist, 1917–1985, joint winner of 1972 Nobel Prize for work related to antibodies.

Porter, Thomas C., English scientist, 1860–1933.
Ferry-Porter law—see under Ferry
Porter law—a principle that critical flicker frequency increases with brightness of stimulus independent of stimulus wavelength.

Porter, W.B.
Porter syndrome—idiopathic benign pericarditis

Porter, William H., Irish surgeon, 1790–1861.
Porter fascia—the layer of fascia investing the infrahyoid muscles and contributing to the formation of the carotid sheath. *SYN:* pretracheal fascia
Porter tugging—tracheal tugging

Porteus, Stanley David, U.S. psychologist, 1883–1972.
Porteus maze—an original intelligence test.
Porteus maze test

Posadas, Alejandro, Argentinian parasitologist, 1870–1902.
Posadas disease—a variable, benign, severe, or fatal systemic mycosis due to inhalation of dust particles containing arthroconidia of *Coccidioides immitis*. *SYN:* coccidioidomycosis

Posner, Carl, German urologist, 1854–1929.
Posner gonioprism
Posner procedure
Posner test—to test for the source of albumin in the urine.

Potain, Pierre C.E., French physician, 1825–1901.
Potain sign—in dilation of the aorta, dullness on percussion.

Pott, Sir Percivall, English surgeon, 1713–1788.

Pott abscess—tuberculous abscess of the spine.

Pott aneurysm—dilation and tortuosity of a vein resulting from an acquired communication with an adjacent artery. *SYN:* aneurysmal varix

Pott curvature—a gibbous deformity, i.e., a sharp angulation of the spine, occurring in Pott disease. *SYN:* angular curvature

Pott disease—tuberculous infection of the spine associated with a sharp angulation of the spine at the point of disease. *SYN:* tuberculous spondylitis

Pott eversion osteotomy

Pott fracture—fracture of the lower part of the fibula and of the malleolus of the tibia, with outward displacement of the foot.

Pott gangrene—dry gangrene occurring in the aged in consequence of occlusion of an artery, particularly affecting the extremities. *SYN:* senile gangrene

Pott I syndrome—*SYN:* Dupuytren fracture

Pott II syndrome—dry gangrene caused by arterial obstruction *SYN:* senile gangrene

Pott paralysis—*SYN:* Pott paraplegia

Pott paraplegia—paralysis of the lower part of the body and the extremities due to pressure on the spinal cord as the result of tuberculous spondylitis. *SYN:* Pott paralysis

Pott puffy tumor—a circumscribed swelling of the scalp indicating an underlying osteitis of the skull or an extradural abscess.

Pott spinal curvature

Potter, Edith L., U.S. perinatal pathologist, *1901.

Potter classification of polycystic kidney

Potter disease—*SYN:* Potter facies

Potter facies—characteristic facies seen in severe renal malformations. *SYN:* Potter disease

Potter syndrome—renal agenesis, with hypoplastic lungs and associated neonatal respiratory distress.

Potter, Irving White, U.S. obstetrician, 1868–1956.

Potter version—obsolete term for an internal version to a breech presentation.

Potts, Willis J., U.S. pediatric surgeon, 1895–1968.

Potts anastomosis—*SYN:* Potts operation

Potts aortic clamp

Potts bronchial forceps

Potts bulldog forceps

Potts cardiovascular clamp

Potts clamp—a fine-toothed, multiple-point, vascular fixation clamp that imparts limited trauma to the vessel while securely holding it.

Potts coarctation clamp

Potts coarctation forceps

(continued)

NOTES

Potts *(continued)*
    Potts dilator
    Potts dissector
    Potts elevator
    Potts expansile dilator
    Potts expansile knife
    Potts forceps
    Potts ligature
    Potts needle
    Potts operation—direct side-to-side anastomosis between the aorta and pulmonary artery as a palliative procedure in congenital malformation of the heart. *Syn:* Potts anastomosis
    Potts patent ductus clamp
    Potts rib shears
    Potts scissors
    Potts shunt
    Potts splint
    Potts tenaculum
    Potts valvulotome
    Potts vascular scissors
    Potts-Smith bipolar forceps

Pötzl, Otto, Austrian psychiatrist, *1877.
    Pötzl phenomenon—an appearance in dreams.
    Pötzl syndrome—a form of alexia.

Poupart, François, French anatomist, 1616–1708.
    Poupart inguinal ligament
    Poupart ligament—a fibrous band that forms the floor of the inguinal canal. *Syn:* inguinal ligament
    Poupart ligament shelving edge
    Poupart line—a vertical line that marks off the hypochondriac, lumbar, and iliac from the epigastric, umbilical, and hypogastric regions, respectively.

Powassan, city in Ontario, Canada, where disease was first reported.
    Powassan encephalitis—an acute disease of children, transmitted by ixodid ticks.
    Powassan virus—virus causing Powassan encephalitis.

Pozzi, Samuel J., French gynecologist and anatomist, 1846–1918.
    Pozzi forceps
    Pozzi muscle—a short extensor muscle of the fingers of rare occurrence, comparable to the short extensor of the toes. *Syn:* extensor digitorum brevis muscle of hand
    Pozzi operation
    Pozzi syndrome—leukorrhea and backache, occasionally affiliated with endometriosis.
    Pozzi tenaculum

Prader, Andrea, Swiss pediatrician, *1919.
    Prader-Willi syndrome—a congenital syndrome of unknown etiology characterized by short stature, mental retardation, polyphagia with marked obesity, and sexual infantilism.

Pratt, Joseph H., U.S. physician, 1872–1956.
    Pratt anoscope
    Pratt curet
    Pratt dilator
    Pratt director
    Pratt forceps
    Pratt hook
    Pratt open reduction
    Pratt probe
    Pratt proctoscope
    Pratt scissors
    Pratt sound
    Pratt speculum
    Pratt symptom—rigidity in the muscles of an injured limb preceding the occurrence of gangrene.
    Pratt T-clamp
    Pratt technique

Prausnitz, Otto Carl, German hygienist, 1876–1963.
    Prausnitz-Küstner antibody—one of the IgE class of antibodies first demonstrated by Prausnitz and Küstner by passive transfer to the skin. *SYN:* atopic reagin
    Prausnitz-Küstner reaction—a test for the presence of immediate hypersensitivity in humans. *SYN:* P-K test
    reversed Prausnitz-Küstner reaction—the appearance of an urticarial reaction at the site of injection when serum containing reaginic antibody is injected into the skin of a person in whom the allergen is already present.

Prehn, D.T., 20th century U.S. physician.
    Prehn sign—a sign to confirm testicular torsion.

Preiser, Georg Karl Felix, German orthopedic surgeon, 1879–1913.
    Preiser disease—atrophy or osteoporosis due to osteoporosis or fracture that has not been properly treated.

Preisz, Hugo von, Hungarian bacteriologist, 1860–1940.
    Preisz-Nocard bacillus—a species found in necrotic areas in sheep kidney, in caseous lymphadenitis in sheep, and in ulcerative lesions in horses, cattle, and other warm-blooded animals. *SYN: Corynebacterium pseudotuberculosis*

Prentice, Charles F., U.S. optician, 1854–1946.
    Prentice rule—each centimeter of decentration of a lens results in 1 prism diopter of deviation of light for each diopter of lens power.

Price, Ernest Arthur, English biochemist, *1882.
    Carr-Price reaction—see under Carr

NOTES

Price-Jones, Cecil, English hematologist, 1863–1943.
    Price-Jones curve—distribution curve of the measured diameters of red blood cells.

Priessnitz, Vinzenz, Silesian peasant, 1799–1851.
    Priessnitz compresses—the use of cold water as packs, showers, or baths as a therapeutic system.
    Priessnitz method of treatment—the use of physical work, fresh air, diet, and exercise, may also include Priessnitz compresses.

Priestley, John Gillies, English physiologist, 1880–1941.
    Haldane-Priestley sample—see under Haldane

Princeteau, L.R., French physician, *1884.
    Princeteau tubercle—a slight prominence on the temporal bone near the apex of the petrous part where the superior petrosal sinus commences.

Pringle, John J., English dermatologist, 1855–1922.
    Bourneville-Pringle disease—see under Bourneville
    Pringle disease—obsolete misnomer for a hamartoma occurring on the face. *SYN:* adenoma sebaceum

Prinzmetal, Myron, U.S. cardiologist, *1908.
    Prinzmetal angina—a form of angina pectoris. *SYN:* angina inversa; variant angina pectoris
    Prinzmetal II syndrome—precordial anginal attacks. *SYN:* angina pectoris variant

Profeta, Giuseppe, Italian dermatologist, 1840–1910.
    Profeta law—the subject of congenital syphilis is immune against the acquired disease.

Profichet, Georges C., French physician, *1873.
    Profichet syndrome—calcareous deposits, primarily affecting extremities. *SYN:* calcinosis circumscripta; calcinosis cutis

Proskauer, Bernhard, German bacteriologist, 1851–1915.
    Voges-Proskauer reaction—see under Voges

Proust, Louis J., French chemist, 1755–1826.
    Proust law—the relative weights of the several elements forming a chemical compound are invariable. *SYN:* law of definite proportions

Proust, T., 19th century French physician.
    Proust space—a pocket formed by the deflection of the peritoneum from the rectum to the bladder in the male. *SYN:* rectovesical pouch

Prowazek, Stanislas J.M. von, German protozoologist, 1876–1915.
    Halberstaedter-Prowazek bodies—*SYN:* Prowazek-Greef bodies
    Prowazek bodies—historic term for either of two types of inclusion bodies associated with certain diseases.
    Prowazek-Greeff bodies—distinctive, complex, intracytoplasmic forms found in the conjunctival epithelial cells of persons in the acute phase of trachoma. *SYN:* trachoma bodies; Halberstaedter-Prowazek bodies
    Prowazekia—a genus of coprozoic flagellate protozoans.

Prusiner, Stanley B., winner of 1997 Nobel Prize for work related to infection.

Prussak, Alexander, Russian otologist, 1839–1897.
  Prussak fibers—elastic and connective tissue fiber bounding the pars flaccida membranae tympani.
  Prussak pouch—*Syn:* superior recess of tympanic membrane
  Prussak space—*Syn:* superior recess of tympanic membrane

Psaume, J., 20th century French physician.
  Papillon-Léage and Psaume syndrome—see under Papillon-Léage

Pudenz, Robert H., U.S. neurosurgeon, *1911.
  Heyer-Pudenz valve—see under Heyer
  Pudenz reservoir
  Pudenz shunt
  Pudenz tube
  Pudenz valve—*Syn:* Heyer-Pudenz valve
  Pudenz ventricular catheter
  Pudenz-Schulte thecoperitoneal shunt

Puestow, Charles B., U.S. surgeon, 1902–1973.
  Puestow anastomosis
  Puestow biliary tract procedure
  Puestow dilator
  Puestow guide wire
  Puestow procedure—longitudinal pancreatic jejunostomy.
  Puestow wire

Punnett, Reginald Crundall, English geneticist, 1875–1967.
  Punnett square—a grid used in genetics. *Syn:* checkerboard

Purdy, Charles Wesley, U.S. physician, 1846–1901.
  Purdy test—urine test for albumin.

Purkinje, Johannes E. von (Jan E. Purkyne), Bohemian anatomist and physiologist, 1787–1869.
  Purkinje afterimage—*Syn:* Bidwell ghost
  Purkinje cells—large nerve cells of the cerebellar cortex with a piriform cell body and dendrites arranged in a plane transverse to the folium. *Syn:* Purkinje corpuscles
  Purkinje conduction—conduction of the cardiac impulse through the Purkinje system.
  Purkinje corpuscles—*Syn:* Purkinje cells
  Purkinje effect—*Syn:* Purkinje phenomenon
  Purkinje fibers—interlacing fibers formed of modified cardiac muscle cells that are the terminal ramifications of the conducting system of the heart found beneath the endocardium of the ventricles.
  Purkinje figures—shadows of the retinal vessels seen as dark lines on a reddish field when a light enters the eye through the sclera and not the pupil.
  Purkinje image tracker

(continued)

P

NOTES

Purkinje *(continued)*
> **Purkinje images**—*SYN:* Purkinje-Sanson images
> **Purkinje layer**—the layer of Purkinje cells between the molecular and granular layers of the cerebellar cortex. *SYN:* piriform neuron layer
> **Purkinje network**—the network formed by Purkinje fibers beneath the endocardium.
> **Purkinje phenomenon**—in the light-adapted eye, the region of maximal brightness is in the yellow; in the dark-adapted eye, the region of maximal brightness is in the green. *SYN:* Purkinje shift; Purkinje effect
> **Purkinje shift**—*SYN:* Purkinje phenomenon
> **Purkinje system**—terminal ramifications in the ventricles of the specialized conducting system of the heart.
> **Purkinje-Sanson images**—the two images formed by the anterior and posterior surfaces of the cornea, and the two images formed by the anterior and posterior surfaces of the lens. *SYN:* catatropic images; Purkinje images; Sanson images

Purmann, Matthaeus G., German surgeon, 1648–1721.
> **Purmann method**—treatment of an aneurysm by extirpation of the sac.

Purtscher, Otmar, German ophthalmologist, 1852–1927.
> **Purtscher disease**—*SYN:* Purtscher retinopathy
> **Purtscher retinopathy**—traumatic retinal angiopathy which causes transient visual impairment. *SYN:* Purtscher disease; Purtscher syndrome
> **Purtscher syndrome**—*SYN:* Purtscher retinopathy

Putnam, James J., U.S. neurologist, 1846–1918.
> **Putnam-Dana syndrome**—*SYN:* subacute combined degeneration of the spinal cord

Putti, Vittorio, Italian surgeon, 1880–1940.
> **Putti approach**
> **Putti arthroplasty gouge**
> **Putti bone rasp**
> **Putti frame**
> **Putti gouge**
> **Putti knee arthrodesis**
> **Putti operation**
> **Putti rasp**
> **Putti shoulder arthrodesis**
> **Putti splint**
> **Putti technique**
> **Putti-Platt arthroplasty**
> **Putti-Platt director**
> **Putti-Platt instrumentation**
> **Putti-Platt operation**—a procedure for recurrent dislocation of shoulder joint. *SYN:* Putti-Platt procedure
> **Putti-Platt procedure**—*SYN:* Putti-Platt operation
> **Putti-Platt shoulder procedure**
> **reverse Putti-Platt procedure**

Pym, Sir William, English physician, 1772–1861.
> **Pym fever**—an infectious but not contagious disease occurring in the Balkan Peninsula and other parts of southern Europe, apparently caused by the bite of the sandfly. *SYN:* phlebotomus fever

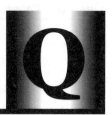

Quain, Sir Richard, English physician, 1816–1898.
Quain fatty heart—fatty tissue around the heart, or fatty degeneration of the heart. *SYN:* cor adiposum

Quant, C.A.J., early 20th century Dutch physician.
Quant sign—a T-shaped depression found in the occipital bone.

Quasimodo, fictional character (deformed bellringer) in the novel, *The Hunchback of Notre Dame.*
Quasimodo complex—personality disorder in which there is abnormal concern about a defect in one's physical appearance.

Quatrefages de Breau, Jean L.A. de, French naturalist, 1810–1892.
Quatrefages angle—an angle formed by the meeting of the prolongation of two lines tangential to the most prominent part of the zygomatic arch and to the parietofrontal suture on each side. *SYN:* parietal angle

Queckenstedt, Hans, German physician, 1876–1918.
Queckenstedt maneuver—*SYN:* Queckenstedt-Stookey test
Queckenstedt phenomenon—*SYN:* Queckenstedt sign
Queckenstedt sign—*SYN:* Queckenstedt phenomenon
Queckenstedt test—*SYN:* Queckenstedt-Stookey test
Queckenstedt-Stookey test—when there is a block of subarachnoid channels, compression of the jugular vein causes little or no increase of pressure in the cerebrospinal fluid. *SYN:* Queckenstedt maneuver; Queckenstedt test

Quénu, Eduard A.V.A., French surgeon and anatomist, 1852–1933.
Quénu hemorrhoidal plexus—lymphatic plexuses in the skin about the anus.
Quénu-Muret sign—in aneurysm, well-maintained collateral circulation is indicated by issue of blood when the main artery of the limb is compressed and a puncture is made at the periphery.

Quervain, Fritz de. See under de Quervain.

Quetelet, Lambert Adolphe Jacques, Belgian mathematician and anthropologist, 1796–1874.
Quetelet index of constitution—weight over height.
Quetelet rule—body weight in kilograms equals height in centimeters minus 100.

Queyrat, L. Auguste, French dermatologist, 1856–1933.
erythroplasia of Queyrat—carcinoma in situ of the glans penis.

(continued)

Queyrat *(continued)*
Queyrat erythroplasia
Queyrat syndrome—painless thickening of external genitalia; has also been described in the mouth and on the tongue.

Quick, Armand J., U.S. physician, 1894–1978.
Quick method—*Syn:* prothrombin test
Quick test—*Syn:* prothrombin test

Quincke, Georg, German physicist, 1834–1924.
Quincke tubes—glass tubes used in the study of hearing thresholds.

Quincke, Heinrich I., German physician, 1842–1922.
Quincke capillary pulsation—*Syn:* Quincke pulse
Quincke disease—*Syn:* Quincke edema
Quincke edema—recurrent large circumscribed areas of subcutaneous edema of sudden onset, usually disappearing within 24 hours. *Syn:* angioedema; Quincke disease; Quincke I syndrome
Quincke I syndrome—*Syn:* Quincke edema
Quincke meningitis—intracranial hypertension of unknown origin.
Quincke needle
Quincke pulse—capillary pulsation, a sign of arteriolar dilation and especially well seen in severe aortic insufficiency. *Syn:* Quincke sign; Quincke capillary pulsation
Quincke puncture—a puncture into the subarachnoid space of the lumbar region to obtain spinal fluid for diagnostic or therapeutic purposes. *Syn:* lumbar puncture
Quincke sign—*Syn:* Quincke pulse
Quincke spinal needle

Quinquad, Charles E., French physician, 1842–1894.
Quinquad disease—pustules of the scalp's hair follicles.
Quinquad phenomenon—sideways movement of the fingers seen in those with tremors. *Syn:* Quinquad sign
Quinquad sign—*Syn:* Quinquad phenomenon

Quinton, Wayne E., 20th century U.S. nephrologist.
Quinton biopsy catheter
Quinton catheter
Quinton dual lumen catheter
Quinton Q-Port catheter
Quinton Q-Port vascular access port
Quinton tube
Quinton-Scribner shunt—an arteriovenous shunt inserted for hemodialysis.

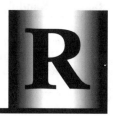

Radford, Edward P., Jr., U.S. physiologist, *1922.
> **Radford nomogram**—used to predict necessary tidal volume for artificial respiration on the basis of respiratory rate, body weight, and sex.

Radovici, André, 20th century French physician.
> **Marinesco-Radovici reflex**—*SYN:* Radovici sign
> **Radovici reflex**—*SYN:* Radovici sign
> **Radovici sign**—chin twitching that is caused by scratching the palm. *SYN:* palm-chin reflex; palmomental reflex; Marinesco-Radovici reflex; Radovici reflex

Raeder, Georg Johan, Norwegian ophthalmologist, 1889–1956.
> **Raeder paratrigeminal syndrome**—a postganglionic Horner syndrome associated with trigeminal nerve dysfunction, caused by involvement of the carotid sympathetic plexus.

Rahe, Richard H., U.S. psychiatrist, *1936.
> **Holmes-Rahe questionnaire**—*SYN:* Rahe-Holmes questionnaire
> **Rahe-Holmes questionnaire**—a survey to measure the stressfulness of various life events. *SYN:* Holmes-Rahe questionnaire

Rahn, Hermann, U.S. respiratory physiologist, *1912.
> **Rahn-Otis sample**—an approximation of alveolar gas continuously provided by a simple device that admits just the latter part of each expiration.

Raimiste, Johann M., early 20th century German neurologist.
> **Raimiste sign**—indicates paresis of the hand.

Rainey, George, English anatomist, 1801–1884.
> **Rainey corpuscles**—spores or bradyzoites found within the elongated cysts of the protozoan *Sarcocystis.*
> **Rainey tube**—sarcocyst. *SYN:* Rainey tubule
> **Rainey tubule**—*SYN:* Rainey tube

Ralfe, Charles Henry
> **Ralfe test**—a test for acetone in the urine.

Raman, Sir Chandrasekhara Venkata, Indian physicist and Nobel laureate, 1888–1970.
> **Raman effect**—a change in frequency undergone by monochromatic light scattered in passage through a transparent substance whose characteristics determine the amount of change. *SYN:* Raman shift

(continued)

Raman *(continued)*
> **Raman shift**—*Syn:* Raman effect
> **Raman spectrum**—the characteristic array of light produced by the Raman effect.

Ramon, Gaston, French bacteriologist, 1886–1963.
> **Ramon flocculation test**—a test to determine amount of antitoxin necessary to neutralize a toxin. *Syn:* Ramon test
> **Ramon test**—*Syn:* Ramon flocculation test

Ramond, Louis, French internist, 1879–1952.
> **Ramond point**
> **Ramond sign**—a rigidity in the erectus spinae muscle, which occurs with effusive pleurisy.

Ramsden, Jesse, English optician, 1735–1800.
> **Ramsden eyepiece**
> **Ramsden ocular**—an eyepiece of a microscope, consisting of two planoconvex lenses with convexities turned to each other.

Ramstedt, Conrad, German surgeon, 1867–1963.
> **Fredet-Ramstedt operation**—*Syn:* Ramstedt operation
> **Ramstedt clamp**
> **Ramstedt dilator**
> **Ramstedt operation**—longitudinal incision through the anterior wall of the pyloric canal to the level of the submucosa, to treat hypertrophic pyloric stenosis. *Syn:* pyloromyotomy; Fredet-Ramstedt operation; Ramstedt pyloromyotomy; Ramstedt procedure
> **Ramstedt procedure**—*Syn:* Ramstedt operation
> **Ramstedt pyloromyotomy**—*Syn:* Ramstedt operation
> **Ramstedt pyloroplasty**

Rancho Los Amigos Hospital, medical facility in Downey, California.
> **Rancho Los Amigos feeder**
> **Rancho Los Amigos Level of Cognitive Functioning Scale**
> **Rancho Los Amigos orthosis**
> **Rancho Los Amigos splint**

Rand, Gertrude, U.S. visual psychologist, 1886–1970.
> **Hardy-Rand-Ritter test**—see under Hardy, LeGrand

Rand, M.J.
> **Burn and Rand theory**—see under Burn, J.H.

Randall, Alexander, U.S. urologist, 1885–1951.
> **Randall curet**
> **Randall endometrial biopsy curet**
> **Randall operation**
> **Randall plaques**—minute stones of urinary salts found on erosions of renal papillae.
> **Randall stone forceps**—a forceps with variably curved slender blades and serrated jaws, used to extract calculi from the renal pelvis or calices.

Randolph, Nathaniel Archer, U.S. physician, 1858–1887.
> **Randolph test**—a test for peptones in the urine.

Ranke, Johannes, German anthropologist and physician, 1836–1916.
Ranke angle—a facial angle.

Ranke, Karl E. von, German chemist, 1870–1926.
Ranke complex
Ranke formula—for determining the amount of albumin in serous fluid.
Ranke stage

Rankin, Fred Wharton, U.S. surgeon, 1886–1954.
Rankin clamp—a three-bladed clamp used in resection of colon.
Rankin forceps
Rankin hemostat
Rankin hemostatic forceps
Rankin intestinal clamp
Rankin operation
Rankin prostatic retractor
Rankin retractor
Rankin suture

Rankine, William J. McQ., Scottish physicist, 1820–1870.
Rankine scale—a thermometer scale with its zero point at absolute zero.

Ransohoff, Joseph, U.S. surgeon, 1853–1921.
Ransohoff sign—yellow pigmentation in the umbilical region in rupture of the common bile duct.

Ranvier, Louis A., French pathologist, 1835–1922.
nodes of Ranvier—short intervals in the myelin sheaths of nerve fibers. *SYN:* Ranvier nodes
Ranvier crosses—black or brown figures in the shape of a cross, marking Ranvier nodes in the longitudinal section of a nerve stained with silver nitrate.
Ranvier disks—tactile nerve endings of cupped disklike form in the skin. *SYN:* Ranvier tactile disks
Ranvier membrane
Ranvier nodes—*SYN:* nodes of Ranvier
Ranvier plexus—a subbasal stroma plexus of the cornea.
Ranvier segment—the portion of a myelinated nerve fiber between two successive nodes. *SYN:* internodal segment
Ranvier tactile disks—*SYN:* Ranvier disks

Raoult, François, M., French physicist, 1830–1899.
Raoult law—the vapor pressure exerted by a component in a solution is directly proportional to its mole-fraction in the solution.

Rapoport, Abraham, Canadian urologist, *1926.
Rapoport test—a differential ureteral catheterization test used to evaluate suspected renovascular hypertension.

Rapoport, Samuel Mitja, Russian biochemist, *1912.
Rapoport-Luebering shunt—part of the glycolytic pathway characteristic of human erythrocytes.

NOTES

R

Rapp, R.S.
> **Rapp-Hodgkin syndrome**—autosomal dominant inheritance, with cleft palate and lip deformities. *SYN:* anhidrotic ectodermal dysplasia

Rappaport, Henry, U.S. pathologist, *1913.
> **Rappaport classification**—a classification of non-Hodgkin lymphomas.

Rapunzel, legendary woman whose long hair allowed her to escape from a tower in which she was held captive.
> **Rapunzel syndrome**—internal matter that has formed a compact body that occasionally assumes the appearance of strands of twisted hair that extend from the bezoar through the intestine. *SYN:* bezoar

Rasmussen, Fritz W., Danish physician, 1834–1881.
> **Rasmussen aneurysm**—aneurysmal dilation of a branch of a pulmonary artery in a tuberculous cavity.

Rastelli, Gian Carlo, Italian cardiovascular surgeon, 1933–1970.
> **Rastelli graft**
> **Rastelli implant**
> **Rastelli operation**—for repair of transposition of the great arteries.
> **Rastelli prosthesis**

Rathbone, Josephine Langworthy Rathbone-Karpovich, U.S. physical educator, 1899–1982.
> **Rathbone relaxation method**—a method of relaxation used in physical education.

Rathke, Martin H., German anatomist, physiologist, and pathologist, 1793–1860.
> **Rathke bundles**—muscular bundles on the lining walls of the ventricles of the heart. *SYN:* trabeculae carneae
> **Rathke cleft cyst**—an intrasellar or suprasellar cyst lined by cuboidal epithelium derived from remnants of Rathke pouch. *SYN:* Rathke cyst
> **Rathke column**
> **Rathke cyst**—*SYN:* Rathke cleft cyst
> **Rathke diverticulum**—a tubular outgrowth of ectoderm from the stomodeum of the embryo. *SYN:* pituitary diverticulum; Rathke pocket; Rathke pouch
> **Rathke duct**
> **Rathke fold**—two fetal folds of mesoderm.
> **Rathke pocket**—*SYN:* Rathke diverticulum
> **Rathke pouch**—*SYN:* Rathke diverticulum
> **Rathke pouch tumor**—a suprasellar neoplasm, usually cystic, that develops from the nests of epithelium derived from Rathke pouch. *SYN:* craniopharyngioma
> **Rathke punch**

Rau, Johann J., Dutch anatomist, 1668–1719.
> **processus ravii**—*SYN:* Rau process
> **Rau process**—a slender spur running anterior from the neck of the malleus toward the petrotympanic fissure. *SYN:* anterior process of malleus; processus ravii

Rauber, August A., German anatomist, 1841–1917.
> **Rauber layer**—the thinned-out trophoblastic membrane over the embryonic disk in developing carnivores and ungulates.

Rauch, S.
    Rauch syndrome—occurs in young women at onset of puberty; bilateral swelling of parotid and occasionally of submandibular glands, with slow progression of obesity over a five-year period.

Rauchfuss, Karl Andreyevich, Russian pediatrician, 1835–1915.
    Rauchfuss sling
    Rauchfuss sling splint
    Rauchfuss triangle—an area of dullness affiliated with Grocco sign.

Rauscher, F.J., 20th century U.S. oncologist.
    Rauscher leukemia virus—an RNA retrovirus associated with leukemia in rodents. *Syn:* Rauscher virus
    Rauscher virus—*Syn:* Rauscher leukemia virus

Ravenna, F.
    Ravenna syndrome—evident at birth or within the third year of life; slow growth eventually determining mild disproportionate dwarfism. *Syn:* atypical achondroplasia

Ray, Isaac, U.S. psychiatrist, 1807–1881.
    Ray mania—moral insanity.

Rayer, Pierre F., French physician, 1793–1867.
    Rayer disease—xanthomatosis with hypercholesterolemia, resulting from biliary cirrhosis. *Syn:* biliary xanthomatosis

Rayleigh, Lord John W.S., English physicist and Nobel laureate, 1842–1919.
    Rayleigh equation—a ratio of red to green required by each observer to match spectral yellow. *Syn:* Rayleigh test
    Rayleigh test—*Syn:* Rayleigh equation

Raymond, Fulgence, French neurologist, 1844–1910.
    Raymond apoplexy—a type of stroke in evolution.
    Raymond syndrome

Raynaud, Maurice, French physician, 1834–1881.
    Raynaud disease—*Syn:* Raynaud syndrome
    Raynaud gangrene—*Syn:* Raynaud phenomenon
    Raynaud phenomenon—spasm of the digital arteries, with blanching and numbness or pain of the fingers, often precipitated by cold.
    Raynaud sign—*Syn:* acrocyanosis
    Raynaud syndrome—idiopathic paroxysmal bilateral cyanosis of the digits. *Syn:* Raynaud disease; Raynaud gangrene; symmetric asphyxia

Réaumur, René A.F. de, French physicist, 1683–1757.
    Réaumur scale—a thermometer scale.

Rebeitz, J.J.
    Rebeitz-Kolodny-Richardson syndrome—possible metabolic failure at the cellular level, clumsiness or slowness of limbs, impairment in control of muscle movements, with involuntary muscle movement.

NOTES

R

Récamier, Joseph C.A., French gynecologist, 1774–1852.
Récamier curet
Récamier operation—curettage of the uterus.
Récamier procedure

Recklinghausen, Friedrich D. von, German histologist and pathologist, 1833–1910.
central Recklinghausen disease type II—congenital disorder characterized by café-au-lait spots, intertriginous freckling, iris hamartomas, and multiple skin neurofibromas.
Recklinghausen disease of bone—increased osteoclastic resorption of calcified bone with replacement by fibrous tissue, due to primary hyperparathyroidism or other causes of the rapid mobilization of mineral salts. *SYN:* osteitis fibrosa cystica
Recklinghausen disease type I—*SYN:* von Recklinghausen disease
Recklinghausen disease type II—*SYN:* von Recklinghausen disease
Recklinghausen tonometer
Recklinghausen tumor—a small benign tumor of the male epididymis and female genital tract. *SYN:* adenomatoid tumor
Recklinghausen-Applebaum disease—a condition of hemochromatosis.
von Recklinghausen disease—two distinct major hereditary disorders: type I (neurofibromatosis type II), and central type II (neurofibromatosis type I). *SYN:* neurofibromatosis
von Recklinghausen neurofibromatosis

Redlich, Emil, Austrian neurologist, 1866–1930.
Obersteiner-Redlich line—*SYN:* Obersteiner-Redlich zone
Obersteiner-Redlich zone—see under Obersteiner

Reed, Dorothy M., U.S. pathologist, 1874–1964.
Dorothy Reed cells—*SYN:* Reed-Sternberg cells
Reed cells—*SYN:* Reed-Sternberg cells
Reed-Sternberg cells—large transformed lymphocytes, generally regarded as pathognomonic of Hodgkin disease. *SYN:* Reed cells; Sternberg cells; Sternberg-Reed cells; Dorothy Reed cells
Sternberg-Reed cells—*SYN:* Reed-Sternberg cells

Reenstierna, John, Swedish dermatologist, *1882.
Ito-Reenstierna test—*SYN:* Ducrey test

Rees, George Owen, English physician, 1813–1889.
Rees test—a test for albumin.

Rees, H. Maynard, 20th century U.S. physician.
Rees-Ecker fluid—an aqueous solution of sodium citrate, sucrose, and brilliant cresyl blue used in platelet counts.

Reese, Algernon B., U.S. ophthalmologist, 1896–1981.
Cogan-Reese syndrome—see under Cogan
Reese dermatome
Reese forceps
Reese knife
Reese ptosis operation

Refetoff, S.
Refetoff syndrome—a condition characterized by goiter and elevated

serum level of thyroid hormones, without manifestations of
thyrotoxicosis.

Refsum, Sigvald, Norwegian neurologist, *1907.
> **Refsum disease**—a rare hereditary degenerative disorder characterized by
> retinitis pigmentosa, demyelinating polyneuropathy, deafness, nystagmus,
> and cerebellar signs. *SYN:* Refsum syndrome; heredopathia atactica
> polyneuritiformis
> **Refsum syndrome**—*SYN:* Refsum disease

Regaud, Claude, French radiologist, 1870–1940.
> **Regaud fixative**—used to preserve mitochondria but not fat.
> **residual body of Regaud**—the excess cytoplasm that separates from the
> spermatozoon during spermiogenesis.

Regen, Eugene M., U.S. orthopedic surgeon, *1900.
> **Regen exercise**—exercise done to emphasize the convexity of the lumbar
> spine. *SYN:* squatting exercise
> **Regen flexion exercise**

Rehfuss, Martin E., U.S. physician, 1887–1964.
> **Rehfuss method**—fractional method to test gastric activity.
> **Rehfuss stomach tube**—a tube with a calibrated syringe.

Reichel, Friedrich P., German gynecologist and surgeon, 1858–1934.
> **Reichel chondromatosis**
> **Reichel cloacal duct**
> **Reichel-Pólya stomach resection**—retrocolic anastomosis of the full
> circumference of the open stomach to the jejunum.

Reichel, P.
> **Reichel syndrome**—swelling and motion limitation of knee, hip, elbow, or
> shoulder. *SYN:* synovial chondromatosis

Reichert, F.L.
> **Reichert syndrome**—paroxysm of stabbing pain in the external auditory
> meatus associated with other pain in the face and postauricular area. *SYN:*
> Jacobson neuralgia

Reichert, Karl B., German anatomist, 1811–1884.
> **Reichert camera**
> **Reichert canal**
> **Reichert cartilage**—embryonic cartilage.
> **Reichert cochlear recess**—*SYN:* cochlear recess
> **Reichert radius gauge**
> **Reichert scar**
> **Reichert slit lamp**
> **Reichert substance**—one of several steroids.
> **Reichert tonometer**
> **Reichert-Meissl number**—an index of the volatile acid content of a fat.

NOTES

R

Reichstein, Tadeus, joint winner of 1950 Nobel Prize for work related to adrenal cortex hormones.

Reid, Robert W., Scottish anatomist, 1851–1939.
>**Reid base line**—a line drawn from the inferior margin of the orbit to the auricular point and extending backward to the center of the occipital bone.

Reifenstein, Edward C. Jr., U.S. endocrinologist, 1908–1975.
>**Reifenstein syndrome**—a familial form of male pseudohermaphroditism.

Reil, Johann C., German physician, neurologist, and histologist, 1759–1813.
>**circular sulcus of Reil**—a semicircular fissure. *SYN:* circular sulcus of insula; limiting sulcus of Reil
>**island of Reil**—an oval region of the cerebral cortex overlying the extreme capsule, lateral to the lenticular nucleus, buried in the depth of the fissura lateralis cerebri (sylvian fissure). *SYN:* insula; insular area; insular cortex
>**limiting sulcus of Reil**—*SYN:* circular sulcus of Reil
>**Reil ansa**—a complex fiber bundle. *SYN:* ansa peduncularis
>**Reil band**—*SYN:* septomarginal trabecula; medial lemniscus
>**Reil ribbon**—*SYN:* medial lemniscus
>**Reil triangle**—*SYN:* lemniscal trigone

Reinke, Friedrich B., German anatomist, 1862–1919.
>**Reinke crystalloids**—rod-shaped crystal-like structures with pointed or rounded ends present in the interstitial cells of the testis (Leydig cells) and ovary.
>**Reinke edema**

Reinsch, Adolf, German physician, 1862–1916.
>**Reinsch test**—a test for arsenic.

Reisseisen, Franz D., German anatomist, 1773–1828.
>**Reisseisen muscles**—microscopic smooth muscle fibers in the smallest bronchial tubes.

Reissner, Ernst, German anatomist, 1824–1878.
>**Reissner fiber**—a rodlike, highly refractive fiber running caudally from the subcommissural organ throughout the length of the central canal of the brainstem and spinal cord.
>**Reissner membrane**—the membrane separating the cochlear duct from the vestibular canal. *SYN:* vestibular membrane

Reitan, Ralph M., U.S. psychologist, *1922.
>**Halstead-Reitan battery**—see under Halstead

Reiter, Hans, German bacteriologist, 1881–1969.
>**Fiessinger-Leroy-Reiter syndrome**—*SYN:* Reiter syndrome
>**Reiter disease**—*SYN:* Reiter syndrome
>**Reiter syndrome**—the association of urethritis, iridocyclitis, mucocutaneous lesions, and arthritis. *SYN:* Reiter disease; Fiessinger-Leroy-Reiter syndrome
>**Reiter test**—a complement-fixation test for syphilis.

Remak, Ernst J., German neurologist, 1848–1911.
>**Remak reflex**—plantar flexion of the first three toes with extension of the

knee induced by stroking of the upper anterior surface of the thigh that occurs when the conducting paths in the cord are interrupted.

Remak sign—dissociation of the sensations of touch and of pain in tabes dorsalis.

Remak, Robert, Polish-German anatomist and histologist, 1815–1865.

Remak band

Remak fibers—nerve fibers (axons) lacking a myelin sheath but, in common with others, enveloped by a sheath of Schwann cells. *SYN:* unmyelinated fibers

Remak ganglia—(1) groups of nerve cells in the wall of the venous sinus where it joins the right atrium of the heart; (2) autonomic ganglia in nerves of the stomach.

Remak nuclear division—direct division of the nucleus and cell, without the changes in the nucleus that occur in the ordinary process of cell reproduction. *SYN:* amitosis

Remak plexus—a gangliated plexus of unmyelinated nerve fibers, derived chiefly from the superior mesenteric plexus, ramifying in the intestinal submucosa. *SYN:* submucosal plexus

Remondini, D.S.

Osebold-Remondini syndrome—see under Osebold

Rendu, Henri J.L.M., French physician, 1844–1902.

Rendu-Osler-Weber syndrome—a disease marked by multiple small telangiectases and dilated venules that develop slowly on the skin and mucous membranes. *SYN:* hereditary hemorrhagic telangiectasia

Renpenning, H., 20th century Canadian physician.

Renpenning syndrome—x-linked mental retardation with short stature and microcephaly.

Renshaw, Birdsey, 20th century U.S. neurophysiologist.

Renshaw cells—inhibitory interneurons.

Renwick, T.K., English physician.

Fisch-Renwick syndrome—see under Fisch

Renwick-Fisch syndrome—*SYN:* Fisch-Renwick syndrome

Restorff, Hedwig von. See under von Restorff.

Rett, Andreas, 20th century Austrian pediatrician.

Rett syndrome—a progressive syndrome of autism, dementia, ataxia, and purposeless hand movements.

Retzius, Anders A., Swedish anatomist and anthropologist, 1796–1860.

cavum retzii—*SYN:* space of Retzius

Retzius cavity—*SYN:* space of Retzius

Retzius fibers—stiff fibers in Deiters cells.

(continued)

NOTES

R

Retzius *(continued)*

Retzius gyrus—the intralimbic gyrus in the cortical portion of the rhinencephalon.

Retzius ligament—the deep attachment of the inferior extensor retinaculum in the tarsal sinus. *Syn:* fundiform ligament of foot

Retzius space—*Syn:* space of Retzius

Retzius veins—portacaval anastomoses. *Syn:* Ruysch veins

space of Retzius—the area of loose connective tissue between the bladder with its related fascia and the pubis and anterior abdominal wall. *Syn:* cavum retzii; Retzius cavity; Retzius space; retropubic space

Retzius, Magnus G., Swedish anatomist and anthropologist, 1842–1919.

calcification lines of Retzius—incremental lines of rhythmic deposition of successive layers of enamel matrix during development. *Syn:* lines of Retzius

foramen of Key-Retzius—see under Key, Ernst

Key-Retzius corpuscles—see under Key, Ernst

lines of Retzius—*Syn:* calcification lines of Retzius

Retzius foramen—*Syn:* lateral aperture of the fourth ventricle

Retzius striae—dark concentric lines crossing the enamel prisms of the teeth, seen in axial cross sections of the enamel. *Syn:* brown striae; striae parallelae

sheath of Key and Retzius—see under Key

Reuss, August von, Austrian ophthalmologist, 1841–1924.

Reuss color chart—*Syn:* Reuss color table

Reuss color table—obsolete charts in test for deficient color vision. *Syn:* Stilling color table; Reuss color chart; Reuss table

Reuss formula—a means of estimating the percentage of albumin in a fluid.

Reuss table—*Syn:* Reuss color table

Reuss test—a test for atropine.

Reverdin, Jacques L., Swiss surgeon, 1842–1929.

Reverdin abdominal spatula

Reverdin bunionectomy

Reverdin epidermal free graft

Reverdin graft—small bits of skin of partial or full thickness removed from a healthy area and seeded in a site to be covered. *Syn:* pinch graft

Reverdin holder

Reverdin implant

Reverdin method

Reverdin needle

Reverdin operation

Reverdin osteotomy

Reverdin prosthesis

Reverdin skin graft

Reverdin suture needle

Revilliod, Léon, Swiss physician, 1835–1919.

Revilliod sign—in hemiplegia, inability to voluntarily close the eye on the paralyzed side except in conjunction with closure of the other eye. *Syn:* sign of the orbicularis

Reye, Ralph Douglas Kenneth, 20th century Australian pathologist.
Reye syndrome—an acquired encephalopathy of young children that follows an acute febrile illness, usually influenza or varicella infection.

Ribbert, Moritz W.H., German pathologist, 1855–1920.
Ribbert theory—that a neoplasm may result when a reduction in tension (exerted by adjacent tissues) leads to conditions favorable to uncontrolled growth of cell rests.

Ribes, François, French physician, 1765–1845.
Ribes ganglion—a small sympathetic ganglion situated on the anterior communicating artery of the brain.

Ricci, Vincenzo, Italian physician.
Cacchi-Ricci syndrome—see under Cacchi
Ricci-Cacchi syndrome—*SYN:* Cacchi-Ricci syndrome

Riccò, Annibale, Italian astrophysicist, 1844–1919.
Riccò law—for small images, light intensity times area equals constant for the threshold.

Rich, Arnold R., U.S. pathologist, 1893–1968.
Hamman-Rich syndrome—*SYN:* usual interstitial pneumonia of Liebow

Richard, Felix Adolphe, Paris surgeon, 1822–1872.
Richard fringes—*SYN:* fimbriae of uterine tube

Richards, Barry W., 20th century English physician.
Richards-Rundle syndrome—a nervous system disorder that begins in early childhood.

Richards, Dickinson W., joint winner of 1956 Nobel Prize for work related to circulation and heart catheterization.

Richardson, E.P.
Rebeitz-Kolodny-Richardson syndrome—see under Rebeitz

Richardson, John Clifford, Canadian neurologist, *1909.
Richardson rod
Steele-Richardson-Olszewski disease—*SYN:* Steele-Richardson-Olszewski syndrome
Steele-Richardson-Olszewski syndrome—see under Steele

Riches, Sir Eric William, English urological surgeon.
Riches bladder syringe
Riches diathermy forceps

Richet, Charles Robert, 1913 Nobel Prize winner for work related to anaphylaxis.

Richet, Didier Dominique Alfred, French surgeon, 1816–1891.
Richet aneurysm
Richet bandage

(continued)

R

NOTES

Richet *(continued)*
> **Richet dressing**
> **Richet operation**

Richter, August G., German surgeon, 1742–1812.
> **Monro-Richter line**—see under Monro, Alexander, Jr.
> **Richter forceps**
> **Richter hernia**—a hernia in which only a portion of the wall of the intestine is engaged. *SYN:* parietal hernia
> **Richter operation**
> **Richter retractor**
> **Richter scissors**
> **Richter-Monro line**—*SYN:* Monro-Richter line

Richter, Maurice N., U.S. pathologist, *1897.
> **Richter syndrome**—a high-grade lymphoma developing during the course of chronic lymphocytic leukemia.

Ricketts, Howard T., U.S. pathologist, 1871–1910.
> *Rickettsia akari*—a species causing human rickettsialpox.
> *Rickettsia australis*—a species causing a spotted fever.
> *Rickettsia conorii*—an African species probably causing boutonneuse fever.
> *Rickettsia prowazekii*—a species causing epidemic typhus.
> *Rickettsia rickettsii*—the agent of Rocky Mountain spotted fever.
> *Rickettsia sibirica*—the agent of Siberian or North Asian tick typhus.
> *Rickettsia tsutsugamushi*—a species causing tsutsugamushi disease and scrub typhus.
> *Rickettsia typhi*—a species causing murine or endemic typhus fever.
> **rickettsial**—pertaining to or caused by rickettsiae.
> **rickettsialpox**—an acute disease caused by *Rickettsia akari*; transmitted by the mite.
> **rickettsiosis**—infection with rickettsiae.
> **rickettsiostatic**—an agent inhibitory to the growth of Rickettsia.

Rickles, Norman H., U.S. oral pathologist, *1920.
> **Rickles test**—a colorimetric test for predicting dental caries activity.

Rideal, Samuel, English chemist and bacteriologist, 1863–1929.
> **Rideal-Walker coefficient**—a figure expressing the disinfecting power of any substance. *SYN:* hygienic laboratory coefficient; phenol coefficient
> **Rideal-Walker method**

Ridgway, Robert, U.S. ornithologist, 1850–1929.
> **Ridgway color system**—method of organizing colors based on the natural color of bird feathers.

Ridley, Humphrey, English anatomist, 1653–1708.
> **circulus venosus ridleyi**—*SYN:* circular sinus
> **Ridley circle**—*SYN:* circular sinus
> **Ridley sinus**—the anterior and posterior anastomoses between the cavernous sinuses. *SYN:* intercavernous sinuses

Riedel, Bernhard M.C.L., German surgeon, 1846–1916.
> **Riedel disease**—*SYN:* Riedel thyroiditis
> **Riedel frontal ethmoidectomy**

Riedel lobe—an occasional tongue-like process extending downward from the right lobe of the liver lateral to the gallbladder. *SYN:* lobus appendicularis; lobus linguiformis

Riedel struma—*SYN:* Riedel thyroiditis

Riedel syndrome—*SYN:* Riedel thyroiditis

Riedel thyroiditis—a rare fibrous induration of the thyroid, with adhesion to adjacent structures, which may cause tracheal compression. *SYN:* Riedel disease; ligneous struma; Riedel struma; chronic fibrous thyroiditis; ligneous thyroiditis; Riedel syndrome

Rieder, Hermann, German pathologist, 1858–1932.

Rieder cell leukemia—a form of acute granulocytic leukemia.

Rieder cells—abnormal myeloblasts frequently observed in acute leukemia.

Rieder lymphocyte—an abnormal form of lymphocyte with a greatly indented nucleus, usually observed in certain examples of chronic lymphocytic leukemia.

Riegel, Franz, German physician, 1843–1904.

Riegel pulse—a pulse that diminishes in volume during expiration.

Rieger, Herwigh, German ophthalmologist, 1898–1986.

Rieger anomaly—mesodermal dysgenesis of cornea and iris, producing pupillary anomalies, posterior embryotoxon, and secondary glaucoma. *SYN:* iridocorneal mesodermal dysgenesis

Rieger syndrome—Rieger anomaly combined with hypodontia or anodontia and maxillary hypoplasia.

Riehl, Gustav, Austrian dermatologist, 1855–1943.

Riehl melanosis—a brown pigmentary condition of the exposed portions of the skin of the neck and face. *SYN:* Riehl syndrome

Riehl syndrome—*SYN:* Riehl melanosis

Rieux, Léon, 19th century French surgeon.

Rieux hernia—a retrocecal hernia.

Riga, Antonio, Italian physician, 1832–1919.

Fede-Riga disease—*SYN:* Riga-Fede disease

Riga-Fede disease—ulceration of the lingual frenum in teething infants. *SYN:* Fede-Riga disease

Riggs, John Mankey, U.S. dentist, 1810–1885.

Riggs disease—periodontitis.

Riley, Conrad M., U.S. pediatrician, *1913.

Riley-Day syndrome—a congenital syndrome, with specific disturbances of the nervous system and aberrations in autonomic nervous system function. *SYN:* familial dysautonomia

Riley, Harris D., Jr., U.S. physician, *1925.

Smith-Riley syndrome—see under Smith, William

NOTES

Rindfleisch, Georg E., German physician, 1836–1908.
  Rindfleisch cells—obsolete term for eosinophilic leukocyte.
  Rindfleisch folds—semilunar folds of the serous surface of the pericardium, embracing the beginning of the aorta.

Ringer, Sydney, English physiologist, 1835–1910.
  Krebs-Ringer solution—see under Krebs
  lactated Ringer injection—a sterile solution of calcium chloride, potassium chloride, sodium chloride, and sodium lactate in water for injection.
  Locke-Ringer solution—see under Locke
  Ringer injection—a sterile solution of sodium chloride, potassium chloride, and calcium chloride, used intravenously as a fluid and electrolyte replenisher.
  Ringer solution—a solution resembling the blood serum in its salt constituents.

Riniker, P., Swiss pediatrician.
  Glanzmann and Riniker lymphocytophthisis—see under Glanzmann

Rinne, Friedrich Heinrich A., German otologist, 1819–1868.
  Rinne test—a hearing test using a vibrating tuning fork.

Riolan, Jean, French anatomist and botanist, 1577–1657.
  Riolan anastomosis—the specific portion of the marginal artery of the colon connecting the middle and left colic arteries. *SYN:* Riolan arc (3)
  Riolan arc—(1) *SYN:* intestinal arterial arcades; (2) *SYN:* marginal artery of colon; (3) *SYN:* Riolan anastomosis
  Riolan arcades—*SYN:* intestinal arterial arcades
  Riolan bones—several small sutural bones sometimes present in the petro-occipital suture.
  Riolan bouquet—the muscles and ligaments arising from the styloid process.
  Riolan muscle—*SYN:* cremaster muscle

Ripault, Louis H.A., French physician, 1807–1856.
  Ripault sign—a sign of death consisting of a permanent change in the shape of the pupil produced by unilateral pressure on the eyeball.

Risley, Samuel D., U.S. ophthalmologist, 1845–1920.
  Risley pliers
  Risley rotary prism—a rotating prism used in examination of ocular muscle imbalance.

Risser, Joseph C., U.S. orthopedic surgeon, 1892–1942.
  Risser cast
  Risser cast table
  Risser frame
  Risser grade
  Risser jacket—a scoliosis plaster jacket.
  Risser localizer scoliosis cast
  Risser method
  Risser sign
  Risser stage
  Risser technique
  Risser turnbuckle cast

Ritgen, Ferdinand August Marie Franz von, German obstetrician, 1787–1867.
  Ritgen maneuver—delivery of a child's head by pressure on the perineum while controlling the speed of delivery by pressure with the other hand on the head.

Ritter, Gottfried Ritter von Rittershain, German physician, 1820–1883.
  Ritter disease—*SYN:* Lyell disease
  Ritter syndrome—*SYN:* Lyell disease

Ritter, Johann W., German physicist, 1776–1810.
  Ritter law—a nerve is stimulated at both the opening and the closing of an electrical current.
  Ritter opening tetanus—the tetanic contraction that occasionally occurs when a strong current passing through a long stretch of nerve is suddenly interrupted.
  Ritter-Rollet phenomenon—on equal electrical stimulation of motor nerve trunks, the flexor and abductor muscle groups react more readily than the extensors and adductors.

Rivero-Carvallo, José Manuel, Mexican cardiologist, *1905.
  Carvallo sign—an increase in the intensity of the pansystolic murmur of tricuspid regurgitation during or at the end of inspiration distinguishes tricuspid from mitral involvement.
  Rivero-Carvallo effect—inspiratory increase in the systolic murmur of tricuspid insufficiency.

Rivers, William H., English physician, 1864–1922.
  Rivers cocktail—an intravenous slow injection used in acute alcoholism. *SYN:* Philadelphia cocktail

Rivière, Lazare (Lazarus), French physician, 1589–1655.
  Rivière salt—a deliquescent powder used as a diuretic, diaphoretic, expectorant, systemic, and urinary alkalizer. *SYN:* potassium citrate

Roach, F. Ewing, U.S. prosthodontist, 1868–1960.
  Roach clasp—part of a denture or retainer. *SYN:* bar clasp

Roaf, R.
  Roaf syndrome—a nonhereditary craniofacial-skeletal disorder characterized by multiple defects.

Robbins, Frederick Chapman, joint winner of 1954 Nobel Prize for work related to poliomyelitis virus.

Robert, César Alphonse, French surgeon, 1801–1862.
  Robert ligament

Robert, Heinrich, L.F., German gynecologist, 1814–1878.
  Robert pelvis—obsolete term for a pelvis narrowed transversely in consequence of the almost entire absence of the alae of the sacrum.

Roberts, John B., U.S. physician, 1852–1924.
  Roberts syndrome—autosomal recessive inheritance, with multiple defects.

NOTES

R

411

Roberts, Richard J., joint winner of 1993 Nobel Prize for work related to split genes.

Roberts, Sir William, English physician, 1830–1899.
  Roberts test—test for albumin.

Robertshaw, Frank L., 20th century English anesthesiologist.
  Robertshaw tube—a variation of Carlen tube.

Robertson, Douglas M.C.L. Argyll, Scottish ophthalmologist, 1837–1909.
  Argyll Robertson pupil—a form of reflex iridoplegia often present in tabetic neurosyphilis. *Syn:* Robertson pupil
  Robertson pupil—*Syn:* Argyll Robertson pupil

Robertson, William Egbert, U.S. physician, 1869–1956.
  Robertson sign—(1) a contraction over the area of the heart of the pectoralis muscle signalling pending death from cardiac disease; (2) signals malingering when pupillary dilatation is absent upon placing pressure on areas identified as painful; (3) demonstrated when the patient has ascites.

Robin, Charles P., French physician, 1821–1885.
  Virchow-Robin space—see under Virchow

Robin, Pierre, French pediatrician, 1867–1950.
  Pierre Robin syndrome—micrognathia and abnormal smallness of the tongue, often with cleft palate, severe myopia, congenital glaucoma, and retinal detachment. *Syn:* Robin syndrome
  Robin syndrome—*Syn:* Pierre Robin syndrome

Robinow, Meinhard, U.S. physician, *1909.
  Robinow dwarfism—*Syn:* Robinow syndrome
  Robinow mesomelic dysplasia
  Robinow syndrome—dwarfism associated with several facial anomalies. *Syn:* Robinow dwarfism; fetal face syndrome

Robinson, Andrew, U.S. dermatologist, 1845–1924.
  Robinson disease—obsolete term for hidrocystoma(s) occurring in the skin of the face, especially in the region of the eyes.

Robinson, Brian F., 20th century English cardiologist.
  Robinson index—an index used to calculate heart work load.

Robinson, E.M.
  Robinson syndrome—dysmenorrhea that begins shortly after menarche. *Syn:* dysmenorrhea; unilateral genital atresia

Robinson, Frederick Byron, U.S. anatomist, 1857–1910.
  Robinson circle—a circle of arteries formed by anastomosing the abdominal aorta, common iliac, hypogastric, uterine, and ovarian arteries.

Robinson, G.C.
  Robinson syndrome—sensorineural deafness and other anomalies. *Syn:* familial ectodermal dysplasia

Robinson, Robert A., U.S. orthopedic surgeon, *1914.
  Robinson anterior cervical diskectomy
  Robinson artificial apparatus

Robinson morcellation
Robinson pocket arthrometer
Robinson prosthesis
Robinson spinal arthrodesis
Smith-Robinson operation—see under Smith, G. W.

Robison, Robert, English chemist, 1884–1941.
Robison ester—*Syn:* D-glucose 6-phosphate
Robison ester dehydrogenase—a deficiency of this enzyme can lead to severe hemolytic anemia and favism. *Syn:* glucose 6-phosphate dehydrogenase
Robison-Embden ester—a key intermediate in glycolysis, glycogenolysis, pentose phosphate shunt, etc. *Syn:* D-glucose 6-phosphate

Robles, Rudolfo (Valverde), Guatemalan dermatologist, 1878–1939.
Robles disease—onchocerciasis.

Rocher, Henri Gaston Louis, French surgeon, *1876.
Rocher sign—the forward or backward sliding of the tibia indicating laxity or tear of the anterior or posterior cruciate ligaments of the knee. *Syn:* drawer sign

Rocky Mountains, mountains in the United States and Canada.
Rocky Mountain spotted fever—an acute infectious disease of high mortality, characterized by frontal and occipital headache, intense lumbar pain, malaise, a moderately high continuous fever, and a rash on wrists, palms, ankles, and soles from the second to the fifth day, later spreading to all parts of the body; it occurs in the spring of the year primarily in the southeast U.S. and the Rocky Mountain region.

Rodbell, Martin, joint winner of 1994 Nobel Prize for work related to G-proteins.

Roenheld, L.
Roenheld syndrome—atypical chest pain and palpitations following a meal. *Syn:* postprandial cardiogastritis

Roenne, Henning K.T., Danish ophthalmologist, 1878–1947.
Roenne nasal step—a visual field defect seen in glaucoma.

Roentgen, Wilhelm K., German physicist and Nobel laureate, 1845–1923.
roentgen—the international unit of exposure dose for x-rays or gamma rays.
roentgen ray—*Syn:* x-ray
roentgenograph—*Syn:* radiograph

Roger, Georges Henri, French physiologist, 1860–1946.
Roger reflex—salivation caused by irritation of the lower end of the esophagus. *Syn:* esophagosalivary reflex

NOTES

R

Roger, Henri L., French physician, 1809–1891.
　bruit de Roger—*SYN:* Roger murmur
　maladie de Roger—*SYN:* Roger disease
　Roger disease—a congenital cardiac anomaly consisting of a small, isolated, asymptomatic defect of the interventricular septum. *SYN:* maladie de Roger
　Roger murmur—a loud pansystolic murmur maximal at the left sternal border, caused by a small ventricular septal defect. *SYN:* bruit de Roger

Rogers, L.E.
　Rogers syndrome—*SYN:* thiamine-responsive megaloblastic anemia

Rogers, Oscar H., U.S. physician, 1857–1941.
　Rogers sphygmomanometer—an sphygmomanometer with an aneroid barometer gauge.

Rohr, Karl, Swiss embryologist and gynecologist, *1863.
　Rohr stria—layer of fibrinoid in the intervillous spaces of the placenta.

Rokitansky, Karl Freiherr von, Austrian pathologist, 1804–1878.
　Mayer-Rokitansky-Küster-Hauser syndrome—see under Mayer
　Rokitansky disease—(1) *SYN:* acute yellow atrophy of the liver; (2) Chiari syndrome.
　Rokitansky diverticulum
　Rokitansky hernia—a separation of the muscular fibers of the bowel allowing protrusion of a sac of the mucous membrane.
　Rokitansky kidney
　Rokitansky pelvis—*SYN:* spondylolisthetic pelvis
　Rokitansky tumor
　Rokitansky-Aschoff sinuses—small outpocketings of the mucosa of the gallbladder which extend through the muscular layer.
　Rokitansky-Küster-Hauser syndrome—*SYN:* Mayer-Rokitansky-Küster-Hauser syndrome

Rolando, Luigi, Italian anatomist, 1773–1831.
　fissure of Rolando—a double S-shaped fissure extending obliquely upward and backward on the lateral surface of each cerebral hemisphere at the boundary between frontal and parietal lobes. *SYN:* central sulcus
　rolandic epilepsy—a benign autosomal dominant form of epilepsy occurring in children.
　Rolando angle—the angle which the fissure of Rolando (central sulcus) makes with the midplane.
　Rolando area—the region of the cerebral cortex most immediately influencing movements of the face, neck and trunk, arm, and leg. *SYN:* motor cortex
　Rolando cells—the nerve cells in Rolando gelatinous substance of the spinal cord.
　Rolando column—a slight ridge on either side of the medulla oblongata related to the descending trigeminal tract and nucleus.
　Rolando gelatinous substance—the apical part of the posterior horn of the spinal cord's gray matter, composed largely of very small nerve cells. *SYN:* gelatinous substance
　Rolando tubercle—a longitudinal prominence on the dorsolateral surface

of the medulla oblongata along the lateral border of the tuberculum cuneatum. *SYN:* tuberculum cinereum

Rolf, Ida, PhD, U.S. biochemist and physical therapist, 1896–1979.
rolfing—deep massage technique

Roller, Christian F.W., German neurologist and psychiatrist, 1844–1978.
Roller nucleus—lateral nucleus of the accessory nerve.

Rolleston, Sir Humphry D., English physician, 1862–1944.
Rolleston rule—the ideal adult systolic blood pressure is 100 plus half the age, whereas the maximal physiologic pressure is 100 plus the age.

Rollet, Alexander, Austrian physiologist, 1834–1903.
Ritter-Rollet phenomenon—see under Ritter, Johann
Rollet stroma—the colorless stroma of the red blood cells.

Rollier, Auguste, Swiss physician, 1874–1954.
Rollier formula—formula used to regulate progressive exposure to natural or artificial ultraviolet radiation.

Romaña, Cecilio, Argentinian physician in Brazil, *1899.
Romaña sign—marked edema of one or both eyelids, thought to be a sensitization response to the bite of a triatomine bug infected with *Trypanosoma cruzi,* and a strong suggestion of acute Chagas disease.

Romano, C., Italian physician, *1923.
Romano-Ward syndrome—a prolonged Q-T interval in the electrocardiogram in children subject to ventricular arrhythmias, including ventricular fibrillation. *SYN:* Ward-Romano syndrome
Ward-Romano syndrome—*SYN:* Romano-Ward syndrome

Romanowsky, Dimitri L., Russian physician, 1861–1921.
Romanowsky stain

Romberg, E.
Romberg-Wood syndrome—dyspnea, angina pectoris, shortness of breath in otherwise healthy individuals after exertion, cold exposure, and/or excitement. *SYN:* primary pulmonary hypertension

Romberg, Moritz H., German physician, 1795–1873.
facial hemiatrophy of Romberg—*SYN:* Romberg syndrome
Romberg disease—facial hemiatrophy.
Romberg sign—a sign of sensory ataxia if a patient standing with heels touching cannot maintain balance on closing eyes. *SYN:* rombergism; Romberg symptom (1); Romberg test; station test
Romberg symptom—(1) *SYN:* Romberg sign; (2) *SYN:* Romberg-Howship symptom.
Romberg syndrome—atrophy, usually progressive, affecting the tissues of one side of the face. *SYN:* facial hemiatrophy of Romberg; Romberg trophoneurosis

(continued)

NOTES

Romberg *(continued)*
    Romberg test—*Syn:* Romberg sign
    Romberg trophoneurosis—*Syn:* Romberg syndrome
    Romberg-Howship symptom—in cases of incarcerated obturator hernia, lancinating pains along the inner side of the thigh to the knee, or down the leg to the foot; caused by compression of the obturator nerve. *Syn:* Romberg symptom (2)
    rombergism—*Syn:* Romberg sign

Römer, Paul H., German bacteriologist, 1876–1916.
    Römer test—a test for tuberculosis.

Rood, Margaret S., 20th century U.S. occupational/physical therapist.
    Rood method of exercise—therapeutic exercises enhanced by cutaneous stimulation for patients with neuromuscular dysfunction.
    Rood technique

Rorschach, Hermann, Swiss psychiatrist, 1884–1922.
    Behn-Rorschach Test—see under Behn
    Rorschach test—a projective psychological test. *Syn:* inkblot test

Roscoe, Sir Henry E., English chemist, 1833–1915.
    Bunsen-Roscoe law—see under Bunsen
    Roscoe-Bunsen law—*Syn:* Bunsen-Roscoe law

Rose, Edmund, German physician, 1836–1914.
    Rose cephalic tetanus—a type of local tetanus that follows wounds to the face and head. *Syn:* cephalic tetanus
    Rose position—the patient lies supine with the head falling down over the end of the table, for operations within the mouth or pharynx.

Rose, H.M., U.S. microbiologist, *1906.
    Rose-Waaler test—a test of historical interest to demonstrate rheumatoid arthritis.

Rosenbach, Anton Julius Friedrich, German pathologist, 1842–1923.
    erysipeloid of Rosenbach—skin infection.

Rosenbach, Ottomar, German physician, 1851–1907.
    Rosenbach disease—(1) *Syn:* Heberden nodes; (2) exostoses on the terminal phalanges of the fingers in osteoarthritis; a specific, usually self-limiting, cellulitis of the hand caused by *Erysipelothrix rhusiopathiae.* *Syn:* erysipeloid.
    Rosenbach law—in affections of the nerve trunks or nerve centers, paralysis of the flexor muscles appears later than that of the extensors; in cases of abnormal stimulation of organs with rhythmical functional periodicity.
    Rosenbach sign—loss of the abdominal reflex in cases of acute inflammation of the viscera.
    Rosenbach test—a test for bile in the urine.
    Rosenbach-Gmelin test—*Syn:* Gmelin test

Rosenberg, Edward Frank, U.S. physician, *1908.
    Hench-Rosenberg syndrome—see under Hench
    Rosenberg-Hench syndrome—*Syn:* Hench-Rosenberg syndrome

Rosenberg, L.E.
    Rowley-Rosenberg syndrome—see under Rowley

Rosenmüller, Johann C., German anatomist, 1771–1820.
    organ of Rosenmüller—a collection of rudimentary tubules in the mesosalpinx between the ovary and the uterine tube. *SYN:* epoöphoron
    Rosenmüller fossa—*SYN:* Rosenmüller recess
    Rosenmüller gland—*SYN:* node of Cloquet
    Rosenmüller node—*SYN:* node of Cloquet
    Rosenmüller recess—a slitlike depression in the membranous pharyngeal wall extending posterior to the opening of the auditory (eustachian) tube. *SYN:* pharyngeal recess; Rosenmüller fossa
    Rosenmüller valve—a fold of mucous membrane guarding the lower opening of the nasolacrimal duct. *SYN:* lacrimal fold

Rosenthal, Curt, 20th century German psychiatrist.
    Melkersson-Rosenthal syndrome—see under Melkersson
    Rosenthal effect—type of self-fulfilling prophecy. *SYN:* pygmalion effect
    Rosenthal syndrome—sleep paralysis that occurs at the moment one falls asleep or awakens.

Rosenthal, Friedrich C., German anatomist, 1780–1829.
    basal vein of Rosenthal—a large vein passing along the medial surface of the temporal lobe, from which it receives tributaries. *SYN:* Rosenthal vein; vena basalis
    Rosenthal aspiration needle
    Rosenthal canal—the winding tube of the bony labyrinth which makes two and a half turns about the modiolus of the cochlea. *SYN:* cochlear canal
    Rosenthal vein—*SYN:* basal vein of Rosenthal

Rosenthal, Robert L., U.S. hematologist, *1923.
    Rosenthal syndrome—inherited hemorrhagic condition that is caused by coagulation Factor XI deficiency.

Roser, Wilhelm, German surgeon, 1817–1888.
    Roser-Nélaton line—*SYN:* Nélaton line

Ross, Sir George W., Canadian physician, 1841–1931.
    Ross-Jones test—a test for an excess of globulin in the cerebrospinal fluid.

Ross, Sir Ronald, English physician and Nobel laureate, 1857–1932.
    Ross cycle—the life cycle of the malaria parasite.

Rossolimo, Grigoriy (Grigorij) I., Russian neurologist, 1860–1928.
    Rossolimo reflex—a stretch reflex of the flexors of the toes seen in lesions of the pyramidal tracts. *SYN:* plantar muscle reflex; Rossolimo sign
    Rossolimo sign—*SYN:* Rossolimo reflex

Rotch, Thomas M., U.S. physician, 1848–1914.
    Rotch sign—in pericardial effusion, percussion dullness in the fifth intercostal space on the right.

NOTES

R

Roth, Moritz, Swiss physician and pathologist, 1839–1914.
   Roth spots—a round white retina spot surrounded by hemorrhage in bacterial endocarditis and in other retinal hemorrhagic conditions.
   vas aberrans of Roth—an occasional diverticulum of the rete testis or of the efferent ductules of the testis.

Roth, Vladimir K., Russian neurologist, 1848–1916.
   Bernhardt-Roth syndrome—*SYN:* Bernhardt disease
   Roth disease—*SYN:* Bernhardt disease
   Roth-Bernhardt disease—*SYN:* Bernhardt disease

Roth, W.
   Roth-Bielschowsky syndrome—complete paralysis of conjugate movements of the eyes in one or more direction, except those under labyrinthine control. *SYN:* pseudo-ophthalmoplegia

Rothera, Arthur C.H., English biochemist, 1880–1915.
   Rothera nitroprusside test—a test for ketone bodies.

Rothmund, August von, German physician, 1830–1906.
   Rothmund syndrome—atrophy, pigmentation, and telangiectasia of the skin, usually with juvenile cataract, saddle nose, congenital bone defects, disturbance of hair growth and hypogonadism. *SYN:* poikiloderma atrophicans and cataract; poikiloderma congenitale; Rothmund-Thomson syndrome
   Rothmund-Thomson syndrome—*SYN:* Rothmund syndrome

Rothschild, Henri Jacques Nathanial Charles de, French physician, 1872–1923.
   Rothschild sign—(1) loss of eyebrow hair seen in hypothyroidism; (2) sternal angle sign seen in tuberculosis.

Rotor, Arturo B., 20th century Philippine internist.
   Rotor syndrome—jaundice appearing in childhood due to impaired biliary excretion.

Rouget, Antoine D., 19th century French physiologist.
   Rouget bulb—a venous plexus on the surface of the ovary.

Rouget, Charles M.B., French physiologist, 1824–1904.
   Rouget cell—a cell with several slender processes that embraces the capillary wall in amphibia. *SYN:* capillary pericyte
   Rouget muscle—the circular fibers of the ciliary muscle. *SYN:* circular fibers
   Rouget-Neumann sheath—the amorphous ground substance between an osteocyte and the lacunar or canalicular wall.

Roughton, Francis J.W., English scientist, 1899–1972.
   Roughton-Scholander apparatus—a syringe-like device for analyzing the respiratory gases in a small sample of blood. *SYN:* Roughton-Scholander syringe
   Roughton-Scholander syringe—*SYN:* Roughton-Scholander apparatus

Rougnon de Magny, Nicholas F., French physician, 1727–1799.
   Rougnon-Heberden disease—*SYN:* Heberden angina

Rous, F. Peyton, U.S. pathologist and Nobel laureate, 1879–1970.
   Rous sarcoma—a fibrosarcoma caused by certain viruses of family Retroviridae. *SYN:* avian sarcoma; Rous tumor

Rous sarcoma virus—a sarcoma-producing virus of the avian leukosis-sarcoma complex identified by Rous in 1911.

Rous tumor—*SYN:* Rous sarcoma

Rous-associated virus—a leukemia virus.

Roussy, Gustave, French pathologist, 1874–1948.

Dejerine-Roussy syndrome—see under Dejerine

Roussy-Cornil syndrome—occasional lancinating pains, with peripheral weakness, fasciculation, visual disturbance, and ataxia. *SYN:* interstitial hypertrophic neuropathy

Roussy-Lévy disease—a type of cerebellar ataxia regularly associated with wasting of the calves and intrinsic muscles of the hands, with absent tendon reflexes. *SYN:* Roussy-Lévy syndrome

Roussy-Lévy syndrome—*SYN:* Roussy-Lévy disease

Rouviere, Henri, French anatomist and embryologist, *1875.

node of Rouviere—one of the lateral group of retropharyngeal lymph nodes.

Roux, César, Swiss surgeon, 1857–1934.

Roux-en-Y anastomosis—a Y-shaped surgical anastomosis involving the small intestine. *SYN:* Roux-en-Y operation

Roux-en-Y gastrectomy

Roux-en-Y gastrojejunostomy

Roux-en-Y hepatic jejunostomy

Roux-en-Y incision

Roux-en-Y loop

Roux-en-Y operation—*SYN:* Roux-en-Y anastomosis

Roux-en-Y pancreatic jejunostomy

Roux, Philibert J., French surgeon, 1780–1854.

Roux method—division of the inferior maxilla in the median line, to facilitate the operation of ablation of the tongue.

Roux sign

Roux, Pierre P.E., French bacteriologist, 1853–1933.

Roux spatula—a very small nickeled steel spatula used to transfer bits of infected material to culture tubes.

Roux stain—a double stain for diphtheria bacilli which employs crystal violet or dahlia and methyl green.

Rovighi, Alberto, Italian physician, 1856–1919.

Rovighi sign—fremitus felt on palpation of hepatic hydatid cyst.

Rovsing, Niels T., Danish surgeon, 1862–1927.

Rovsing operation

Rovsing sign—pain at McBurney point induced in cases of appendicitis by exerting pressure over the descending colon.

Rowland Payne, CME

Rowland Payne syndrome—pain and weakness in the shoulder; change in voice in women with metastatic breast cancer.

NOTES

R

Rowley, P.T.
>**Rowley-Rosenberg syndrome**—growth retardation; reduced muscle and adipose tissue; various degrees of recurrent pulmonary infections; right ventricular hypertrophy.

Rowntree, Leonard G., U.S. physician, 1883–1959.
>**Rowntree and Geraghty test**—*SYN:* phenolsulfonphthalein test

Rozenzweig, Saul, U.S. psychologist, *1907.
>**Rosenzweig picture-frustration study**—a projective test used by psychologists.

Rubarth, Sven, Swedish veterinarian, *1905.
>**Rubarth disease**—a disease of dogs caused by canine adenovirus 1. *SYN:* infectious canine hepatitis
>**Rubarth disease virus**—a virus causing infectious canine hepatitis in dogs. *SYN:* canine adenovirus 1

Rubin, Edgar J.
>**Rubin figure**—a figure which some see as one goblet; others as two facing profiles. *SYN:* goblet figure

Rubin, Isidor C., U.S. gynecologist, 1883–1958.
>**Rubin test**—an obsolete test of patency of the fallopian tubes.

Rubinstein, Jack H., U.S. child psychiatrist and pediatrician, *1925.
>**Rubinstein-Taybi syndrome**—mental retardation, facial deformities, and cardiac anomaly.

Rubner, Max, German hygienist and biochemist, 1854–1932.
>**Rubner laws of growth**—the rate of growth is proportional to the intensity of the metabolic processes.
>**Rubner test**—a test for lactose or glucose in the urine.

Rud, Einar, Danish physician, *1892.
>**Rud syndrome**—ichthyosiform erythroderma associated with acanthosis nigricans, dwarfism, hypogonadism, and epilepsy.

Ruffini, Angelo, Italian histologist, 1864–1929.
>**flower-spray organ of Ruffini**—one of the two types of sensory nerve ending (the other being the annulospiral ending) associated with the neuromuscular spindle. *SYN:* flower-spray ending
>**Ruffini corpuscles**—sensory end-structures in the subcutaneous connective tissues of the fingers, consisting of an ovoid capsule within which the sensory fiber ends with numerous collateral knobs.
>**Ruffini papillary endings**—papillary endings of the skin's nerve endings.

Rukavinas, J.B.
>**Rukavinas syndrome**—peripheral neuropathy most severely affecting the upper limbs; scleroderma-like changes in the skin of hands and arms; vitreous opacities in the eyes.

Rumpel, Theodor, German physician, 1862–1923.
>**Leede-Rumpel phenomenon**—*SYN:* Rumpel-Leede phenomenon
>**Rumpel-Leede phenomenon**—appearance of petechiae in an area following application of vascular constriction due to capillary fragility or abnormal platelet numbers or function. *SYN:* Leede-Rumpel phenomenon

Rumpel-Leede sign—*SYN:* Rumpel-Leede test
Rumpel-Leede test—a tourniquet test for capillary fragility. *SYN:* bandage sign; Rumpel-Leede sign; Hess test

Rumpf, Theodor, German physician, 1851–1923.
Rumpf sign—neurasthenia reaction.

Rundle, A.T., 20th century English physician.
Richards-Rundle syndrome—see under Richards, Barry

Rundles, Ralph W., U.S. internist, *1911.
Rundles-Falls syndrome—weakness, tiredness, occasional leg pain and paresthesias of the feet and associated with pyridoxine deficiency.

Runeberg, Johan W., Finnish physician, 1843–1918.
Runeberg anemia
Runeberg formula—a formula for estimating the percentage of albumin in a serous fluid.

Runyon, Ernest H., 20th century U.S. microbiologist.
Runyon classification—mycobacteria classification. *SYN:* Runyon group
Runyon group—*SYN:* Runyon classification

Rushton, Martin, English pathologist.
Rushton bodies—linear or curved hyaline bodies found within the epithelial lining of odontogenic cysts.

Russell, Albert L., U.S. dentist, *1905.
Russell Periodontal Index—an index that estimates the degree of periodontal disease.

Russell, Alexander, 20th century English pediatrician.
Russell syndrome—failure of infants and young children to thrive due to suprasellar lesions, commonly astrocytomas of the anterior third ventricle.
Russell-Silver dwarfism—*SYN:* Silver-Russell syndrome
Silver-Russell dwarfism—*SYN:* Silver-Russell syndrome
Silver-Russell syndrome—see under Silver, Henry

Russell, G.F.M., 20th century English physician.
Russell sign—abrasions and scars on the back of the hands of individuals with bulimia, usually due to manual attempts at self-induced vomiting.

Russell, James S. Risien, English physician, 1863–1939.
hooked bundle of Russell—*SYN:* uncinate bundle of Russell
uncinate bundle of Russell—fastigial efferent fibers that terminate in the vestibular nuclei and the reticular formation of the pons and medulla. *SYN:* hooked bundle of Russell; uncinate fasciculus of Russell
uncinate fasciculus of Russell—*SYN:* uncinate bundle of Russell

NOTES

R

421

Russell, Patrick, Irish physician in India, 1727–1805.
Russell viper—characteristically marked, highly venomous snake of southeastern Asia. *Syn:* daboia
Russell viper venom—a venom used as a coagulant in the arrest of hemorrhage from accessible sites in hemophilia.

Russell, R. Hamilton, Australian surgeon, 1860–1933.
Russell fibular head autograft
Russell skeletal traction
Russell splint
Russell traction—an improvement of Buck extension that permits the resultant vector of the applied traction force to be changed, for fractures of the femur.
Russell-Taylor classification
Russell-Taylor delta tibial nail
Russell-Taylor femoral interlocking nail system
Russell-Taylor interlocking medullary nail
Russell-Taylor nail
Russell-Taylor rod
Russell-Taylor screw
split Russell skeletal traction

Russell, William James, English chemist, 1830–1909.
Russell effect—the ability of an agent, other than light, to make a developable latent image in a photographic film emulsion. *Syn:* photechic effect

Russell, William, Scottish physician, 1852–1940.
Russell bodies—small, discrete hyaline bodies that occur frequently in plasma cells in chronic inflammation. *Syn:* fuchsin bodies

Russo, Mario, 19th century Italian physician.
Russo reaction—urine reaction to Russo test in typhoid patients.
Russo test

Rust, Johann N., German surgeon, 1775–1840.
Rust disease—tuberculosis of the two upper cervical vertebrae and their articulations. *Syn:* malum vertebrale suboccipitale; spondylarthrocace; spondylocace
Rust phenomenon—in cancer of the upper cervical vertebrae, the patient will always support the head by the hands when changing from the recumbent to the sitting posture or the reverse.
Rust sign

Rutishauser, E., Swiss physician.
Martin du Pan-Rutishauser syndrome—see under Martin du Pan

Ruysch, Frederik, Dutch anatomist, 1638–1731.
Ruysch membrane—the internal layer of the choroidea of the eye, composed of a very close capillary network. *Syn:* choriocapillary layer
Ruysch muscle—the muscular tissue of the fundus of the uterus.
Ruysch tube—a minute tubular cavity opening in the nasal septum.
Ruysch veins—*Syn:* Retzius veins

Ryle, John A., English physician, 1889–1950.
Ryle tube—a thin rubber tube, with about the lumen of a #8 catheter, and an olive-tipped extremity, used in the giving of a test meal.

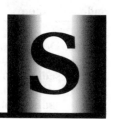

Sabin, Albert B., Polish-U.S. virologist, 1906–1993.
> **Sabin vaccine**—an orally administered vaccine containing live, attenuated strains of poliovirus.
> **Sabin-Feldman dye test**—a method for the detection of anti-toxoplasma antibody in serum.

Sabouraud, Raymond J.A., French dermatologist, 1864–1938.
> **Sabouraud agar**—a culture medium for fungi. *SYN:* French proof agar
> **Sabouraud pastils**—disks that undergo a color change when exposed to x-rays, previously used to indicate the administered dose.
> **Sabouraud syndrome**—progressively thinning hair during first 2 months of life; may occur again in adult life. *SYN:* beaded hair
> **Sabouraud-Noiré instrument**—an obsolete device for measuring the quantity of x-rays.

Sacher-Masoch, Leopold von, Austrian attorney and writer, 1836–1895.
> **masochism**—a form of perversion in which a person experiences pleasure in being abused, humiliated, or mistreated.
> **masochist**—the passive party in the practice of masochism.

Sachs, Bernard, U.S. neurologist, 1858–1944.
> **Tay-Sachs disease**—see under Tay

Sachs, Hans, German bacteriologist, 1877–1945.
> **Sachs-Georgi test**—the first precipitin test for syphilis of diagnostic practicality.

Sachs, M.
> **Ghon-Sachs bacillus**—*SYN:* Sachs bacillus
> **Sachs bacillus**—a species found in malignant edema of animals, in human war wounds, and in cases of appendicitis. *SYN: Clostridium septicum;* Ghon-Sachs bacillus

Sachs, Maurice D., U.S. radiologist, *1909.
> **Hill-Sachs lesion**—see under Hill, Harold

Sacks, Benjamin, U.S. physician, 1896–1939.
> **Libman-Sacks endocarditis**—see under Libman
> **Libman-Sacks syndrome**—*SYN:* Libman-Sacks endocarditis
> **Sacks QuickStick catheter**
> **Sacks Single-Step catheter**
> **Sacks-Vine gastrostomy kit**
> **Sacks-Vine PEG system**
> **Sacks-Vine type PEG**

Sade, Donatien Alphonse Francois, Comte de, French soldier, writer, and libertine, 1740–1814.

> **sadism**—a form of perversion in which a person finds pleasure in inflicting abuse and maltreatment.
> **sadist**—one who practices sadism.

Saemisch, Edwin T., German ophthalmologist, 1833–1909.

> **Saemisch operation**
> **Saemisch section**—procedure of transfixing the cornea beneath an ulcer and then cutting from within outward through the base.
> **Saemisch ulcer**—a form of serpiginous keratitis, frequently accompanied by hypopyon.

Saenger, Alfred, German neurologist, 1860–1921.

> **Saenger pupil**
> **Saenger reflex**
> **Saenger sign**—a lost light reflex of the pupil returns after a short time in the dark.

Saenger, M., Czech obstetrician, 1853–1903.

> **Saenger macula**—a spot of red brighter than the surrounding membrane, at the congested orifice of the duct of Bartholin gland. *SYN:* macula gonorrhoica
> **Saenger operation**—cesarean section followed by careful closure of the uterine wound by three tiers of sutures.
> **Saenger ovum forceps**
> **Saenger suture**
> **Saenger ulcer**

Saint, Charles F.M., South African radiologist, *1886.

> **Saint triad**—the concurrence of hiatal hernia, diverticulosis, and cholelithiasis.

Sakmann, Bert, joint winner of 1991 Nobel Prize for work related to ion channels in the cell.

Salah, M., 20th century Egyptian surgeon.

> **Salah sternal puncture needle**—a wide-bore needle for obtaining samples of red marrow from the sternum.

Salk, Jonas, U.S. immunologist, 1914–1995.

> **Salk polio vaccine**—*SYN:* Salk vaccine
> **Salk vaccine**—the original poliovirus vaccine. *SYN:* Salk polio vaccine

Salmon, Daniel Elmer, U.S. pathologist, 1850–1914.

> *Salmonella enteritidis*—*SYN:* Gärtner bacillus
> *Salmonella gallinarum*—occasionally causes food poisoning or gastroenteritis.
> *Salmonella hirschfeld*—a species causing enteric fever.
> *Salmonella paratyphi*—a species causing enteric fever.
> *Salmonella schottmülleri*—a species causing enteric fever. *SYN:* Schottmüeller bacillus
> *Salmonella typhi*—*SYN:* Eberth bacillus
> *Salmonella typhimurium*—a species causing food poisoning.

S

Salter, Robert, 20th century Canadian orthopedist.
    Salter fracture (I-VI)
    Salter innominate osteotomy
    Salter operation
    Salter osteotomy
    Salter technique
    Salter-Harris classification of epiphysial plate injuries—the classification correlates with different prognoses.
    Salter-Harris epiphyseal injury

Salter, Sir Samuel J.A., English dentist, 1825–1897.
    Salter incremental lines—transverse lines sometimes seen in dentin due to improper calcification.

Salus, Robert, Bohemian ophthalmologist, *1877.
    Koerber-Salus-Elschnig syndrome—*SYN:* Parinaud I syndrome

Salzmann, Maximilian, German ophthalmologist, 1862–1954.
    Salzmann nodular corneal degeneration—prominent nodules of a solid opaque material that stand out from the surface of the cornea.

Sampson, John Albertson, U.S. gynecologist, 1873–1946.
    Sampson cyst—a cyst that results from local hemorrhage. *SYN:* chocolate cyst

Samuelsson, Bengt I., joint winner of 1982 Nobel Prize for work related to prostaglandins.

Sanarelli, Giuseppe, Italian bacteriologist, 1864–1940.
    Sanarelli phenomenon—*SYN:* generalized Shwartzman phenomenon
    Sanarelli-Shwartzman phenomenon—*SYN:* generalized Shwartzman phenomenon

Sanchez Salorio, Manuel, Spanish ophthalmologist, *1930.
    Sanchez Salorio syndrome—a syndrome characterized by retinal pigmentary dystrophy, cataract, hypotrichosis of the lashes, mental deficiencies, and retarded somatic development.

Sanctis, Carlo De. See under De Sanctis.

Sanders, Clarence Elmer, U.S. physician, 1885–1949.
    Sanders oscillating bed—a rocking bed designed to treat patients with peripheral vascular and cardiovascular disease.

Sandhoff, K., contemporary German biochemist.
    Sandhoff disease—a lysosomal storage disease. *SYN:* Sandhoff syndrome
    Sandhoff syndrome—*SYN:* Sandhoff disease

Sandison, J. Calvin, U.S. surgeon, *1899.
    Sandison-Clark chamber—a chamber that can be fitted over a hole punched in a rabbit's ear so that tissue will grow to fill the defect between two transparent plates.

NOTES

Sandow, Eugene, 1867–1925.
Sandow apparatus—an elastic extensor apparatus used primarily for upper limb and shoulder girdle exercises.
Sandow method—method of muscular training. *SYN:* Sandow system
Sandow system—*SYN:* Sandow method

Sandström, I., Swedish anatomist, 1852–1889.
Sandström bodies

Sanfilippo, Sylvester J., 20th century U.S. pediatrician.
Sanfilippo syndrome—*SYN:* type III mucopolysaccharidosis

Sanger, Frederick, English biochemist and twice Nobel laureate, *1918.
Sanger method—sequencing of DNA by employing an enzyme that can polymerase DNA and labeled nucleotides.
Sanger reagent—*SYN:* fluoro-2,4-dinitrobenzene

Sansom, Arthur E., English physician, 1838–1907.
Sansom sign—in mitral stenosis, apparent duplication of the second heart sound.

Sanson, Louis J., French physician, 1790–1841.
Purkinje-Sanson images—see under Purkinje
Sanson images—*SYN:* Purkinje-Sanson images

Santorini, Giandomenico (Giovanni Domenico), Italian anatomist, 1681–1737.
concha santorini
incisurae santorini—*SYN:* notches in cartilage of external acoustic meatus
papilla of Santorini—*SYN:* Vater tubercle
Santorini canal—*SYN:* Santorini duct
Santorini cartilage—a conical nodule of elastic cartilage surmounting the apex of each arytenoid cartilage. *SYN:* corniculate cartilage
Santorini concha—a small concha frequently present on the posterosuperior part of the lateral nasal wall. *SYN:* supreme nasal concha
Santorini duct—the excretory duct of the head of the pancreas. *SYN:* accessory pancreatic duct; Santorini canal
Santorini fissures—(usually) two vertical fissures in the anterior portion of the cartilage of the external auditory meatus, filled by fibrous tissue. *SYN:* notches in cartilage of external acoustic meatus
Santorini incisures—*SYN:* notches in cartilage of external acoustic meatus
Santorini labyrinth—a venous plexus arising chiefly from the dorsal vein of the penis, situated below the base of the bladder at the sides of the prostate. *SYN:* prostatic venous plexus
Santorini major caruncle—point of opening of the common bile duct and pancreatic duct into the duodenum. *SYN:* major duodenal papilla
Santorini minor caruncle—the site of the opening of the accessory pancreatic duct into the duodenum, located anterior to and slightly superior to the major papilla. *SYN:* minor duodenal papilla
Santorini muscle—draws angle of mouth laterally. *SYN:* risorius muscle
Santorini tubercle—a rounded eminence on the posterior part of the aryepiglottic fold, formed by the underlying corniculate cartilages. *SYN:* corniculate tubercle
Santorini vein—the vein that connects the superior sagittal sinus with the tributaries of the superficial temporal vein and other veins of the scalp. *SYN:* parietal emissary vein

Sappey, Marie P.C., French anatomist, 1810–1896.
   Sappey fibers—nonstriated muscular fibers in the check ligaments of the eyeball.
   Sappey plexus—a network of lymphatics in the areola of the nipple.
   Sappey veins—several small veins arising from cutaneous veins about the umbilicus running along the round ligament of the liver and terminating as accessory portal veins. *SYN:* paraumbilical veins

Sarason, Seymour Bernard, U.S. psychologist, *1919.
   Sarason test anxiety scale—test used in psychiatry.

Satchmo, nickname of Louis Armstrong, U.S. jazz musician, 1900–1971.
   Satchmo syndrome—rupture of orbicularis oris muscle frequently occurring in musicians who play wind instruments.

Sattler, Hubert, Austrian ophthalmologist, 1844–1928.
   Sattler elastic layer—the middle layer of the choroid.
   Sattler veil—a diffuse edema of the corneal epithelium that may develop after wearing contact lenses.

Saturday, day of the week.
   Saturday night palsy syndrome—*SYN:* alcoholic neuropathy
   Saturday night paralysis—musculospiral paralysis.

Saundby, Robert, English physician, 1849–1918.
   Saundby test—a test for blood in the stool.

Savage, Henry, English anatomist and gynecologist, 1810–1900.
   Savage perineal body—the fibromuscular mass between the anal canal and the urogenital diaphragm. *SYN:* central tendon of perineum

Savage, Paul Thwaites, English surgeon.
   Savage decompressor

Sayre, George P., U.S. ophthalmologist, *1911.
   Kearns-Sayre syndrome—see under Kearns

Sayre, Lewis A., U.S. surgeon, 1820–1900.
   Sayre apparatus
   Sayre bandage
   Sayre elevator
   Sayre jacket—a plaster-of-Paris jacket applied while the patient is suspended by the head and axillae.
   Sayre sling—sling used for head suspension.
   Sayre splint
   Sayre suspension apparatus—obsolete term for Sayre suspension traction.
   Sayre suspension traction—spinal traction obtained by vertical suspension of the patient by means of a head halter.

NOTES

Scanzoni, Friedrich W., German obstetrician, 1821–1891.
  Scanzoni maneuver—forceps rotation and traction in a spiral course, with reapplication of forceps for delivery.
  Scanzoni second os—a constriction in the uterus resulting from obstructed labor, one of the classic signs of threatened rupture of the uterus. *SYN:* pathologic retraction ring

Scardino, Peter L., U.S. urologist, *1915.
  Scardino ureteropelvioplasty
  Scardino vertical flap pyeloplasty—a reconstructive technique for correction of uteropelvic obstruction.

Scarff, John E., U.S. neurosurgeon, *1898.
  Stookey-Scarff operation—see under Stookey

Scarpa, Antonio, Italian anatomist, orthopedist, and ophthalmologist, 1747–1832.
  canals of Scarpa—separate canals for the nasopalatine nerves and vessels.
  fossa scarpae major—*SYN:* femoral triangle
  Scarpa fascia—the deeper membranous or lamellar part of the subcutaneous tissue of the lower abdominal wall. *SYN:* membranous layer of superficial fascia
  Scarpa fluid—the fluid contained within the membranous labyrinth of the inner ear. *SYN:* endolymph
  Scarpa foramina—two openings in the line of the intermaxillary suture that transmit the nasopalatine nerve.
  Scarpa ganglion—a collection of bipolar nerve cell bodies forming a swelling on the vestibular part of the eighth nerve in the internal acoustic meatus. *SYN:* vestibular ganglion
  Scarpa habenula—*SYN:* Haller habenula
  Scarpa hiatus—a semilunar opening at the apex of the cochlea through which the scala vestibuli and the scala tympani of the cochlea communicate with one another. *SYN:* helicotrema
  Scarpa liquor—the fluid contained within the membranous labyrinth of the inner ear. *SYN:* endolymph
  Scarpa membrane—the membrane closing the fenestra cochleae or rotunda. *SYN:* secondary tympanic membrane
  Scarpa method—cure of an aneurysm by ligation of the artery at some distance above the sac.
  Scarpa sheath—one of the coverings of the spermatic cord, formed of delicate connective tissue and of muscular fibers derived from the internal oblique muscle. *SYN:* cremasteric fascia
  Scarpa staphyloma—a bulging near the posterior pole of the eyeball due to degenerative changes in severe myopia. *SYN:* posterior staphyloma
  Scarpa triangle—the branches of the femoral nerve are distributed within the femoral triangle. *SYN:* femoral triangle; fossa scarpae major

Scatchard, George, U.S. chemist and biochemist, 1892–1973.
  Scatchard plot—a graphical representation used in the analysis of binding phenomena.

Schacher, Polycarp G., German physician, 1674–1737.
  Schacher ganglion—a small parasympathetic ganglion lying in the orbit between the optic nerve and the lateral rectus muscle. *SYN:* ciliary ganglion

S

Schaeffer, Max, German neurologist, 1852–1923.
   Schaeffer reflex—great toe dorsiflexion produced by pinching the Achilles tendon.

Schäfer, Sir Edward A. Sharpey, English physiologist and histologist, 1850–1935.
   Schäfer method—an obsolete method of resuscitation in cases of drowning or asphyxia.

Schäffer, var. of Schaeffer

Schally, Andrew V., joint winner of 1977 Nobel Prize for work related to production of peptide hormone.

Schamberg, Jay F., U.S. dermatologist, 1870–1934.
   Schamberg dermatitis—chronic purpura, especially of the legs of men, spreading to form brownish patches. SYN: progressive pigmentary dermatosis

Schanz, Alfred, German orthopedic surgeon, 1868–1931.
   Schanz angulation osteotomy
   Schanz brace
   Schanz collar—a tube of material stuffed with cellulose and wound in 3 loops around the neck, forming a collar.
   Schanz collar brace
   Schanz femoral osteotomy
   Schanz operation
   Schanz osteotomy
   Schanz pin
   Schanz screw
   Schanz syndrome—spinal muscle weakness, pain on pressure over the spinous processes, and a tendency to curvature of the spine.

Schapiro, Heinrich, Russian physician, 1852–1901.
   Schapiro sign—in myocardial weakness, no slowing of the pulse occurs when the patient lies down.

Schardinger, Franz, 19th century Austrian scientist.
   Schardinger dextrins—the result of action of *Bacillus macerans* on starch.
   Schardinger enzyme—a flavoprotein containing molybdenum. SYN: xanthine oxidase
   Schardinger reaction—an example of oxidation in the absence of O_2 with an organic hydrogen acceptor.

Schatzki, Richard, U.S. radiologist, 1901–1992.
   Schatzki ring—a contraction ring or incomplete mucosal diaphragm in the lower third of the esophagus, which is occasionally symptomatic. SYN: Schatzki syndrome
   Schatzki syndrome—SYN: Schatzki ring

Schaudinn, Fritz R., German bacteriologist, 1871–1906.
   Schaudinn fixative—a solution of mercuric chloride, sodium chloride, alcohol, and glacial acetic acid, used on wet smears for cytologic fixation.

NOTES

Schaumann, Jörgen, Swedish physician, 1879–1953.
   Besnier-Boeck-Schaumann disease—*SYN:* Besnier-Boeck disease
   Besnier-Boeck-Schaumann syndrome—*SYN:* Besnier-Boeck disease
   Schaumann bodies—concentrically laminated calcified bodies found in granulomas, particularly in sarcoidosis. *SYN:* conchoidal bodies
   Schaumann lymphogranuloma—obsolete term for sarcoidosis.
   Schaumann syndrome—*SYN:* Besnier-Boeck disease

Schauta, Friedrich, Austrian gynecologist, 1849–1919.
   Schauta operation—an extensive extirpation of the uterus and the adnexa, using the vaginal approach facilitated by Schuchardt operation.
   Schauta radical vaginal hysterectomy
   Schauta-Amreich operation
   Schauta-Wertheim operation

Schede, Max, German surgeon, 1844–1902.
   Schede clot
   Schede method—filling of the defect in bone after removal of a sequestrum or scraping away carious material by allowing the cavity to fill with blood which may become organized.
   Schede osteotomy

Scheele, Karl W., Swedish chemist, 1742–1786.
   Scheele green—*SYN:* cupric arsenite

Scheffé, Henry, U.S. mathematician, *1907.
   Scheffé test—a test which compares the difference between means in the analysis of variance.

Scheibe, A., U.S. physician, *1875.
   Scheibe deafness—congenital deafness.

Scheie, Harold G., U.S. ophthalmologist, 1909–1990.
   Scheie blade
   Scheie cannula
   Scheie cataract aspiration
   Scheie cautery
   Scheie electrocautery
   Scheie knife
   Scheie needle
   Scheie operation
   Scheie syndrome—error of mucopolysaccharide related to Hurler syndrome. *SYN:* type IS mucopolysaccharidosis
   Scheie trephine

Scheiner, Christoph, German physicist, 1575–1650.
   Scheiner experiment—a demonstration of accommodation.

Schellong, Fritz, German physician, 1891–1953.
   Schellong test—a test for circulatory function.
   Schellong-Strisower phenomenon—a reduction of the systolic blood pressure, accompanied sometimes by vertigo, on rising from the horizontal to the erect posture.

Schenck, Benjamin R., U.S. surgeon, 1873–1920.
   Schenck disease—fungal infection with lymphatic spread to involve

S

musculoskeletal system, gastrointestinal system, and nervous system. *SYN:* sporotrichosis; Beuermann disease; Beuermann-Gourgerot disease

Scheuermann, Holger W., Danish surgeon, 1877–1960.
    Scheuermann disease—epiphysial aseptic necrosis of vertebral bodies. *SYN:* adolescent round back; juvenile kyphosis; osteochondritis deformans juvenilis dorsi; Scheuermann syndrome
    Scheuermann juvenile kyphosis
    Scheuermann syndrome—*SYN:* Scheuermann disease

Schick, Bela, Austrian pediatrician in U.S., 1877–1967.
    Schick method—*SYN:* Schick test
    Schick sign
    Schick test—a test for susceptibility to *Corynebacterium diphtheriae* toxin. *SYN:* Schick method
    Schick test toxin—*SYN:* diagnostic diphtheria toxin

Schiff, Hugo, German chemist in Florence, 1834–1915.
    Kasten fluorescent Schiff reagents—used to detect DNA, polysaccharides, and proteins.
    ninhydrin-Schiff stain for proteins
    periodic acid-Schiff stain—a tissue-staining procedure. *SYN:* PAS stain
    Schiff base—condensation products of aldehydes and ketones with primary amine. *SYN:* aldimine
    Schiff reagent—used for aldehydes and in histochemistry to detect polysaccharides, DNA, and proteins.

Schiff, Moritz, German physiologist, 1823–1896.
    Schiff-Sherrington phenomenon—when the spinal cord is transected in the midthoracic region or a little lower, the stretch and other postural reflexes of the upper extremity become exaggerated; if the transection is made in the sacral cord, a similar effect is observed in the lower limbs.

Schilder, Paul Ferdinand, Austrian neurologist, 1886–1940.
    Addison-Schilder disease—*SYN:* Schilder disease
    Flatau-Schilder disease—*SYN:* Schilder disease
    Schilder disease—encephalitis periaxialis diffusa; progressive demyelinating disorder in adults; early symptom is visual impairment with mental deterioration. *SYN:* Addison-Schilder disease; Flatau-Schilder disease; Schilder syndrome
    Schilder encephalitis
    Schilder syndrome—*SYN:* Schilder disease

Schiller, Walter, Austrian pathologist in U.S., 1887–1960.
    Schiller test—a test for early carcinoma of the cervix.
    Schiller tumor

Schilling, Victor, German hematologist, 1883–1960.
    Schilling band cell—any cell of the granulocytic (leukocytic) series that has
(continued)

NOTES

Schilling *(continued)*

a nucleus that could be described as a curved or coiled band. *SYN:* band cell

Schilling blood count—a method of counting blood. *SYN:* Schilling index

Schilling index—*SYN:* Schilling blood count

Schilling test—a procedure for determining the amount of vitamin B$_{12}$ excreted in the urine using cyanocobalamin tagged with a radioisotope of cobalt.

Schilling type of monocytic leukemia

Schiötz, Hjalmar, Norwegian physician, 1850–1927.

Schiötz tonometer—an instrument that measures ocular tension by indicating the ease with which the cornea is indented.

Schirmer, Otto W.A., German ophthalmologist, 1864–1917.

Schirmer test—a test for tear production using a strip of filter paper; a measurement of basal and reflex lacrimal gland function.

Schlatter, Carl, Swiss surgeon, 1864–1934.

Osgood-Schlatter disease—see under Osgood

Schlatter disease—*SYN:* Osgood-Schlatter disease

Schlatter-Osgood disease—*SYN:* Osgood-Schlatter disease

Schlemm, Friedrich, German anatomist, 1795–1858.

Schlemm canal—the vascular structure encircling the anterior chamber of the eye and through which the aqueous is returned to the blood circulation. *SYN:* sinus venosus sclerae

Schlesinger, Hermann, Austrian physician, 1868–1934.

Pool-Schlesinger sign—*SYN:* Pool phenomenon

Schlesinger cervical punch

Schlesinger cervical rongeur

Schlesinger clamp

Schlesinger forceps

Schlesinger Gigli saw guide

Schlesinger instrument

Schlesinger punch

Schlesinger rongeur

Schlesinger sign—*SYN:* Pool phenomenon

Schmid, Rudi, Swiss-U.S. internist and biochemist, *1922.

McArdle-Schmid-Pearson disease—*SYN:* McArdle syndrome

Schmid, W.

Schmid-Fraccaro syndrome—iris colobomas and anal atresia, associated with an additional acrocentric chromosome. *SYN:* cat's-eye syndrome

Schmidel, Kasimir C., German anatomist, 1718–1792.

Schmidel anastomoses—abnormal channels of communication between the caval and portal venous systems.

Schmidt, Gerhard, U.S. biochemist, *1900.

Schmidt-Thannhauser method—a method for fractionation of nucleic acid.

Schmidt, Henry D., U.S. anatomist and pathologist, 1823–1888.

Schmidt-Lanterman clefts—*SYN:* Schmidt-Lanterman incisures

Schmidt-Lanterman incisures—funnel-shaped interruptions in the regular

S

structure of the myelin sheath of nerve fibers. *Syn:* Schmidt-Lanterman clefts; Lanterman incisures

Schmidt, Johann F.M., German laryngologist, 1838–1907.
Schmidt syndrome—unilateral paralysis of a vocal cord, the velum palati, trapezius, and sternocleidomastoid.

Schmidt, Martin Benno, German physician, 1863–1949.
Schmidt syndrome—the association of primary hypothyroidism, primary adrenocortical insufficiency, and insulin-dependent diabetes mellitus.

Schmorl, Christian G., German pathologist, 1861–1932.
Schmorl bacillus—a bacterial species causing or associated with several necrotic conditions in animals and occasionally in humans. *Syn: Fusobacterium necrophorum*
Schmorl body
Schmorl ferric-ferricyanide reduction stain—a stain to test for reducing substances in tissues.
Schmorl furrow
Schmorl groove
Schmorl jaundice—kernicterus.
Schmorl nodes
Schmorl nodule—prolapse of the nucleus pulposus through the vertebral body endplate into the spongiosa of the vertebra.
Schmorl picrothionin stain—a stain for compact bone.

Schneider, Conrad V., German anatomist, 1614–1680.
schneiderian membrane—*Syn:* nasal mucosa

Schneider, Franz C., German chemist, 1813–1897.
Schneider carmine—a stain consisting of a 10% solution of carmine in 45% acetic acid, used for fresh chromosome preparations.

Schneider, Richard C., U.S. neurologist.
Schneider catheter
Schneider driver
Schneider extractor
Schneider fixation
Schneider hip arthrodesis
Schneider hip fusion
Schneider intramedullary nail
Schneider medullary nail
Schneider nail driver
Schneider nail shaft reamer
Schneider pelvimeter
Schneider pin
Schneider raspatory
Schneider rod

(continued)

NOTES

Schneider (continued)
Schneider self-broaching pin
Schneider syndrome—cervical spine injury resulting in upper extremity paralysis.
Schneider-Shiley catheter

Scholander, Per F., Norwegian physiologist, 1905–1980.
Roughton-Scholander apparatus—see under Roughton
Roughton-Scholander syringe—*Syn:* Roughton-Scholander apparatus
Scholander apparatus—a device used for determining the oxygen and carbon dioxide percentage in 0.5 ml of a respiratory gas.

Scholz, Willibald, German neurologist, *1889.
Scholz disease—obsolete term for the juvenile form of metachromatic leukodystrophy.

Schönbein, Christian F., German chemist, 1799–1868.
Schönbein test—*Syn:* Almén test for blood

Schönlein, Johann L., German physician, 1793–1864.
Henoch-Schönlein purpura—see under Henoch
Henoch-Schönlein syndrome—*Syn:* Henoch-Schönlein purpura
Schönlein disease—*Syn:* Henoch-Schönlein purpura
Schönlein purpura—*Syn:* Henoch-Schönlein purpura
Schönlein-Henoch syndrome—*Syn:* Henoch-Schönlein purpura

Schott, Theodor, German physician, 1850–1921.
Schott treatment—*Syn:* Nauheim treatment

Schottmueller, Hugo A.G., German physician, 1867–1936.
Schottmueller bacillus—a species causing enteric fever. *Syn: Salmonella schottmülleri*
Schottmueller disease—an acute infectious disease with symptoms and lesions resembling those of typhoid fever. *Syn:* paratyphoid fever

Schreger, Christian H.T., German anatomist and chemist, 1768–1833.
Hunter-Schreger bands—see under Hunter, John
Hunter-Schreger lines—*Syn:* Hunter-Schreger bands
Schreger lines—*Syn:* Hunter-Schreger bands

Schridde, Hermann, German pathologist, *1875.
Schridde cancer hairs—thick lusterless hairs scattered in the beard and the temporal region.

Schroeder, Karl L.E., German gynecologist, 1838–1887.
Schroeder curet
Schroeder operation—excision of diseased endocervical mucosa.
Schroeder scissors
Schroeder tenaculum
Schroeder tenaculum loop
Schroeder uterine sound

Schrötter, Leopold von, Austrian laryngologist, 1837–1908.
Paget-von Schrötter syndrome—see under Paget, Sir James

Schuchardt, Karl A., German surgeon, 1856–1901.
Schuchardt incision

S

Schuchardt operation—a surgical technique making the upper vagina accessible for fistula closure or radical surgery via the vagina.
Schuchardt-Pfeifer operation

Schüffner, Wilhelm, German pathologist in Sumatra, 1867–1949.
Schüffner dots—fine, round, uniform dots characteristically observed in erythrocytes infected with *Plasmodium vivax* and *P. ovale. SYN:* Schüffner granules
Schüffner granules—*SYN:* Schüffner dots

Schüller, Artur, Austrian neurologist, 1874–1958.
Hand-Schüller-Christian disease—see under Hand
Schüller disease—*SYN:* Hand-Schüller-Christian disease
Schüller phenomenon—in cases of functional hemiplegia, the patient usually turns to the sound side in walking, but in cases of organic lesion, to the affected side.
Schüller syndrome—*SYN:* Hand-Schüller-Christian disease

Schüller, Karl H.L.A. Max, German surgeon, 1843–1907.
Schüller ducts—inconstant ducts along the side of the female urethra that convey the mucoid secretion of Skene glands to the vestibule. *SYN:* paraurethral ducts

Schultes, var. of Schultetus

Schultz, Arthur R.H., German physician, *1890.
Schultz reaction
Schultz stain—a stain for cholesterol.

Schultz, Johann Heinrich, German neurologist and psychiatrist, 1884–1970.
Schultz autogenic training—system of relaxation and awareness of one's body parts and their degree of warmth.

Schultz, Werner, German internist, 1878–1947.
Schultz-Charlton phenomenon—*SYN:* Schultz-Charlton reaction
Schultz-Charlton reaction—the specific blanching of a scarlatina rash at the site of intracutaneous injection of scarlatina antiserum. *SYN:* Schultz-Charlton phenomenon
Schultz-Dale reaction—the contraction of an excised intestinal loop or of an excised strip of virginal uterus from a sensitized animal, which occurs when the tissue is exposed to the specific antigen. *SYN:* Dale reaction

Schultze, Bernhard, German obstetrician, 1827–1919.
Schultz method
Schultze fold—*SYN:* amniotic fold
Schultze knife
Schultze mechanism—expulsion of the placenta with the fetal surface foremost.

(continued)

NOTES

Schultze *(continued)*
> **Schultze phantom**—a model of a female pelvis used in demonstrating the mechanism of childbirth and the application of forceps.
>
> **Schultze placenta**—a placenta that appears at the vulva with the glistening fetal surface presenting.

Schultze, Max J., German histologist and zoologist, 1825–1874.
> **comma bundle of Schultze**—a compact bundle composed of descending branches of posterior root fibers located near the border between the fasciculi gracilis and cuneatus of the cervical and thoracic spinal cord. *SYN:* semilunar fasciculus; comma tract of Schultze
>
> **comma tract of Schultze**—*SYN:* comma bundle of Schultze
>
> **Schultze cells**—*SYN:* olfactory receptor cells
>
> **Schultze membrane**—the specialized olfactory receptive area. *SYN:* region of olfactory mucosa
>
> **Schultze sign**—in latent tetany, tapping the tongue causes its depression with a concave dorsum. *SYN:* tongue phenomenon

Schütz, Erich, German biochemist, *1902.
> **Schütz law**—*SYN:* Schütz rule
>
> **Schütz rule**—the rate of an enzyme reaction is proportional to the square root of the enzyme concentration. *SYN:* Schütz law

Schütz, Hugo, early 20th century German neurologist anatomist.
> **Schütz bundle**—a bundle of thin, poorly myelinated nerve fibers reciprocally connecting the periventricular zone of the hypothalamus with ventral parts of the central gray substance of the midbrain. *SYN:* dorsal longitudinal fasciculus

Schwabach, Dagobert, German otologist, 1846–1920.
> **Schwabach test**—a hearing test using a series of five tuning forks of different tones.

Schwalbe, Gustav A., German anatomist, 1844–1916.
> **Schwalbe corpuscle**—*SYN:* taste bud
>
> **Schwalbe fissure**
>
> **Schwalbe foramen**
>
> **Schwalbe membrane**
>
> **Schwalbe nucleus**
>
> **Schwalbe ring**—the periphery of the cornea. *SYN:* anterior limiting ring
>
> **Schwalbe sheath**
>
> **Schwalbe spaces**—the spaces within the internal sheath of the optic nerve filled with cerebrospinal fluid and continuous with the subarachnoid space. *SYN:* intervaginal space of optic nerve

Schwann, Theodor, German histologist and physiologist, 1810–1882.
> **Schwann cell unit**—a single Schwann cell and all of the axons lying in troughs indenting its surface.
>
> **Schwann cells**—cells of ectodermal (neural crest) origin that compose a continuous envelope around each nerve fiber of peripheral nerves. *SYN:* neurilemma cells; neurolemma cells
>
> **Schwann tumor**
>
> **Schwann white substance**—the lipid material present in the myelin sheath of nerve fibers; the medulla of bones and other organs.
>
> **schwannoma**—*SYN:* neurilemoma; neuroschwannoma

sheath of Schwann—a cell that enfolds one or more axons of the peripheral nervous system. *SYN:* neurilemma

Schwartz, Henry, U.S. neurosurgeon, *1909.
Schwartz tractotomy—a medullary spinothalamic tractotomy.

Schwartz, Oscar, U.S. pediatrician, *1919.
Schwartz syndrome—multiple congenital disorders.

Schwartz, R. Plato, orthopedic surgeon, 1892–1965.
Schwartz method—system of locomotor exercises for children with cerebral palsy.

Schweigger-Seidel, Franz, German physiologist, 1834–1871.
sheath of Schweigger-Seidel—(1) a spherical or spindle-shaped condensation of phagocytic macrophages in a reticular stroma investing the wall of the splenic arterial capillaries; (2) the outer end of the inner segment of the retinal rods and cones. *SYN:* ellipsoid

Schweninger, Ernst, German dermatologist, 1850–1924.
Schweninger method—a method suggested to reduce obesity by restricting intake of fluid.
Schweninger-Buzzi anetoderma—sudden appearance of bluish-white balloon-like lesions, soft and readily indented.

Scott, Bruce A., U.S. orthotist at Craig Rehabilitation Hospital, Englewood, CO.
Scott-Craig orthosis—a hip stabilizing knee-ankle-foot orthosis.

Scott, Charles I., Jr., U.S. pediatrician, *1934.
Aarskog-Scott syndrome—see under Aarskog

Scott, H. William, U.S. surgeon, *1916.
Scott operation—a jejunoileal bypass for morbid obesity.

Scott-Wilson, H., English scientist.
Scott-Wilson reagent—an alkaline solution of mercuric cyanide and silver nitrate used in the detection of acetone.

Scottish Rite, Scottish Rite Hospitals for Children, located throughout the U.S., owned by a division of the Masonic membership.
Scottish Rite brace
Scottish Rite hip orthosis
Scottish Rite splint

Scribner, Belding H., U.S. nephrologist, *1921.
Quinton-Scribner shunt—see under Quinton
Scribner shunt—connection of an artery, customarily the radial, to the cephalic vein via a short extracorporeal catheter.

Scultetus, originally Schultes, Johann, German surgeon, 1595–1645.
Scultetus bandage—applied to the thorax or abdomen. *SYN:* many-tailed bandage
Scultetus binder
Scultetus position—a supine position on an inclined plane, with head low.

NOTES

Seashore, Carl Emil, U.S. psychologist, 1866–1949.
> **Seashore measures of musical talent tests**—series of tests given to determine the components of musical aptitude.
> **Seashore test**—a test in which the individual must discriminate between two sounds.

Sebileau, Pierre, French anatomist, 1860–1953.
> **Sebileau hollow**—depression between the inferior aspect of the tongue and the sublingual glands.
> **Sebileau muscle**—deep fibers of the dartos tunic that pass into the scrotal septum.

Seckel, Helmut P.G., German physician, 1900–1960.
> **Seckel dwarfism**—*SYN:* Seckel syndrome
> **Seckel syndrome**—an autosomal recessive disorder. *SYN:* Seckel dwarfism

Secrétan, H., Swiss surgeon, 1856–1916.
> **Secrétan syndrome**—traumatic, recurrent edema or hemorrhage of the dorsum of the hand.

Seeligmüller, Otto L.G.A., German neurologist, 1837–1912.
> **Seeligmüller sign**—contraction of the pupil on the affected side in facial neuralgia.

Seessel, Albert, U.S. embryologist, 1850–1910.
> **Seessel pocket**—the part of the embryonic foregut extending cephalad to the level of the oral plate and caudal to the pituitary diverticulum. *SYN:* preoral gut
> **Seessel pouch**

Séguin, Edouard, French-U.S. psychiatrist, 1812–1880.
> **Séguin formboard**—a board with cutouts into which corresponding-shaped blocks of geometric forms are placed.

Seidel, Erich, German ophthalmologist, 1882–1946.
> **Seidel scotoma**—a form of Bjerrum scotoma.
> **Seidel sign**—a sickle-shaped scotoma appearing as an upward or downward extension of the blind spot.

Seignette, Pierre, French apothecary, 1660–1719.
> **Seignette salt**—a mild saline cathartic, used as an ingredient in compound effervescent powders. *SYN:* potassium sodium tartrate

Seiler, Carl, Swiss laryngologist and anatomist in U.S., 1849–1905.
> **Seiler cartilage**—a small rod of cartilage attached to the vocal process of the arytenoid cartilage.
> **Seiler knife**
> **Seiler tonsillar knife**

Seip, Martin, 20th century Scandinavian physician.
> **Lawrence-Seip syndrome**—see under Lawrence

Seitelberger, Franz, Austrian neuropathologist, *1916.
> **Seitelberger disease**—demyelination of the pyramidal tracts. *SYN:* neuroaxonal degeneration; Seitelberger syndrome
> **Seitelberger syndrome**—*SYN:* Seitelberger disease

Seldinger, Sven Ivar, Swedish radiologist, *1921.
    Seldinger cardiac catheterization
    Seldinger catheter
    Seldinger intubation technique
    Seldinger method
    Seldinger needle
    Seldinger retrograde wire
    Seldinger technique—a method of percutaneous insertion of a catheter
      into an artery or vein.
    Seldinger wire

Selivanoff, Feodor, Russian chemist, *1859.
    Selivanoff test—a test for fructosuria. *SYN:* resorcinol test

Seliwanow, var. of Selivanoff

Sellick, Brian A., 20th century English anesthetist.
    Sellick maneuver—pressure applied to the cricoid cartilage to prevent
      regurgitation during tracheal intubation in the anesthetized patient.

Selye, Hans, Austrian endocrinologist in Canada, 1907–1982.
    adaptation syndrome of Selye—general nonspecific adaptation of the
      organism in response to specific stimuli, which trigger physiological
      changes in the endocrine and other organ systems due to prolonged and
      intense stress. *SYN:* Selye syndrome
    Selye syndrome—*SYN:* adaptation syndrome of Selye

Semon, Richard W., German biologist, 1859–1908.
    Semon-Hering theory—the theory that stimuli leave definite traces on the
      protoplasm of the animal or plant that persist after the stimuli cease.
      SYN: mnemic hypothesis

Semon, Sir Felix, German laryngologist in England, 1849–1921.
    Gerhardt-Semon law—see under Gerhardt, Carl
    Semon law—an obsolete law regarding injury to the recurrent laryngeal
      nerve.

Semple, Sir David, English physician, 1856–1937.
    Semple vaccine—a modification of the original rabies vaccine.

Senear, Francis E., U.S. dermatologist, 1889–1958.
    Senear-Usher disease—*SYN:* Senear-Usher syndrome
    Senear-Usher syndrome—an eruption involving sun-exposed skin,
      especially the face. *SYN:* pemphigus erythematosus; Senear-Usher disease

Sengstaken, Robert W., U.S. neurosurgeon, *1923.
    Sengstaken-Blakemore tube—a tube with three lumens used for
      emergency treatment of bleeding esophageal varices.

Sergent, Emile, French physician, 1867–1943.
    Bernard-Sergent syndrome—see under Bernard, Claude

(continued)

NOTES

Sergent *(continued)*

Sergent white line—a pale streak appearing within 30 to 60 seconds after stroking the skin with a fingernail and lasting for several minutes, a sign of diminished arterial tension. *Syn:* white line

Serres, Antoine E.R.A., French anatomist, 1786–1868.

rests of Serres—remnants of dental lamina epithelium entrapped within the gingiva.

Serres angle—the angle between the pterygoid processes and the base of the skull. *Syn:* metafacial angle

Serres glands—epithelial cell rests found in the subepithelial connective tissue in the palate of the newborn, similar to those found in the gingivae.

Sertoli, Enrico, Italian histologist, 1842–1910.

Sertoli cell tumor—a testicular tumor. *Syn:* androblastoma

Sertoli cells—elongated cells in the seminiferous tubules to which spermatids are attached during spermiogenesis. *Syn:* nurse cells

Sertoli columns

Sertoli-cell-only syndrome—the absence from the seminiferous tubules of the testes of germinal epithelium, Sertoli cells alone being present. *Syn:* Del Castillo syndrome

Servetus, Miguel, Spanish anatomist and theologian, 1511–1553.

Servetus circulation—obsolete term for the pulmonary circulation.

Sever, James Warren, U.S. surgeon, 1878–1964.

Sever disease—calcaneoapophysitis.

Sever modification of Fairbank technique

Sever operation

Severinghaus, John W., U.S. physiologist and anesthesiologist, *1922.

Severinghaus electrode—commonly used to analyze arterial blood samples. *Syn:* carbon dioxide electrode

Sézary, A., French dermatologist, 1880–1956.

Sézary cell—an atypical T lymphocyte seen in the peripheral blood in Sézary syndrome.

Sézary erythroderma—*Syn:* Sézary syndrome

Sézary syndrome—a variant of mycosis fungoides. *Syn:* Sézary erythroderma

Shaffer, A., U.S. biochemist, 1881–1960.

Shaffer-Hartmann method—an obsolete method for the quantitative determination of glucose in biological fluids, based on the reduction of copper by the reducing group of the sugar.

Sharp, Phillip A., joint winner of 1993 Nobel Prize for work related to split genes.

Sharpey, William, Scottish physiologist and histologist, 1802–1880.

Sharpey fibers—bundles of collagenous fibers that pass into the outer circumferential lamellae of bone or the cementum of teeth. *Syn:* perforating fibers

Shaver, Cecil Gordon, Canadian physician, *1901.
   Shaver disease—a condition due to the occupational inhalation of bauxite
      fumes. *SYN:* bauxite pneumoconiosis

Sheehan, Harold L., English pathologist, *1900.
   Sheehan syndrome—hypopituitarism arising from a severe circulatory
      collapse postpartum, with resultant pituitary necrosis. *SYN:* postpartum
      pituitary necrosis syndrome; thyrohypophysial syndrome

Sheldon, Joseph H., English pediatrician, 1920–1964.
   Freeman-Sheldon syndrome—see under Freeman

Sheldon, William H., U.S. psychologist, 1898–1970.
   Sheldon constitutional theory of personality—theory used in psychology/
      psychiatry.

Shenton, Edward W.H., English radiologist, 1872–1955.
   Shenton line—a curved line formed by the top of the obturator foramen
      and the inner side of the neck of the femur, seen on an anteroposterior
      frontal x-ray of a normal hip joint.

Shepherd, Francis J., Canadian surgeon, 1851–1929.
   Shepherd fracture—a fracture of the posterior process of the talus,
      sometimes mistaken for a displacement of the os trigonum.

Sherman, H.M. O'Neill, U.S. surgeon, 1854–1921.
   Sherman block test
   Sherman bone plate
   Sherman bone screw
   Sherman knife
   Sherman plate
   Sherman plates and screws
   Sherman screw
   Sherman screwdriver
   Sherman suction tube

Sherman, Henry C., U.S. biochemist, 1875–1955.
   Sherman unit—unit of vitamin C, minimum protective dose.
   Sherman-Bourquin unit of vitamin B$_2$—equivalent to 1 to 7 μg (0.001 to
      0.007 mg) of riboflavin.
   Sherman-Munsell unit—a rat growth unit.

Sherren, James, English surgeon, 1872–1946.
   Oschner-Sherren regime
   Sherren triangle—an area of skin hyperesthesia found in acute
      appendicitis.

Sherrington, Sir Charles, English physiologist and Nobel laureate, 1857–1952.
   Liddell-Sherrington reflex—see under Liddell
   Schiff-Sherrington phenomenon—see under Schiff, Moritz

(continued)

NOTES

Sherrington *(continued)*
   Sherrington law—every dorsal spinal nerve root supplies a particular area of the skin.
   Sherrington phenomenon—after the muscles of the leg have been deprived of their motor innervation, stimulation of the sciatic nerve causes slow contraction of the muscles.

Shiga, Kiyoshi, Japanese bacteriologist, 1870–1957.
   Shigella boydii—a species found in feces of symptomatic individuals.
   Shigella dysenteriae—a species causing dysentery in humans and in monkeys. *SYN:* Shiga bacillus; Shiga-Kruse bacillus
   Shigella flexneri—a species found in the feces of symptomatic individuals and of convalescents or carriers. *SYN:* Flexner bacillus; paradysentery bacillus
   Shigella sonnei—a species causing mild dysentery and also summer diarrhea in children. *SYN:* Sonne bacillus
   Shigella—a genus of nonmotile, aerobic to facultatively anaerobic bacteria (family Enterobacteriaceae), all of whose species produce dysentery.
   Shiga bacillus—*SYN: Shigella dysenteriae*
   Shiga-Kruse bacillus—*SYN: Shigella dysenteriae*
   shigellosis—bacillary dysentery caused by bacteria of the genus *Shigella*.

Shiley, D.B., U.S. engineer, 20th century.
   Schneider-Shiley catheter
   Shiley cardioplegia system
   Shiley catheter
   Shiley catheter distention system
   Shiley cuffless fenestrated tube
   Shiley cuffless tracheostomy tube
   Shiley decannulation plug
   Shiley distention kit
   Shiley endotracheal tube
   Shiley guiding catheter
   Shiley heart valve
   Shiley Infusaid pump
   Shiley JL-4 guiding catheter
   Shiley JR-4 guiding catheter
   Shiley laryngectomy tube
   Shiley low-pressure cuffed tracheostomy tube
   Shiley MultiPro catheter
   Shiley neonatal tracheostomy tube
   Shiley oxygenator
   Shiley pediatric tracheostomy tube
   Shiley pressure-relief adapter
   Shiley sump tube
   Shiley tracheostomy tube
   Shiley valve

Shipley, Walter C., U.S. psychiatrist, *1903.
   Shipley-Hartford scale—a test of intellectual and conceptual aptitude.

Shirodkar, N.V., Indian obstetrician and gynecologist, 1900–1971.
   Shirodkar needle

Shirodkar operation—a cerclage procedure done by pursestring suturing of an incompetent cervical os with a nonabsorbent suture material.
Shirodkar probe
Shirodkar suture

Shokeir, M.K.H.
    Pena-Shokeir II syndrome—see under Pena

Shone, John D., 20th century English cardiologist.
    Shone anomaly—coarctation of the aorta, subaortic stenosis, and stenosing ring of the left atrium found in association with a parachute mitral valve.
    Shone complex—an obstructive lesion of the mitral valve complex, with left ventricular outflow obstruction and coarctation of the aorta.
    Shone syndrome—the association of obstructive lesions of the mitral valve complex, with left ventricular outflow obstruction and coarctation of the aorta.

Shope, Richard E., U.S. pathologist, 1902–1966.
    Shope fibroma—a connective tissue tumor of cottontail rabbits caused by a poxvirus of the genus *Leporipoxvirus*. *SYN:* rabbit fibroma
    Shope fibroma virus—a poxvirus of the genus *Leporipoxvirus*, closely related to vaccinia and myxoma viruses, that causes Shope fibroma. *SYN:* rabbit fibroma virus
    Shope papilloma—a papillomatous growth found in wild cottontail rabbits.
    Shope papilloma virus—a papillomavirus infecting wild cottontail rabbits.

Short, D.S.
    Short syndrome—alternating bradycardia tachycardia.

Shrapnell, Henry J., English anatomist, 1761–1841.
    Shrapnell membrane—triangular part of tympanic membrane between the malleolar folds. *SYN:* flaccid part of tympanic membrane

Shulman, Lawrence E., U.S. rheumatologist, *1919.
    Shulman syndrome—induration and edema of the connective tissues of the extremities, usually appearing following exertion. *SYN:* eosinophilic fasciitis

Shwartzman, Gregory, Russian bacteriologist in U.S., 1896–1965.
    generalized Shwartzman phenomenon—death occurs in an animal that has been injected with a primary injection of endotoxin-containing filtrate and secondary injection given intravenously 24 hours apart. *SYN:* Sanarelli phenomenon; Sanarelli-Shwartzman phenomenon
    Sanarelli-Shwartzman phenomenon—*SYN:* generalized Shwartzman phenomenon
    Shwartzman phenomenon—a rabbit injected intradermally with a small quantity of endotoxin followed by a second intravenous injection 24 hours later will develop a hemorrhagic and necrotic lesion at the site of the first injection. *SYN:* Shwartzman reaction
    Shwartzman reaction—*SYN:* Shwartzman phenomenon

NOTES

Shy, G. Milton, U.S. neurologist, 1919–1967.
Shy-Drager syndrome—a progressive disorder involving the autonomic system, characterized by hypotension, external ophthalmoplegia, iris atrophy, incontinence, anhidrosis, impotence, tremor, and muscle wasting.

Siamese twins, named for Eng and Chang (1811–1874) who were born in Siam (now Thailand).

Sibson, Francis, English anatomist, 1814–1876.
Sibson aortic vestibule—the anterosuperior portion of the left ventricle of the heart immediately below the aortic orifice. *SYN:* aortic vestibule
Sibson aponeurosis—*SYN:* suprapleural membrane
Sibson fascia—*SYN:* suprapleural membrane
Sibson groove—a groove occasionally seen on the outer side of the thorax, formed by the prominent lower border of the pectoralis major muscle.
Sibson muscle—an occasional independent muscular fasciculus between the scalenus anterior and medius, and having the same action and innervation. *SYN:* scalenus minimus muscle

Sicard, Jean Anasthase, French physician, 1872–1929.
Collet-Sicard syndrome—see under Collet

Siegert, Ferdinand, German pediatrician, 1865–1946.
Siegert sign—shortness and inward curvature of the terminal phalanges of the fifth fingers in Down syndrome.

Siegle, Emil, German otologist, 1833–1900.
Siegle otoscope—an ear speculum.

Siemens, Hermann Werner, German dermatologist, 1891–1969.
Christ-Siemens-Touraine syndrome—see under Christ

Siemerling, Ernst, German physician, 1857–1931.
Siemerling nucleus—a subdivision of the oculomotor nucleus complex.

Siggaard-Andersen, Ole, Danish clinical biochemist, *1932.
Siggaard-Andersen nomogram—a nomogram used to predict acid-base composition of blood.

Signorelli, Angelo, Italian physician, 1876–1952.
Signorelli sign—tenderness on pressure in the glenoid fossa in front of the mastoid process in meningitis.

Silber, Robert H., U.S. biochemist, *1915.
Porter-Silber chromogens—see under Porter, Curt
Porter-Silber chromogens test—see under Porter, Curt
Porter-Silber reaction—see under Porter, Curt

Silver, Henry K., U.S. pediatrician, *1918.
Russell-Silver dwarfism—*SYN:* Silver-Russell syndrome
Silver-Russell dwarfism—*SYN:* Silver-Russell syndrome
Silver-Russell syndrome—a disorder characterized by low birth weight, late closure of the anterior fontanel, bilateral bodily asymmetry, clinodactyly of the fifth fingers, triangular facies, and carp mouth. *SYN:* Silver-Russell dwarfism; Russell-Silver dwarfism

Silverman, Leslie, U.S. engineer, 1914–1966.
Silverman-Lilly pneumotachograph—measures flow in terms of the

S

proportional pressure drop across a resistance consisting of a very fine mesh screen.

Silverman, William A., 20th century U.S. pediatrician.
  Caffey-Silverman syndrome—*SYN:* Caffey syndrome
  Silverman score

Silverskiöld, Nils G., Swedish orthopedist, 1888–1957.
  Silverskiöld syndrome—osteochondrodystrophy, with only slight vertebral changes but with shortened and curved long bones of the extremities.

Silvester, Henry Robert, English physician, 1829–1908.
  Silvester method—an artificial respiration technique.

Simmonds, Franklin Adin, English orthopedic surgeon.
  Simmonds test—tests the Achilles tendon.

Simmonds, Morris, German physician, 1855–1925.
  Simmonds disease—anterior pituitary insufficiency due to trauma, vascular lesions, or tumors. *SYN:* hypophysial cachexia; pituitary cachexia; Simmonds syndrome
  Simmonds syndrome—*SYN:* Simmonds disease

Simmons, J.S., U.S. bacteriologist, 1890–1954.
  Simmons citrate medium—a diagnostic medium used in the differentiation of species of Enterobacteriaceae, based on their ability to utilize sodium citrate as the sole source of carbon.

Simon, Charles E., U.S. physician, 1866–1927.
  Simon sign—the movements of the diaphragm that are dissociated from those of the thorax in incipient meningitis in children.

Simon, Gustav, German surgeon, 1824–1876.
  Simon incision
  Simon perineorrhaphy
  Simon position—a position for vaginal examination.
  Simon speculum

Simon, Théodore, French physician, 1873–1961.
  Binet-Simon scale—see under Binet

Simonart, Pierre J.C., Belgian obstetrician, 1817–1847.
  Simonart bands—weblike band of tissue partially filling the gap between the medial and lateral portions of a cleft lip.
  Simonart ligaments—*SYN:* Simonart threads
  Simonart threads—strands of amniotic tissue adherent to the embryo or fetus. *SYN:* amniotic bands; Simonart ligaments

Simons, Arthur, German physician, *1877.
  Simons disease—*SYN:* Barraquer disease

Simpson, J.L., U.S. physician.
  Simpson syndrome—X-linked dysmorphia syndrome. *SYN:* bulldog syndrome

NOTES

Simpson, Sir James Y., Scottish obstetrician, 1811–1870.
    Simpson forceps—obstetrical forceps.
    Simpson uterine sound—a slender flexible metal rod.

Sims, J. Marion, U.S. gynecologist, 1813–1883.
    Sims anoscope
    Sims cannula
    Sims curet
    Sims dilator
    Sims double-ended retractor
    Sims double-ended speculum
    Sims knife
    Sims needle
    Sims plug
    Sims position—a position to facilitate a vaginal examination. *SYN:* English position; lateral recumbent position; semiprone position
    Sims probe
    Sims proctoscope
    Sims retractor
    Sims scissors
    Sims sound
    Sims speculum
    Sims suction tip
    Sims suture
    Sims tenaculum
    Sims uterine sound—a slender flexible sound.
    Sims vaginal decompressor
    Sims vaginal speculum

Singleton, Edward B., U.S. radiologist.
    Singleton-Merten syndrome—calcification of the aortic arch, with enlargement of the heart.

Sipple, John H., U.S. physician, *1930.
    Sipple syndrome—pheochromocytoma, medullary carcinoma of the thyroid, and neural tumors. *SYN:* multiple endocrine neoplasia, type 2

Sippy, Bertram W., U.S. physician, 1866–1924.
    sippy diet—a diet formerly used in the initial stages of treatment of peptic ulcer.

Siris, Evelyn, U.S. radiologist, *1914.
    Coffin-Siris syndrome—see under Coffin

Sister Mary Joseph Dempsey, Superintendent at Saint Mary's hospital, Mayo Clinic, and surgical assistant to Dr. William Mayo, c. 1928, 1856–1929.
    Sister Joseph nodule—malignant intraabdominal neoplasm metastatic to the umbilicus. *SYN:* Sister Mary Joseph nodule
    Sister Mary Joseph nodule—*SYN:* Sister Joseph nodule

Sistrunk, Walter Ellis, U.S. surgeon, 1880–1933.
    Sistrunk band retractor
    Sistrunk dissecting scissors
    Sistrunk double-ended retractor
    Sistrunk operation—excision of the thyroglossal cyst and duct, including

the midportion of the hyoid bone through or near which the duct traverses.
Sistrunk procedure
Sistrunk retractor
Sistrunk scissors

Siwe, Sture A., Swedish pediatrician, 1897–1966.
Letterer-Siwe disease—see under Letterer

Sjögren, Henrik C., Swedish ophthalmologist, *1899.
Gougerot-Sjögren disease—*SYN:* Sjögren syndrome
Sjögren disease—*SYN:* Sjögren syndrome
Sjögren syndrome—keratoconjunctivitis sicca, dryness of mucous membranes, telangiectasias or purpuric spots on the face, and bilateral parotid enlargement, seen in menopausal women. *SYN:* Gougerot-Sjögren disease; Sjögren disease; sicca syndrome

Sjögren, Torsten, Swedish physician, 1859–1939.
Marinesco-Sjögren-Garland syndrome—see under Marinesco
Sjögren syndrome—*SYN:* Marinesco-Sjögren syndrome
Sjögren-Larsson syndrome—congenital ichthyosis in association with oligophrenia and spastic paraplegia.
Torsten Sjögren syndrome—*SYN:* Marinesco-Sjögren-Garland syndrome
Torsten syndrome—*SYN:* Marinesco-Sjögren syndrome

Sjöqvist, O., Swedish neurosurgeon, 1901–1954.
Sjöqvist tractotomy—division of the descending fibers of the trigeminal tract in the medulla. *SYN:* trigeminal tractotomy

Skene, Alexander J.C., U.S. gynecologist, 1838–1900.
ducts of Skene glands—inconstant ducts along the side of the female urethra that convey the mucoid secretion of Skene glands to the vestibule. *SYN:* paraurethral ducts
Skene glands—numerous mucous glands in the wall of the female urethra. *SYN:* glands of the female urethra
Skene tubules—the embryonic urethral glands that are the female homologue of the prostate.

Skillern, Penn Gaskell, U.S. surgeon, *1882.
Skillern cannula
Skillern forceps
Skillern fracture—fracture of distal radius with greenstick fracture of neighboring portion of ulna.
Skillern phimosis forceps
Skillern probe
Skillern punch
Skillern sinus curet
Skillern sphenoid cannula
Skillern sphenoid probe

NOTES

Skinner, Burrhus F., U.S. psychologist, 1904–1990.
> **Skinner box**—an experimental apparatus in which an animal presses a lever to obtain a reward or receive punishment.
> **skinnerian conditioning**—an experimenter waits for the target response to be conditioned to occur spontaneously, immediately after which the organism is given a reinforcer reward. *Syn:* operant conditioning

Sklowsky, E.L., 20th century German physician.
> **Sklowsky symptom**—the rupture of a varicella vesicle on very slight pressure with the finger.

Skoda, Joseph, Bohemian clinician in Vienna, 1805–1881.
> **Skoda rale**—a rale in a bronchus heard through an area of consolidated tissue in pneumonia.
> **Skoda sign**—*Syn:* skodaic resonance
> **Skoda tympany**—*Syn:* skodaic resonance
> **skodaic resonance**—a peculiar, high-pitched sound, less musical than that obtained over a cavity, elicited by percussion just above the level of a pleuritic effusion. *Syn:* Skoda sign; Skoda tympany

Slater, Robert James, Canadian-U.S. pediatrician, *1923.
> **Bearn-Kunkel-Slater syndrome**—*Syn:* Bearn-Kunkel syndrome

Sluder, Greenfield, U.S. laryngologist, 1865–1928.
> **Sluder guillotine tonsillectomy**

Slyke, Donald D. Van. See under Van Slyke.

Smellie, William, English obstetrician, 1697–1763.
> **Smellie scissors**—obsolete term for lance-pointed shears with external cutting edges, used for fetal craniotomy.

Smith, David W., U.S. pediatrician, 1926–1981.
> **Smith-Lemli-Opitz syndrome**—mental retardation, small stature, anteverted nostrils, ptosis, male genital anomalies, and syndactyly of the second and third toes.

Smith, G.W., U.S. neurosurgeon, 1917–1964.
> **Smith aneurysmal clip**
> **Smith-Robinson anterior approach**
> **Smith-Robinson anterior cervical diskectomy**
> **Smith-Robinson anterior fusion**
> **Smith-Robinson cervical disk approach**
> **Smith-Robinson cervical fusion**
> **Smith-Robinson interbody arthrodesis**
> **Smith-Robinson interbody fusion**
> **Smith-Robinson operation**—interbody spinal fusion through an anterior cervical approach.
> **Smith-Robinson technique**

Smith, Hamilton O., joint winner of 1978 Nobel Prize for work related to restriction enzymes.

Smith, Henry, Irish born English military surgeon in India, 1862–1948.
> **Smith cataract extraction**
> **Smith cataract knife**
> **Smith eye speculum**

Smith hook
Smith intraocular implant lens
Smith lens
Smith lens expressor
Smith lid expressor
Smith lid retracting hook
Smith operation—*Syn:* Smith-Indian operation
Smith orbital floor implant
Smith-Indian operation—a surgical technique for removal of cataract within the capsule. *Syn:* Smith operation
Smith-Leiske cross-action intraocular lens forceps

Smith, M.J.V., 20th century U.S. urologist.
Smith pessary

Smith, Robert W., Irish surgeon, 1807–1873.
Smith fracture—fracture of the radius near its lower articular surface, with displacement of the fragment toward the volar aspect.

Smith, Sir Thomas, English orthopedic surgeon, 1833–1909.
Tom Smith arthritis—a septic arthritic condition that occurs in infancy.

Smith, Theobald, U.S. pathologist, 1859–1934.
Theobald Smith phenomenon—guinea pigs that had survived use for diphtheria antitoxin standardization were highly susceptible to subsequent inoculation of horse serum.

Smith, William R., 20th century U.S. physician.
Smith-Riley syndrome—multiple hemangiomas, macrocephaly, and blurred optic disks.

Smith-Petersen, Marius N., U.S. surgeon, 1886–1953.
Smith ankle prosthesis
Smith bone clamp
Smith clamp
Smith dislocation
Smith drill
Smith flexor pollicis longus abductor plasty
Smith fracture
Smith physical capacities evaluation
Smith prosthesis
Smith scissors
Smith STA-peg
Smith technique
Smith-Petersen acromioplasty
Smith-Petersen approach
Smith-Petersen cannulated nail
Smith-Petersen capsule retractor
Smith-Petersen cervical fusion

(continued)

NOTES

Smith-Petersen *(continued)*
    Smith-Petersen chisel
    Smith-Petersen cup
    Smith-Petersen cup arthroplasty
    Smith-Petersen curved gouge
    Smith-Petersen curved osteotome
    Smith-Petersen fracture pin
    Smith-Petersen hammer
    Smith-Petersen hemiarthroplasty
    Smith-Petersen hip cup prosthesis
    Smith-Petersen incision
    Smith-Petersen laminectomy rongeur
    Smith-Petersen mallet
    Smith-Petersen nail—a flanged nail for pinning a fracture of the neck of the femur.
    Smith-Petersen nail with Lloyd adapter
    Smith-Petersen osteotome
    Smith-Petersen osteotomy
    Smith-Petersen pin
    Smith-Petersen plate
    Smith-Petersen prosthesis
    Smith-Petersen reamer
    Smith-Petersen rongeur
    Smith-Petersen sacroiliac joint fusion
    Smith-Petersen spatula
    Smith-Petersen straight gouge
    Smith-Petersen straight osteotome
    Smith-Petersen synovectomy
    Smith-Petersen technique
    Smith-Petersen transarticular nail
    Smith-Petersen tucker

Sneddon, Ian B., English dermatologist, *1923.
    Sneddon syndrome—a cerebral arteriopathy of unknown etiology, characterized by noninflammatory intimal hyperplasia of medium-size vessels.
    Sneddon-Wilkinson disease—a chronic pruritic annular eruption of sterile vesicles and pustules beneath the stratum corneum. *SYN:* subcorneal pustular dermatosis

Snell, George D., joint winner of 1980 Nobel Prize for work related to cell structures and regulation of immunological reactions.

Snell, Simeon, English ophthalmologist, 1851–1909.
    Snell law—for two given media, the sine of the angle of incidence bears a constant relation to the sine of the angle of refraction. *SYN:* law of refraction

Snellen, Hermann, Dutch ophthalmologist, 1834–1908.
    Snellen chart—used to test visual acuity.
    Snellen conventional reform implant
    Snellen entropion forceps
    Snellen eye implant

Snellen letters
Snellen operation
Snellen reform eye
Snellen sign—bruit heard on auscultation over the eye in a patient with Graves disease.
Snellen soft contact lens
Snellen suture
Snellen test types—square black symbols employed in testing the acuity of distant vision.
Snellen vectis

Snyder, Marshall L., U.S. microbiologist, *1907.
Snyder test—a colorimetric test for determining dental caries activity or susceptibility. *Syn:* colorimetric caries susceptibility test

Soave, F., 20th century Italian pediatric surgeon.
Soave operation—endorectal pull-through for treatment of congenital megacolon.

Soemmerring, Samuel Thomas von, German anatomist, 1755–1830.
ring of Soemmerring—a mass of lenticular fibers enclosed between the anterior and posterior portion of the lenticular capsule, leaving the pupillary area relatively free.
Soemmerring ganglion—a large cell mass extending forward over the dorsal surface of the crus cerebri from the rostral border of the pons into the subthalamic region. *Syn:* substantia nigra
Soemmerring ligament—small fibers attaching the lacrimal gland to the periorbita.
Soemmerring muscle—a fasciculus occasionally passing from the thyrohyoid muscle to the isthmus of the thyroid gland. *Syn:* levator muscle of thyroid gland
Soemmerring spot—an oval area of the sensory retina at the center of which is the central fovea, which contains only retinal cones. *Syn:* macula retinae

Soffer, Louis J., U.S. internist, *1904.
Sohval-Soffer syndrome—see under Sohval

Sohval, Arthur R., U.S. internist, 1904–1985.
Sohval-Soffer syndrome—hypogonadism, gynecomastia, skeletal anomalies, and mental retardation, without chromosomal abnormality.

Somogyi, Michael, U.S. biochemist, 1883–1971.
Somogyi effect—in diabetes, a rebound phenomenon of reactive hyperglycemia in response to a preceding period of relative hypoglycemia.
Somogyi method
Somogyi unit—a measure of the level of activity of amylase in blood serum.

NOTES

Sondermann, R., 20th century German ophthalmologist.
Sondermann canal—a blind outpouching of Schlemm canal, extending toward the anterior chamber of the eye.

Sonne, Carl, Danish bacteriologist, 1882–1948.
Sonne bacillus—*Syn: Shigella sonnei*
Sonne dysentery—dysentery due to infection by *Shigella sonnei.*

Sörensen, Sören P.L., Danish chemist, 1868–1939.
Sörensen scale—the negative logarithm of the hydrogen ion concentration, used as a scale for expressing acidity and alkalinity. *Syn:* pH scale

Soret, Charles, French radiologist, 1854–1931.
Soret band—the absorption band of all porphyrins at about 400 nm.
Soret phenomenon—in a solution kept in a long, upright tube at room temperature, the upper part being the warmer, is also the more concentrated.

Sorsby, Arnold, English ophthalmologist, 1900–1980.
Sorsby macular degeneration—hereditary macular degeneration that occurs during the fifth decade of life. *Syn:* familial pseudoinflammatory macular degeneration
Sorsby syndrome—congenital macular coloboma and apical dystrophy of the extremities.

Sotos, Juan F., U.S. pediatrician, *1927.
Sotos syndrome—cerebral gigantism and generalized large muscles in childhood, with mental retardation and defective coordination.

Sottas, Jules, French neurologist, 1866–1943.
Dejerine-Sottas disease—see under Dejerine
Dejerine-Sottas neuropathy—*Syn:* Dejerine-Sottas disease

Soulier, Jean Pierre, French hematologist, *1915.
Bernard-Soulier syndrome—see under Bernard, Jean

Southern, M.E., 20th century English biologist.
Southern blot analysis—a procedure to separate and identify DNA sequences.

Southey, Reginald, English physician, 1835–1899.
Southey tubes—obsolete cannulas of small caliber thrust by a trocar into the subcutaneous tissues to drain the fluid of anasarca.

Souttar, Sir Henry Sessions, English surgeon, 1875–1964.
Souttar tube

Spallanzani, Lazaro, Italian priest and scientist, 1729–1799.
Spallanzani law—the younger the individual, the greater is the regenerative power of its cells.

Spatz, Hugo, German neurologist and psychiatrist, 1888–1969.
Hallervorden-Spatz disease—*Syn:* Hallervorden-Spatz syndrome
Hallervorden-Spatz syndrome—see under Hallervorden

Spee, Ferdinand Graf von, German embryologist, 1855–1937.
curve of Spee—the anatomic curvature of the mandibular occlusal plane. *Syn:* von Spee curve

Spee embryo
von Spee curve—*SYN:* curve of Spee

Spencer Wells, Sir Thomas, English surgeon, 1818–1897.
Spencer Wells forceps

Spens, Thomas, Scottish physician, 1764–1842.
Spens syndrome—*SYN:* Adams-Stokes syndrome

Sperry, Roger Wolcott, U.S. researcher and 1981 Nobel Prize winner for medicine and physiology, *1994.

Spiegelberg, Otto, German gynecologist, 1830–1881.
Spiegelberg criteria—for differentiating ovarian from other ectopic pregnancies.

Spiegler, Eduard, Austrian dermatologist, 1860–1908.
Spiegler-Fendt pseudolymphoma—a soft red to violaceous skin nodule often involving the head, caused by dense infiltration of the dermis by lymphocytes and histiocytes. *SYN:* benign lymphocytoma cutis; Spiegler-Fendt sarcoid
Spiegler-Fendt sarcoid—*SYN:* Spiegler-Fendt pseudolymphoma

Spielmeyer, Walter, German neurologist, 1879–1935.
Spielmeyer acute swelling—a form of degeneration of nerve cells in which the cell body and its processes swell and stain palely and diffusely.
Spielmeyer-Stock disease—retinal atrophy in amaurotic familial idiocy.
Spielmeyer-Vogt disease—*SYN:* Batten disease
Vogt-Spielmeyer disease—*SYN:* Batten disease

Spigelius, Adrian (van der Spieghel), Flemish anatomist in Padua, 1578–1625.
spigelian hernia—abdominal hernia through the semilunar line. *SYN:* lateral ventral hernia
Spigelius line—the slight groove in the external abdominal wall parallel to the lateral edge of the rectus sheath. *SYN:* linea semilunaris
Spigelius lobe—a small lobe of the liver situated posteriorly between the sulcus for the vena cava and the fissure for the ligamentum venosum. *SYN:* lobus caudatus

Spiller, William G., U.S. neurologist, 1864–1940.
Frazier-Spiller operation—see under Frazier

Spinelli, Pier G., Italian gynecologist, 1862–1929.
Spinelli operation—an operation splitting the anterior wall of the prolapsed uterus and reversing the organ preliminary to reduction.

Spitz, Sophie, U.S. pathologist, *1910.
Spitz nevus—a benign, slightly pigmented or red superficial small skin tumor. *SYN:* epithelioid cell nevus; spindle cell nevus

Spitzer, Alexander, Austrian anatomist, 1868–1943.
Spitzer theory—an interpretation of the partitioning of the heart of mammalian embryos, primarily on the basis of recapitulations of the adult structural pattern of lower forms.

NOTES

Spitzka, Edward C., U.S. neurologist, 1852–1914.
column of Spitzka-Lissauer—*Syn:* Spitzka marginal tract
Spitzka marginal tract—a longitudinal bundle of thin, unmyelinated and poorly myelinated fibers capping the apex of the posterior horn of the spinal gray matter. *Syn:* dorsolateral fasciculus; Spitzka marginal zone; column of Spitzka-Lissauer
Spitzka marginal zone—*Syn:* Spitzka marginal tract
Spitzka nucleus—*Syn:* Perlia nucleus

Spitzy, Hans, Austrian orthopedic surgeon, 1872–1956.
Spitzy button—a device used in correction of postural defect. *Syn:* Spitzy spike
Spitzy spike—*Syn:* Spitzy button

Spix, Johann B., German anatomist, 1781–1826.
Spix spine—a pointed tongue of bone overlapping the mandibular foramen, giving attachment to the sphenomandibular ligament. *Syn:* lingula of mandible

Splendore, A., 20th century Italian physician.
Lutz-Splendore-Almeida disease—see under Lutz
Splendore-Hoeppli phenomenon—radiating or annular eosinophilic deposits of host-derived materials and possibly of parasite antigens, which form around fungi, helminths, or bacterial colonies in tissue.

Sprengel, Otto G.K., German surgeon, 1852–1915.
Sprengel anomaly
Sprengel deformity—*Syn:* Sprengel shoulder
Sprengel shoulder—congenital elevation of the scapula. *Syn:* Sprengel syndrome; Sprengel deformity
Sprengel syndrome—*Syn:* Sprengel shoulder

Spurway, John, 19th century English physician.
Spurway syndrome—osteogenesis imperfecta.

Squire, Truman Hoffman, U.S. surgeon, 1823–1899.
Squire catheter
Squire sign

Ssabanejew, Ivan, 19th century Russian surgeon.
Ssabanejew-Frank operation—a method of performing gastrostomy.

St. Clair, St. Clare of Assisi, patron saint of eyes, television, telegraph, and telephone.
St. Clair forceps

St. Helenia's Island, site where first cases were observed.
St. Helenia cellulitis syndrome—intense burning in legs, headache and rigor accompany.

St. Jude, patron saint of desperate situations and hospitals.
St. Jude bileaflet prosthetic valve
St. Jude composite valve graft
St. Jude mitral valve prosthesis
St. Jude valve

S

St. Louis, Missouri, where first observed in 1933.
  St. Louis syndrome—encephalitis. *Syn:* St. Louis encephalitis

St. Luke, patron saint of physicians, surgeons, artists, sculptors, painters, notaries, glass workers, butchers, and brewers.
  St. Luke retractor
  St. Luke rongeuer

St. Mark, patron saint of notaries, Egypt, and Venice, Italy.
  St. Mark clamp
  St. Mark excision
  St. Mark incision

St. Vincent, patron saint of charitable organizations.
  St. Vincent forceps
  St. Vincent tube clamp

Stader, Otto, U.S. veterinary surgeon, *1894.
  Stader pin
  Stader pin guide
  Stader splint—a splint used primarily in veterinary medicine.

Staderini, Rutilio, 19th century Italian neuroanatomist.
  Staderini nucleus—a small collection of nerve cells in the medulla oblongata lying lateral to the hypoglossal nucleus. *Syn:* intercalated nucleus

Stafne, Edward C., U.S. oral pathologist, *1894.
  Stafne bone cyst—an indentation on the lingual surface of the mandible within which a portion of the submandibular gland lies. *Syn:* lingual salivary gland depression

Stahl, Friedrich K., German physician, 1811–1873.
  Stahl ear—a deformed external ear regarded as a stigma of degenerate constitution.

Stähli, Jean, Swiss ophthalmologist, *1890.
  Hudson-Stähli line—see under Hudson, Arthur

Stanger, J., German tanner.
  Stanger bath—a hydrogalvanic bath.

Stanley, Edward, English surgeon, 1793–1862.
  Stanley cervical ligaments—fibers of the capsule of the hip joint reflected onto the neck of the femur.

Stannius, Herman F., German biologist, 1808–1883.
  Stannius ligature

Stargardt, Karl, German ophthalmologist, 1875–1927.
  Stargardt disease—juvenile macular degeneration. *Syn:* Stargardt syndrome
  Stargardt syndrome—*Syn:* Stargardt disease

NOTES

Starling, Ernest H., English physiologist, 1866–1927.
>   **Frank-Starling curve**—*Syn:* Starling curve
>   **Starling curve**—a graph in which cardiac output or stroke volume is plotted against mean atrial or ventricular end-diastolic pressure. *Syn:* Frank-Starling curve
>   **Starling equilibrium**
>   **Starling hypothesis**
>   **Starling law**—the energy liberated by the heart when it contracts is a function of the length of its muscle fibers at the end of diastole. *Syn:* law of the heart
>   **Starling reflex**—tapping the volar surfaces of the fingers causes flexion.

Starr, Albert, U.S. physician, *1926.
>   **Starr ball heart prosthesis**
>   **Starr ball heart valve**
>   **Starr fixation forceps**
>   **Starr forceps**
>   **Starr valve**—*Syn:* Starr-Edwards valve
>   **Starr-Edwards aortic valve prosthesis**
>   **Starr-Edwards ball valve prosthesis**
>   **Starr-Edwards ball-cage valve**
>   **Starr-Edwards disk valve prosthesis**
>   **Starr-Edwards heart valve**
>   **Starr-Edwards hermetically sealed pacemaker**
>   **Starr-Edwards mitral prosthesis**
>   **Starr-Edwards pacemaker**
>   **Starr-Edwards prosthesis**
>   **Starr-Edwards prosthetic aortic valve**
>   **Starr-Edwards prosthetic mitral valve**
>   **Starr-Edwards Silastic valve**
>   **Starr-Edwards silicone rubber ball valve**
>   **Starr-Edwards valve**—a cage and ball artificial cardiac valve with high reliability and durability, first used to replace the mitral valve. *Syn:* Starr valve

Stas, Jean-Servais, Belgian chemist, 1813–1891.
>   **Stas-Otto method**—a method of extraction of alkaloids from plants and animal bodies.

Staub, Hans, Swiss internist, 1890–1967.
>   **Staub-Traugott effect**—in normal persons, a drop in blood glucose which follows a second oral dose of glucose given 30 minutes or so after the first. *Syn:* Staub-Traugott phenomenon
>   **Staub-Traugott phenomenon**—*Syn:* Staub-Traugott effect

Stearns, A. Warren, U.S. physician, 1885–1959.
>   **Stearns alcoholic amentia**—a temporary alcoholic mental disorder resembling delirium tremens but lasting for a longer time and showing a greater degree of amnesia and other mental defects.

Steele, John C., 20th century Canadian neurologist.
>   **Steele-Richardson-Olszewski disease**—*Syn:* Steele-Richardson-Olszewski syndrome
>   **Steele-Richardson-Olszewski syndrome**—a progressive neurologic disorder

characterized by a supranuclear paralysis of vertical gaze, retraction of eyelids, exophoria under cover, dysarthria, and dementia. *SYN:* progressive supranuclear palsy; Steele-Richardson-Olszewski disease

Steell, Graham, English physician, 1851–1942.
 Graham Steell murmur—an early diastolic murmur of pulmonic insufficiency secondary to pulmonary hypertension. *SYN:* Steell murmur
 Steell murmur—*SYN:* Graham Steell murmur

Steenbock, Harry, U.S. physiologist and chemist, 1886–1967.
 Steenbock unit—a unit of vitamin D.

Steidele, Raphael J., 18th century Austrian physician.
 Steidele complex—*SYN:* Steidele syndrome
 Steidele syndrome—absence of the aortic arch. *SYN:* Steidele complex

Stein, Irving F., U.S. gynecologist, *1887.
 Stein-Leventhal syndrome—a condition commonly characterized by hirsutism, obesity, menstrual abnormalities, infertility, and enlarged ovaries. *SYN:* polycystic ovary syndrome

Stein, Stanislav A.F. von, Russian otologist, *1855.
 Stein test—in cases of labyrinthine disease the patient is unable to stand or to hop on one foot with his/her eyes shut.

Steinberg, I.
 Steinberg thumb sign—in Marfan syndrome, when the thumb is held across the palm of the same hand it projects well beyond the ulnar surface of the hand.

Steinbrinck, W., 20th century Germany physician.
 Chédiak-Steinbrinck-Higashi anomaly—*SYN:* Chédiak-Steinbrinck-Higashi syndrome
 Chédiak-Steinbrinck-Higashi syndrome—see under Chédiak

Steindler, Arthur, U.S. orthopedic surgeon, 1878–1959.
 Steindler arthrodesis
 Steindler effect
 Steindler elbow arthrodesis
 Steindler flexorplasty
 Steindler matrixectomy
 Steindler operation
 Steindler procedure
 Steindler release
 Steindler stripping
 Steindler technique
 Steindler wrist fusion

Steinert, Hans, German physician, *1875.
 Steinert disease—a chronic, slowly progressing disease marked by atrophy
(continued)

NOTES

457

Steinert *(continued)*
of the muscles, failing vision, lenticular opacities, ptosis, slurred speech, and general muscular weakness. *SYN:* myotonic dystrophy
Steinert myotonic dystrophy
Steinert syndrome

Steinhert, var. of Steinert

Steinmann, Fritz, Swiss surgeon, 1872–1932.
Steinmann calibrated pin
Steinmann extension
Steinmann fixation pin
Steinmann holder
Steinmann nail
Steinmann pin—a pin that is used to transfix bone for traction or fixation.
Steinmann pin chuck
Steinmann pin fixation
Steinmann pin with ball bearing
Steinmann pin with Crowe pilot point
Steinmann pin with pin chuck
Steinmann test
Steinmann traction
Steinmann tractor

Stellwag, Carl von C., Austrian ophthalmologist, 1823–1904.
Stellwag sign—infrequent and incomplete blinking in Graves disease.

Stender, Wilhelm P., 19th century German manufacturer of scientific apparatus.
Stender dish—a flat shallow vessel used in staining sections.

Stensen, Niels, Danish anatomist, 1638–1686.
Stensen canal
Stensen duct—*SYN:* parotid duct
Stensen experiment—an experiment on an animal in which the blood supply is cut off from the lumbar region of the spine.
Stensen foramen—*SYN:* incisive foramen
Stensen plexus—the parotid duct's venous structure.
Stensen veins—*SYN:* vortex veins

Stent, C., English dentist, d. 1901.
Stent graft—an inlay skin graft, or a skin graft held in place by a tie-over dressing.

Stern, Heinrich, U.S. physician, 1868–1918.
Stern posture—a supine position, with the head extended and lowered over the end of the table.

Sternberg, George M., U.S. bacteriologist, 1838–1915.
Reed-Sternberg cells—see under Reed, Dorothy
Sternberg cells—*SYN:* Reed-Sternberg cells
Sternberg-Reed cells—*SYN:* Reed-Sternberg cells

Stevens, Albert M., U.S. pediatrician, 1884–1945.
Stevens-Johnson syndrome—a bullous form of erythema multiforme. *SYN:* erythema multiforme exudativum; ectodermosis erosiva pluriorificialis; erythema multiforme bullosum; erythema multiforme major

Stevens, Stanley Smith, U.S. psychophysicist, 1906–1973.
  Stevens power law—a logarithm used in psychology/psychiatry.

Stewart, Fred Waldorf, U.S. physician, *1894.
  Stewart-Treves syndrome—angiosarcoma arising in arms, affected by postmastectomy lymphedema.

Stewart, George N., Canadian-U.S. scientist, 1860–1930.
  Stewart test—estimation (by means of a calorimeter) of the amount of collateral circulation in case of an aneurysm of the main artery of a limb.
  Stewart-Hamilton method—a method for measuring cardiac output. *SYN:* Hamilton-Stewart method; indicator dilution method; Hamilton-Stewart formula

Stewart, James Purves, English physician, 1869–1949.
  Stewart-Holmes sign—in cerebellar disease, the inability to check a movement when passive resistance is suddenly released. *SYN:* rebound phenomenon

Stewart, R.M., 20th century English neurologist.
  Stewart-Morel syndrome—*SYN:* Morgagni syndrome

Sticker, Georg, German physician, 1860–1960.
  Sticker disease—a mild infectious exanthema of childhood caused by Parvovirus B19. *SYN:* erythema infectiosum

Stickler, Gunnar B., 20th century U.S. physician.
  Stickler syndrome—*SYN:* hereditary progressive arthro-ophthalmopathy

Stieda, Alfred, German surgeon, 1869–1945.
  Pellegrini-Stieda disease—*SYN:* Pellegrini disease
  Stieda disease
  Stieda fracture

Stieda, Ludwig, German anatomist, 1837–1918.
  Stieda process—a projection of the talus bearing medial and lateral tubercles. *SYN:* posterior process of talus

Stierlin, Eduard, German surgeon, 1878–1919.
  Stierlin sign—repeated emptying of the cecum seen radiographically.

Stiles, Walter, English physicist, *1901.
  Stiles-Crawford effect—light that enters through the center of the pupil produces a greater visual effect than light that enters obliquely.

Still, Sir George F., English physician, 1868–1941.
  Still disease—a form of juvenile chronic arthritis.
  Still murmur—an innocent musical murmur.
  Still-Chauffard syndrome—*SYN:* Chauffard syndrome

Stiller, Berthod, Hungarian physician, 1837–1922.
  Stiller rib—*SYN:* Stiller sign
  Stiller sign—floating tenth rib. *SYN:* Stiller rib; costal stigma

NOTES

Stilling, Benedict, German anatomist, 1810–1879.
  Stilling canal—a minute canal running through the vitreous from the discus nervi optici to the lens. *Syn:* hyaloid canal
  Stilling column—*Syn:* Stilling nucleus
  Stilling gelatinous substance—the central gray matter of the spinal cord surrounding the central canal. *Syn:* central and lateral intermediate substance
  Stilling nucleus—a column of large neurons located in the base of the posterior gray column of the spinal cord, extending from the first thoracic through the second lumbar segment. *Syn:* thoracic nucleus; Stilling column
  Stilling raphe—the transverse interdigitations of fiber bundles across the anterior median fissure of the medulla oblongata at the decussation of the pyramidal tracts.

Stilling, Jakob, German ophthalmologist, 1842–1915.
  Stilling color table—*Syn:* Reuss color table
  Stilling test—test used in ophthalmology.

Stirling, William, English histologist and physiologist, 1851–1932.
  Stirling modification of Gram stain—a stable aniline-crystal violet stain.

Stock, Wolfgang, German ophthalmologist, 1874–1956.
  Spielmeyer-Stock disease—see under Spielmeyer
  Stock eye trephine
  Stock operation

Stocker, Frederick William, U.S. ophthalmologist, 1893–1974.
  Stocker cyclodiathermy needle
  Stocker line—a fine line of pigment in the corneal epithelium near the head of a pterygium.
  Stocker operation

Stoerk, Karl, Austrian laryngologist, 1832–1899.
  Stoerk blennorrhea—chronic catarrh of the upper air passages with hypertrophy of the mucous membrane and submucosa.

Stoffel, Adolf, German orthopedic surgeon, 1880–1937.
  Stoffel operation—division of certain motor nerves for the relief of spastic paralysis.

Stokes, Sir George Gabriel, English physicist and mathematician, 1819–1903.
  stoke—A unit of kinematic viscosity.
  Stokes law—a relationship of the rate of fall of a small sphere in a viscous fluid.

Stokes, Sir William, Irish surgeon, 1839–1900.
  Gritti-Stokes amputation—see under Gritti
  Stokes amputation—a modification of the Gritti-Stokes amputation so that the line of section of the femur is slightly higher.

Stokes, William, Irish physician, 1804–1878.
  Adams-Stokes disease—*Syn:* Adams-Stokes syndrome
  Adams-Stokes syncope—see under Adams, Robert
  Cheyne-Stokes breathing—*Syn:* Cheyne-Stokes respiration
  Cheyne-Stokes psychosis—see under Cheyne

Cheyne-Stokes respiration—see under Cheyne
Morgagni-Adams-Stokes syndrome—*SYN:* Adams-Stokes syndrome
Stokes law—a muscle lying above an inflamed mucous or serous
  membrane is frequently the seat of paralysis.
Stokes-Adams disease—*SYN:* Adams-Stokes syndrome
Stokes-Adams syndrome—*SYN:* Adams-Stokes syndrome

Stookey, Byron, U.S. neurosurgeon, 1887–1966.
  Queckenstedt-Stookey test—see under Queckenstedt
  Stookey cranial rongeur
  Stookey reflex
  Stookey retractor
  Stookey-Scarff operation—an operation to establish an opening from the
  third ventricle to the prechiasmal and interpeduncular cisterns. *SYN:* third
  ventriculostomy

Strandberg, James Victor., Swedish dermatologist, *1883.
  Grönblad-Strandberg syndrome—see under Grönblad

Strassburg, Gustav A., German physiologist, *1848.
  Strassburg test—a test for bile in the urine.

Strassman, Paul F., German gynecologist, 1866–1938.
  Strassman phenomenon—obsolete term for failure of placental
  detachment in the third stage of labor.

Stratton, George Malcolm, U.S. psychologist, 1865–1957.
  Stratton experiment—visual and tactual motor study technique.

Straus, Isidore, French physician, 1845–1896.
  Straus reaction—a diagnostic test for glanders.
  Straus sign—in facial paralysis, if an injection of pilocarpine is followed by
  sweating on the affected side later than on the other, the lesion is
  peripheral.

Strauss, Alfred A., psychologist.
  Strauss syndrome—behavioral characteristics of brain-injured children.

Strauss, Lotte, U.S. pathologist, *1913.
  Churg-Strauss syndrome—see under Churg

Streeter, George L., U.S. embryologist, 1873–1948.
  Streeter bands—strands of amniotic tissue adherent to the embryo or
  fetus. *SYN:* amniotic bands
  Streeter developmental horizon(s)—a term borrowed from geology and
  archeology by Streeter to define 23 developmental stages in young
  human embryos, from fertilization through the first 2 months.
  Streeter dysplasia

Streiff, Enrico Bernard, Swiss ophthalmologist, *1908.
  Hallermann-Streiff syndrome—see under Hallermann
  Hallermann-Streiff-François syndrome—*SYN:* Hallermann-Streiff syndrome

NOTES

Stroganoff, Vasili V., Russian obstetrician, 1857–1938.
    Stroganoff method—obsolete term for treatment of eclampsia.

Strong, Edward K., Jr., U.S. psychologist, *1884.
    Strong vocational interest test—a test that matches an individual's specific likes, dislikes, and interests to those characteristic of persons working in each of a number of vocations.

Stroop, J.R., psychologist.
    Stroop test—test used in psychology/psychiatry.

Stroud, Bert B., 19th century U.S. physiologist, anatomist, and zoologist.
    Stroud pectinated area—obsolete term for the area of the anal canal lying just below the rectal columns.

Strümpell, Ernst Adolf von, German physician, 1853–1925.
    Fleischer-Strümpell ring—*SYN:* Kayser-Fleischer ring
    Marie-Strümpell disease—*SYN:* Strümpell-Marie disease
    Strümpell disease—arthritis and osteitis deformans involving the spinal column. *SYN:* spondylitis deformans; acute epidemic leukoencephalitis
    Strümpell phenomenon—dorsal flexion of the great toe in a paralyzed limb when the limb is drawn up against the body, flexing both knee and hip. *SYN:* tibial phenomenon
    Strümpell reflex—stroking the abdomen or thigh causes flexion of the leg and adduction of the foot.
    Strümpell-Marie disease—arthritis of the spine, resembling rheumatoid arthritis, that may progress to bony ankylosis. *SYN:* Marie-Strümpell disease; ankylosing spondylitis
    Strümpell-Westphal disease—*SYN:* Wilson disease
    Westphal-Strümpell pseudosclerosis—*SYN:* Wilson disease

Struthers, Sir John, Scottish anatomist, 1823–1899.
    ligament of Struthers—a fibrous band located on the medial aspect of the distal humerus.

Stryker, Garold V., U.S. pathologist, *1896.
    Stryker-Halbeisen syndrome—reddish, scaling, macular eruption on the head and upper trunk due to vitamin B complex deficiency.

Stryker, Homer H., U.S. orthopedic surgeon, 1894–1980.
    mini-Stryker power drill
    Stryker bed—*SYN:* Stryker frame
    Stryker cast cutter
    Stryker CircOlectric bed
    Stryker drill
    Stryker fracture frame
    Stryker fracture table
    Stryker frame—a frame that holds the patient and permits turning in various planes without individual motion of parts. *SYN:* Stryker bed
    Stryker leg exerciser
    Stryker power instrumentation
    Stryker saw—a rapidly oscillating saw used for cutting bone or plaster casts.
    Stryker screw

Sturge, William A., English physician, 1850–1919.
    Sturge syndrome
    Sturge-Kalischer-Weber syndrome—*Syn:* Sturge-Weber syndrome
    Sturge-Weber disease—*Syn:* Sturge-Weber syndrome
    Sturge-Weber syndrome—a triad of 1) congenital cutaneous angioma (flame nevus) in the distribution of the trigeminal nerve, usually unilateral; 2) homolateral meningeal angioma with intracranial calcification and neurologic signs; and 3) angioma of the choroid, often with secondary glaucoma. *Syn:* Sturge-Weber disease; cephalotrigeminal angiomatosis; encephalotrigeminal angiomatosis; Sturge-Kalischer-Weber syndrome

Sturm, Johann C., Germany physician and mathematician, 1635–1703.
    Sturm conoid—in optics, the pattern of rays formed after passage through a spherocylindrical combination.
    Sturm interval—the distance between the anterior and posterior focal lines in a spherocylindrical lens combination.

Sturmdorf, A., U.S. gynecologist, 1861–1934.
    Sturmdorf amputation of the cervix
    Sturmdorf colporrhaphy
    Sturmdorf needle
    Sturmdorf operation—conical removal of the endocervix.
    Sturmdorf reamer
    Sturmdorf suture

Sucquet, J.P., French anatomist, 1840–1870.
    Sucquet anastomoses—*Syn:* Sucquet-Hoyer canals
    Sucquet canals—*Syn:* Sucquet-Hoyer canals
    Sucquet-Hoyer anastomoses—*Syn:* Sucquet-Hoyer canals
    Sucquet-Hoyer canals—arteriovenous anastomoses controlling blood flow in the glomus bodies in the digits. *Syn:* Hoyer anastomoses; Sucquet anastomoses; Hoyer canals; Sucquet canals; Sucquet-Hoyer anastomoses

Sudeck, Paul H.M., German surgeon, 1866–1938.
    Sudeck atrophy—atrophy of bones, commonly of the carpal or tarsal bones, following a slight injury such as a sprain. *Syn:* acute reflex bone atrophy; posttraumatic osteoporosis; Sudeck syndrome
    Sudeck critical point—region in the colon between the supply of the sigmoid arteries and that of the superior rectal artery.
    Sudeck disease
    Sudeck syndrome—*Syn:* Sudeck atrophy

Sugiura, M., 20th century Japanese surgeon.
    Sugiura procedure—esophageal transection with paraesophageal devascularization for esophageal varices.

Suker, George Franklin, 20th century U.S. ophthalmologist.
    Suker cyclodialysis spatula

(continued)

NOTES

Suker *(continued)*
 Suker iris forceps
 Suker knife
 Suker sign—sign seen in Graves disease.

Sulkowitch, Hirsh W., U.S. physician, *1906.
 Sulkowitch reagent—a reagent for the detection of calcium in the urine.
 Syn: Sulkowitch test
 Sulkowitch test—*Syn:* Sulkowitch reagent

Sulzberger, Marion B., U.S. dermatologist, 1895–1983.
 Bloch-Sulzberger disease—see under Bloch, Bruno
 Bloch-Sulzberger syndrome—*Syn:* Bloch-Sulzberger disease
 Sulzberger-Garbe disease—disease resembling an exudative form of
 eczema described in Jewish males with oval lesions on the penis, trunk,
 and face. *Syn:* Sulzberger-Garbe syndrome
 Sulzberger-Garbe syndrome—*Syn:* Sulzberger-Garbe disease

Sumner, Franklin W., 20th century English surgeon.
 Sumner sign—a slight increase in tonus of the abdominal muscles, an early
 indication of inflammation of the appendix, stone in the kidney or ureter,
 or a twisted pedicle of an ovarian cyst.

Sutherland, Jr., Earl W., winner of 1971 Nobel Prize in medicine or physiology
for work related to hormones.

Sutton, Richard Lightburn, Jr., U.S. dermatologist, *1908.
 Sutton disease—*Syn:* Sutton nevus
 Sutton nevus—a benign melanocytic nevus in which involution occurs with
 a central brown mole surrounded by a uniformly depigmented zone or
 halo. *Syn:* halo nevus; Sutton disease
 Sutton ulcer—a solitary, deep, painful ulcer of the buccal or genital
 mucous membrane.

Suzanne, Jean G., French physician, *1859.
 Suzanne gland—a small mucous gland in the floor of the mouth.

Svedberg, Theodor, Swedish chemist and Nobel laureate, 1884–1971.
 Svedberg equation
 Svedberg unit—a sedimentation constant.

Swan, Harold James C., U.S. cardiologist, *1922.
 Swan discission knife
 Swan lancet
 Swan needle
 Swan-Ganz balloon flotation catheter
 Swan-Ganz bipolar pacing catheter
 Swan-Ganz catheter—a thin (5-Fr), flexible, flow-directed catheter using a
 balloon to carry it through the heart to a pulmonary artery.
 Swan-Ganz flow-directed catheter
 Swan-Ganz pacing TD catheter

Swediauer, Francois X., Austrian physician, 1748–1824.
 Swediauer disease—*Syn:* Albert disease

Swedish, named for the country of its origin, Sweden.
 Swedish massage—traditional massage.

S

Sweet, Robert Douglas, 20th century English dermatologist.
    Sweet disease—*SYN:* acute febrile neutrophilic dermatosis; Sweet
      syndrome
    Sweet syndrome—*SYN:* Sweet disease

Swift, H., Australian physician, 1858–1937.
    Swift disease—*SYN:* Feer disease

Swindle, Percy Ford, U.S. physiologist, 1889–1916.
    Swindle ghost—prolonged afterimage.

Swyer, Paul R., U.S. pediatrician, *1921.
    Swyer-James syndrome—(1) radiographic evidence that density of one
      lung (or one lobe) is markedly less than the other(s) because of the
      presence of air trapped during expiration. *SYN:* Macleod syndrome; (2)
      hyperlucency of one lung from obliterating bronchiolitis. *SYN:* Swyer-
      James-Macleod syndrome.
    Swyer-James-Macleod syndrome—*SYN:* Swyer-James syndrome (2)

Sydenham, Thomas, English physician, 1624–1689.
    Sydenham chorea—a postinfectious chorea appearing several months after
      a streptococcal infection, with subsequent rheumatic fever. *SYN:*
      Sydenham disease; Sydenham syndrome
    Sydenham cough
    Sydenham disease—*SYN:* Sydenham chorea
    Sydenham syndrome—*SYN:* Sydenham chorea

Sylvest, Ejnar, Norwegian physician, 1880–1931.
    Sylvest disease—an acute infectious disease usually occurring in epidemic
      form. *SYN:* epidemic pleurodynia

Sylvius, Franciscus, Dutch physician, 1614–1672.
    aqueduct of Sylvius
    fossa of Sylvius
    sylvian angle
    sylvian fissure—*SYN:* lateral cerebral sulcus
    sylvian line
    sylvian point
    sylvian valve—*SYN:* valve of inferior vena cava
    sylvian ventricle—*SYN:* cavity of septum pellucidum
    vallecula sylvii

Syme, James, Scottish surgeon, 1799–1870.
    Syme amputation—amputation of the foot at the ankle joint. *SYN:* Syme
      operation
    Syme amputation prosthesis
    Syme ankle disarticulation amputation
    Syme foot prosthesis
    Syme operation—*SYN:* Syme amputation
    Syme procedure

(continued)

NOTES

Syme *(continued)*
Syme prosthesis
Syme prosthetic foot
terminal Syme procedure
two-stage Syme amputation

Symington, Johnson, Scottish anatomist, 1851–1924.
Symington anococcygeal body—a musculofibrous band that passes between the anus and the coccyx. *Syn:* anococcygeal ligament

Symmers, Douglas, U.S. pathologist, 1879–1952.
Brill-Symmers disease—see under Brill

Symmers, W. St. C., English pathologist, 1863–1937.
Symmers clay pipestem fibrosis—a characteristic pipe-shaped fibrosis formed around hepatic portal veins. *Syn:* pipestem fibrosis

Symonds, Percival Mallon, U.S. psychologist, 1893–1960.
Symonds picture-study test—projective test for adolescents, used in psychology/psychiatry.

Syms, Parker, U.S. surgeon, 1860–1933.
Syms traction
Syms tractor—a collapsible rubber bag and tube used to draw an enlarged prostate into an operative wound.

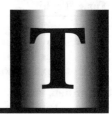

Taenzer, Paul R., German dermatologist, 1858–1919.
    Taenzer stain—an orcein solution used for staining elastic tissue. *SYN:* Unna-Taenzer stain
    Unna-Taenzer stain—*SYN:* Taenzer stain

Tagliacozzi, Gaspare, Italian surgeon, 1546–1599.
    tagliacotian operation—Italian method of rhinoplasty utilizing a flap from the arm. *SYN:* Italian rhinoplasty

Tait, Robert L., English gynecologist, 1845–1899.
    Tait law—an obsolete dictum that an exploratory laparotomy should be performed in every case of obscure pelvic or abdominal disease that threatens health or life.

Takahara, Shigeo, 20th century Japanese otolaryngologist.
    Takahara disease—*SYN:* Takahara syndrome
    Takahara syndrome—chronic severe mouth infection. *SYN:* Takahara disease; acatalasia

Takayama, Masao, Japanese physician, *1872.
    Takayama stain—a stain used for identification of blood stains.

Takayashu, Mikito, Japanese surgeon, 1860–1938.
    Takayashu disease—*SYN:* Takayashu pulseless disease
    Takayashu pulseless disease—obliterative arteritis, primarily of the carotid and subclavian arteries. *SYN:* Takayashu disease; Takayashu syndrome
    Takayashu syndrome—*SYN:* Takayashu pulseless disease

Talbot, William Henry Fox, English scientist, 1800–1877.
    Plateau-Talbot law—see under Plateau

Tamm, Igor, U.S. virologist, *1922.
    Tamm-Horsfall mucoprotein—the matrix of urinary casts derived from the secretion of renal tubular cells.
    Tamm-Horsfall protein

Tanner, Norman Cecil, English surgeon.
    Tanner incision
    Tanner slide

Tapia, Antonio, Spanish otolaryngologist, 1875–1950.
    Tapia syndrome—unilateral paralysis of the larynx, velum palati, and tongue, with atrophy of the latter.
    Tapia vagohypoglossal palsy

Tar, Aloys, Hungarian physician, *1886.
> **Tar symptom**—the low lung borders lie as deeply with moderate exhalation as in the upright position of the lungs with deep inhalation.

Tardieu, Auguste A., French physician, 1818–1879.
> **Tardieu ecchymoses**—subpleural and subpericardial petechiae or ecchymoses (or both), as observed in the tissues of persons who have been asphyxiated. *SYN:* Tardieu petechiae; Tardieu spots
> **Tardieu petechiae**—*SYN:* Tardieu ecchymoses
> **Tardieu spots**—*SYN:* Tardieu ecchymoses
> **Tardieu test**

Tarin, Pierre, French anatomist, 1725–1761.
> **Tarin space**—a dilation of the subarachnoid space in front of the pons. *SYN:* interpeduncular cistern
> **Tarin tenia**—a slender, compact fiber bundle that connects the amygdala with the hypothalamus and other basal forebrain regions. *SYN:* terminal stria
> **Tarin valve**—a thin sheet of white matter hidden by the cerebellar tonsil and attached along the peduncle of the flocculus and to the nodulus of the vermis. *SYN:* inferior medullary velum

Tarlov, Isadore Max, U.S. surgeon, 1905–1977.
> **Tarlov cyst**—a perineural cyst found in the proximal radicles of the lower spinal cord.
> **Tarlov nerve elevator**

Tarnier, Étienne Stephane, French obstetrician, 1828–1897.
> **Tarnier forceps**—a type of axis-traction forceps.

Tatum, Edward Lawrie, joint winner of 1958 Nobel Prize for work related to genetics.

Taussig, Helen B., U.S. pediatrician, 1898–1986.
> **Blalock-Taussig operation**—see under Blalock
> **Blalock-Taussig shunt**—see under Blalock
> **Taussig-Bing disease**—*SYN:* Taussig-Bing syndrome
> **Taussig-Bing syndrome**—complete transposition of the aorta with a left-sided pulmonary artery overriding the left ventricle and ventricular septal defect, right ventricular hypertrophy, anteriorly situated aorta, and posteriorly situated pulmonary artery. *SYN:* Taussig-Bing disease

Tawara, K. Sunao, Japanese pathologist, 1873–1952.
> **His-Tawara system**—see under His, Wilhelm, Jr.
> **node of Aschoff and Tawara**—see under Aschoff
> **Tawara node**—*SYN:* node of Aschoff and Tawara

Tay, Warren, English physician, 1843–1927.
> **Tay cherry-red spot**—the ophthalmoscopic appearance of the normal choroid beneath the fovea centralis. *SYN:* cherry-red spot
> **Tay-Sachs disease**—cerebral sphingolipidosis, infantile type. *SYN:* infantile G_{M2} gangliosidosis

Taybi, Hooshang, U.S. pediatrician and radiologist, *1919.
> **Rubinstein-Taybi syndrome**—see under Rubinstein
> **Taybi syndrome**

Taylor, Charles F., U.S. orthopedic surgeon, 1827–1899.
    Taylor apparatus—*Syn:* Taylor back brace
    Taylor back brace—a steel spinal support. *Syn:* Taylor apparatus; Taylor splint
    Taylor clavicle support
    Taylor procedure
    Taylor retractor
    Taylor spinal frame
    Taylor spine brace
    Taylor splint—*Syn:* Taylor back brace
    Taylor technique
    Taylor thoracolumbosacral orthosis
    Taylor-Knight brace

Taylor, H.C., Jr.
    Taylor syndrome—various areas of congestive dysfunction, possibly psychogenic in origin.

Taylor, Robert W., U.S. dermatologist, 1842–1908.
    Taylor disease—diffuse idiopathic cutaneous atrophy.

Teale, Thomas P., English surgeon, 1801–1868.
    Teale amputation—amputation of the forearm, thigh, or leg.

Teichmann, Ludwig, German histologist, 1823–1895.
    Teichmann crystals—used in microscopic detection of blood. *Syn:* chlorohemin crystals

TeLinde, Richard W., U.S. gynecologist, *1894.
    TeLinde operation—*Syn:* modified radical hysterectomy

Temin, Howard Martin, joint winner of 1975 Nobel Prize for work related to tumor viruses and cell material.

ten Horn, C., 20th century Dutch surgeon.
    ten Horn sign—pain caused by gentle traction on the right spermatic cord, indicative of appendicitis.

Tenon, Jacques R., French pathologist and oculist, 1724–1816.
    Tenon capsule—*Syn:* fascial sheath of eyeball
    Tenon space—the space between the fascial sheath of the eyeball and the sclera. *Syn:* episcleral space

Terman, Lewis Madison, U.S. psychologist, 1877–1956.
    Terman-McNemar test of mental ability—a group intelligence scale.

Terrey, Mary, 20th century U.S. physician.
    Lowe-Terrey-MacLachlan syndrome—*Syn:* Lowe syndrome

Terrien, Felix, French ophthalmologist, *1872.
    Terrien marginal degeneration—a form of marginal corneal degeneration.
    Terrien-Viel syndrome—recurrent glaucoma, unilateral.

NOTES

Terrien, Louis-Felix, French surgeon, 1837–1908.
   Terrien valve—a valvelike fold between the gallbladder and the cystic duct.

Terry, Theodore L., U.S. ophthalmologist, 1899–1946.
   Terry syndrome—*SYN:* retinopathy of prematurity

Terson, Albert, French ophthalmologist, 1867–1935.
   Terson forceps
   Terson glands—*SYN:* conjunctival glands
   Terson speculum
   Terson syndrome—hemorrhage into the vitreous of the eye.

Tesla, Nikola, Serbian-U.S. electrical engineer, 1856–1943.
   tesla—in the SI system, the unit of magnetic flux density.
   Tesla current—*SYN:* high-frequency current
   Tesla magnet
   Tesla measurement

Tessier, French physician.
   Tessier bone bender
   Tessier craniofacial instruments
   Tessier craniofacial operation
   Tessier elevator
   Tessier facial dysostosis operation
   Tessier osteotomy

Teutleben, F.E.K. von, German anatomist, *1842.
   Teutleben ligament—*SYN:* pulmonary ligament

Thal, Alan P., U.S. surgeon, *1925.
   Thal procedure—correction of a benign stricture of the lower esophagus.

Thane, Sir George D., English anatomist, 1850–1930.
   Thane method—a method for indicating the position of the central sulcus (Rolando fissure) of the brain.

Thayer, J.D.
   Thayer-Martin agar—used for transport and primary isolation of *Neisseria gonorrhoeae* and *Neisseria meningitides*. *SYN:* Thayer-Martin medium
   Thayer-Martin medium—*SYN:* Thayer-Martin agar

Thebesius, Adam C., German physician, 1686–1732.
   thebesian foramina—a number of fossae in the wall of the right atrium containing the openings of minute intramural veins. *SYN:* foramina of the venae minimae
   thebesian valve—a delicate fold of endocardium at the opening of the coronary sinus into the right atrium. *SYN:* valve of coronary sinus
   thebesian veins—numerous small valveless venous channels that open directly into the chambers of the heart from the capillary bed in the cardiac wall, enabling a form of collateral circulation unique to the heart. *SYN:* venae cordis minimae

Theden, Johann C.A., German surgeon, 1714–1797.
   Theden method—treatment of aneurysms or of large sanguineous effusions by compression of the entire limb with a roller bandage.

Theile, Friedrich W., German anatomist, 1801–1879.

    Theile canal—a passage in the pericardial sac between the origins of the great vessels, formed as a result of the flexure of the heart tube. *SYN:* transverse pericardial sinus

    Theile glands—small, mucous, tubuloalveolar glands in the mucosa of the larger bile ducts and especially in the neck of the gallbladder. *SYN:* glands of biliary mucosa

    Theile muscle—*SYN:* superficial transverse perineal muscle

Theiler, Max, South African microbiologist in the U.S. and Nobel laureate, 1899–1972.

    Theiler disease—(1) *SYN:* mouse encephalomyelitis; (2) *SYN:* equine serum hepatitis.

    Theiler mouse encephalomyelitis virus—a virus in the family Picornaviridae. *SYN:* Theiler virus

    Theiler virus—*SYN:* Theiler mouse encephalomyelitis virus

Theobald Smith, see under Smith.

Theorell, Axel Hugo Theodor, winner of 1955 Nobel Prize for work related to oxidation enzymes.

Thier, Carl Jörg, German physician.

    Weyers-Thier syndrome—see under Weyers

Thiers, Joseph, French physician, *1885.

    Achard-Thiers syndrome—see under Achard

Thiersch, Karl, German surgeon, 1822–1895.

    Ollier-Thiersch graft—*SYN:* Ollier graft

    Thiersch canaliculi—minute channels in newly formed reparative tissue.

    Thiersch graft—*SYN:* Ollier graft

    Thiersch graft operation—*SYN:* Thiersch operation

    Thiersch implant

    Thiersch knife

    Thiersch medium split free graft

    Thiersch method

    Thiersch operation—the application of a partial thickness skin graft. *SYN:* Thiersch graft operation

    Thiersch prosthesis

    Thiersch suture

    Thiersch thin split free graft

    Thiersch wire

Thiry, Ludwig, Austrian physiologist, 1817–1897.

    Thiry fistula—*SYN:* Thiry-Vella fistula

    Thiry-Vella fistula—experimental isolation of a segment of intestine in a dog or other animal. *SYN:* Vella fistula; Thiry fistula

NOTES

Thoma, Richard, German histologist, 1847–1923.

Thoma ampulla—a dilation of the arterial capillary beyond the sheathed artery of the spleen.

Thoma fixative—nitric acid in 95% alcohol, used for decalcifying bone in the preparation of histologic specimens.

Thoma laws—the development of blood vessels is governed by dynamic forces acting on their walls.

Thomas, André Antoine Henri, French neurologist, 1867–1963.

André Thomas sign

Thomas, E. Donnall, joint winner of 1990 Nobel Prize for work related to cell and organ transplantation.

Thomas, Hugh Owen, English surgeon, 1834–1891.

Thomas Allis forceps
Thomas brace
Thomas cervical collar brace
Thomas classification
Thomas collar
Thomas collar cervical orthosis
Thomas extrapolated bar graft
Thomas fracture frame
Thomas full-ring splint
Thomas heel
Thomas hinged splint
Thomas hyperextension frame
Thomas Kapsule instruments
Thomas knee splint
Thomas Kodel sling
Thomas posterior splint
Thomas procedure
Thomas ring
Thomas sign
Thomas splint—a long leg splint extending from a ring at the hip to beyond the foot.
Thomas splint with Pearson attachment
Thomas suspension splint
Thomas test
Thomas test of function
Thomas walking brace
Thomas wrench

Thompson, Frederick R., U.S. orthopedic surgeon, 1907–1983.

Thompson anterolateral approach
Thompson anteromedial approach
Thompson approach
Thompson arthroplasty
Thompson excision
Thompson femoral head prosthesis
Thompson femoral neck prosthesis
Thompson fracture frame
Thompson frame

Thompson hemiarthroplasty hip prosthesis
Thompson hip endoprosthesis system
Thompson hip prosthesis
Thompson hip prosthesis forceps
Thompson modification of Denis Browne splint
Thompson posterior radial approach
Thompson prosthesis
Thompson quadriceps plasty
Thompson resection
Thompson sign
Thompson splint
Thompson squeeze test of Achilles tendon
Thompson telescoping V osteotomy
Thompson test

Thompson, Sir Henry, English surgeon, 1820–1904.
   bandaletta of Thompson—thickened inferior margin of the transversalis fascia. *SYN:* iliopubic tract
   Thompson test—for extent of gonorrheal infection. *SYN:* two-glass test

Thomsen, Asmus J., Danish physician, 1815–1896.
   Thomsen disease—a hereditary disease marked by tonic spasms that occur when voluntary movement is attempted. *SYN:* Thomsen myotonia congenita
   Thomsen myotonia congenita—*SYN:* Thomsen disease

Thomson, Frederick H., English physician, 1867–1938.
   Thomson sign—*SYN:* Pastia sign

Thomson, Matthew Sidney, English dermatologist, 1894–1969.
   Rothmund-Thomson syndrome—*SYN:* Rothmund syndrome

Thormählen, Johann, 19th century German physician.
   Thormählen test—a test for melanin.

Thorn, George W., U.S. physician, *1906.
   Thorn syndrome—a rare disorder resulting from renal tubular damage of a variety of etiologies. *SYN:* salt-losing nephritis
   Thorn test—putative test of adrenal cortical function.

Thorndike, Edward Lee, U.S. psychologist and lexicographer, 1874–1949.
   Thorndike handwriting scale—a series of handwriting samples that compares an individual's handwriting.
   Thorndike trial and error learning—a theory used in psychology.

Thornwaldt, var. of Tornwaldt

Thygeson, Phillips, U.S. ophthalmologist, *1903.
   Thygeson disease—epithelial punctate keratitis associated with viral conjunctivitis. *SYN:* superficial punctate keratitis

NOTES

Tièche, Max, Swiss dermatologist, 1878–1938.
    Jadassohn-Tièche nevus—see under Jadassohn

Tiedemann, Friedrich, German anatomist, 1781–1861.
    Tiedemann gland—one of two mucoid-secreting tubuloalveolar glands on either side of the lower part of the vagina. *SYN:* greater vestibular gland
    Tiedemann nerve—a sympathetic nerve accompanying the central artery of the retina in the optic nerve.
    Tiedemann rongeur

Tietze, Alexander, German surgeon, 1864–1927.
    Tietze disease—*SYN:* Tietze syndrome
    Tietze syndrome—inflammation and painful nonsuppurative swelling of a costochondral junction. *SYN:* peristernal perichondritis; Tietze disease

Tillaux, Paul J., French surgeon, 1834–1904.
    spiral of Tillaux—an imaginary line connecting the insertions of the recti muscles of the eye.
    Tillaux disease
    Tillaux fracture

Tinbergen, Nikolaas, joint winner of 1973 Nobel Prize for work related to social behavior.

Tinel, Jules, French neurologist, 1879–1952.
    Tinel sign—a sensation of tingling felt in the distal extremity of a limb with percussion over the site of an injured nerve, indicating a partial lesion or early regeneration in the nerve. *SYN:* Tinel test
    Tinel suture
    Tinel test—*SYN:* Tinel sign

Tiselius, Arne, Swedish biochemist and Nobel laureate, 1902–1971.
    Tiselius apparatus—used to separate proteins in solution by electrophoresis.
    Tiselius electrophoresis cell—the special container in a Tiselius apparatus containing the solution to be analyzed electrophoresis.

Tissot, Jules, early 20th century French physiologist.
    Tissot spirometer—a large water-sealed spirometer designed for accumulating expired gas over a long period of time.

Tizzoni, Guido, Italian physician, 1853–1932.
    Tizzoni stain—a stain used as a test for iron in tissue.

Tobey, George L., Jr., U.S. otolaryngologist, 1881–1947.
    Ayer-Tobey test
    Tobey-Ayer test

Tod, David, English surgeon, 1794–1856.
    Tod muscle—*SYN:* oblique auricular muscle

Todaro, Francesco, Italian anatomist, 1839–1918.
    Todaro tendon—an inconstant tendinous structure that extends from the right fibrous trigone of the heart toward the valve of the inferior vena cava.

Todd, Robert B., English physician, 1809–1860.
    Todd paralysis—paralysis of temporary duration that occurs in the limb(s)

involved in jacksonian epilepsy after the seizure. *Syn:* Todd postepileptic paralysis

Todd postepileptic paralysis—*Syn:* Todd paralysis

Toison, J., French histologist, 1858–1950.
Toison stain—a blood dilutent and leukocyte stain also used for erythrocyte counts.

Toldt, Karl, Austrian anatomist, 1840–1920.
Toldt fascia—continuation of Treitz fascia behind the body of the pancreas.
Toldt membrane—the anterior layer of the renal fascia.
white line of Toldt—junction of parietal peritoneum with Denonvillieri fascia.

Tolman, Edward Chase, U.S. psychologist, 1886–1959.
Tolman purposive behaviorism—combination of Gestalt concepts.

Tolosa, Eduardo S., 20th century Spanish neurosurgeon.
Tolosa-Hunt syndrome—cavernous sinus syndrome produced by an idiopathic granuloma.

Tomes, Sir Charles S., English dentist, 1846–1928.
Tomes processes—processes of the enamel cells.

Tomes, Sir John, English dentist and anatomist, 1815–1895.
Tomes fibers—the processes of the pulpal cells which are contained within the dentinal tubules. *Syn:* dentinal fibers
Tomes granular layer—a thin layer of dentin adjacent to the cementum.

Tomkins, Silvan S., U.S. psychologist, *1911.
Tomkins-Horn picture arrangement test—test in which an individual arranges three sketches in a sensible sequence.

Tommaselli, Salvatore, Italian physician, 1834–1906.
Tommaselli disease—hemoglobinuria and pyrexia due to quinine intoxication.

Tonegawa, Susumu, winner of 1987 Nobel Prize for work related to antibodies.

Tooth, Howard H., English physician, 1856–1925.
Charcot-Marie-Tooth disease—see under Charcot

Töpfer, Alfred E., German physician, *1858.
Töpfer test—an obsolete test for free hydrochloric acid in the gastric contents.

Topinard, Paul, French anthropologist, 1830–1912.
Topinard facial angle—ophryospinal facial angle.
Topinard line—a line running between the glabella and the mental point.

Topolanski, Alfred, Austrian ophthalmologist, 1861–1960.
Topolanski sign—congestion of the pericorneal region of the eye in Graves disease.

NOTES

Torek, Franz J.A., U.S. surgeon, 1861–1938.
    Keetley-Torek operation—*Syn:* Torek operation
    Torek operation—a two-stage operation for bringing down an undescended testicle. *Syn:* Keetley-Torek operation

Torkildsen, Arne, Norwegian neurosurgeon, *1899.
    Torkildsen operation
    Torkildsen shunt—a ventriculocisternal shunt.
    Torkildsen shunt procedure
    Torkildsen ventriculocisternostomy

Tornwaldt, Gustavus Ludwig, German physician, 1843–1910.
    Tornwaldt abscess—chronic infection of the pharyngeal bursa.
    Tornwaldt cyst—a cystic notochordal remnant found inconstantly in the posterior wall of the nasopharynx at the lower end of the pharyngeal tonsil. *Syn:* pharyngeal bursa
    Tornwaldt disease—inflammation or obstruction of the pharyngeal bursa or an adenoid cleft with the formation of a cyst containing pus.
    Tornwaldt syndrome—nasopharyngeal discharge, occipital headache, and stiffness of posterior cervical muscles, with halitosis due to chronic infection of the pharyngeal bursa.

Torrance, Ellis Paul, U.S. psychologist, *1915.
    Torrance tests of creative thinking—batteries of test items that use creative thinking with words, pictures, and sounds.

Torre, Douglas P., U.S. dermatologist, *1919.
    Muir-Torre syndrome—*Syn:* Torre syndrome
    Torre syndrome—multiple sebaceous gland neoplasms associated with multiple visceral malignancies. *Syn:* Muir-Torre syndrome

Touraine, Albert, French dermatologist, 1883–1961.
    Christ-Siemens-Touraine syndrome—see under Christ

Tournay, Auguste, French ophthalmologist, 1878–1969.
    Tournay phenomenon—dilation of the pupil in the abducting eye on extreme lateral gaze. *Syn:* Tournay sign; Gianelli sign
    Tournay sign—*Syn:* Tournay phenomenon

Tourtual, Kaspar, Prussian anatomist, 1802–1865.
    Tourtual membrane—the elastic fibra membrane that extends from the ventricular fold of the larynx upward to the aryepiglottic fold. *Syn:* quadrangular membrane
    Tourtual sinus—the interval between the palatoglossal and palatopharyngeal arches above the tonsil, most obvious after the tonsil has regressed in the adult. *Syn:* supratonsillar fossa

Touton, Karl, German dermatologist, 1858–1934.
    Touton giant cell—a xanthoma cell in which the multiple nuclei are grouped around a small island of nonfoamy cytoplasm.

Tovell, Ralph M., U.S. anesthesiologist, 1901–1967.
    Tovell tube—a tracheal tube.

Towne, Edward B., U.S. otolaryngologist, 1883–1957.
    Towne projection—anteroposterior radiographic projection devised to permit demonstration of the entire occipital bone, foramen magnum, and

dorsum sellae, as well as the petrous ridges. *Syn:* half-axial view; half-axial projection; Towne view

Towne view—*Syn:* Towne projection

Toynbee, Joseph, English otologist, 1815–1866.

Toynbee corpuscles—connective tissue cells found between the laminae of fibrous tissue in the cornea. *Syn:* corneal corpuscles

Toynbee muscle—draws the handle of the malleus medialward, tensing the tympanic membrane to protect it from excessive vibration by loud sounds. *Syn:* tensor tympani muscle

Toynbee tube—a tube by which an otologist can listen to the sounds in a patient's ear during politzerization.

Trantas, Alexios, Greek ophthalmologist, 1867–1960.

Horner-Trantas dots—see under Horner, Johann

Trantas dots—pale, grayish red, uneven nodules of gelatinous aspect at the limbal conjunctiva in vernal conjunctivitis.

Trapp, Julius, Russian pharmacist, 1815–1908.

Trapp formula—*Syn:* Häser formula

Trapp-Häser formula—*Syn:* Häser formula

Traube, Ludwig, German physician and pathologist, 1818–1876.

Traube bruit—a triple cadence to the heart sounds at rates of 100 beats per minute or more, usually indicative of serious disease. *Syn:* gallop

Traube corpuscle—a hypochromic, crescent-shaped erythrocyte, probably resulting from artifactual rupture of a red cell with loss of hemoglobin. *Syn:* achromocyte

Traube double tone—a double sound heard on auscultation over the femoral vessels in cases of aortic and tricuspid insufficiency.

Traube dyspnea—obsolete term for inspiratory dyspnea with maximal expansion of the chest and a slow respiratory rhythm.

Traube plugs—*Syn:* Dittrich plugs

Traube semilunar space—a crescentic space about 12 cm wide, just above the costal margin.

Traube sign—a double sound or murmur heard in auscultation over arteries in significant aortic regurgitation.

Traube-Hering curves—rhythmical variations in blood pressure. *Syn:* Traube-Hering waves

Traube-Hering waves—*Syn:* Traube-Hering curves

Traugott, Carl, German internist, *1885.

Staub-Traugott effect—see under Staub

Staub-Traugott phenomenon—*Syn:* Staub-Traugott effect

Trautmann, Moritz F., German otologist, 1832–1902.

Trautmann triangular space—the area of the temporal bone bounded by the sigmoid sinus, the superior petrosal sinus, and a tangent to the posterior semicircular canal. *Syn:* triangle of Trautmann

triangle of Trautmann—*Syn:* Trautmann triangular space

NOTES

Treacher Collins, See under Collins.

Treitz, Wenzel, Bohemian pathologist, 1819–1872.
> **Treitz arch**—a sickle-shaped fold of peritoneum that forms the anterior boundary of the paraduodenal recess. *SYN:* paraduodenal fold
> **Treitz fascia**—fascia behind the head of the pancreas.
> **Treitz fossa**—an inconstant depression in the peritoneum extending posterior to the cecum. *SYN:* subcecal fossa
> **Treitz hernia**—a hernia in the subperitoneal tissues. *SYN:* duodenojejunal hernia
> **Treitz ligament**—*SYN:* suspensory muscle of duodenum
> **Treitz muscle**—*SYN:* suspensory muscle of duodenum

Trélat, Ulysse, French surgeon, 1828–1890.
> **Leser-Trélat sign**—see under Leser
> **Trélat sign**—an obsolete sign.
> **Trélat stools**—stools streaked with blood, occurring in proctitis.

Trenaunay, Paul, French physician, *1875.
> **Klippel-Trenaunay-Weber syndrome**—see under Klippel

Trendelenburg, Friedrich, German surgeon, 1844–1924.
> **Brodie-Trendelenburg test**—see under Brodie
> **reverse Trendelenburg position**—supine position, without flexing or extending, in which the head is higher than the feet.
> **steep Trendelenburg position**
> **Trendelenburg cannula**
> **Trendelenburg gait**
> **Trendelenburg limp**
> **Trendelenburg lurch**
> **Trendelenburg operation**—pulmonary embolectomy.
> **Trendelenburg position**—a supine position on the operating table, used during and after operations in the pelvis or for shock.
> **Trendelenburg sign**—in congenital dislocation of the hip or in hip abductor weakness, the pelvis will sag on the side opposite to the dislocation when the hip and knee of the normal side is flexed.
> **Trendelenburg symptom**—a waddling gait in paresis of the gluteal muscles, as in progressive muscular dystrophy. *SYN:* Trendelenburg waddle
> **Trendelenburg tampon**
> **Trendelenburg test**—a test of the valves of the leg veins.
> **Trendelenburg vein ligation**
> **Trendelenburg waddle**—*SYN:* Trendelenburg symptom

Tresilian, Frederick J., English physician, 1862–1926.
> **Tresilian sign**—a reddish prominence at the orifice of Stenson duct, noted in mumps.

Trethowan, W.H., English orthopedic surgeon, 1882–1934.
> **Trethowan line**—along the upper border of the femoral neck on hip x-ray, failure to enter the head indicates slipped upper femoral epiphysis.
> **Trethowan metatarsal osteotomy**

Treves, Norman, U.S. surgeon, 1894–1964.
> **Stewart-Treves syndrome**—see under Stewart, Fred

Treves, Sir Frederick, English surgeon, 1853–1923.
bloodless field of Treves
Treves fold—a fold of peritoneum bounding the ileocecal or
ileoappendicular fossa. *Syn:* ileocecal fold
Treves intestinal clamp

Trevor, David, English orthopedic surgeon, 1906–1988.
Trevor disease—epiphysealis hemimelica, affects ankles and knees leading
to limitation of motion. *Syn:* tarsoepiphyseal aclasis

T

Tripier, Léon, French surgeon, 1842–1891.
Tripier amputation—a modification of Chopart amputation, in that a part
of the calcaneus is also removed.

Troisier, Charles-Emile, French physician, 1844–1919.
Troisier ganglion—lymph node immediately above the clavicle, palpably
enlarged as the result of a metastasis from a malignant neoplasm. *Syn:*
Troisier node
Troisier node—*Syn:* Troisier ganglion
Troisier sign—Troisier ganglion enlargement.

Trolard, Paulin, French anatomist, 1842–1910.
Trolard vein—a large communicating vein between the superficial middle
cerebral vein and the superior sagittal sinus. *Syn:* superior anastomotic
vein
vein of Trolard

Tröltsch, Anton F. von, German otologist, 1829–1890.
Tröltsch corpuscles—minute spaces resembling corpuscles between the
radial fibers of the drum membrane of the ear.
Tröltsch fold—one of two ligamentous bands that mark the boundary
between the tense and the flaccid portions of the tympanic membrane.
Syn: mallear fold
Tröltsch pockets—*Syn:* Tröltsch recesses
Tröltsch recesses—slitlike spaces on the tympanic wall between the
anterior and posterior malleolar folds and the tympanic membrane. *Syn:*
anterior recess of tympanic membrane; posterior recess of tympanic
membrane; Tröltsch pockets

Trömner, Ernest L.O., German neurologist, 1868–1949.
Trömner reflex—a modified Rossolimo reflex, seen in pyramidal tract
lesions, with moderate spasticity.

Trotter, W.
Trotter syndrome—nasopharyngeal tumor.

Trousseau, Armand, French physician, 1801–1867.
Trousseau point—a painful point in neuralgia at the spinous process of the
vertebra below which arises the offending nerve.

(continued)

NOTES

Trousseau (*continued*)

Trousseau sign—in latent tetany, the occurrence of carpopedal spasm accompanied by paresthesia, elicited when the upper arm is compressed.

Trousseau spot—a line of redness resulting from drawing a point across the skin, especially notable in cases of meningitis. *Syn:* meningitic streak

Trousseau syndrome—thrombophlebitis migrans associated with visceral cancer. *Syn:* Nygaard-Brown syndrome

Trousseau-Lallemand bodies—*Syn:* Lallemand bodies (2)

Trunecek, Karel, Czech physician, *1865.

Trunecek sign—palpable impulse of the subclavian artery near the point of origin of the sternomastoid muscle in cases of aortic sclerosis.

Tubbs, Oswald Sydney, English surgeon.

Tubbs dilator

Tucker, Ervin Alden, U.S. obstetrician, 1862–1902.

Tucker-McLean forceps—a type of axis-traction forceps.

Tuffier, Marin Théodore, French surgeon, 1857–1929.

Tuffier test—*Syn:* Hallion test

Tulp, Nicholas (Nicolaus), Dutch anatomist, 1593–1674.

Tulp valve—the bilabial prominence of the terminal ileum into the large intestine at the cecocolic junction as seen in cadavers. *Syn:* ileocecal valve

Tuohy, Edward B., 20th century U.S. anesthesiologist.

Tuohy aortography needle

Tuohy needle—a needle used to place catheters into the subarachnoid or epidural space.

Tuohy-Borst adapter

Tuohy-Borst introducer

Türck, Ludwig, Austrian neurologist, 1810–1868.

Türck bundle—uncrossed fibers forming a small bundle in the pyramidal tract. *Syn:* Türck tract; Türck column

Türck column—*Syn:* Türck bundle

Türck degeneration—degeneration of a nerve fiber and its sheath distal to the point of injury or section of the axon.

Türck tract—*Syn:* Türck bundle

Türk, Siegmund, 20th century Swiss ophthalmologist.

Ehrlich-Türk line—see under Ehrlich

Türk, Wilhelm, Austrian hematologist, 1871–1916.

Türk cell—a relatively large immature cell found in circulating blood only in pathologic conditions. *Syn:* irritation cell; Türk leukocyte

Türk leukocyte—*Syn:* Türk cell

Turner, George Grey, English surgeon, 1877–1951.

Grey Turner sign—local areas of discoloration about the umbilicus and in the region of the loins, in acute hemorrhagic pancreatitis and other causes of retroperitoneal hemorrhage.

Turner, Henry H., U.S. endocrinologist, 1892–1970.

Turner syndrome—a syndrome with chromosome count 45 and only one X chromosome. *Syn:* XO syndrome

Turner, Joseph G., English dentist, d. 1955.
Turner tooth—enamel hypoplasia involving a solitary permanent tooth.

Turner, Sir William, English anatomist, 1832–1916.
intraparietal sulcus of Turner—*Syn:* Turner sulcus
Turner sulcus—a horizontal sulcus that divides the parietal lobe into superior and inferior parietal lobules. *Syn:* intraparietal sulcus of Turner

Turner, U.C., U.S. surgeon.
Hefke-Turner sign—see under Hefke
Turner pin
Turner prosthesis
Turner-Hefke sign—*Syn:* Hefke-Turner sign

Tuttle, James P., U.S. surgeon, 1857–1913.
Tuttle proctoscope—a tubular rectal speculum illuminated at its distal extremity.

Tweed, Charles H., U.S. orthodontist, 1895–1970.
Tweed edgewise treatment
Tweed triangle—a triangle defined by facial and dental landmarks.

Twort, Frederick W., English bacteriologist, 1877–1950.
Twort phenomenon—*Syn:* Twort-d'Herelle phenomenon
Twort-d'Herelle phenomenon—the lysis of bacteria by bacteriophage. *Syn:* d'Herelle phenomenon; Twort phenomenon; bacteriophagia

Tyndall, John, English physicist, 1820–1893.
Tyndall effect—*Syn:* Tyndall phenomenon
Tyndall light—light that is reflected by gas- or liquid-suspended particles.
Tyndall phenomenon—the visibility of floating particles in gases or liquids when illuminated by a ray of sunlight and viewed at right angles to the illuminating ray. *Syn:* Tyndall effect
tyndallization—exposure to a temperature of 100°C (flowing steam) for a definite period, usually an hour, on each of several days. *Syn:* fractional sterilization

Tyrode, Maurice V., U.S. pharmacologist, 1878–1930.
Tyrode solution—a modified Locke solution used to irrigate the peritoneal cavity.

Tyrrell, Frederick, English anatomist and surgeon, 1797–1843.
Tyrrell fascia—a fascial layer that extends superiorly from the central tendon of the perineum to the peritoneum between the prostate and rectum. *Syn:* rectovesical septum

Tyson, Edward, English anatomist, 1649–1708.
Tyson glands—sebaceous glands of the corona glandis and inner surface of the prepuce, which produce smegma. *Syn:* preputial glands

Tzanck, Arnault, Russian dermatologist, 1886–1954.
Tzanck cells—acantholytic epithelial cells seen in the Tzanck test.
Tzanck test—the examination of fluid from a bullous lesion for Tzanck cells.

NOTES

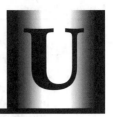

Uehlinger, E., Swiss pathologist, *1899.
  Meyenburg-Altherr-Uehlinger syndrome—*SYN:* Meyenburg disease

Uffelmann, Jules, German physician, 1837–1894.
  Uffelmann reagent—a 2% solution of phenol in water and aqueous ferric chloride.

Uhl, Henry S.M., internist, *1921.
  Uhl anomaly—*SYN:* Uhl syndrome
  Uhl syndrome—congenital malformation of the heart. *SYN:* Uhl anomaly

Uhthoff, Wilhelm, German ophthalmologist, 1853–1927.
  Uhthoff sign—*SYN:* Uhthoff symptom
  Uhthoff symptom—a damaged nerve that often has a lowered shut-down temperature. *SYN:* Uhthoff sign

Ullmann, Emerich, Hungarian surgeon, 1861–1937.
  Ullmann line—the line of displacement in spondylolisthesis.
  Ullmann syndrome—a systemic angiomatosis due to multiple arteriovenous malformations.

Ullrich, Otto, German physician, 1894–1957.
  Morquio-Ullrich disease—*SYN:* Morquio syndrome
  Ullrich drill guard
  Ullrich forceps
  Ullrich laminectomy retractor
  Ullrich self-retaining retractor
  Ullrich tubing clamp

Ultzmann, Robert, German urologist, 1842–1889.
  Ultzmann test—a test for bile pigments.

Umber, Friedrich, German physician, 1871–1946.
  Umber test—a test to determine scarlet fever.

Underwood, Michael, English pediatrician, 1737–1820.
  Underwood disease—*SYN:* Underwood syndrome
  Underwood syndrome—neonatal sclerema. *SYN:* Underwood disease

Unna, Marie
  Marie Unna syndrome—childhood hair loss. *SYN:* Unna syndrome
  Unna syndrome—*SYN:* Marie Unna syndrome

Unna, Paul G., German dermatologist and staining expert, 1850–1929.
  Unna disease—*SYN:* seborrheic dermatitis

(continued)

Unna *(continued)*

Unna mark—a pale vascular birthmark found on the nape of the neck in 25 to 50% of normal persons. *SYN:* nape nevus

Unna stain—an alkaline methylene blue stain for plasma cells.

Unna syndrome—*SYN:* seborrheic dermatitis

Unna-Pappenheim stain—a contrast stain used to detect RNA and DNA in tissue sections; used to demonstrate plasma cells during chronic inflammation.

Unna-Taenzer stain—*SYN:* Taenzer stain

Unschuld, Paul, German internist, 1835–1905.

Unschuld sign—a tendency toward cramps in the calves of the legs.

Unverricht, Heinrich, German physician, 1853–1912.

Unverricht disease—a progressive myoclonic epilepsy. *SYN:* Unverricht syndrome

Unverricht syndrome—*SYN:* Unverricht disease

Urbach, Erich, dermatologist, 1893–1946.

Urbach-Wiethe disease—a disturbance of lipid metabolism. *SYN:* lipoid proteinosis

Urban, Jerome A., surgeon, *1914.

Urban operation—extended radical mastectomy, including en bloc resection of internal mammary lymph nodes, part of the sternum, and costal cartilages.

Urban retractor

Usher, Barney, Canadian dermatologist, *1899.

Senear-Usher disease—*SYN:* Senear-Usher syndrome

Senear-Usher syndrome—see under Senear

Usher, Charles Howard, English ophthalmologist, 1865–1942.

Usher syndrome—sensorineural hearing loss and retinitis pigmentosa.

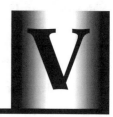

Vaduz, city in Liechtenstein.

    Vaduz hand—below-the-elbow prosthesis with a myoelectric hand. *SYN:* French electric hand

Valentin, Gabriel G., German-Swiss physiologist, 1810–1883.

    Valentin corpuscles—small bodies, probably amyloid, found occasionally in nerve tissue.

    Valentin ganglion—a ganglion on the superior alveolar nerve.

    Valentin nerve—a nerve that connects the pterygopalatine ganglion with the abducens nerve.

Valentine, Ferdinand C., U.S. surgeon, 1851–1909.

    Valentine irrigation tube

    Valentine irrigator

    Valentine position—a supine position on a table used to facilitate urethral irrigation.

    Valentine test—the bladder is emptied by passing urine into a series of 3-ounce test tubes, and the contents of the first and the last are examined. *SYN:* three-glass test

    Valentine tube

Valleix, François L. I., French physician, 1807–1855.

    Valleix points—various points in the course of a nerve, pressure upon which is painful in cases of neuralgia.

Valsalva, Antonio M., Italian anatomist, 1666–1723.

    aneurysm of sinus of Valsalva—a congenital thin-walled tubular outpouching usually in the right or noncoronary sinus with an entirely intracardiac course.

    teniae of Valsalva—the three bands in which the longitudinal muscular fibers of the large intestine, except the rectum, are collected. *SYN:* teniae coli

    Valsalva antrum—a cavity in the petrous portion of the temporal bone. *SYN:* mastoid antrum

    Valsalva ligaments—the three ligaments that attach the auricle to the side of the head. *SYN:* auricular ligaments

    Valsalva maneuver—any forced expiratory effort against a closed airway.

    Valsalva muscle—a band of vertical muscular fibers on the outer surface of the tragus of the ear. *SYN:* tragicus muscle

    Valsalva sinus—the space between the superior aspect of each cusp of the aortic valve and the dilated portion of the wall of the ascending aorta. *SYN:* aortic sinus

(continued)

Valsalva *(continued)*
> **Valsalva test**—when the heart is monitored during the Valsalva maneuver, there is a characteristic complex sequence of cardiocirculatory events, departure from which indicates disease or malfunction.

van Bogaert, Ludo, Belgian neurologist, *1897.
> **Canavan-van Bogaert-Bertrand disease**—*SYN:* Canavan disease
> **Nyssen-van Bogaert-Meyer syndrome**—see under Nyssen
> **van Bogaert disease**
> **van Bogaert encephalitis**—a rare chronic, progressive encephalitis that affects primarily children and young adults, caused by the measles virus. *SYN:* subacute sclerosing panencephalitis

van Buchem, Francis Steven Peter, Dutch internist, *1897.
> **van Buchem syndrome**—an inherited skeletal dysplasia. *SYN:* generalized cortical hyperostosis

van Buren, William H., U.S. surgeon, 1819–1883.
> **van Buren disease**—*SYN:* Peyronie disease
> **van Buren sound**—a standard sound used for urethral calibration or dilation.

van Creveld, S., Dutch pediatrician, *1894.
> **Ellis-van Creveld syndrome**—see under Ellis, Richard

van Deen, Izaak A., Dutch physiologist, 1804–1869.
> **van Deen test**—*SYN:* Almén test for blood

van den Bergh, A.A. Hymans, Dutch physician, 1869–1943.
> **van den Bergh reaction**—*SYN:* van den Bergh test
> **van den Bergh test**—a test for bilirubin. *SYN:* van den Bergh reaction

van der Kolk, Jacobus L.C.S., Dutch physician, 1797–1862.
> **van der Kolk law**—in a mixed nerve, the sensory fibers are distributed to the parts moved by the muscles controlled by the motor fibers.

van der Velden, Reinhardt, German physician, 1851–1903.
> **van der Velden test**—a test for free hydrochloric acid.

van der Waals, Johannes D., Dutch physicist and Nobel laureate, 1837–1923.
> **van der Waals forces**—explains deviations from ideal gas behavior seen in real gases. *SYN:* London forces

van Ekenstein, W.A., 19th century scientist.
> **Lobry de Bruyn-van Ekenstein transformation**—see under Lobry de Bruyn

van Ermengen, Emile P., Belgian bacteriologist, 1851–1932.
> **van Ermengen stain**—a method for staining flagella.

van Gieson, Ira, U.S. histologist and bacteriologist, 1865–1913.
> **van Gieson stain**—a mixture of acid fuchsin in saturated picric acid solution, used in collagen staining.

van Helmont, Jean B., Flemish physician and chemist, 1577–1644.
> **van Helmont mirror**—obsolete term for central tendon of diaphragm.

van Horne, Jan (Johannes), Dutch anatomist, 1621–1670.
    van Horne canal—the largest lymph vessel in the body, beginning at the cisterna chyli at about the level of the second lumbar vertebra. *Syn:* thoracic duct

Van Slyke, Donald D., U.S. biochemist, 1883–1971.
    slyke—a unit of buffer value, the slope of the acid-base titration curve of a solution.
    Van Slyke apparatus—an apparatus for determining the amounts of respiratory gases in the blood.
    Van Slyke formula—the value obtained when the square root of the urine flow is multiplied by the urine urea concentration and divided by the whole blood urea concentration. *Syn:* standard urea clearance

van't Hoff, Jacobus H., Dutch chemist and Nobel laureate, 1852–1911.
    Le Bel-van't Hoff rule—see under Le Bel
    van't Hoff equation—equation for osmotic pressure of dilute solutions for any reaction.
    van't Hoff law—in stereochemistry, all optically active substances have one or more multivalent atoms united to four different atoms or radicals so as to form in space an unsymmetrical arrangement.
    van't Hoff theory—that substances in dilute solution obey the gas laws.

Vane, Sir John R., joint winner of 1982 Nobel Prize for work related to prostaglandins.

Vaquez, Louis H., French physician, 1860–1936.
    Vaquez disease—a chronic form of polycythemia characterized by bone marrow hyperplasia. *Syn:* polycythemia vera

Varmus, Harold E., joint winner of 1989 Nobel Prize for work related to oncogenes.

Varolius, Constantius (Costanzio), Italian anatomist and physician, 1543–1575.
    pons varolii—(1) in neuroanatomy, the pons varolii or pons cerebelli; (2) any bridgelike formation connecting two more or less disjoined parts of the same structure or organ. *Syn:* pons
    valve of Varolius—the bilabial prominence of the terminal ileum into the large intestine at the cecocolic junction as seen in cadavers. *Syn:* ileocecal valve

Vater, Abraham, German anatomist and botanist, 1684–1751.
    Vater ampulla—the dilation within the major duodenal papilla that normally receives both the common bile duct and the main pancreatic duct. *Syn:* hepatopancreatic ampulla
    Vater corpuscles—small oval bodies in the skin of the fingers, in the mesentery, tendons, and elsewhere sensitive to pressure. *Syn:* lamellated corpuscles; pacinian corpuscles; Vater-Pacini corpuscles
    Vater fold—a fold of mucous membrane in the duodenum just above the greater duodenal papilla.

(continued)

NOTES

Vater *(continued)*
    Vater tubercle—duodenal papilla. *SYN:* papilla of Santorini
    Vater-Pacini corpuscles—*SYN:* Vater corpuscles

Vella, Luigi, Italian physiologist, 1825–1886.
    Thiry-Vella fistula—see under Thiry
    Vella fistula—*SYN:* Thiry-Vella fistula

Velpeau, Alfred A.L.M., French surgeon, 1795–1867.
    Velpeau axillary lateral view
    Velpeau axillary radiograph
    Velpeau bandage—a bandage which serves to immobilize arm to chest wall, with the forearm positioned obliquely across and upward on front of chest.
    Velpeau canal—passage through the layers of the lower abdominal wall that transmits the spermatic cord in the male and the round ligament in the female. *SYN:* inguinal canal
    Velpeau cast
    Velpeau deformity
    Velpeau dressing
    Velpeau fossa—a wedge-shaped space with its base toward the perineum. *SYN:* ischiorectal fossa
    Velpeau hernia—femoral hernia in which the intestine is in front of the blood vessels.
    Velpeau shoulder immobilizer
    Velpeau sling
    Velpeau stockinette
    Velpeau tendon transfer
    Velpeau wrap

Venable, Charles Scott, U.S. surgeon.
    Venable plates and screws
    Venable screw
    Venable-Stuck fracture pin
    Venable-Stuck nail

Venn, John, English logician and philosopher, 1834–1923.
    Venn diagram—pictorial representation of the extent to which two or more quantities or concepts are mutually inclusive and exclusive.

Venturi, Giovanni B., Italian physicist, 1746–1822.
    Venturi apparatus
    Venturi aspiration vitrectomy device
    Venturi bobbin myringotomy tube
    Venturi collar button myringotomy tube
    Venturi effect—term applied to the operation of a Venturi tube and similar systems.
    Venturi grommet myringotomy tube
    Venturi insufflator
    Venturi mask
    Venturi meter—a device for measuring flow of a fluid.
    Venturi pediatric myringotomy tube
    Venturi spirometer

Venturi tube—a tube with a specially streamlined constriction.
Venturi ventilator

Verbrugge, Jean, Belgian orthopedic surgeon, 1896–1964.
    Verbrugge bone-holding clamp
    Verbrugge clamp
    Verbrugge forceps
    Verbrugge needle
    Verbrugge retractor

Verga, Andrea, Italian neurologist, 1811–1895.
    cavum vergae—*SYN:* Verga ventricle
    Verga ventricle—an inconstant, horizontal, slitlike space between the posterior one-third of the corpus callosum and the underlying commissura fornicis resulting from failure of these two commissural plates to fuse completely during fetal development. *SYN:* cavum vergae; cavum psalterii; sixth ventricle

V

Verheyen, Philippe, Flemish anatomist, 1648–1710.
    stellulae verheyenii—*SYN:* venulae stellatae
    Verheyen stars—the star-shaped groups of venules in the renal cortex. *SYN:* venulae stellatae

Verhoeff, Frederick H., U.S. ophthalmologist, 1874–1968.
    Verhoeff advancement
    Verhoeff capsule forceps
    Verhoeff cataract forceps
    Verhoeff dissecting scissors
    Verhoeff elastic tissue stain
    Verhoeff expressor
    Verhoeff operation
    Verhoeff scissors
    Verhoeff sclerotomy
    Verhoeff suture

Verner, John, U.S. internist, *1927.
    Verner-Morrison syndrome—watery diarrhea, hypokalemia, and achlorhydria associated with secretion of vasoactive intestinal polypeptide by a pancreatic islet-cell tumor in the absence of gastric hypersecretion. *SYN:* WDHA syndrome

Vernet, Maurice, French neurologist, *1887.
    Vernet syndrome—paralysis of the motor components of the glossopharyngeal, vagus, and accessory cranial nerves, most commonly the result of head injury.

Verneuil, Aristide A., French surgeon, 1823–1895.
    hidradenitis axillaris of Verneuil—an axillary abscess.
    Verneuil neuroma—a nodular enlargement of the cutaneous nerves.

NOTES

Vernier, Pierre, French mathematician, 1580–1637.
    Vernier acuity—detection of displacement of a portion of a line.

Verocay, José, Czech pathologist, 1876–1927.
    Verocay bodies—hyalinized acellular areas seen microscopically in neurilemomas.

Vesalius, Andreas (Andre), Flemish anatomist, 1514–1564.
    Vesalius bone—the tuberosity of the fifth metatarsal bone sometimes existing as a separate bone. *SYN:* os vesalianum
    Vesalius foramen—a minute inconstant foramen in the greater wing of the sphenoid bone. *SYN:* foramen venosum
    Vesalius vein—the emissary vein passing through the foramen venosum.

Vicat, L.J., French engineer, 1786–1861.
    Vicat needle—a device for obtaining the setting time of plaster and other materials.

Vicq d'Azyr, Félix, French anatomist, 1748–1794.
    Vicq d'Azyr bundle—a compact, thick bundle of nerve fibers that passes from the mamillary body to terminate in the anterior nucleus of the thalamus. *SYN:* mamillothalamic fasciculus
    Vicq d'Azyr centrum semiovale—the great mass of white matter composing the interior of the cerebral hemisphere. *SYN:* centrum semiovale
    Vicq d'Azyr foramen—a small triangular depression at the lower boundary of the pons that marks the upper limit of the median fissure of the medulla oblongata. *SYN:* foramen cecum medullae oblongatae

Vidal, Jean Baptiste Emile, French dermatologist, 1825–1893.
    Vidal disease—obsolete term for lichen simplex chronicus.

Vidius, Guidi (Guido), Italian anatomist and physician, 1500–1569.
    vidian artery—*SYN:* artery of pterygoid canal
    vidian canal—an opening through the base of the medial pterygoid process of the sphenoid bone through which pass the artery, vein, and nerve of the pterygoid canal. *SYN:* pterygoid canal
    vidian nerve—the nerve constituting the parasympathetic and sympathetic root of the pterygopalatine ganglion. *SYN:* nerve of pterygoid canal
    vidian vein—a vein accompanying the nerve and artery through the pterygoid canal and emptying into the pharyngeal venous plexus. *SYN:* vein of pterygoid canal

Viel, P.
    Terrien-Viel syndrome—see under Terrien

Vierordt, Karl, German physiologist, 1818–1884.
    Vierordt law—principle used to determine two-point threshold for a stimulus.

Vierra, J.P., 20th century Brazilian dermatologist.
    Vierra sign—yellowing and canalization of the nail.

Vieussens, Raymond de, French anatomist, 1641–1715.
    valve of Vieussens—a prominent valve in the great cardiac vein where it turns around the obtuse margin to become the coronary sinus.
    Vieussens annulus—*SYN:* Vieussens ring

Vieussens ansa—*Syn:* Vieussens loop

Vieussens centrum—the great mass of white matter composing the interior of the cerebral hemisphere. *Syn:* centrum semiovale

Vieussens foramina—a number of fossae in the wall of the right atrium, containing the openings of minute intramural veins. *Syn:* foramina of the venae minimae

Vieussens ganglia—the largest and highest group of prevertebral sympathetic ganglia, located on the superior part of the abdominal aorta, on either side of the origin of the celiac artery. *Syn:* celiac ganglia

Vieussens isthmus—*Syn:* Vieussens ring

Vieussens limbus—*Syn:* Vieussens ring

Vieussens loop—a nerve cord connecting the middle cervical and stellate sympathetic ganglia, forming a loop around the subclavian artery. *Syn:* ansa subclavia; Vieussens ansa

Vieussens ring—a muscular ring surrounding the fossa ovalis in the wall of the right atrium of the heart. *Syn:* limbus fossae ovalis; Vieussens annulus; Vieussens isthmus; Vieussens limbus

Vieussens valve—the thin layer of white matter stretching between the two superior cerebellar peduncles forming the roof of the superior recess of the fourth ventricle. *Syn:* superior medullary velum

Vieussens veins—the small superficial veins of the heart. *Syn:* innominate cardiac veins

Vieussens ventricle—a slitlike fluid-filled space of variable width between the left and right transparent septum. *Syn:* cavity of septum pellucidum

Vigotsky, Lev Semionovich, Russian psychologist, 1896–1934.

Vigotsky test—used to study thinking and concept formation process; also used to detect ability to think in abstract and to detect thought disturbance.

Vincent, Henri, French physician, 1862–1950.

Vincent angina—an ulcerative infection of the oral soft tissues, including the tonsils and pharynx, caused by fusiform and spirochetal organisms.

Vincent bacillus—probably *Fusobacterium nucleatum.*

Vincent disease—*Syn:* necrotizing ulcerative gingivitis

Vincent spirillum—the spirillum or spirochete found in association with Vincent bacillus. *Fusobacterium nucleatum* is frequently the only bacillus isolated.

Vincent tonsillitis—angina limited chiefly to the tonsils, caused by Vincent organisms (bacillus and spirillum).

Vincent white mycetoma—mycetoma caused by *Actinomadura madurae* and occurring in North Africa, India, Argentina, and Cuba.

Vineberg, Arthur M., Canadian thoracic surgeon, *1903.

Vineberg procedure—implantation of the internal mammary artery into the myocardium to improve blood flow to the heart.

Vinson, Porter P., U.S. surgeon, 1890–1959.

Plummer-Vinson syndrome—see under Plummer

NOTES

Vipond, French physician.

Vipond sign—generalized adenopathy occurring during the period of incubation of various exanthemas of childhood.

Virchow, Rudolf, German pathologist and politician, 1821–1902.

Virchow angle—an angle formed by the meeting of a line drawn from the middle of the nasofrontal suture to the base of the anterior nasal spine, with a line drawn from this last point to the center of the external auditory meatus. *SYN:* Virchow-Holder angle

Virchow cells—(1) the lacunae in osseous tissue containing the bone cells; also the bone cells themselves; (2) connective tissue cells between the laminae of fibrous tissue in the cornea. *SYN:* corneal corpuscles; Virchow corpuscles

Virchow corpuscles—*SYN:* Virchow cells (2)

Virchow crystals—yellow-brown, amber, or burnt orange crystals of hematoidin, frequently observed in extravasated blood in tissues.

Virchow disease—acute congenital encephalitis, a condition in which the head is abnormally large. *SYN:* megacephaly

Virchow law—there is no special or distinctive neoplastic cell inasmuch as the component cells of neoplasms originate from preexisting forms.

Virchow node—a firm, palpable supraclavicular lymph node that may be the first recognized presumptive evidence of a malignant neoplasm in one of the viscera. *SYN:* signal node

Virchow psammoma—a firm, cellular neoplasm derived from fibrous tissue of the meninges, choroid plexus, and certain other brain structures. *SYN:* psammomatous meningioma

Virchow triad—factors predisposing vascular thrombosis.

Virchow-Hassall bodies—*SYN:* Hassall bodies

Virchow-Holder angle—*SYN:* Virchow angle

Virchow-Robin space—a tunnel-like extension of the subarachnoid space surrounding blood vessels that pass into the brain or spinal cord from the subarachnoid space. *SYN:* His perivascular space

Vladimiroff, Vladimir D., Russian surgeon, 1837–1903.

Mikulicz-Vladimiroff amputation—see under Mikulicz

Vladimiroff-Mikulicz amputation—*SYN:* Mikulicz-Vladimiroff amputation

Voges, Daniel Wilhelm Otto, German physician, *1867.

Voges-Proskauer reaction—a chemical reaction used in testing for the production of acetyl methyl carbinol by various bacteria.

Vogt, Alfred, Swiss ophthalmologist, 1879–1943.

Vogt-Koyanagi syndrome—bilateral uveitis with iritis and glaucoma, premature graying of the hair, alopecia, vitiligo, and dysacusia. *SYN:* oculocutaneous syndrome; uveocutaneous syndrome

Vogt, Cécile, 1875–1962 and Oskar, 1870–1959, German neurologists.

Vogt syndrome—a type of cerebral palsy. *SYN:* double athetosis

Vogt, Heinrich, German neurologist, *1875.

Spielmeyer-Vogt disease—*SYN:* Batten disease

Vogt-Spielmeyer disease—*SYN:* Batten disease

Vogt, Karl, German physiologist, 1817–1895.

Vogt angle—a craniometric angle formed by the nasobasilar and alveolonasal lines.

Got a Good Word for STEDMAN'S?

Help us keep STEDMAN'S products fresh and up-to-date with new words and new ideas!

Do we need to add or revise any items? Is there a better way to organize the content?

Be specific! How can we make this STEDMAN'S product the best medical word reference possible for you? Fill in the lines below with your thoughts and recommendations. Attach a separate sheet of paper if you need to— *you* are our most important contributor and we want to know what's on *your* mind. Thanks!

(PLEASE TYPE OR PRINT CAREFULLY)

Terms you believe are incorrect:

Appears as: Suggested revision:

_____   _____

_____   _____

_____   _____

New terms you would like us to add:

_____

_____

Other comments:

_____

_____

_____

All done? Great, just mail this card in today. No postage necessary, and thanks again!

Name / Title:

Facility / Company:

Address:

City / State / Zip:

Day Telephone No. (   )

Lippincott Williams & Wilkins
351 West Camden Street
Baltimore, Maryland 21201-2436

To order or to receive a catalog
call toll free 1-800-527-5597.

BUSINESS REPLY MAIL

FIRST CLASS   PERMIT NO. 724   BALTIMORE, MD

POSTAGE WILL BE PAID BY ADDRESSEE

ATTN: STEDMAN'S EDITORIAL TEAM
LIPPINCOTT WILLIAMS & WILKINS
351 W. CAMDEN STREET
BALTIMORE   MD   21201-9801

Voigt, Christian A., Austrian anatomist, 1809–1890.
  Voigt lines—*SYN:* Futcher line

Volhard, Franz, German physician, 1872–1950.
  Volhard test—a test for renal function.

Volkmann, Alfred W., German physiologist, 1800–1877.
  Volkmann canals—vascular canals in compact bone that are not
  surrounded by concentric lamellae of bone.
  Volkmann membrane

Volkmann, Richard, German surgeon, 1830–1889.
  Volkmann bone curet
  Volkmann bone hook
  Volkmann cheilitis—an acquired disorder, of unknown etiology of the
  lower lip, characterized by swelling, ulceration, crusting, mucous gland
  hyperplasia, abscesses, and sinus tracts. *SYN:* cheilitis glandularis
  Volkmann claw hand deformity
  Volkmann contracture—ischemic contracture resulting from irreversible
  necrosis of muscle tissue, produced by a compartment syndrome.
  Volkmann fracture
  Volkmann ischemia
  Volkmann ischemic contracture
  Volkmann ischemic paralysis
  Volkmann rake retractor
  Volkmann splint
  Volkmann spoon—a sharp spoon for scraping away carious bone or other
  diseased tissue.
  Volkmann subluxation

Vollmer, Herman, U.S. pediatrician, 1896–1959.
  Vollmer test—a tuberculin patch test.

Volpe, Anthony R., U.S. dentist, *1932.
  Volpe-Manhold Index—an index for comparing the amount of dental
  calculus in individuals.

Voltolini, Friedrich E.R., German laryngologist, 1819–1889.
  Voltolini disease—disease of the labyrinth leading to deaf-mutism in
  young children.

von Behring, Emil A. See under Behring.

von Békésy, Georg. See under Békésy.

von Brunn, Albert. See under Brunn.

von Bruns, Ludwig. See under Bruns.

von Ebner, Victor, Austrian histologist, 1842–1925.
  Ebner glands—serous glands of the tongue opening in the bottom of the
  trough surrounding the circumvallate papillae.

(continued)

NOTES

von Ebner *(continued)*
    Ebner reticulum—a network of nucleated cells in the seminiferous tubules.
    imbrication lines of von Ebner—incremental lines in the dentin of the tooth that reflect variations in mineralization during dentin formation. *SYN:* incremental lines of von Ebner
    incremental lines of von Ebner—*SYN:* imbrication lines of von Ebner

von Economo, Constantin, Austrian neurologist, 1876–1931.
    Economo disease—*SYN:* von Economo disease
    von Economo disease—the basis for postencephalitic parkinsonism, suspected to be of viral origin. *SYN:* polioencephalitis infectiva; encephalitis lethargica; sleeping sickness; Economo disease

von Gierke, Edgar. See under Gierke.

von Graefe, Albrecht. See under Graefe.

von Hansemann, D.P., German pathologist, 1858–1920.
    Hansemann macrophages—large cells associated with a granulomatous condition primarily affecting the urinary tract.

von Heine, Jacob, German orthopedist, 1800–1879.
    Heine-Medin disease—poliomyelitis or infantile paralysis.

von Hippel, Eugen, German ophthalmologist, 1867–1939.
    Hippel keratoplasty
    Hippel trephine
    von Hippel disease—retinal hemangiomatosis.
    von Hippel-Lindau syndrome—a type of phacomatosis, consisting of hemangiomas of the retina associated with hemangiomas or hemangioblastomas primarily of the cerebellum and walls of the fourth ventricle, occasionally involving the spinal cord. *SYN:* cerebroretinal angiomatosis; Lindau disease

von Kossa, Julius, 19th century Austrian-Hungarian pathologist.
    Kossa stain—*SYN:* von Kossa stain
    von Kossa stain—a stain for calcium in mineralized tissue. *SYN:* Kossa stain

von Linné, Carl. See under Linné.

von Meyenburg, H. See under Meyenburg.

von Recklinghausen, Friedrich D. See under Recklinghausen.

von Restorff, Hedwig, German psychologist.
    von Restorff effect—memory process theory.

von Schrötter, Leopold. See under Schrötter.

von Spee, Ferdinand Graf. See under Spee.

von Willebrand, Erik A., Finnish physician, 1870–1949.
    von Willebrand disease—a hemorrhagic diathesis characterized by the tendency to bleed primarily from mucous membranes.

Voorhoeve, N., Dutch radiologist, 1879–1927.
    Voorhoeve disease—linear striations seen radiographically in the metaphyses of long and flat bones. *SYN:* osteopathia striata

Vossius, Adolf, German pathologist, 1855–1925.

Vossius lenticular ring—a ring-shaped opacity found on the anterior lens capsule after contusion of the eye.

Vulpian, Edme F.A., French physician, 1826–1887.

Vulpian atrophy—progressive spinal muscular atrophy beginning in the shoulder. *Syn:* scapulohumeral atrophy

V

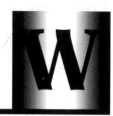

Waage, P., Norwegian chemist, 1833–1900.
  Guldberg-Waage law—see under Guldberg

Waaler, Erik, 20th century Norwegian biologist.
  Rose-Waaler test—see under Rose, H.M.

Waardenburg, Petrus Johannes, Dutch ophthalmologist, 1886–1979.
  Waardenburg syndrome—*SYN:* type IV acrocephalosyndactyly

Wachendorf, Eberhard J., German botanist and anatomist, 1702–1758.
  Wachendorf membrane—the protoplasmic boundary of all cells that
    controls permeability and may serve other functions through surface
    specializations. *SYN:* cell membrane; pupillary membrane

Wachstein, Max, U.S. histologist and pathologist, 1905–1965.
  Wachstein-Meissel stain for calcium-magnesium-ATPase—enzyme activity
    is generally demonstrated at cell membranes.

Wachter, Herman J.G., German pathologist, *1878.
  Bracht-Wachter bodies—see under Bracht
  Bracht-Wachter lesion—see under Bracht

Wada, John A., Japanese-Canadian neurosurgeon, *1924.
  Wada test—unilateral internal carotid injection of amobarbital to
    determine the laterality of speech.

Wadsworth, Guy W. Jr., U.S. psychologist, *1901.
  Humm-Wadsworth Temperament Scale—personality inventory.

Wagner, Hans, Swiss ophthalmologist, *1905.
  Wagner disease—progressive liquefaction and destruction of the vitreous
    humor with grayish-white preretinal membranes, myopia, cataract, retinal
    detachment, and hyperpigmentation and hypopigmentation. *SYN:*
    hyaloideoretinal degeneration; Wagner syndrome
  Wagner syndrome—*SYN:* Wagner disease

Wagner-Jauregg, Julius, 1927 Nobel Prize winner for work related to malaria
  inoculation for treating dementia paralytica.

Wagstaffe, William, English surgeon, 1843–1910.
  Wagstaffe fracture—fracture with displacement of the medial malleolus.

Waksman, Selman Abraham, winner of 1952 Nobel Prize for discovery of
  streptomycin.

Walcher, Gustav A., German obstetrician, 1856–1935.
  Walcher position—obsolete term for a supine position of the parturient
    woman with the lower extremities falling over the edge of the table.

Wald, George, joint winner of 1967 Nobel Prize for work related to the eye.

Waldenström, Jan G., Swedish physician, *1906.
Waldenström macroglobulinemia—*SYN:* hyperglobulinemic purpura; Waldenström purpura; Waldenström syndrome
Waldenström purpura—*SYN:* Waldenström macroglobulinemia
Waldenström syndrome—*SYN:* Waldenström macroglobulinemia
Waldenström test—a test for porphyrin in the urine.

Waldeyer, Heinrich G. von, German anatomist and pathologist, 1836–1921.
Waldeyer fascia—rectal fascia.
Waldeyer fluid
Waldeyer forceps
Waldeyer fossae
Waldeyer glands—glands near the margins of the eyelids.
Waldeyer sheath—*SYN:* Waldeyer space
Waldeyer space—the tubular space between the bladder wall and the intramural portion of the ureter. *SYN:* Waldeyer sheath
Waldeyer sulcus
Waldeyer throat ring—the broken ring of lymphoid tissue, formed of the lingual, faucial, and pharyngeal tonsils. *SYN:* lymphoid ring
Waldeyer tract—*SYN:* Waldeyer zonal layer
Waldeyer zonal layer—a longitudinal bundle of thin, unmyelinated and poorly myelinated fibers capping the apex of the posterior horn of the spinal gray matter. *SYN:* dorsolateral fasciculus; Waldeyer tract

Walker, Arthur Earl, U.S. neurologist, *1907.
Dandy-Walker syndrome—see under Dandy
Walker tractotomy—a mesencephalic spinothalamic tractotomy.
Walker-Warburg syndrome—a congenital disorder, usually fatal before age one.

Walker, J.T. Ainslie, English chemist, 1868–1930.
Rideal-Walker coefficient—see under Rideal
Rideal-Walker method

Walker, James, English gynecologist, *1916.
Walker chart—a system of plotting the relative fetal and placental sizes.

Wallace, Alexander Burns, Scottish plastic surgeon, *1903.
Wallace rule of nines—a guide to assist estimating proportion of body surface affected by burns.

Wallenberg, Adolf, German physician, 1862–1949.
Wallenberg syndrome—a syndrome due usually to thrombosis. *SYN:* posterior inferior cerebellar artery syndrome

Waller, Augustus V., English physiologist, 1816–1870.
wallerian degeneration—degenerative changes in the distal segment of a peripheral nerve fiber when its continuity with its cell body is interrupted by a focal lesion. *SYN:* orthograde degeneration; secondary degeneration

Walshe, J.J., U.S. physician.
Magoss-Walshe syndrome—see under Magoss

Walthard, Max, Swiss gynecologist, 1867–1933.
> **Walthard cell rest**—a nest of epithelial cells occurring in the peritoneum of the uterine tubes or ovary.

Walther, August F., German anatomist, 1688–1746.
> **Walther canals**—from 8 to 20 small ducts of the sublingual salivary gland that open into the mouth on the surface of the sublingual fold. *SYN:* minor sublingual ducts; Walther ducts
> **Walther ducts**—*SYN:* Walther canals
> **Walther ganglion**—the most inferior, unpaired ganglion of the sympathetic trunk. *SYN:* ganglion impar
> **Walther plexus**—the portion of the internal carotid plexus in the cavernous sinus. *SYN:* intracavernous plexus

Walther, Augustine Friedrich, German surgeon and gynecologist, 1688–1746.
> **Walther catheter**
> **Walther clamp**
> **Walther dilator**
> **Walther forceps**
> **Walther sound**
> **Walther tissue forceps**
> **Walther trocar**

Wang, Chung T., Chinese pathologist, 1889–1931.
> **Wang test**—a quantitative test for indican.

Wangensteen, Owen H., U.S. surgeon, 1898–1981.
> **Wangensteen apparatus**
> **Wangensteen awl**
> **Wangensteen carrier**
> **Wangensteen clamp**
> **Wangensteen colostomy**
> **Wangensteen dissector**
> **Wangensteen drain**
> **Wangensteen drainage**—continuous drainage by suction through an indwelling gastric or duodenal tube.
> **Wangensteen dressing**
> **Wangensteen duodenal tube**
> **Wangensteen forceps**
> **Wangensteen herniorrhaphy**
> **Wangensteen needle**
> **Wangensteen needle holder**
> **Wangensteen suction**—a modified siphon that maintains constant negative pressure, used with a duodenal tube for the relief of gastric and intestinal distention. *SYN:* Wangensteen tube
> **Wangensteen tissue inverter**
> **Wangensteen trocar**
> **Wangensteen tube**—*SYN:* Wangensteen suction

W

NOTES

Warburg, Mette, 20th century Danish physician.
  Walker-Warburg syndrome—see under Walker, Arthur

Warburg, Otto, German biochemist and Nobel laureate, 1883–1970.
  Barcroft-Warburg apparatus—*SYN:* Warburg apparatus
  Barcroft-Warburg technique—*SYN:* Warburg apparatus
  Warburg apparatus—an apparatus for measuring the oxygen consumption of incubated tissue slices by manometric measurement of changes in gas pressure produced by oxygen absorption in an enclosed flask. *SYN:* Barcroft-Warburg apparatus; Barcroft-Warburg technique
  Warburg old yellow enzyme—a flavoprotein oxidizing NADPH to NADP$^+$. *SYN:* NADPH dehydrogenase
  Warburg respiratory enzyme—a system of cytochromes and their oxidases that participate in respiratory processes. *SYN:* Atmungsferment
  Warburg theory—that the development of cancer is due to irreversible damage to the respiratory mechanism of cells, leading to the selective multiplication of cells with increased glycolytic metabolism, both aerobic and anaerobic.
  Warburg-Lipmann-Dickens-Horecker shunt—*SYN:* Dickens shunt

Ward, Frederick O., English osteologist, 1818–1877.
  Ward triangle—an area of diminished density in the trabecular pattern of the neck of the femur, evident by x-ray as well as by direct inspection.

Ward, O.C., 20th century Irish pediatrician.
  Romano-Ward syndrome—see under Romano
  Ward-Romano syndrome—*SYN:* Romano-Ward syndrome

Wardrop, James, English surgeon, 1782–1869.
  Wardrop disease—acute onychia occurring spontaneously in debilitated patients, or in response to slight trauma. *SYN:* onychia maligna
  Wardrop method—for treatment of aneurysm.

Warfarin, Wisconsin Alumni Research Foundation (WARF).
  Warfarin—oral anticoagulant, named for the foundation.

Warm Springs, Georgia Warm Springs Foundation, where the crutch was made.
  Warm Springs crutch—*SYN:* Everett crutch

Warren, W. Dean, U.S. surgeon, 1924–1989.
  Warren flap
  Warren incision
  Warren shunt—anastomosis of the splenic end of the divided splenic vein to the left renal vein. *SYN:* distal splenorenal shunt
  Warren-Mack rotating drill

Wartenberg, Robert, German neurologist, 1887–1956.
  Wartenberg sign –inability to adduct 5th digit
  Wartenberg symptom—intense pruritus of the tip of the nose and nostrils in cases of cerebral tumor.

Warthin, Aldred S., U.S. pathologist, 1866–1931.
  Warthin area
  Warthin tumor—a benign glandular tumor, usually arising in the parotid gland. *SYN:* adenolymphoma
  Warthin-Finkeldey cells—giant cells with multiple overlapping nuclei,

found in lymphoid tissue in measles, especially during the prodromal stage. *SYN:* Finkeldey cells

Warthin-Starry silver stain—a stain for spirochetes in which preparations are incubated in 1% silver nitrate solution followed by a developer.

Warthin-Starry staining method

Wasmann, Adolphus, 19th century German anatomist.
Wasmann glands—branched tubular glands lying in the mucosa of the fundus and body of the stomach. *SYN:* gastric glands

Wassermann, August P. von, German bacteriologist, 1866–1925.
provocative Wassermann test—an obsolete test of historical interest only.
Wassermann antibody—antibody evoked during syphilitic infections.
Wassermann reaction—*SYN:* Wassermann test
Wassermann test—a complement-fixation test used in the diagnosis of syphilis. *SYN:* Wassermann reaction

Waterhouse, Rupert, English physician, 1873–1958.
Friderichsen-Waterhouse syndrome—*SYN:* Waterhouse-Friderichsen syndrome
Waterhouse-Friderichsen syndrome—a condition characterized by vomiting, diarrhea, extensive purpura, cyanosis, tonic-clonic convulsions, and circulatory collapse. *SYN:* acute fulminating meningococcal septicemia; Friderichsen-Waterhouse syndrome; Friderichsen syndrome

Waters, Charles Alexander, U.S. radiologist, 1888–1961.
Waters view radiograph—*SYN:* maxillary sinus radiograph

Waters, Edward G., U.S. obstetrician and gynecologist, *1898.
Waters operation—an extraperitoneal cesarean section with a supravesical approach.
Waters position

Waterston, David J., English thoracic and pediatric surgeon, *1910.
Waterston operation—a surgically created anastomosis between the pulmonary artery and the ascending aorta to palliate adult tetralogy of Fallot.
Waterston shunt—creation of a narrow opening between the ascending aorta and the subjacent right pulmonary artery.

Watson, James D., U.S. geneticist and Nobel laureate, *1928.
Watson-Crick helix—the helical structure assumed by two strands of deoxyribonucleic acid. *SYN:* DNA helix; double helix; twin helix

Watson-Jones, Sir Reginald, English orthopedic surgeon, 1902–1972.
Watson-Jones anterior approach
Watson-Jones approach
Watson-Jones arthrodesis
Watson-Jones bone gouge
Watson-Jones bone lever

W

(continued)

NOTES

Watson-Jones *(continued)*
    Watson-Jones classification of tibial tubercle avulsion fracture
    Watson-Jones dressing
    Watson-Jones elevator
    Watson-Jones fracture repair
    Watson-Jones frame
    Watson-Jones gouge
    Watson-Jones guide pin
    Watson-Jones incision
    Watson-Jones lateral approach
    Watson-Jones ligament reconstruction
    Watson-Jones nail
    Watson-Jones operation
    Watson-Jones procedure
    Watson-Jones reconstruction
    Watson-Jones repair
    Watson-Jones tibial fracture classification
    Watson-Jones traction
    Watson-Jones tractor

Way, Stanley, English obstetrician-gynecologist.
    Stanley Way procedure—a radical vulvectomy.
    Way operation

Weber, Ernst H., German physiologist and anatomist, 1795–1878.
    Fechner-Weber law—*Syn:* Weber-Fechner law
    Weber experiment—if the peripheral end of the divided vagus nerve is stimulated, the heart is arrested in diastole.
    Weber glands—muciparous glands at the border of the tongue on either side posteriorly.
    Weber law—*Syn:* Weber-Fechner law
    Weber paradox—if a muscle is loaded beyond its power to contract, it may elongate.
    Weber test for hearing—using a vibrating tuning fork.
    Weber-Fechner law—the intensity of a sensation varies by a series of equal increments as the strength of the stimulus is increased geometrically. *Syn:* Fechner-Weber law; Weber law

Weber, Frederick Parkes, English physician, 1863–1962.
    Klippel-Trenaunay-Weber syndrome—see under Klippel
    Rendu-Osler-Weber syndrome—see under Rendu
    Sturge-Kalischer-Weber syndrome—*Syn:* Sturge-Weber syndrome
    Sturge-Weber disease—*Syn:* Sturge-Weber syndrome
    Sturge-Weber syndrome—see under Sturge
    Weber-Christian disease—a group of conditions with recurrent subcutaneous nodules, with or without fever or suppuration, followed by depression of the overlying skin. *Syn:* nodular nonsuppurative panniculitis; Christian disease (2)
    Weber-Cockayne syndrome—epidermolysis bullosa of the hands and feet.

Weber, Moritz I., German anatomist, 1795–1875.
    Weber organ—a minute pouch in the prostate opening on the summit of the seminal colliculus. *Syn:* prostatic utricle

Weber, Sir Hermann, English physician, 1823–1918.
    Weber sign—*SYN:* Weber syndrome
    Weber syndrome—midbrain tegmentum lesion characterized by ipsilateral oculomotor nerve paresis and contralateral paralysis of the extremities, face, and tongue. *SYN:* Weber sign

Weber, Wilhelm E., German physicist, 1804–1891.
    Weber point—a point situated 1 cm below the promontory of the sacrum, believed by Weber to represent the center of gravity of the body.
    Weber triangle—an area on the sole of the foot.

Webster, John C., U.S. gynecologist, 1863–1950.
    Webster operation—*SYN:* Baldy operation

Webster, John, English chemist, 1878–1927.
    Webster test—a test for trinitrotoluene in the urine.

Wechsler, David, U.S. psychologist, *1896.
    Wechsler Adult Intelligence Scale—modification of the Wechsler-Bellevue scale.
    Wechsler Intelligence Scale for Children—intelligence test for children between the ages of 5 years to 15 years, 11 months.
    Wechsler Intelligence Scale for Children-Revised
    Wechsler intelligence scales—scales for the measurement of general intelligence in children and adults.
    Wechsler Memory Scale
    Wechsler Preschool and Primary Scale of Intelligence—intelligence test for children between the ages 4 years to 6 years, 6 months.
    Wechsler-Bellevue scale—a measure of general intelligence superseded by the Wechsler adult intelligence scale and its subsequent revision.

Wecker, Louis H. de. See under de Wecker.

Wedensky, Nikolai I., Russian neurophysiologist, 1852–1922.
    Wedensky effect—a relatively long enhancing effect following application of a maximal shock or stimulus to a neuromuscular preparation.
    Wedensky facilitation—the additive effect of a series of electric shocks.
    Wedensky inhibition—inhibition of muscle response as a result of a series of rapidly repeated stimuli to the motor nerve.

Weeks, John E., U.S. ophthalmologist, 1853–1949.
    Koch-Weeks bacillus—see under Koch, Robert
    Weeks bacillus—*SYN:* Koch-Weeks bacillus

Wegener, Friedrich, German pathologist, 1907–1990.
    Wegener granulomatosis—characterized by necrotizing granulomas and ulceration of the upper respiratory tract, with purulent rhinorrhea, nasal obstruction, and sometimes with otorrhea, hemoptysis, pulmonary infiltration and cavitation, and fever.

NOTES

Wegner, Friedrich R.G., German pathologist, 1843–1917.
    Wegner disease—inflammation of the epiphyseal line associated with congenital syphilis. *SYN:* syphilitic osteochondritis
    Wegner line—a narrow whitish line at the junction of the epiphysis and diaphysis of a long bone, related to syphilitic epiphysitis.

Weibel, Ewald R., 20th century Swiss physician.
    Weibel-Palade bodies—rod-shaped bundles of microtubules seen by electron microscopy in vascular endothelial cells.

Weichselbaum, Anthony, Austrian pathologist, 1845–1920.
    Fraenkel-Weichselbaum pneumococcus—*SYN:* Fraenkel pneumococcus
    Weichselbaum coccus—a species found in the human nasopharynx, the causative agent of meningococcal meningitis. *SYN: Neisseria meningitidis*

Weidel, Hugo, Austrian chemist, 1849–1899.
    Weidel reaction—a reaction showing the presence of xanthine.

Weigert, Carl, German pathologist, 1845–1904.
    Weigert iodine solution—an iodine-potassium iodide mixture used as a reagent to alter crystal and methyl violet so that they are retained by certain bacteria and fungi.
    Weigert iron hematoxylin stain
    Weigert law—the loss or destruction of a part or element in the organic world is likely to result in compensatory replacement and overproduction of tissue during the process of regeneration or repair. *SYN:* overproduction theory
    Weigert stain—dye used in the study of myelinated axons.
    Weigert stain for actinomyces
    Weigert stain for elastin
    Weigert stain for fibrin
    Weigert stain for myelin
    Weigert stain for neuroglia
    Weigert-Gram stain—a stain for bacteria in tissues in which sections are stained in alum-hematoxylin, then in eosin, aniline methyl violet, and Lugol solution.

Weigl, Egon, Romanian born psychologist.
    Weigl-Goldstein-Scheerer test—a concept formation test.

Weil, Adolf, German physician, 1848–1916.
    Larrey-Weil disease—*SYN:* Weil disease
    Weil disease—leptospirosis. *SYN:* Larrey-Weil disease; infectious icterus; infectious jaundice

Weil, Edmund, Austrian physician, 1880–1922.
    Weil-Felix reaction—*SYN:* Weil-Felix test
    Weil-Felix test—a test for the presence and type of rickettsial disease. *SYN:* Weil-Felix reaction

Weil, Ludwig A., German dentist, 1849–1895.
    Weil basal layer—the layer beneath the odontoblasts of the tooth. *SYN:* Weil basal zone
    Weil basal zone—*SYN:* Weil basal layer

Weill, Georges, French ophthalmologist, 1866–1952.
Weill syndrome—*Syn:* Adie syndrome
Weill-Marchesani syndrome—*Syn:* Marchesani syndrome

Weill, Jean A., French physician, *1903.
Leri-Weill disease—*Syn:* dyschondrosteosis
Leri-Weill syndrome—*Syn:* dyschondrosteosis

Weinberg, Michel, French pathologist, 1868–1940.
Weinberg reaction—a complement fixation test of the presence of hydatid disease.

Weinberg, Wilhelm, German physician, 1862–1937.
Hardy-Weinberg equilibrium—see under Hardy, Godfrey
Hardy-Weinberg law—see under Hardy, Godfrey

Weir, Robert F., U.S. surgeon, 1838–1927.
Weir operation—obsolete term for appendicostomy.

Weisbach, Albin, Austrian anthropologist, 1837–1914.
Weisbach angle—a craniometric angle formed by the junction at the alveolar point of lines passing from the basion and from the middle of the frontonasal suture.

Weiss, Nathan, Austrian physician, 1851–1883.
Weiss gold dilator
Weiss sign—*Syn:* Chvostek sign

Weiss, Soma, U.S. physician, 1898–1942.
Charcot-Weiss-Baker syndrome—see under Charcot
Mallory-Weiss lesion—see under Mallory, G. Kenneth
Mallory-Weiss syndrome—see under Mallory, G. Kenneth
Mallory-Weiss tear—*Syn:* Mallory-Weiss lesion

Weitbrecht, Josias, German-Russian anatomist in St. Petersburg, 1702–1747.
Weitbrecht cartilage—the articular disk of fibrocartilage usually found between the acromial end of the clavicle and the medial border of the acromion. *Syn:* articular disc of acromioclavicular joint
Weitbrecht cord—*Syn:* Weitbrecht ligament
Weitbrecht fibers—one of several longitudinal folds of the articular capsule of the hip joint. *Syn:* retinaculum capsulae articularis coxae
Weitbrecht foramen—an opening in the articular capsule of the shoulder joint, communicating with the subtendinous bursa of the subscapularis muscle.
Weitbrecht ligament—a slender band extending from the lateral part of the coronoid process of the ulna distad and laterad to the radius immediately distal to the bicipital tuberosity. *Syn:* oblique ligament of elbow joint; Weitbrecht cord

Welander, Lisa, Swedish neurologist, *1909.
Kugelberg-Welander disease—see under Kugelberg

(continued)

NOTES

W

Welander *(continued)*
Welander myopathy
Wohlfart-Kugelberg-Welander disease—*Syn:* Kugelberg-Welander disease

Welch, William H., U.S. pathologist, 1850–1934.
Clostridium welchii—*Syn:* Welch bacillus
Welch bacillus—the chief causative agent of gas gangrene, also one of the most common causes of food poisoning in the U.S. *Syn: Clostridium perfringens; Clostridium welchii*

Welcker, Hermann, German anthropologist and anatomist, 1822–1898.
Welcker angle—the anterior inferior angle of the parietal bone. *Syn:* sphenoidal angle of parietal bone

Weller, Thomas Huckle, joint winner of 1954 Nobel Prize for work related to the poliomyelitis virus.

Wells, G.C., 20th century English dermatologist.
Wells syndrome—recurrent cellulitis followed by brawny edematous skin lesions. *Syn:* eosinophilic cellulitis

Wells, Michael Vernon, 20th century English physician.
Muckle-Wells syndrome—see under Muckle

Wenckebach, Karel F., Dutch internist, 1864–1940.
Wenckebach block—*Syn:* Wenckebach phenomenon
Wenckebach period—a sequence of cardiac cycles in the electrocardiogram ending in a dropped beat due to A-V block.
Wenckebach phenomenon—progressive lengthening of conduction time in cardiac tissue, with ultimate dropping of a beat. *Syn:* Wenckebach block

Wenzel, Joseph, German anatomist and physiologist, 1768–1808.
Wenzel ventricle—a slitlike, fluid-filled space of variable width between the left and right transparent septum. *Syn:* cavity of septum pellucidum

Wepfer, Johann J., 1620–1695.
Wepfer glands—small, branched, coiled tubular glands in the duodenum that secrete an alkaline mucoid substance that serves to neutralize gastric juice. *Syn:* duodenal glands

Werdnig, Guido, Austrian neurologist, 1862–1919.
Werdnig-Hoffmann disease—*Syn:* Werdnig-Hoffmann muscular atrophy
Werdnig-Hoffmann muscular atrophy—progressive dysfunction of the anterior horn cells in the spinal cord and brainstem cranial nerves, with profound weakness and bulbar dysfunction. *Syn:* Werdnig-Hoffmann disease; infantile spinal muscular atrophy

Wermer, Paul, U.S. internist, 1898–1975.
Wermer syndrome—Zollinger-Ellison syndrome with additional endocrine and glandular disorders.

Wernekinck, Friedrich C.G., German anatomist and physician, 1798–1835.
Wernekinck commissure—the decussation of the brachia conjunctiva before their entrance into the red nucleus of the tegmentum.
Wernekinck decussation—the decussation of the left and right superior cerebellar peduncles in the tegmentum of the caudal mesencephalon. *Syn:* decussation of superior cerebellar peduncles

Werner, F.F., early 20th century German chemist.
　　Werner test—*SYN:* thyroid suppression test
Werner, Otto, German physician, 1879–1936.
　　Werner disease—hereditary disorder characterized by premature aging.
　　SYN: Werner syndrome; progeria adultorum
　　Werner syndrome—a disorder consisting of scleroderma-like skin changes,
　　bilateral juvenile cataracts, progeria, hypogonadism, and diabetes
　　mellitus.
Wernicke, Karl, German neurologist, 1848–1905.
　　Gayet-Wernicke syndrome—*SYN:* Wernicke syndrome
　　Wernicke aphasia—aphasia in which there is impairment in the
　　comprehension of spoken and written words. *SYN:* sensory aphasia;
　　Bastian aphasia
　　Wernicke area—*SYN:* Wernicke center
　　Wernicke center—the region of the cerebral cortex thought to be essential
　　for understanding and formulating coherent, propositional speech. *SYN:*
　　Wernicke zone; Wernicke area; sensory speech center; Wernicke field;
　　Wernicke region
　　Wernicke cramp—psychogenic muscle cramp. *SYN:* cramp neurosis
　　Wernicke disease—*SYN:* Wernicke syndrome
　　Wernicke encephalopathy—*SYN:* Wernicke syndrome
　　Wernicke field—*SYN:* Wernicke center
　　Wernicke radiation—the massive, fanlike fiber system passing from the
　　lateral geniculate body of the thalamus to the visual cortex. *SYN:* optic
　　radiation
　　Wernicke reaction—in hemianopia, a reaction due to damage of the optic
　　tract, consisting in loss of pupillary constriction when the light is directed
　　to the blind side of the retina. *SYN:* Wernicke sign
　　Wernicke region—*SYN:* Wernicke center
　　Wernicke sign—*SYN:* Wernicke reaction
　　Wernicke syndrome—a condition encountered in chronic alcoholics,
　　largely due to thiamin deficiency and characterized by disturbances in
　　ocular motility, pupillary alterations, nystagmus, and ataxia with tremors.
　　SYN: superior hemorrhagic polioencephalitis; Wernicke disease; Wernicke
　　encephalopathy; Gayet disease; Gayet-Wernicke syndrome
　　Wernicke zone—*SYN:* Wernicke center
　　Wernicke-Korsakoff encephalopathy
　　Wernicke-Korsakoff syndrome—the coexistence of Wernicke and
　　Korsakoff syndromes.
　　Wernicke-Mann hemiplegia—extremity hemiplegia that is partial. *SYN:*
　　Wernicke-Mann paralysis
　　Wernicke-Mann paralysis—*SYN:* Wernicke-Mann hemiplegia
Wertheim, Ernst, Austrian gynecologist, 1864–1920.
　　Wertheim clamp
　　Wertheim deep surgery scissors

W

(continued)

NOTES

Wertheim *(continued)*
Wertheim forceps
Wertheim hysterectomy
Wertheim needle holder
Wertheim operation—a radical operation for carcinoma of the uterus.
Wertheim vaginal forceps

Werther, J., 20th century German physician.
Werther disease—recurrent eruption of vesicles, papules, and papulonecrotic lesions on the buttocks and extensor surfaces of the extremities, accompanied by fever, sore throat, diarrhea, and eosinophilia. *Syn:* dermatitis nodularis necrotica

West, Charles, English physician, 1816–1898.
West syndrome—an encephalopathy in infancy characterized by infantile spasms, arrest of psychomotor development, and hypsarhythmia.

Westberg, Friedrich, 19th century German physician.
Westberg space—the space surrounding the origin of the aorta which is invested with the pericardium.

Westergren, Alf, Swedish physician, *1891.
Westergren method—a procedure for estimating the sedimentation rate of red blood cells in fluid blood.
Westergren sedimentation rate

Westphal, Karl F.O., German neurologist, 1833–1890.
Edinger-Westphal nucleus—see under Edinger
Erb-Westphal sign—see under Erb
Strümpell-Westphal disease—*Syn:* Wilson disease
Westphal ataxia—*Syn:* Westphal-Leyden syndrome
Westphal disease—*Syn:* Wilson disease
Westphal phenomenon—*Syn:* Erb-Westphal sign
Westphal pseudosclerosis—*Syn:* Wilson disease
Westphal pupillary reflex—*Syn:* Piltz sign
Westphal sign—*Syn:* Erb-Westphal sign
Westphal-Erb sign—*Syn:* Erb-Westphal sign
Westphal-Leyden syndrome—absence of knee jerk reflex characteristic of neurosyphilitic disease. *Syn:* Leyden ataxia; Westphal ataxia
Westphal-Piltz phenomenon—*Syn:* Piltz sign
Westphal-Strümpell pseudosclerosis—*Syn:* Wilson disease

Wetzel, Norman C., U.S. pediatrician, 1897–1984.
Wetzel grid—chart of growth, plotting height, weight, physical fitness and related aspects of young and adolescent children during growth.

Wever, Ernest Glen, U.S. psychologist, *1902.
Wever-Bray effect—*Syn:* Wever-Bray phenomenon
Wever-Bray phenomenon—action potentials in the acoustic nerve that correspond to auditory stimuli reaching the cochlea. *Syn:* Wever-Bray effect

Weyers, Helmut, 20th century German pediatrician.
Weyers-Thier syndrome—microphthalmia, colobomas, or anophthalmia with small orbit, twisted face due to unilateral dysplasia of maxilla, macrostomia with malformed teeth and malocclusion, vertebral

malformations, and branched and hypoplastic ribs. *Syn:* oculovertebral dysplasia

Wharton, Thomas, English anatomist and physician, 1614–1673.
Wharton duct—of the salivary gland. *Syn:* submandibular duct
Wharton jelly—the mucous connective tissue of the umbilical cord.

Wheatstone, Charles, English physicist, 1802–1875.
Wheatstone bridge—an apparatus for measuring electrical resistance.

Wheeler, Henry Lord, U.S. chemist, 1867–1914.
Wheeler-Johnson test—cystosine or uracil when treated with bromine yields dialuric acid which gives a green color with excess of barium hydroxide.

Wheeler, John M., U.S. ophthalmologist, 1879–1938.
Wheeler cyclodialysis system
Wheeler cystotome
Wheeler discission knife
Wheeler eye implant
Wheeler eye sphere implant
Wheeler graft material
Wheeler halving procedure
Wheeler incision
Wheeler knife
Wheeler malleable-shape knife
Wheeler method—a surgical procedure for correction of cicatricial ectropion.
Wheeler prosthesis
Wheeler spatula
Wheeler vessel forceps

Wheelhouse, Claudius G., English surgeon, 1826–1909.
Wheelhouse operation—obsolete term for external urethrotomy via an external opening in the perineum or penile skin. *Syn:* external urethrotomy

Whipple, Allen O., U.S. surgeon, 1881–1963.
Whipple incision
Whipple operation—excision of all or part of the pancreas together with the duodenum. *Syn:* pancreatoduodenectomy
Whipple pancreatectomy

Whipple, George H., U.S. pathologist and Nobel laureate, 1878–1976.
Whipple disease—a rare disease characterized by steatorrhea, frequently generalized lymphadenopathy, arthritis, fever, and cough.

White, Paul Dudley, U.S. cardiologist, 1886–1973.
Lee-White method—see under Lee, Roger
Wolff-Parkinson-White syndrome—see under Wolff

W

NOTES

Whitehead, Walter, English surgeon, 1840–1913.
    Whitehead deformity—circumferential mucosal ectropion at the anus following Whitehead operation.
    Whitehead operation—excision of hemorrhoids by two circular incisions above and below involved veins, allowing normal mucosa to be pulled down and sutured to anal skin.

Whitfield, Arthur, English dermatologist, 1867–1947.
    Whitfield ointment

Whitman, Royal, U.S. surgeon, 1857–1946.
    Whitman arch support
    Whitman arthroplasty
    Whitman femoral neck reconstruction
    Whitman fracture appliance
    Whitman fracture frame
    Whitman frame—a frame similar to the Bradford frame, but with curved sides.
    Whitman operation
    Whitman osteotomy
    Whitman paralysis
    Whitman plate
    Whitman talectomy procedure
    Whitman technique

Whitmore, Alfred, English surgeon, 1876–1946.
    Whitmore bacillus—a species found in cases of melioidosis in humans and other animals and in soil and water in tropical regions. *SYN: Pseudomonas pseudomallei*
    Whitmore disease—an infectious disease of rodents in India and Southeast Asia that is caused by *Pseudomonas pseudomallei* and is communicable to humans. *SYN:* melioidosis

Whitnall, Samuel E., English anatomist, 1876–1952.
    Whitnall tubercle—*SYN:* orbital tubercle of zygomatic bone

Wickham, Louis-Frédéric, French dermatologist, 1861–1913.
    Wickham striae—fine whitish lines, having a network arrangement, on the surface of lichen planus papules.

Widal, Georges F.I., French physician, 1862–1929.
    Gruber-Widal reaction—*SYN:* Widal reaction
    Hayem-Widal syndrome—see under Hayem
    Widal reaction—agglutination reaction as applied to the diagnosis of typhoid. *SYN:* Gruber reaction; Gruber-Widal reaction
    Widal syndrome—*SYN:* Hayem-Widal syndrome

Wiedemann, Hans Rudolf, German pediatrician, *1915.
    Beckwith-Wiedemann syndrome—see under Beckwith
    Maroteaux-Spranger-Wiedemann syndrome—see under Maroteaux
    Wiedemann syndrome—deformities in neonates caused by thalidomide ingestion during pregnancy.

Wiener, H.
    tract of Münzer and Wiener—see under Münzer

Wieschaus, Eric F., joint winner of 1995 Nobel Prize for work related to genetics and early development of embryo.

Wiesel, Torsten N., joint winner of 1981 Nobel Prize for work related to vision.

Wigand, J. Heinrich, German obstetrician and gynecologist, 1766–1817.
  Wigand maneuver—assisted breech delivery with pressure above the symphysis while the fetus lies astraddle the operator's other arm.
  Wigand version

Wilbrand, H. German neuro-ophthalmologist, 1851–1935.
  Charcot-Wilbrand syndrome—see under Charcot

Wilcoxon, Frank, U.S. chemist and statistician, 1892–1962.
  Wilcoxon test—nonparametric test.

Wilde, Sir William R.W., Irish oculist and otologist, 1815–1876.
  Wilde cords—transverse markings on the corpus callosum.
  Wilde triangle—a triangular area at the anterior inferior part of the tympanic membrane. *SYN:* pyramid of light

Wilder, Helenor C., 20th century U.S. scientist.
  Wilder stain for reticulum—a silver impregnation technique in which reticulum appears as black, well-defined fibers without beading and with a relatively clear background.

W

Wilder, Joseph, U.S. neuropsychiatrist, *1895.
  Wilder law of initial value—the direction of response of a body function to any agent depends to a large degree on the initial level of that function. *SYN:* law of initial value

Wilder, William H., U.S. ophthalmologist, 1860–1935.
  Wilder band spreader
  Wilder dilating forceps
  Wilder dilator
  Wilder lens hook
  Wilder lens loop
  Wilder lens scoop
  Wilder loupe
  Wilder retractor
  Wilder scleral depressor
  Wilder scleral self-retaining retractor
  Wilder sign—a slight twitch of the eyeball when changing its movement from abduction to adduction or the reverse, noted in Graves disease.
  Wilder trephine

Wildermuth, Hermann A., German psychiatrist, 1852–1907.
  Wildermuth ear—an ear in which the helix is turned backward and the anthelix is prominent.

NOTES

Wildervanck, L.S., 20th century Dutch geneticist.
Wildervanck syndrome—a congenital short neck on girls associated with paralysis of the external ocular muscles and with perceptive deafness. *SYN:* cervico-oculoacoustic syndrome

Wilhelmy, Ludwig F., German scientist, 1812–1864.
Wilhelmy balance—a device for measuring surface tension used in a Langmuir trough to study pulmonary surfactant.

Wilkie, David P.D., Scottish surgeon, 1882–1938.
Wilkie artery—the right colic artery when it occasionally crosses the duodenum.
Wilkie disease—partial or complete block of the superior mesenteric artery. *SYN:* superior mesenteric artery syndrome
Wilkie syndrome

Wilkinson, Daryl Sheldon, 20th century English dermatologist.
Sneddon-Wilkinson disease—see under Sneddon

Willebrand, Erik A. von. See under von Willebrand.

Willett, J. Abernethy, English obstetrician, 1872–1932.
Willett clamp
Willett forceps—obsolete term for a traction forceps used to treat placenta previa.

Willi, Heinrich, Swiss pediatrician, 1900–1971.
Prader-Willi syndrome—see under Prader

Williams, Anna, U.S. bacteriologist, 1863–1955.
Park-Williams bacillus—see under Park, William H.
Park-Williams fixative—see under Park, William H.
Williams stain—a stain for Negri bodies.

Williams, J.C.P., 20th century New Zealand cardiologist.
Williams syndrome—multiple congenital disorders.

Williams, Paul C., U.S. orthopedic surgeon, 1900–1978.
Williams back brace—a thoracolumbosacral brace.
Williams brace
Williams diskectomy
Williams diskography
Williams flexion exercise
Williams interlocking Y nail
Williams orthosis
Williams procedure
Williams rod
Williams screwdriver
Williams self-retaining retractor

Williamson, Carl S., U.S. surgeon, 1896–1952.
Mann-Williamson operation—see under Mann, Frank
Mann-Williamson ulcer

Willis, Thomas, English physician, 1621–1675.
accessorius willisii—nerve that arises by two sets of roots: cranial, emerging from the side of the medulla, and spinal, emerging from the

ventrolateral part of the first five cervical segments of the spinal cord. *Syn:* accessory nerve

chordae willisii—*Syn:* Willis cords

circle of Willis—an anastomotic circle of arteries (roughly pentagonal in outline) at the base of the brain. *Syn:* arterial circle of cerebrum

Willis centrum nervosum—the largest and highest group of prevertebral sympathetic ganglia, located on the superior part of the abdominal aorta. *Syn:* celiac ganglia

Willis cords—several fibrous cords crossing the superior sagittal sinus. *Syn:* chordae willisii

Willis pancreas—a portion of the head of the pancreas formed by the superior mesteric artery and abdominal aorta. *Syn:* uncinate process of pancreas

Willis paracusis—the apparent increase in auditory acuity of a deaf person to conversation in noisy surroundings due to a companion's unconscious voice raising. *Syn:* false paracusis

Willis pouch—obsolete term for lesser omentum.

Williston, Samuel Wendell, U.S. paleontologist, 1852–1918.
Williston law—as the vertebrate scale is ascended, the number of bones in the skull is reduced.

Wilms, Max, German surgeon, 1867–1918.
Wilms syndrome—*Syn:* Wilms tumor
Wilms tumor—a malignant renal tumor of young children. *Syn:* nephroblastoma; adenomyosarcoma; embryoma of the kidney; Wilms syndrome

Wilson, Clifford, English physician, *1906.
Kimmelstiel-Wilson disease—*Syn:* Kimmelstiel-Wilson syndrome
Kimmelstiel-Wilson syndrome—see under Kimmelstiel

Wilson, Frank Norman, U.S. cardiologist, 1890–1952.
Wilson block—the most common form of right bundle-branch block.

Wilson, James, English anatomist, physiologist, and surgeon, 1765–1821.
Wilson muscle—(1) certain fibers of the levator ani; (2) *Syn:* sphincter urethrae

Wilson, Miriam G., U.S. pediatrician, *1922.
Wilson-Mikity syndrome—a respiratory disorder occurring in small, premature infants. *Syn:* pulmonary dysmaturity syndrome

Wilson, Samuel A. Kinnier, English neurologist, 1878–1937.
Wilson disease—(1) disorder characterized by cirrhosis, degeneration in the basal ganglia of the brain, and deposition of green pigment in the periphery of the cornea. *Syn:* Westphal-Strümpell pseudosclerosis; Strümpell-Westphal disease; Westphal disease; Wilson syndrome; Westphal pseudosclerosis. (2) generalized exfoliation with scaling of the skin and usually with erythema. *Syn:* exfoliative dermatitis.
Wilson syndrome—*Syn:* Wilson disease

NOTES

Wilson, Sir William J.E., English dermatologist, 1809–1884.
Wilson lichen—eruption of flat-topped, shiny, violaceous papules on flexor surfaces, male genitalia, and buccal mucosa of unknown cause. *SYN:* lichen planus

Wimshurst, James, English engineer, 1822–1903.
Wimshurst machine—generates static electricity.

Winiwarter, Felix von, German surgeon, 1852–1931.
Winiwarter-Buerger disease—*SYN:* Buerger disease

Winkler, Max, Swiss physician, 1875–1952.
Winkler disease—a benign, chronic, small, painful nodule on the helix of the ear in elderly white males, which may occasionally become ulcerated. *SYN:* chondrodermatitis nodularis chronica helicis; Winkler syndrome
Winkler syndrome—*SYN:* Winkler disease

Winslow, Jacob B., Danish anatomist, physicist, and surgeon in Paris, 1669–1760.
stellulae winslowii—capillary whorls in the lamina choroidocapillaris from which arise the venae vorticosae. *SYN:* Winslow stars
Winslow foramen—the passage, below and behind the portal hepatis, connecting the two sacs of the peritoneum. *SYN:* epiploic foramen
Winslow ligament—the cordlike ligament that passes from the lateral epicondyle of the femur to the head of the fibula. *SYN:* fibular collateral ligament
Winslow pancreas—a portion of the head of the pancreas formed by the superior mesteric artery and abdominal aorta. *SYN:* uncinate process of pancreas
Winslow stars—*SYN:* stellulae winslowii

Winterbottom, Thomas M., English physician, 1765–1859.
Winterbottom sign—swelling of the posterior cervical lymph nodes, characteristic of early stages of African trypanosomiasis.

Winternitz, Wilhelm, Austrian physician, 1835–1917.
Winternitz sound—a double-current catheter in which water at any desired temperature circulates.

Wintersteiner, Hugo, Austrian ophthalmologist, 1865–1918.
Wintersteiner rosettes—rosettes found only in retinal embryonic tumors.

Wirsung, Johann G., German anatomist in Padua, 1600–1643.
Wirsung canal—*SYN:* Wirsung duct
Wirsung duct—the excretory duct of the pancreas. *SYN:* pancreatic duct; Wirsung canal

Wiskott, Alfred, 20th century German pediatrician.
Wiskott-Aldrich syndrome—a fatal X-linked immunodeficiency disorder occurring in male children. *SYN:* Aldrich syndrome

Wissler, Hans, Swiss pediatrician, *1906.
Wissler syndrome—high intermittent fever and rash in children and adolescents.
Wissler-Fanconi syndrome—toxic allergic hypersensitivity.

Wistar, Caspar, U.S. biologist, 1760–1818, after whom the Wistar Institute is named.
    Wistar rats—an inbred strain of rats used for research.

Wohlfart, Gunnar, Swedish neurologist, 1910–1961.
    Wohlfart-Kugelberg-Welander disease—*SYN:* Kugelberg-Welander disease

Wolf, A., 20th century U.S. pathologist.
    Wolf-Orton bodies—intranuclear inclusion bodies seen in cells of malignant neoplasms, especially those of glial cell origin.

Wolfe, John R., Scottish ophthalmologist, 1824–1904.
    Krause-Wolfe graft—*SYN:* Krause graft
    Wolfe eye forceps
    Wolfe graft—a full-thickness skin graft without any subcutaneous fat. *SYN:* Wolfe-Krause graft
    Wolfe method
    Wolfe prosthesis
    Wolfe ptosis operation
    Wolfe-Krause graft—*SYN:* Wolfe graft

Wolff, Julius, German anatomist, 1836–1902.
    Wolff law—changes in bone function are followed by changes in internal architecture.
    Wolff vasogenic theory

W

Wolff, Kaspar F., German embryologist in Russia, 1733–1794.
    wolffian body—one of three excretory organs appearing in the evolution of vertebrates. *SYN:* mesonephros
    wolffian cyst—a cyst lying in the broad ligaments of the uterus and arising from any mesonephric structures.
    wolffian duct—a duct in the embryo draining the mesonephric tubules. *SYN:* mesonephric duct
    wolffian rest—remnants of the wolffian duct in the female genital tract that give rise to cysts. *SYN:* mesonephric rest
    wolffian ridge—one of the paired longitudinal ridges developing in the dorsal body wall of the embryo. *SYN:* urogenital ridge
    wolffian tubules—*SYN:* Kobelt tubules

Wolff, Louis, U.S. cardiologist, 1898–1972.
    Wolff-Chaikoff block—blocking of the organic binding of iodine and its incorporation into hormone caused by large doses of iodine. *SYN:* Wolff-Chaikoff effect
    Wolff-Chaikoff effect—*SYN:* Wolff-Chaikoff block
    Wolff-Parkinson-White syndrome—an electrocardiographic pattern sometimes associated with paroxysmal tachycardia. *SYN:* preexcitation syndrome

Wölfler, Anton, Bohemian surgeon, 1850–1917.
    Wölfler gland—*SYN:* accessory thyroid gland

NOTES

Wolfring, Emilj F. von, Polish ophthalmologist, 1832–1906.
 Wolfring glands

Wollaston, William H., English physician and physicist, 1766–1828.
 Wollaston doublet—a combination of two planoconvex lenses in the eyepiece of a microscope designed to correct the chromatic aberration.
 Wollaston theory—a theory that the semidecussation of the optic nerves at the chiasm is proved by the homonymous hemianopia seen in brain lesions.

Wolman, Moske, Israeli neuropathologist, *1914.
 Wolman disease—lipidosis caused by deficiency of liposomal acid lipase activity. *SYN:* cholesterol ester storage disease
 Wolman xanthomatosis

Woltman, Henry W., U.S. neurologist, 1889–1964.
 Kernohan-Woltman syndrome—see under Kernohan
 Woltman-Kernohan syndrome—*SYN:* Kernohan-Woltman syndrome

Wood, origin unknown.
 Romberg-Wood syndrome—see under Romberg

Wood, Robert, U.S. physicist, 1868–1955.
 Wood glass—a glass containing nickel oxide, used in Wood lamp.
 Wood lamp—an ultraviolet lamp used to detect by fluorescence hairs infected with species of *Microsporum*.
 Wood light—ultraviolet light produced by Wood lamp.

Woodworth, Robert Sessions, U.S. psychologist, 1869–1962.
 Woodworth-Mathews personal data sheet—a personality inventory.

Woolf, B., 20th-century English biochemist.
 Woolf-Lineweaver-Burk plot—a graphical representation of enzyme kinetic data. *SYN:* double-reciprocal plot

Woolner, Thomas, English sculptor, 1826–1892.
 Woolner tip—a point projecting upward and posteriorly from the free outcurved margin of the helix a little posterior to its upper end. *SYN:* tip of auricle

Woringer, Frédéric, French dermatologist, 1903–1964.
 Woringer-Kolopp disease—a benign localized form of lymphoma. *SYN:* pagetoid reticulosis

Worm, Ole, Danish anatomist, 1588–1654.
 wormian bones—small irregular bones found along the sutures of the cranium, particularly related to the parietal bone. *SYN:* sutural bones

Wormley, Theodore G., U.S. chemist, 1826–1897.
 Wormley test—a test for alkaloids.

Worth, Claud, English ophthalmologist, 1869–1936.
 Worth amblyoscope—the original amblyoscope.
 Worth strabismus forceps

Woulfe, Peter, English chemist, 1727–1803.
 Woulfe bottle—a bottle with two or three necks, used in a series, connected with tubes, for working with gases.

Wright, Basil Martin, 20th century English physician.
    Wright peak flow meter
    Wright respirometer—an inferential meter used to measure tidal and minute volume.

Wright, James Homer, U.S. pathologist, 1871–1928.
    Wright stain—a staining mixture of eosinates of polychromed methylene blue used in staining of blood smears.

Wright, Marmaduke Burr, U.S. obstetrician, 1803–1879.
    Wright version—a cephalic version employed in cases of shoulder presentation.

Wrisberg, Heinrich A., German anatomist and gynecologist, 1739–1808.
    nerve of Wrisberg
    Wrisberg cartilage—a small nonarticulating rod of elastic cartilage. *SYN:* cuneiform cartilage
    Wrisberg ganglia—parasympathetic ganglia of the cardiac plexus. *SYN:* cardiac ganglia
    Wrisberg lesion
    Wrisberg ligament—the band that passes posterior to the posterior cruciate ligament. *SYN:* posterior meniscofemoral ligament
    Wrisberg ligament type of discoid meniscus
    Wrisberg nerve—*SYN:* medial brachial cutaneous nerve; nervus intermedius
    Wrisberg tubercle—a rounded eminence on the posterior part of the aryepiglottic fold. *SYN:* cuneiform tubercle

Wucherer, Otto, German physician, 1820–1873.
    Wuchereria bancrofti—the bancroftian filaria.
    Wuchereria—genus of filarial nematodes.
    wuchereriasis—infection with worms of the genus *Wuchereria*.

Wunderlich, Carl R.A., German physician, 1815–1877.
    Wunderlich syndrome—traumatic perirenal hematoma.

Wundt, Wilhelm Max, German psychologist/physiologist, 1932–1920.
    Wundt curve—an illusion in which straight lines appear to be curved.

Wurster, Casimir, German chemist, 1856–1913.
    Wurster reagent—filter paper impregnated with tetramethyl-*p*-phenylenediamine, which turns blue in the presence of ozone or hydrogen peroxide.
    Wurster test—a test for tyrosine.

Wyatt, W.
    Brushfield-Wyatt disease—see under Brushfield

Wyburn-Mason, Roger, 20th century English physician.
    Wyburn-Mason syndrome—arteriovenous malformation on the cerebral cortex, retinal arteriovenous angioma and facial nevus.

Wyman, Jeffries, U.S. biochemist, *1901.
    Monod-Wyman-Changeux model—see under Monod

W

NOTES

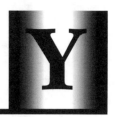

Yerkes, Robert Mearns, U.S. psychobiologist, 1876–1956.
    Yerkes discrimination box—a box used to study visual discrimination in animals.
    Yerkes-Dodson law—rule regarding task performance.

Yersin, Alexandre Émil Jean, Swiss bacteriologist and surgeon, 1863–1943.
    Yersinia enterocolitica—a species causing yersiniosis.
    Yersinia pestis—a species causing plague.
    Yersinia pseudotuberculosis—a species causing pseudotuberculosis in birds and rodents; rarely in humans.
    yersiniosis—infectious disease caused by *Yersinia enterocolitica*.

Young, Hugh H., U.S. urologist, 1870–1945.
    Young approach
    Young clamp
    Young cystoscope
    Young dilator
    Young dissector
    Young epispadias repair—*SYN:* Young operation (2)
    Young operation—(1) perineal prostatectomy. *SYN:* Young perineal prostatectomy; (2) epispadias repair. *SYN:* Young epispacias repair.
    Young perineal prostatectomy—*SYN:* Young operation (1)
    Young prostatic tractor
    Young vastectomy

Young, J.
    Young-Paxson syndrome—traumatic uteroplacental damage.

Young, Thomas, English physician and physicist, 1773–1829.
    Young modulus—a type of modulus of elasticity.
    Young rule—an obsolete rule to determine a child's medication dose.
    Young-Helmholtz theory of color vision—a theory that there are three color-perceiving elements in the retina: red, green, and blue. *SYN:* Helmholtz theory of color vision

Young, William John, 20th century Australian biochemist.
    Harden-Young ester—see under Harden

Yvon, Paul, French physician and chemist, 1848–1913.
    Yvon test—for alkaloids.

Z

Zaffaroni, Alejandro, Uruguayan-U.S. chemist and biochemist, *1923.
Zaffaroni system—a chromatographic system for the separation of steroids.

Zaglas, John, 19th century anatomist's assistant in Edinburgh, Scotland.
Zaglas ligament—a short, thick, fibrous band extending from the posterior superior spine of the ilium to the second transverse tubercle of the sacrum.

Zahn, Friedrich W., German pathologist, 1845–1904.
lines of Zahn—riblike markings seen by the naked eye on the surface of antemortem thrombi. *SYN:* striae of Zahn
striae of Zahn—*SYN:* lines of Zahn
Zahn infarct—a pseudoinfarct of the liver due to obstruction of a branch of the portal vein.

Zahorsky, John, U.S. physician, 1871–1963.
Zahorsky disease—a skin disorder.

Zambusch, Leo von, 20th century German physician.
generalized pustular psoriasis of Zambusch—an extensive exacerbation of psoriasis. *SYN:* pustular psoriasis

Zander, Jonas Gustav Wilhelm, Swedish physician, 1835–1920.
Zander apparatus—equipment used for exercise therapy.
Zander exercise—passive, active, or resistive exercise.

Zang, Christoph Bonifacius, Austrian surgeon, 1772–1835.
Zang metatarsal cap
Zang metatarsal cap implant
Zang space—supraclavicular fossa.

Zange, Johannes, German otorhinolaryngologist, 1880–1969.
Kindler-Zange syndrome—*SYN:* Zange-Kindler syndrome
Zange-Kindler syndrome—neurological disorder resulting from blockage of cerebrospinal fluid in the cisterna magna. *SYN:* Kindler-Zange syndrome

Zappert, Julius, Austrian physician, 1867–1942.
Zappert counting chamber—a special standardized glass slide used for counting cells and other particulate material in a measured volume of fluid.

Zaufal, Emanuel, Czech physician, 1833–1910.
Zaufal bone rongeur
Zaufal sign—saddle-nose defect.

Zeeman, Pieter, Dutch physicist and Nobel laureate, 1865–1943.
> **Zeeman effect**—the splitting of spectral lines into three or more symmetrically placed lines when the light source is subjected to a magnetic field.

Zeis, Eduard, Dresden ophthalmologist, 1807–1868.
> **Zeis glands**—sebaceous glands opening into the follicles of the eyelashes.
> **zeisian sty**—inflammation of one of the Zeis glands.

Zellweger, Hans U., U.S. pediatrician, *1909.
> **Zellweger syndrome**—*SYN:* cerebrohepatorenal syndrome

Zenker, Friedrich A., German pathologist, 1825–1898.
> **formol-Zenker fixative**—Zenker fixative in which glacial acetic acid has been replaced by formalin.
> **Zenker degeneration**—a form of severe hyaline degeneration or necrosis in skeletal muscle, occurring in severe infections. *SYN:* Zenker necrosis; waxy degeneration
> **Zenker diverticulum**—common diverticulum of the esophagus, arises between the inferior pharyngeal constrictor and the cricopharyngeus muscle. *SYN:* pharyngoesophageal diverticulum
> **Zenker fixative**—a rapid fixative.
> **Zenker necrosis**—*SYN:* Zenker degeneration
> **Zenker paralysis**—paresthesia and paralysis in the area of the external popliteal nerve.

Ziegler, S. Louis, U.S. ophthalmologist, 1861–1925.
> **Ziegler blade**
> **Ziegler cautery**
> **Ziegler cilia forceps**
> **Ziegler dilator**
> **Ziegler ectropion repair**
> **Ziegler eye speculum**
> **Ziegler forceps**
> **Ziegler iridectomy**
> **Ziegler iris knife**
> **Ziegler lacrimal probe**
> **Ziegler needle**
> **Ziegler operation**
> **Ziegler probe**
> **Ziegler puncture**
> **Ziegler wash bottle**

Ziehen, Georg T., German psychiatrist, 1862–1950.
> **Ziehen-Oppenheim disease**—a disorder beginning in childhood or adolescence marked by muscular contractions that distort the spine and hips. *SYN:* dystonia musculorum deformans

Ziehl, Franz, German bacteriologist, 1857–1926.
> **Ziehl stain**—a carbol-fuchsin solution of phenol and basic fuchsin used to demonstrate bacteria and cell nuclei.
> **Ziehl-Neelsen stain**—a method for staining acid-fast bacteria.

Zielke, K., 20th century German orthopedic surgeon.
> **Zielke bifid hook**